Health Informatics
(formerly Computers in Health Care)

Kathryn J. Hannah   Marion J. Ball
Series Editors

For other titles published in this series, go to
www.springer.com/series/1114

William Hersh

Information Retrieval: A Health and Biomedical Perspective

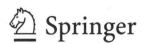 Springer

William Hersh, M.D.
Professor and Chair
Department of Medical Informatics
    & Clinical Epidemiology
Oregon Health & Science University
3181 SW Sam Jackson Park Rd.
BICC
Portland, OR, USA 97239

Series Editors
Kathryn J. Hannah
Adjunct Professor,
Department of Community Health Science
Faculty of Medicine
The University of Calgary
Calgary, Alberta T2N 4N1, Canada

Marion J. Ball, Ed.D
Fellow, Center for Healthcare Management
IBM Research
Professor Emerita, Johns Hopkins
    University School of Nursing
7506 Coley Court
Baltimore Maryland 21210
USA

ISBN 978-0-387-78702-2   e-ISBN 978-0-387-78703-9

Library of Congress Control Number: 200893135

To Sally, Becca and Alyssa

Series Preface

This series is directed to healthcare professionals who are leading the transformation of health care by using information and knowledge to advance the quality of patient care. Launched in 1988 as Computers in Health Care, the series offers a broad range of titles: some are addressed to specific professions such as nursing, medicine, and health administration; others to special areas of practice such as trauma and radiology. Still other books in this series focus on interdisciplinary issues, such as the computer-based patient record, electronic health records, and networked healthcare systems.

Renamed Health Informatics in 1998 to reflect the rapid evolution in the discipline now known as health informatics, the series continues to add titles that contribute to the evolution of the field. In this series, eminent experts, serving as editors or authors, offer their accounts of innovation in health informatics. Increasingly, these accounts go beyond hardware and software to address the role of information in influencing the transformation of healthcare delivery systems around the world. The series also increasingly focuses on "peopleware" and the organizational, behavioral, and societal changes that accompany the diffusion of information technology in health services environments.

These changes will shape health services in the new millennium. By making full and creative use of the technology to tame data and to transform information, health informatics will foster the development of the knowledge age in health care. As co-editors, we pledge to support our professional colleagues and the series readers as they share the advances in the emerging and exciting field of health informatics.

Kathryn J. Hannah
Marion J. Ball

Preface

The main goal of this book is to provide an understanding of the theory, implementation, and evaluation of information retrieval (IR) systems in health and biomedicine. There are already a number of excellent "how-to" volumes on searching for health and biomedical information (listed in Chap. 1). Similarly, there are also a number of high-quality basic IR textbooks (also listed in Chap. 1). This volume is different from all of the above in that it covers basic IR as do the latter books, but with a distinct focus on the health and biomedicine domain.

The first two editions of this book were published in 1996 and 2003, respectively. Although subsequent editions of books in many fields represent incremental updates, this edition is profoundly rewritten, and is essentially a new book. The IR world has changed substantially since I wrote the first and second editions of the book. At the time of the first edition, IR systems were available and not too difficult to access if you had the means and expertise. Also in that edition, the Internet was a "special topic" in the very last chapter of the book. By the second edition, the World Wide Web had become the widespread platform for use of information access and delivery, but had not achieved the nearly ubiquitous and saturated use it has now. At present, however, not only health care professionals and biomedical researchers must understand how to use IR systems to be effective in their work, but also patients and consumers must understand them as well to attain optimal health care.

The Web also profoundly altered the way this edition was researched and written. When preparing the first edition, finding an article not in my own collection or the Oregon Health & Science University (OHSU) Library was a chore that entailed either driving to a nearby library at another university or ordering it through interlibrary loan. For the second edition, I was often able to find articles on the Web, either because OHSU or I had a subscription or because the article was freely available. By this edition, with so much information so easily accessible, the biggest challenge was selecting from the overwhelming amount of articles, reports, and other sources. In researching and writing a book like this, I really learned firsthand the value of scientific publishing on the Web.

Another way the Web impacted the second edition and will continue to do so for this third edition is through the maintenance of a Website for errata and updates. The Website http://www.irbook.info/ will identify all errors in the book text as well as provide updates on important new findings in the field as they become available.

The work on this edition also drove home the quality of the IR systems I was using. I must give particular mention to the following resources that provided fast and accurate access to a great deal of information: PubMed and related systems of the National Library of Medicine (NLM), Google, and the multitude of journals and organizations that have opted to electronically publish their full content.

As in the first two editions, the approach is still to introduce all the necessary theories to allow coverage of the implementation and evaluation of IR systems in health and biomedicine. Any book on theoretical aspects must necessarily use technical jargon, and this book is no exception. Although jargon is minimized, it cannot be eliminated without retreating to a more superficial level of coverage. The reader's understanding of the jargon will vary based on their background, but anyone with some background in computers, libraries, health, and/or biomedicine should be able to understand most of the terms used. In any case, an attempt to define all jargon terms is made.

Another approach is to attempt wherever possible to classify topics, whether discussing types of information or models of evaluation. I have always found classification useful in providing an overview of complex topics. One problem, of course, is that everything does not fit into the neat and simple categories of the classification. This occurs repeatedly with IR, and the reader is forewarned.

This book had its origins in a tutorial taught at the former Symposium on Computer Applications in Medicine (SCAMC) meeting. The content continues to grow each year through my annual course taught to biomedical informatics students in the on-campus and distance-learning programs at OHSU. (Students often do not realize that next year's course content is based in part on the new and interesting things they teach me!) The book can be used in either a basic information science course or a health and biomedical informatics course. It should also provide a strong background for others interested in this topic, including those who design, implement, use, and evaluate IR systems.

Interest continues to grow in health and biomedical IR systems. I entered a fellowship in medical informatics at Harvard University in the late 1980s, when the influence of medical artificial intelligence was still strong. I had assumed I would take up the banner of some aspect of that area, such as knowledge representation. But along the way I came across a reference from the field of "information retrieval." It looked interesting, so I looked at the references of that reference. It did not take long to figure out that this was where my real interests lay, and I spent many an afternoon in my fellowship tracing references in the Harvard University and Massachusetts Institute of Technology libraries. Even though I had not yet heard of the field of bibliometrics, I was personally validating all its principles. Like many in the field, I have been amazed to see IR become so "mainstream" with the advent of the Web in recent years.

The book is divided into three sections. The first section covers the basic concepts of IR. Chap. 1 provides basic definitions and models that will be used throughout the book. It also points to resources for the field and introduces evaluation of systems. Chap. 2 provides an overview of health and biomedical information, describing some of the issues in its production, dissemination, and use.

The second section covers the current state of the art in commercial and other widely used retrieval systems. Chap. 3 gives an overview of the great deal of content that is currently available. The next two chapters cover the two fundamental intellectual tasks of IR, indexing and retrieval, with the predominant paradigms of each discussed in detail. Chap. 6 discusses how IR systems are fashioned into digital libraries, addressing the myriad of challenges.

The third section covers the major threads of research and development in efforts to build better IR systems. Chap. 7 focuses on evaluation research that has been done on state-of-the-art systems. Next, Chap. 8 explores research about IR systems and their users. Finally, Chap. 9 covers a group of areas closely related to IR, including information extraction and text mining, categorization, question-answering, and summarization. Throughout this section, a theme of implementation feasibility and evaluation is maintained.

Within each chapter, the goal is to provide a comprehensive overview of the topic, with thorough citations of pertinent references. There is a preference to discuss health and biomedical implementations of principles, but where this is not possible, the original domain of implementation is discussed.

This book would not have been possible without the influence of various mentors, dating back to high school, who nurtured my interests in science generally and/or biomedical informatics specifically, and/or helped me achieve my academic and career goals. The most prominent include: Mr. Robert Koonz (then of New Trier West High School, Northfield, IL), Dr. Darryl Sweeney (University of Illinois at Champaign-Urbana), Dr. Robert Greenes (then of Harvard Medical School), Dr. David Evans (Clairvoyance Corp.), Dr. Mark Frisse (then of Washington University), Dr. J. Robert Beck (then of OHSU), Dr. David Hickam (OHSU), Dr. Brian Haynes (McMaster University), Dr. Lesley Hallick (OHSU), and Dr. Jerris Hedges (then of OHSU). I must also acknowledge the contributions of the late Dr. Gerard Salton (Cornell University), whose writings initiated and sustained my interest in this field.

I also like to note the contributions of institutions and people in the federal government that aided the development of my career and this book. While many Americans increasingly question the abilities of their government to do anything successfully, the NLM, under the directorship of Dr. Donald A. B. Lindberg, has led the growth and advancement of the field of medical informatics. The NLM's fellowship and research funding have given me the skills and experience to succeed in this field. Likewise, the Agency for Healthcare Research and Quality (AHRQ), under the leadership of Dr. Carolyn Clancy, deserves mention for its contributions to my own growth as well as others in the field of medical informatics. I also acknowledge retired Oregon Senator Mark O. Hatfield through his dedication to biomedical research funding that aided myself and many others.

Finally, this book also would not have been possible without the love and support of my family. All of my parents, Mom and Jon, Dad and Gloria, as well as my brother Jeff and sister-in-law Myra, supported the various interests I developed in life and the somewhat different career path I chose. Now as they have become Web users and searchers, they appreciate my interest in this area. And last, but most importantly, has been the contribution of my wife, Sally, and two children, Becca and Alyssa, whose unlimited love and support made this undertaking so enjoyable and rewarding.

William Hersh
Portland, OR

Contents

Part I
Basic Concepts

Chapter 1
Terms, Models, Resources, and Evaluation

The goal of this book is to present the field of *information retrieval* (IR), with an emphasis on the health and biomedical domain. To many, "information retrieval" implies retrieving information of any type from a computer. However, to those working in the field, it has a different, more specific meaning, which is the retrieval of information from databases that predominantly contain textual information. A field at the intersection of information science and computer science, IR concerns itself with the indexing and retrieval of information from heterogeneous and mostly textual information resources. The term was coined by Mooers (1951), who advocated that it be applied to the "intellectual aspects" of description of information and systems for its searching.

The advancement of computer technology, however, has altered the nature of IR. As recently as the 1970s, Lancaster (1978) stated that an IR system does not inform the user about a subject; it merely indicates the existence (or nonexistence) and whereabouts of documents related to an information request. At that time, of course, computers had considerably less power and storage than today's personal computers. As a result, systems were only sufficient to handle bibliographic databases, which contained just the title, source, and a few indexing terms for documents. Furthermore, the high cost of computer hardware and telecommunications usually made it prohibitively expensive for end-users to directly access such systems, so they had to submit requests that were run in batches and returned hours to days later.

In the twenty-first century, however, the state of computers and IR systems is much different. End-user access to massive amounts of information in databases and on the World Wide Web is routine. Not only can IR databases contain the full text of resources, but also they may contain images, sounds, and even video sequences. Indeed, there is continued development of the *digital library*, where books and journals are replaced by powerful file servers that allow high-resolution viewing and printing, and library buildings are augmented by far-reaching computer networks (Witten and Bainbridge, 2003; Lesk, 2005). The notion of the "mass digitization" of information raises a host of issues, many of which we will discuss in this book, such as copyright, optical character recognition (OCR) quality, libraries, long-term ownership, business models for publishers and content sellers, information literacy, standards, and interoperability (Anonymous, 2006e). This is

W. Hersh, *Information Retrieval: A Health and Biomedical Perspective*,
doi: 10.1007/978-0-387-78703-9, © Springer Science + Business Media, LLC 2009

further challenged by our transition to "e-Science" and how individuals access, use, and manage data (Anonymous, 2007b).

Another change in the twenty-first century is a new name that is increasingly used to describe IR, *search*, which has been described as an "integral application" for the modern computing environment (Barrows and Traverso, 2006). Some of the biggest computer industry battles in recent times are for the ability to be a user's search engine (Vogelstein, 2005). Various technology writers speculate on who will develop the "ultimate" next-generation search engine (Hoover, 2007).

The name of the leading Web search engine, Google, has entered the vernacular in a variety of ways, including as a verb (i.e., looking up information about a person is called "Googling" them). The all-knowing nature of Google and the Web content it searches has led one political columnist to ask if it is "God" (Friedman, 2003). Studies published in medical journals note the ability of Google to correctly nominate medical diagnoses (Greenwald, 2005; Tang and Ng, 2006). The Google Zeitgeist (http://www.google.com/press/zeitgeist.html) keeps a tally of the world's interests as measured by what humans collectively type into the Google search engine. In addition, some lament that the "Google generation," i.e., today's legions of technology-savvy young people, are not critical enough in their skills regarding seeking, synthesizing, and critically analyzing information (Anonymous, 2008).

One of the early motivations for IR systems was the ability to improve access to information. Noting that the work of early geneticist Gregor Mendel was undiscovered for nearly 30 years, Vannevar Bush called in the 1960s for science to create better means of accessing scientific information (Bush, 1967). In current times, there is equal if not more concern with "information overload" and how to avoid missing important information. A well-known example occurred when a patient who died in a clinical trial in 2000 might have survived if information about the toxicity of the agent being studied from the 1950s (before the advent of MEDLINE) had been more readily accessible (McLellan, 2001). Indeed, a major challenge in IR is helping users find "what they don't know" (Belkin, 2000).

Just how much information is out there? Table 1.1 shows the amount of computer storage required for various types of information items. Lyman and Varian (2003) have estimated that the sum of information on physical electronic media was about 5 exabytes (or about 5 billion gigabytes) in 2003. This was noted to be equivalent to about one-half million new libraries the size of the US Library of Congress. The majority of this information (72%) was stored on magnetic media, primarily hard disks, with most of the remainder on film and a small proportion on paper (about 1.5 petabytes or 0.001 exabytes). This amounted to about 800 megabytes for each man, woman, and child on Earth. In a given year, the distribution of paper content around the world was estimated to be in the form of office documents (279–1,379 terabytes), newspapers (27–138 terabytes), mass market periodicals (10–52 terabytes), books (8–39 terabytes), and journals (1.3–6 terabytes). Card (2003) notes that information continues to grow exponentially (see Fig. 1.1). Comparatively, online information has now exceeded all human documents generated in the first 40,000 years of human history and is vastly more than all the information on Earth that all humans can learn.

Table 1.1 Relative sizes of information items (adapted from Lesk, 2005)

Size	Example (size)
Kilobytes (10^3 bytes)	Printed page (1)
	Scanned page (30)
	One second of speech (10)
	Small book (500)
Megabytes (10^6 bytes)	Medical X-ray or digital image (1–2)
	The Bible (5)
	Large medical textbook (10)
	Two-hour audio program (50)
	Oxford English Dictionary (500)
Gigabytes (10^9 bytes)	Digital movie (10)
	MEDLINE database (40)
	Books on the floor of a library (100)

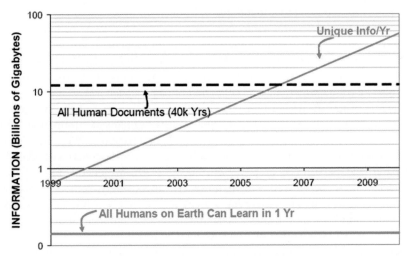

Fig. 1.1 Growth of information and comparison to all human documents and learning (courtesy of Stuart Card)

Gantz et al. (2007) estimated the amount of information in 2006 to be about 161 exabytes, projecting it to grow sixfold annually by 2010 to 988 exabytes (nearly 1 zettabyte). About 70% of the information is generated by individuals but 85% is maintained in some way by various organizations. Most of the growth is fueled by analog-to-digital conversions. For images, about 1 billion devices generate about 250 billion images annually (150 billion on cameras, 100 billion on cell phones), which is projected to double by 2010. The amount of video is also expected to double by 2010. The report also notes that the world has about 1.5 billion email accounts, which consume about 6 exabytes. It also notes that there are about 1.1 billion Internet users now, 60% of whom have broadband access. This is projected to increase to 1.6 billion by 2010. And, perhaps most pertinent to IR,

about 95% of the information is "unstructured," i.e., most appropriately searched
by IR indexing and retrieval techniques.

Nevertheless, IR systems are a unique type of computer application, and their
growing prevalence demands a better understanding of the principles underlying
their operation. This chapter gives an overview of the basic terminology of IR, some
models of systems and their interactions with the rest of the world, a discussion
of available resources, a view of IR on the Internet and the World Wide Web, and
introduction to how IR is evaluated.

1.1 Basic Definitions

There are a number of terms commonly used in IR. An *IR system* consists of
content, computer hardware to store and access that content, and computer software
to process user input in order to retrieve it. Collections of content go by a variety of
terms, including *database*, *collection*, or – in modern Web parlance – *site*.
In conventional database terminology, the items in a database are called *records*.
In IR, however, records are also called *documents*, and an IR database may be
called a *document database*. In modern parlance, items in a Web-based collection
may also be called *pages*, and the collection of pages called a *Web site*.

A view of the IR system is depicted in Fig. 1.2. The goal of the system is to
enable access by the user to content. Content consists of units of information, which
may themselves be an article, a section of a book, or a page on a Web site. Content
databases were easier to describe in the pre-Web era, as the boundaries of nonlinked
databases and persistence of paper documents were, in general, more easy to
delineate. The scope of Web content, however, varies widely: some sites organize
information into long pages covering a great deal of matter, while others break it
down into numerous short pages. The picture is further complicated by multimedia
elements, which may be part of a page or may be found in their own separate file.
In addition, Web pages may be composed of frames, each of which in turn may
contain its own Web page of information. Furthermore, the content of Web pages
may be generated dynamically and undergo constant change.

Users seek content by the input of queries to the system. Content is retrieved by
matching *metadata*, which is meta-information about the information in the content

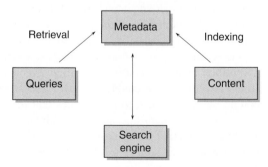

Fig. 1.2 A model of the IR system

collection, common to the user's query and the document. As we will see in Chap. 4, metadata consist of both indexing *terms* and *attributes*. Indexing terms represent the subject of content, i.e., what it is about. They vary from words that appear in the document to specialized terms assigned by professional indexers. Indexing attributes can likewise be diverse. They can, for example, consist of information about the type of a document or page (e.g., a journal article reporting a randomized controlled trial), its source (e.g., citation to its location in the *Journal of the American Medical Informatics Association* and/or its Web page address), or features in an image. A *search engine* is the software application that matches indexing terms and attributes from the query and document to return to the user.

There are two major intellectual or content-related processes in building and accessing IR systems: indexing and retrieval. *Indexing* is the process of assigning metadata to items in the database to facilitate and make efficient their retrieval. The term *indexing language*, sometimes used, refers to the sum of possible terms that can be used in the indexing of terms. There may be, and typically are, more than one set of indexing terms, hence indexing languages, for a collection.

In most bibliographic databases, for example, there are usually two indexing procedures and languages. The first indexing procedure is the assignment of indexing terms from a *controlled vocabulary* or *thesaurus* by human indexers. In this case, the indexing language is the controlled vocabulary itself, which contains a list of terms that describe the important concepts in a subject domain. The controlled vocabulary may also contain nonsubject attributes, such as the document publication type. The second indexing procedure is the extraction of all words that occur (as identified by a computer) in the entire database. Although one tends typically not to think of word extraction as indexing, the words in each document can be viewed as descriptors of the document content, and the sum of all words that occur in all the documents is an indexing language.

Retrieval is the process of interaction with the IR system to obtain documents. The user approaches the system with an *information need*. The user (or a specialized intermediary) formulates the information need into a *query*, which most often consists of terms from one or more of the indexing vocabularies, sometimes (if supported by the system) connected by the Boolean operators AND, OR, or NOT. The query may also contain specified metadata attributes. The search engine then matches the query and returns documents or pages to the user.

1.2   Scientific Disciplines Concerned with IR

The scientific disciplines historically most concerned with IR have been *library and information science* and *computer science*, although in recent years, many other disciplines have focused on search. *Information science* is a multidisciplinary field that studies the creation, use, and flow of information. Information scientists come from a wide variety of backgrounds, including information science itself, library science, computer science, systems science, decision science, and many professional fields. A broad attempt to define information science and the terms used by it was recently undertaken by Zins (2007a, b, c, d). He assembled 57 leading scholars (including this author) and carried them through an online Delphi process. The results are presented on a Web site (http://www.success.co.il/is/overview.html) and revealed 50 definitions of information science and 130 definitions of data, information, and knowledge.

IR has strong relations to computer science as well. Croft (2003) states that IR has always been just a part of the overall computer science field but has a common heritage with database systems. He also notes that the field grew and was validated by the success of Web search engines in the 1990s. Croft describes some known successes of the field:

- Search engines have become a significant means by which society accesses information.
- IR has long championed the "statistical" approach to using language, which has now been adopted by other areas of computer science, such as natural language processing.
- IR has focused on large-scale evaluation more extensively than other areas of computer science, which have come to adopt many of these techniques.
- IR has also focused on the importance of the user and interaction as part of its process.
- The global goals of information access and contextual retrieval are part of the vision of other grand research goals for computer science, as also noted by Gray (2003).

A recent paper by Moffat et al. (2005) provided a list of the most important IR research papers that are "recommended reading" for research students. One paper of note in this collection is the paper by Brin and Page (1998) describing the PageRank algorithm at the heart of Google. This paper was rejected by the leading computer science IR conference as being poorly written and not having evaluation of its efficacy. While these criticisms were no doubt valid, the underlying idea truly transformed IR, at least on the Web.

A collection of leaders in the computer science portion of the IR field held a workshop for defining the research agenda for the IR field in 2003 (Allan, Aslam et al., 2003). This workshop was motivated to offset a notion that current Web search engines were so effective that further research and development in the field was not warranted. However, this workshop noted that while Web searching had become mainstream and successful, there were still other aspects of search warranting research, based on assertions that:

- Web searching and IR are not equivalent: Web searching is at best a part of overall information access.
- Web queries do not represent all information needs: Users do much more than search for the Web pages and other content indexed by Web search engines. For example, while much biomedical content is on the Web, much of it exists (and is usually search) in more specialized databases, such as the medical literature in MEDLINE.

- Web search engines are effective for some types of queries in some contexts: There are many times when users are looking for more specific and/or different information that resides on the Web. For example, the "popularity ranking" that works well in search engines like Google may not be the best strategy (or even work) for a biomedical textbook or an organization's intranet.

The report also outlined what workshop attendees considered to be the major challenge areas for IR research:

- Retrieval models: Web search engines tend to have a "one size fits all" model that does not take into account other tasks that the user wishes to perform, such as answer questions, browse specific collections of information, find certain types of content, etc.
- Cross-language IR: While English was initially the predominant language of the Web, less than half of all pages are in English and at some point in the future, other languages might surpass it. Systems need to find content in other languages when appropriate and provide the user a summary so he/she can determine whether to expend the resources to translate it.
- Web search: While Web search is not the only type of IR application, it is certainly very popular, and further research must continue to improve it.
- User modeling: Different users have diverse needs, even when searching for the same "topic." This is certainly true in healthcare, where a patient, primary care physician, and subspecialist all might want information on the same topic but bring different levels of reading ability, prior knowledge, and so forth to the information-seeking process.

A more recent workshop reached similar conclusions (Callan, Allan et al., 2007). This report noted that despite the success and ubiquity of Web search engines, more research to improve systems is still an imperative. They noted some problems that Web search engines have not solved, such as heterogeneous data (i.e., not everything is Web pages), heterogeneous context (i.e., search is not the "end goal," but users have specific tasks with the information they seek to find), need for information analysis and organization (i.e., helping the user discover relationships and other aspects of the information), and evaluation (i.e., the need to go beyond the "Cranfield paradigm" that has served the field so well and is described below).

The field of biomedical informatics has great interest in IR as well, though like computer science, IR is just a small part of the larger field. The National Library of Medicine (NLM), the leading funder of biomedical informatics research and training in the United States, recently released an update of its long-range plan, which includes four overall goals, all of which are related to IR (Anonymous, 2006a):

1. Seamless, uninterrupted access to expanding collections of biomedical data, medical knowledge, and health information
2. Trusted information services that promote health literacy and the reduction of health disparities worldwide

3. Integrated biomedical, clinical, and public health information systems that promote scientific discovery and speed the translation of research into practice
4. A strong and diverse workforce for biomedical informatics research, systems development, and innovative service delivery

Two leaders of the NLM have laid out a vision for the future of medical libraries 10 years hence, noting that the "place" will be preserved but that most of the information will be interactive and electronic (Lindberg and Humphreys, 2005).

Another growing category of IR system users are biomedical researchers. This is due in large part to new "high-throughput" biotechnologies, such as gene micro-arrays. These technologies not only generate large amounts of data but also identify new information that must be explored, e.g., the microarray experiment that uncovers increased expression of genes previously unknown to be related to a physiological or disease process (Buetow, 2005). There is growing awareness that IR and other techniques, such as text mining, are important tools for researchers (Cohen and Hersh, 2005; Hunter and Cohen, 2006; Jensen, Saric et al., 2006; Roberts, 2006). We will explore these further in Chap. 9.

But even literature retrieval and analysis are difficult for scientists. Barnes and Gary (2003) have said, "Few areas of biological research call for a broader background in biology than the modern approach to genetics. This background is tested to the extreme in the selection of candidate genes for involvement with a disease process... Literature is the most powerful resource to support this process, but it is also the most complex and confounding data source to search." A leading neuroscientist, noting the advances in the Human Genome Project and related areas, has advocated that biology should now be considered an "information science," with many advances likely to come from using data to form and test hypotheses (Insel, Volkow et al., 2003). Meanwhile, pharmaceutical (and likely other) companies fight for information and library talent (Davies, 2006). One such talented individual quotes Harvard University Chemistry Professor Frank Westheimer, who once famously said, "A month in the laboratory can save an hour in the library."

An essential skill for healthcare practice, biomedical research, and anyone in the population staying healthy is *health information literacy*. The Medical Library Association (MLA, http://www.mlanet.org/) has defined health information literacy as the set of abilities needed to:

• Recognize a health information need
• Identify likely information sources and use them to retrieve relevant information
• Assess the quality of the information and its applicability to a specific situation
• Analyze, understand, and use the information to make good health decisions

The MLA has developed a Web site devoted to this topic, which includes a variety of resources and plans for action (http://www.mlanet.org/resources/healthlit/). McCray (2005) recently reviewed health literacy and noted most of it focused on low literacy and its impact on understanding health information but advocated a broader, including attention to:

- Methods to assess literacy and the related topic readability of texts
- The mismatch between the readability of health information and the literacy of those for whom it is intended
- The difficulty patients with low literacy have in the healthcare system, from accessing care to understanding their treatment plans to their worse clinical outcomes
- The impact of new information technologies

1.3   Models of IR

Another way to understand a field is to look at models of the processes that are studied. A model of the IR system has already been presented above. In this section, four models are discussed that depict the overall information world, the user's interaction with an IR system, factors that influence decision making in healthcare, and knowledge acquisition and use.

1.3.1   The Information World

Figure 1.3 depicts the cyclic flow of information from its producers, into the IR system, and on to its users (Meadow, Boyce et al., 2007). Starting from the creation of information, events occur in the world that lead to written observations in the form of books, periodicals, scientific journals, and so on. These are collected by

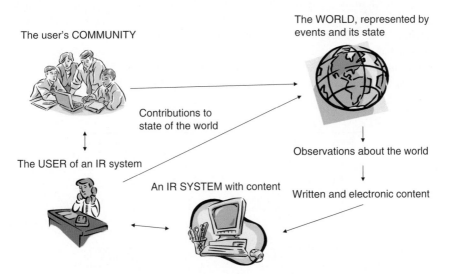

Fig. 1.3 A model of information flow in the world (adapted from Meadow, Boyce et al., 2007)

database producers, who may create a bibliographic database of references to these sources or, as is happening with greater frequency, may create electronic versions of the full text. However a database is constructed, it is then organized into records and loaded into the IR system.

In the system, a file update program stores the data physically. Users, either directly or through trained intermediaries, query the database and retrieve content. Those users not only use the information but also may add value to it, some of which may make its way into new or other existing content. In addition, users also feed back observations to the database producers, who may correct errors or organize it better.

1.3.2 Users

Figure 1.4 shows the information-seeking functions of the user (Marchionini, 1992). The central component is the user defining the problem (or information need). Once this has been done, the user selects the source for searching and articulates the problem (or formulates the query). The user then does the search, examines the results, and extracts information. Many of these tasks are interactive. Any step along the way, for example, may lead the user to redefine the problem. Perhaps, some results obtained have provided new insight that changes the information need. Or, examination of the results may lead the user to change the search strategy. Likewise, information extracted may cause the user to examine the rest of the searching results in a different manner.

A variety of other models of interaction between the user and IR system have been put forth in recent years. Marchionini (2006) has looked beyond fact lookup to "exploratory search," where users also engage in learning and investigation. Downey et al. (2007) have developed a comprehensive model of user search activity that can be used to quantify various aspects of the process. Another view of information seeking focusing on "strategies" and "tactics" for searching, with a focus on the clinical domain, has been put forth by Hung et al. (2008).

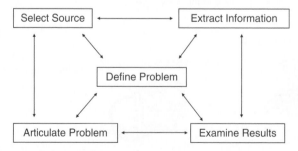

Fig. 1.4 A model of the IR user (adapted from Marchionini, 1992)

1.3.3   Health Decision Making

The ultimate goal of searching for health information is often to make a decision, such whether to order a test or prescribe a treatment. The decision maker may be a patient, his/her family, or a healthcare professional. A variety of factors go into making a health-related decision. The first of these categories is the scientific evidence, which answers the question of whether there has been objective-as-possible science to support a decision. An approach for finding and appraising this sort of information most effectively is called evidence-based medicine (EBM). As discussed in more detail in Chap. 2, EBM provides a set of tools that enable individuals to more effectively find information and apply it to health decisions.

Evidence alone, however, is not sufficient for decisions. Both patients and clinicians may have personal, cultural, or other preferences that influence how evidence will be applied. The healthcare professional may also have limited training or experience to be able to apply evidence, such as a physician not trained as a surgeon or not trained to perform a specific treatment or procedure. There are other constraints on decision making as well. There may be legal or other restrictions on what medical care can be provided. There may also be constraints of time (patient far away from the site at which a specific type of care can be provided) or financial resources (patient or entity responsible for paying for the care cannot afford it).

Figure 1.5 adapted from Mulrow et al. (1997), depicts the relationships among the factors that influence health decision making. The intersection of evidence and preferences provides the knowledge that can be used to make decisions. The intersection of evidence and constraints leads to guidelines. There is a growing interest in practice guidelines, with this specialized type of content discussed in Chap. 3. The ethical dimensions of healthcare lie at the intersection of preferences and constraints. Finally, the intersection of all three represents everything that is considered in a health decision.

1.3.4   Knowledge Acquisition and Use

Another model of information seeking and use is depicted in Fig. 1.6, with the process viewed as a funnel by which the user searches all of the scientific literature using IR systems to obtain a set of possibly relevant literature. In the current state of the art, he/she reviews this literature by hand, selecting which articles are definitely relevant and may become "actionable knowledge," i.e., part of his or her active store of knowledge. However, newer techniques from areas such as information extraction and text mining in the future may provide more automated assistance for determining what is relevant and converting it to actionable knowledge.

It is important to note that Fig. 1.6 also reminds us of the importance of IR systems for aiding processes like information extraction and text mining, which

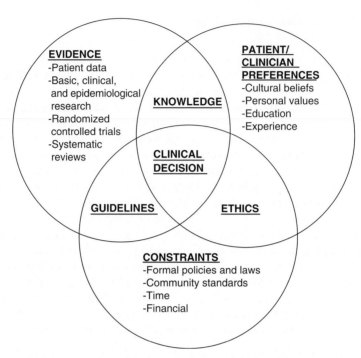

Fig. 1.5 A model of health decision making (adapted from Mulrow, Cook et al., 1997)

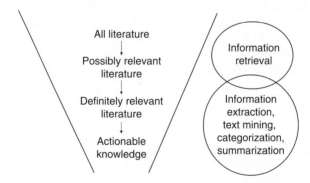

Fig. 1.6 The funnel of knowledge acquisition and use, showing the focus of the information retrieval field vs. information extraction and text mining

tend to apply more intensive processing to understand and create actionable knowledge as opposed to IR, which aims to deliver content to the user. Information extraction and text mining cannot, however, proceed effectively without good output from IR systems to feed their algorithms. We will cover these topics in Chap. 9.

1.4 IR Resources

It has already been noted that IR is a heterogeneous, multidisciplinary field. This section describes the field's organizations and publications. Because of the diversity of this field, the focus is on the organizations and publications most centrally committed to IR. Also included are those from the healthcare field that may not have IR as a central focus but do have an interest in it. The Web addresses of all the organizations, journals, and tools mentioned in this section are listed in Tables 1.2, 1.3, and 1.4, respectively.

1.4.1 Organizations

A number of specialty organizations have interests that overlap with IR. The organization devoted specifically to information science is the *American Society for Information Science and Technology* (ASIST). The largest computer science organization devoted to IR is the *Special Interest Group in Information Retrieval* (SIGIR) of the *Association for Computing Machinery* (ACM). The library science field is closely related to information science, and there is much overlap in personnel, but its central issues are more related to the structure and functioning of libraries. The major library science organization is the *American Library Association* (ALA). Another organization more focused on technical libraries is the *Special Libraries Association* (SLA). There is also a professional group devoted specifically to document indexing, called the *American Society of Indexers* (ASI).

A number of health and biomedical information organizations have IR among their interests. The *American Medical Informatics Association* (AMIA) is devoted to all aspects of information technology in healthcare, biomedical research, and public health, including IR. MLA is concerned with the needs and issues of health science libraries, which of course include IR systems. Another organization that is not a professional society per se but is heavily involved in health-related IR is the

Table 1.2 Information retrieval-related professional organizations

Organization	Web address
American Library Association (ALA)	http://www.ala.org/
American Medical Informatics Association (AMIA)	http://www.amia.org/
American Society for Information Science and Technology (ASIST)	http://www.asist.org/
American Society of Indexers (ASI)	http://www.asindexing.org/
Association for Computing Machinery–Special Interest Group on Information Retrieval (ACM/SIGIR)	http://www.sigir.org/
Medical Library Association (MLA)	http://www.mlanet.org/
National Library of Medicine (NLM)	http://www.nlm.nih.gov/
Special Libraries Association (SLA)	http://www.sla.org/

Table 1.3 Journals noted for coverage of information retrieval

Journal	Web address
General	
ACM Transaction on Information Systems (ACM TOIS)	http://tois.acm.org/
D-Lib Magazine	http://www.dlib.org/
First Monday	http://firstmonday.org/
Journal of the American Society for Information Science and Technology (JASIST)	http://www.asis.org/Publications/ JASIS/jasis.html
Information Processing and Management (IP&M)	http://www.elsevier.com/locate/ infoproman/
Information Research	http://InformationR.net/ir/
Information Retrieval (IR)	http://www.springerlink.com/content/ 1386-4564/
Biomedical	
Biomedical Digital Libraries	http://www.bio-diglib.org/
British Medical Journal (BMJ)	http://www.bmj.com/
Journal of Biomedical Discovery and Collaboration (JBDC)	http://www.j-biomed-discovery.com/
Journal of Biomedical Informatics (JBI)	http://www.elsevier.com/locate/yjbin/
Journal of the American Medical Informatics Association (JAMIA)	http://www.jamia.org/
Journal of Medical Internet Research (JMIR)	http://www.jmir.org/
Journal of the Medical Library Association (JMLA)	http://www.mlanet.org/publications/ jmla/
Methods of Information in Medicine (MIM)	http://www.schattauer.de/index.php? id=704

NLM, the US government agency that not only maintains many important medical databases but also funds research and training in medical informatics.

An additional group of organizations involved in IR are the companies that comprise the growing marketplace for search and retrieval products, which have by now become household names. In addition to the major Web search engines, whose names are household names (e.g., Google, Yahoo, and Microsoft), there are a variety of others that offer more specialized products. In the health and biomedical domain, some well-known names are WebMD (http://www.webmd.com/), Healthline (http://www.healthline.com/), and MedStory (http://www.medstory.com/). The latter was recently acquired by Microsoft.

1.4.2   Journals

There are a variety of scientific journals that are devoted fully or in part to IR research. Table 1.3 divides these into general and biomedically oriented categories. Even general medical journals occasionally publish IR articles. Probably, the most

Table 1.4 Information science tools

Name and description	Web address
Bow: library of code for writing statistical text analysis, language modeling, and information retrieval programs	http://www.cs.cmu.edu/~mccallum/bow/
Frakes and Baeza-Yates: source code from Frakes and Baeza-Yates (Frakes and Baeza-Yates, 1992)	ftp://ftp.vt.edu/pub/reuse/IR.code/
freeWAIS-sf: Wide Area Information Searcher	http://www.is.informatik.uni-duisburg.de/projects/freeWAIS-sf/
Internet Archive: archive of the Internet, including various "snapshots" from specific points in time	http://www.archive.org
IR Framework: object-oriented framework for information retrieval (IR) applications written in Java	http://www.itl.nist.gov/iaui/894.02/projects/irf/irf.html
Lemur Toolkit for Language Modeling and Information Retrieval: supports indexing of large-scale text databases, the construction of simple language models for documents, queries, or subcollections, and the implementation of retrieval systems based on language models as well as a variety of other retrieval models	http://www.lemurproject.org/
Lucene: open source toolkit that is part of the Apache open source Web server platform (Gospodnetic and Hatcher, 2005)	http://lucene.apache.org/
MG: public domain indexing and retrieval system for text, images, and textual images	http://www.ncsi.iisc.ernet.in/raja/netlis/wise/mg/mainmg.html
NCBI: most of the genomic databases of the National Center for Biotechnology Information of the National Library of Medicine are freely available	http://www.ncbi.nlm.nih.gov/Ftp/
NLM: the entire MEDLINE database, MeSH vocabulary, Unified Medical Language System, and other resources are available from the National Library of Medicine	http://www.nlm.nih.gov/databases/leased.html
PRISE: prototype indexing and search engine developed by National Institute of Standards and Technology	http://www-nlpir.nist.gov/works/papers/zp2/zp2.html
Okapi: indexing and retrieval system implementing Okapi weighting scheme	http://okapi.sourceforge.net/
SMART: current version of IR system based on Salton's algorithms	ftp://ftp.cs.cornell.edu/pub/smart/
Terrier: open source retrieval platform for research and applications	http://ir.dcs.gla.ac.uk/terrier/
Zettair: a compact and fast text search engine from a research group focused on query efficiency	http://www.seg.rmit.edu.au/zettair/

notable of these is the *British Medical Journal* (BMJ), which not only publishes articles on the topic but also has been a leader in innovating Web technology in electronic publishing of the journal.

1.4.3 Texts

There are a variety of IR texts. As noted in the Preface, some are of the "how to" variety for searching the medical literature (Edhlund, 2005, 2006; Katcher, 2006). There is also a comprehensive three-volume reference on health and medical information on the Web, available both in print and on CD-ROM from the MLA (Anderson and Allee, 2004). In addition to books on searching MEDLINE and other health resources, additional help can be found in the tutorials and help files on the PubMed site:

- Tutorials: http://www.nlm.nih.gov/bsd/disted/pubmed.html
- Help: http://www.ncbi.nlm.nih.gov/books/bv.fcgi?rid=helppubmed.chapter.pub medhelp

There are also books for how to effectively search the Web generally (Hock, 2004; Poremsky, 2004; Schlein, 2004; Notess, 2006).

Another category of texts consist of general IR books. Among the most recent are those by Baeza-Yates and Ribeiro-Neto (1999), Belew (2000), Rubin (2004), Grossman and Frieder (2004), Meadow et al. (2007), and Agosti (2008). There are also a variety of books devoted to specialized topics, such as image retrieval (DelBimbo, 1999) and information seeking in context (Ingwersen and Jarvelin, 2005; Case, 2006). There are also books that focus on the confluence of IR with natural language processing, information extraction, text categorization, and/or text mining (Jackson and Moulinier, 2002; Tait, 2005; Ananiadou and McNaught, 2006).

Some "classic" texts in the field include Salton and McGill (1983), which was written by the pioneer of "statistical" techniques in IR, and van Rijsbergen (1979), whose text is maintained on the Web (http://www.dcs.gla.ac.uk/Keith/Preface.html). A text designed for those interested in actual computer implementation of IR systems (Frakes and Baeza-Yates, 1992) describes actual algorithms and provides source code in the C programming language for many of them. The book is actually a complement to other IR texts and is oriented toward the actual implementation of IR systems.

Of course, the success of the Google search engine has spawned a variety of books. Some of these are "how to" manuals (Poremsky, 2004; Miller, 2007), while others describe how to take advantage of its advertising (Davis, 2006) and other features (Calishain and Dornfest, 2004). One book focuses on the mathematical details of its PageRank algorithm (Langville and Meyer, 2006). Still others focus on the company's business success (Battelle, 2005; Vise and Malseed, 2005; Arnold, 2007).

1.4.4 Tools

When the first edition of this book was written, access to IR systems was expensive and, in many cases, required specialized software. Now, however, a plethora of search engines are just a mouse click away in anyone's Web browser. For those actually wanting to experiment implementing IR systems, there are many options. Some maintained lists are available at:

- http://www.searchtools.com/tools/tools-opensource.html
- http://compbio.uchsc.edu/corpora/bcresources.html
- http://www.pdg.cnb.uam.es/martink/LINKS/bionlp_tools_links.htm

Some of these tools are listed in Table 1.4, along with a number of other related tools. Probably, the most widely used toolkit is Lucene, which is part of the Apache open source Web server platform (Gospodnetic and Hatcher, 2005). In addition to these systems, there are a number of commercial text retrieval packages available, some of which run on microcomputers and are fairly inexpensive.

1.5   The Internet and World Wide Web

This chapter has already alluded to the profound impact on IR of the Internet and World Wide Web. Indeed, it is telling that in the first edition of this book, the Internet and the Web were described in the last chapter in the "special topics" section. In the second edition, they were introduced here in the first chapter and discussed widely throughout. But in the third edition, along with search in general, they have achieved near ubiquity in the lives of most knowledge professionals (including healthcare professionals and researchers) and assumed a major role in the lives of many who confront personal health issues. These technologies transformed IR from a task done by information professionals and a small number of other computer-savvy individuals to one done by people of all ages, levels of education, and geographic locations.

Few readers of this book are likely to need a description of the Internet and Web. However, it does help to define the key terms and point out some of their attributes relevant to IR. The Internet is the global computer network that connects machines of varying sizes and capacities using a communications protocol called TCP/IP. The Web is a software application that runs on the Internet, with servers making available pages coded in the Hypertext Mark-Up Language (HTML) that are downloaded and displayed on client computers running a Web browser. In the hardware/software distinction of computers, the Internet is the hardware and the Web is the software. But the Web is more than a simple computer application; essentially, it is a platform from which virtually any computer functions can be done, including searching as well as database access and transactions.

1.5.1   Size

Because of its distributed nature (i.e., there is no central server or authority), the total size of the Web cannot be known, nor can it be indexed in its entirety since it is constantly changing. The first published total size of the Web came from Lawrence and Giles (1999), who estimated in 1999 that the Web consisted of 800 million pages, with a total of 6 terabytes (TB) of text residing on 2.8 million servers. This study also found that Web search engines covered less than half of all the available pages on the Web, and there was considerable lack of overlap across different search engines. More recently, the size of the Web has been estimated to be on the order of 25–30 billion pages, with about 100 million Web hosts.

Another commonly measured statistic is the number of people who use the Internet and where they live. There are several Web sites that track Internet use in different countries and languages: comScore (http://www.comscore.com/), Internet World Statistics (http://www.internetworldstats.com/), and Global Reach (http://www.glreach.com/). They all paint a relatively consistent picture: World-wide use of the Internet continues to grow, particularly in emerging economies like India, China, and Russia (Anonymous, 2007w). While the largest number of users still comes from the US (154 million), China is rapidly closing in (87 million) and only 20% of all Internet users worldwide come from the US. Despite its growth, Doyle et al. (2005) have noted that the Internet is "robust yet fragile." In other words, its distributed nature makes it fault-tolerant, but faults do occur frequently.

1.5.2   Usage

Broder (2002) noted that although classic IR is driven by user's needing informa-tion, Web searching is often not informational. Instead, the user's intent might be navigational (e.g., finding a specific page) or transactional (e.g., purchase some-thing, download a file, check the status of an account). He noted that navigational searches are similar to what classic IR calls a "known-item search," where the user is trying to find a particular piece of content, such as an article or image. Broder also states that "hub" pages (see Sect. 1.5.5) with lists of links that get to the target in one click may be acceptable to retrieve in a search. In transactional queries, the user needs not only to reach a site but also to interact with it once he/she gets there.

Broder analyzed the frequency of these types of Web search by users of the AltaVista search engine via two means: a pop-up survey window and a search log analysis. Based on his data, he concluded the following approximate types of Web search and their frequency:

- Information tasks: traditional IR seeking of information in "documents" (39–48%)
- Navigational tasks: finding something, such as the Web site of an institution or a resource such as a database (20–24%)

- Transactional tasks: accessing a service, data (such as an airline schedule), or shopping (30–36%)

In other words, less than half of searches on the Web (at least those entered into the AltaVista search engine at that time) were classical IR informational seeking.

Broder also describes what he calls three generations of search engines on the Web. The first generation uses mostly static HTML pages and is very close to classic IR. The second generation uses off-page, Web-specific data such as link analysis, anchor text, and click-through data. He cites the Google PageRank algorithm as an example of this and notes that it supports informational as well as navigational queries. The third generation attempts to discern the "need behind the query" based on semantic analysis of the user's input and determination of their context. He gives the example of the user entering the name of a city and the system returning a hotel reservation page, map server, weather server, etc. The aim of this generation would be to support all transactional searches in addition to those which are informational and navigational.

Search engine use is very high among Internet users. Data from Fallows et al. (2004) and Rainie and Shermak (2005) have shown that over 84% of all Internet users have used a search engine and that 87% of people say they find what they want most of the time. This research has also shown that the average user performs 33 searches per month, spending about 41 min at search engine sites and that the average visit to a search engine results in 4.4 searches. Search engine users are enthusiastic and trusting of search engines but are also unaware and naive about certain aspects of them (Fallows, 2005). A large majority of users report confidence in their searching abilities (92%) and they have successful searches most of the time (87%). However, 62% are unaware in the differences between paid and unpaid results.

It seems almost like ancient history now, but the original Web (sometimes called Web 1.0) featured a boom and then a bust, i.e., the dot-com era. Some (e.g., O'Reilly, 2005) talk of a new Web now, a "Web 2.0" that is built on sustainable business models and widespread collaboration. A more sound business model gives users what they want and make it more sustainable, e.g., Google Ads, eBay, and Amazon. But Web 2.0 is also more collaborative, e.g., blogging, wikis and Wikipedia, Flickr, and Craig's List. It has been advocated that this "mass collaboration" augments collection and expansion of human knowledge in ways not previously possible (Tapscott and Williams, 2006). Could Web 2.0 impact medicine? One view was put forth by Giustini (2006). Naturally, talk of Web 2.0 has spawned talk of a Web 3.0, which is a Web of interacting data and knowledge, sometimes also called the "Semantic Web" (Fensel, Wahlster et al., 2002; Yu, 2007).

Of course, one irony that few IR "old timers" could ever have fathomed is the need, in the Web era, for the study of "adversarial IR" – in other words, the development of techniques to *prevent* retrieval of certain content. One group of adversarial IR applications is the prevention of "spam" (i.e., unwanted) pages or emails (Metaxas and DeStefano, 2005; Cormack and Lyman, 2007). On the Web, this called "link spam" (Noruzi, 2006). There is now an annual conference devoted to research in this area (http://airweb.cse.lehigh.edu/). Singhal (2004) has noted that there is a continual tit-for-tat battle between those who develop search engines and those who try to "game" them. Indeed, a key modern business strategy is the attempt to drive traffic to one's Web site via search engines and other means, which is called search engine *optimization* or *visibility* (Thurow, 2007).

Another form of adversarial IR involves "filtering," with the usual goal of preventing linkage to pornography sites. As the Internet is usually available on computers where most people work, there is increasing effort to block various sites. Of course, many of these approaches to such filtering are imperfect and can lead to blocking of legitimate medical Web sites (Richardson, Resnick et al., 2002).

Also, a concern about search engines is the growing desire of governments and others to monitor their usage (Hansell, 2006). Ostensibly to thwart the very real threats of terrorism, many are concerned about governments knowing our searching interests. There are also some governments, most notably China, who have required search engines to filter pages containing certain words (such as democracy) and have led to the arrest of political dissidents (MacDonald, 2006). Some express concerns about other entities that monitor search behavior, such as advertisers seeking to sell things to us (Röhle, 2007). At the current time, privacy laws that protect things like email and library checkouts do not protect queries to search engines (Hansell, 2006). Of course, there is potential value in monitoring searches, at least anonymously, for epidemiological surveillance (Johnson, Wagner et al., 2004).

1.5.3   Hypertext and Linking

In both the paper and electronic information worlds, there are two ways of finding information: searching and browsing. In *searching*, information is sought by finding terms in an index that point to locations where material about that term may be. In books, for example, searching is done by looking up topics in the index in the back. Searching in electronic resources is carried out by means of an IR system. *Browsing*, on the other hand, is done by delving into the text itself, navigating to areas that are presumed to hold the content that is sought. In books, browsing is usually started by consulting the table of contents, but the reader may also follow references within the text to other portions of the book. Electronic browsing in early computer systems was difficult if not impossible but has been made easier with the advent of *hypertext*, which is the electronic linking of nonlinear text.

The majority of the chapters of this book focus on searching as the means to find information. But computers also allow a unique form of information seeking that recognizes the nonlinearity of most text, especially scientific and technical reference information. Most paper-based resources allow some nonlinearity by referring to other portions of the text (e.g., "see Chapter X"). Computers allow these linkages to be made explicit.

The person most often credited with originating the notion of hypertext is Vannevar Bush, who proposed in 1945 that the scientist of the future would carry a device called a *memex* that linked all his or her information (Bush, 1945). Another pioneer in the hypertext area was Ted Nelson, who implemented the first systems in the 1970s (Nelson, 1987). The popularity of hypertext did not take hold until the widespread proliferation of computers that used a graphical user interface (GUI) and a mouse pointing device. These systems allowed simple and easy-to-use hypertext interfaces to be built. Although not a true hypertext system, Apple Computer's Hypercard application, released in 1987, brought the concepts of hypertext to the mainstream. Another change brought by computers with GUIs was the ability to display nontextual information, such as images, sounds, video, and other media, often integrated with text. The term *hypermedia* is sometimes used to describe systems that employ hypertext combined with other nontextual information. The Web brought Internet-based hypermedia to the mainstream.

For certain types of content, hypermedia systems offer dynamic ways of viewing it. Consider as an example a hypermedia neurology textbook. Many neurological conditions, such as the abnormal gait seen in Parkinson's disease, are much better viewed in video than described in a narrative. Furthermore, since the pharmacological treatment of this disease can be complex, this textbook may be linked to other sources, such as a pharmacology textbook that described the use and side effects of the medications in more detail than could a neurology textbook. Another valuable link could be to the primary medical literature, where clinical trials with these medications could be accessed.

1.5.4   The Web in Health and Biomedicine

The Web has transformed health and biomedicine and will likely continue to do so. Repeated surveys show that of Americans who use the Web, over 80% have searched for information related to health for themselves, a family member, or close associate (Fox, 2006; Anonymous, 2007m). This means that over 160 million, or more than half, of the US population has searched online for health information. Madden and Fox (2006) found that for over half of all people searching for health information, the most important information was found online. Comparable numbers have been found by the Health Information National Trends Survey (HINTS), funded by the National Cancer Institute (NCI) (Hesse, Nelson et al., 2005). The first report of this survey found that 63.0% of Americans reported going online, with 63.7% of those who did so reporting that they looked for health information for themselves or someone they know in the last 12 months. Eysenbach and Kohler (2004) found that about 4.5% of queries to a major search engine were on health-related topics. The most common topics included healthcare services and organizations (9.6%), medications (8.1%), and diet, nutrition, and weight loss (6.7%).

Unfortunately, it is not clear that all these information seekers are appropriately skilled or skeptical of online health information. Fox (2006) found that three quarters of searchers do not consistently check the source or date of the information they retrieve. In a study of college students, Ivanitskaya et al. (2006) found that only half of a group of college students could identify trustworthy features of health

Web sites. Furthermore, self-reported skills were only weakly correlated with actual skill level as measured by a standardized instrument.

Although physicians were slow to adopt use of the Internet and Web, its use is now nearly 100% (Anonymous, 2005e). Previous research showed that physicians who were more active clinically (i.e., saw more patients per week) spent more time online (Taylor and Leitman, 2001). Older research also showed that the average physician user spent 7.1 h per week online and that about 65% of physicians over 60 years of age were users, showing that use was not limited to younger physicians (Anonymous, 2001a).

1.5.5   Science of the World Wide Web

A growing amount of research has studied the Web and related large-scale networking phenomena, including biology. The originator of the Web, Tim Berners-Lee, recently called for an emerging "science of the Web" (Berners-Lee, Hall et al., 2006). Barabási (2002) has studied complex networks extensively, noting similarities across different types of networks from biological to human-made ones. He has particularly noted this phenomenon in the organization of the living cell (Barabási and Oltvai, 2004).

Kleinberg and Lawrence (2001) proposed a widely cited model for the Web, consisting of hubs and authorities. *Hubs* are catalogs and resource lists of pages that point to *authorities* on given topics. Another view of the Web is to divide into the *visible* and *invisible* Web, as depicted in Fig. 1.7 (Sherman and Price, 2001). The former contains all of the Web content that can be found by fixed or static URLs, while the latter contains content "hidden" behind password-protected sites or in databases (Anonymous, 2002d). In general, the visible Web is searched via general Web search engines. On the other hand, most of the commercial online databases to be described in later chapters reside on the invisible Web.

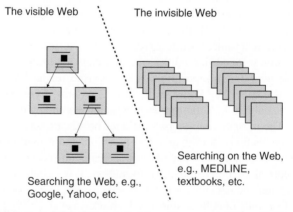

Fig. 1.7   The visible vs. invisible Web (adapted from Sherman and Price, 2001)

1.6   Evaluation

Another important topic to introduce early on concerns evaluation of IR systems, which is important for many reasons. Like any other technology, IR systems are expensive, if not to individuals then the institutions in which they work. And as with many areas of computer use, there is a good deal of hype, marketing and otherwise, about the benefits of the technology. Thus, the main reason to evaluate is to determine whether a system helps the users for whom it is intended. However, after this benefit has been demonstrated, it must also be shown that the system justifies its cost. And ultimately, the system's real-world results should indicate some measure of improvement on the tasks in which it is used. This notion has an analogy in the medical research world to outcomes research, where not only must an intervention demonstrate *efficacy* (benefit in controlled research) but also *effectiveness* (benefit in the real world outside the controlled research setting).

Evaluations of IR systems are often classified as macroevaluations or microevaluations. *Macroevaluations* look at the whole IR system and/or the user's interaction with it. This type of evaluation can take place in either a laboratory or a real-world setting. At times, however, one wishes to evaluate individual components of IR systems. Such evaluations are called *microevaluations*, and the motivations for doing them are to assess individual components of the system, to solve problems that arise with its use, and to determine how changes in the system might impact performance. They are typically performed in a laboratory or other controlled setting.

Another distinction often made when discussing IR evaluation is *system-oriented* vs. *user-oriented*. System-oriented research focuses on evaluation of the system, either by part or as a whole, focusing on how well it performs a set of standardized tasks. The usual approach to system-oriented evaluation in IR is through the use of recall and precision. User-oriented evaluation, on the other hand, focuses on assessing the system in the hands of real users, who themselves may be in a simulated laboratory setting or real-world environment.

1.6.1   Classification of Evaluation

There are many classifications of evaluation or aspects therein that have been developed. One early and widely cited model was developed by Lancaster and Warner (1993), who defined three levels of evaluation, as shown in Table 1.5. The first level is the evaluation of the effectiveness of the system and the user interacting with the system. (Health services researchers would actually state that efficacy and not effectiveness is being studied here, but Lancaster and Warner's own language shall be used.) At this level, the authors identify three general criteria for effectiveness: cost, time, and quality. While issues of cost and time are straightforward, those of quality are considerably more subjective. In fact, what constitutes quality

Table 1.5 Lancaster and Warner's classification of IR evaluation (adapted from Lancaster and Warner, 1993)

I. Evaluation of effectiveness
   A. Cost
      1. Monetary cost to user (per search, document, or subscription)
      2. Other, less tangible, cost considerations
         (a) Effort involved in learning how to use the system
         (b) Effort involved in actual use
         (c) Effort involved in retrieving documents
         (d) Form of output provided by system
   B. Time
      1. Time from submission of request to retrieval of references
      2. Time from submission of request to retrieval of documents
      3. Other time considerations, such as waiting to use system
   C. Quality
      1. Coverage of database
      2. Completeness of output (recall)
      3. Relevance of output (precision)
      4. Novelty of output
      5. Completeness and accuracy of data
II. Evaluation of cost-effectiveness
   A. Unit cost per relevant citation retrieved
   B. Unit cost per new (previously unknown) relevant citation retrieved
   C. Unit cost per relevant document retrieved
III. Cost-benefit evaluation: value of systems balanced against costs of operating or using them

in a retrieval system may be one of the most controversial questions in the IR field. This category also contains the relevance-based measures of recall and precision, which are the most frequently used evaluation measures in IR. The second level of retrieval evaluation in Lancaster and Warner's schema is *cost-effectiveness*. This level measures the unit costs of various aspects of the retrieval system, such as cost per relevant citation or cost per relevant document. The final level of evaluation in the schema is *cost-benefit*, which compares the costs of different approaches directly.

Fidel and Soergel (1983) devised a classification to catalog for researchers all the factors that need to be controlled in IR evaluations. This classification can also, however, be used to review the components that should be studied (or at least considered) in effective IR evaluation. Its items include:

- Setting: where system used, e.g., library, clinic, laboratory, etc.
- User: type of searcher, e.g., researcher vs. clinician, or other attributes about him or her
- Request: type of information need, e.g., background, comprehensive, discussion, fact, update
- Database: content searched, e.g., type, cost, indexing

- System: retrieval system used, e.g., how accessed, cost, help provided, user interface
- Searcher: who did the search, e.g., intermediary vs. end-user
- Process: how searches done experimentally, e.g., in batch process or an operational setting
- Outcome: results of search and their value to the user and his or her information need

While both Lancaster and Warner as well as Fidel and Soergel had "outcome" in their classifications, it may be desirable to expand what it means. In particular, there are (at least) six questions one can ask related to an IR resource (system or information collection) in a particular setting. These questions were developed for a systematic review assessing how well physicians use IR systems (Hersh and Hickam, 1998), but they could be applied to other users and settings. These questions were developed for a systematic review assessing how well physicians use IR systems (Hersh and Hickam, 1998), but they can be applied to other users and settings.

1.6.1.1   Was the System Used?

An important question to ask about an IR resource is whether it was actually used by those for whom it was provided. Measurement of system or collection use can be gleaned from user questionnaires, preferably, however, it is done directly by system logging software. It is important to know how frequently people used a resource, since to be installed in the first place, someone had to have thought it would be beneficial to users. The nonuse of a system or collection is a telling evaluation of its (non)value to users.

1.6.1.2   For What Was the System Used?

A related concern is knowing the tasks for which the system was being used. One might want to know what information collections were used (if there were more than one) and what types of questions were posed. In a clinical setting, there might be interest in what kind(s) of clinical problem led to use of which resource. Likewise, it may be important to know whether the system was used as a primary information resource or to obtain references for library lookup.

1.6.1.3   Were the Users Satisfied?

The next question to ask is whether users were satisfied with the IR system. User satisfaction is an important question both for administrators who make decisions to install and maintain systems and for researchers trying to determine the role of systems for users. It is also relatively straightforward to assess, with the use of instruments such as questionnaires, direct observation, and focus groups.

A well-known instrument for assessing computer software is the Questionnaire for User Interface Satisfaction (QUIS) (Chin, Diehl et al., 1988).

1.6.1.4   How Well Was the System Used?

Once it has been determined that systems were used and with satisfaction, the next issue is how effectively they were actually used. Whereas frequency of use and user satisfaction are relatively simple concepts, the notion of "how well" someone uses a system is more complex. Does one operate at the level of counting the number of relevant documents obtained, perhaps over a given time period? Or are larger issues assessed, such as whether use of the system results in better patient care outcomes? An example of the latter would be showing that the system had led a practitioner to make better decisions or had resulted in better patient outcomes. This issue will be addressed further shortly.

While many studies have focused on a wide variety of performance measures, the most widely used are still the relevance-based measures of recall and precision. These were first defined decades ago by Kent et al. (1955) and achieved prominence by their use in the Cranfield studies of the 1960s (Cleverdon and Keen, 1966). Indeed, many consider them to be the "gold standard" of retrieval evaluation and call their use the "Cranfield paradigm." Yet as we see in this and other chapters, their use has some serious limitations, especially when they are the sole measurements in an evaluation. It is not that they are unimportant conceptually, but rather that they are difficult to measure in operational settings and do not necessarily correlate with the success of using an IR system. In acknowledgment of their prevalence, however, we will cover them separately in Sect. 1.6.2.

1.6.1.5   What Factors Were Associated with Successful or Unsuccessful Use of the System?

Whether an IR system works well, or does not work well, there are likely explanations for the result. A variety of factors (e.g., demographic, cognitive, experiential) can be measured and correlated with the outcome of system use. Furthermore, if the system did not perform well, a researcher might wish to ask why. The assessment of system failure, called *failure analysis*, typically involves retrospectively determining the problems and ascertaining whether they were due to indexing, retrieval, user error, or some combination of these.

1.6.1.6   Did the System Have an Impact?

The final, and obviously most important question, is whether the system had an impact. In the case of clinical users, this might be measured by some type of improved healthcare delivery outcome, such as care of better quality or reduced cost. This item which is addressed in the schemas of both Lancaster and Warner and Fidel and Soergel takes on increased pertinence in healthcare, given the emphasis on quality of care and the desire to control costs. Of course, demonstrating that a computer system has an impact in actual patient outcome is difficult, because this effect is often indirect (Friedman and Wyatt, 2006). This is particularly true of IR systems, where not only is use for a given patient optional but also each new patient on whose behalf the system is used is likely to require a different kind of use. As such, there have been few studies of patient outcomes as related to IR systems. Such studies are easier to do for computer-based decision support systems, where the same function (e.g., recommended drug dose, alert for an abnormal laboratory test) is used for the same situation each time (Garg, Adhikari et al., 2005).

1.6.2 Relevance-Based Evaluation

Relevance-based measures are so prevalent in their usage and important concep- tually that we will explore them further. Certainly, a major goal of using an IR system is to find relevant documents. We measure how well systems do that through the measures of recall and precision. Furthermore, these two measures can be aggregated into a single measure using a number of different approaches, including the *F*-measure, the recall–precision table, and mean average precision (MAP). For all of these measures, a system is assessed by calculating the average or mean across a set of topics in a given evaluation study.

1.6.2.1 Recall and Precision

Recall and precision quantify the number of relevant documents retrieved by the user from the database and in his or her search. Ignoring for a moment the subjective nature of relevance, we can see in Fig. 1.8 that for a given user query

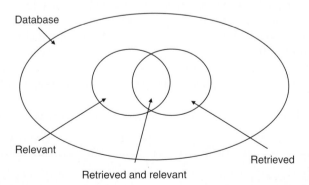

Fig. 1.8 Graphical depiction of the elements necessary to calculate recall and precision

on a topic, there are relevant documents (Rel), retrieved documents (Ret), and retrieved documents that are also relevant (Retrel). Recall is the proportion of relevant documents retrieved from the database:

$$\text{Recall} = \frac{\text{Retrel}}{\text{Rel}} \tag{1.1}$$

In other words, recall answers the question: For a given search, what fraction of all the relevant documents have been obtained from the database?

One problem with (1.1) is that the denominator implies that the total number of relevant documents for a query is known. For all but the smallest of databases, however, it is unlikely, perhaps even impossible, for one to succeed in identifying all relevant documents in a database. Thus, most studies use the measure of *relative recall*, where the denominator is redefined to represent the number of relevant documents identified by multiple searches on the query topic.

Precision is the proportion of relevant documents retrieved in the search:

$$\text{Precision} = \frac{\text{Retrel}}{\text{Ret}} \tag{1.2}$$

This measure answers the question: For a search, what fraction of the retrieved documents are relevant?

A sample recall and precision matrix is shown in Table 1.6. The database contains a total of one million documents. For this particular query, there are 50 known relevant documents. The searcher has retrieved 100 documents, of which 30 are relevant to the query. The proportion of all relevant documents obtained, or recall, is 30/50, or 60%. The fraction of relevant documents from the set retrieved is 30/100, or 30%.

Table 1.6 is very similar to the matrix used to calculate the diagnostic test performance measures of sensitivity and specificity. In fact, if "relevance" is changed to "presence of disease" and "number retrieved" is changed to "number with positive test result," then recall is identical to sensitivity, while precision is the same as positive predictive value. (Specificity would be a much less useful number in IR research, since the numbers of both relevant and retrieved articles for a given query tend to be small. With large databases, therefore, specificity would almost always approach 100%.)

It is known in medical testing that there is a tradeoff between sensitivity and specificity. That is, if the threshold is changed for a positive test, it will change not

Table 1.6 Table of retrieved and/or relevant documents for a query to calculate recall and precision

	Relevant	Not relevant	Total
Retrieved	30	70	100
Not retrieved	20	999,880	999,900
Total	50	999,950	1,000,000

only the proportion of people correctly diagnosed but also the proportion incorrectly diagnosed. If the threshold for diagnosis is lowered, then the test not only will usually identify more true positive cases of the disease (and thus raise sensitivity) but also will identify more false positive instances. The relationship between sensitivity (recall) and positive predictive value (precision) is not quite so direct, but it usually occurs in IR systems. The tradeoff can be demonstrated qualitatively by comparing searchers of different types, such as researchers and clinicians. A researcher would more likely want to retrieve everything on a given topic. This searcher (or an intermediary) would thus make the query statement broad to be able to retrieve as many relevant documents as possible. As a result, however, this searcher would also tend to retrieve a high number of nonrelevant documents as well. Conversely, a clinician searching for a small number of good articles on a topic is much less concerned with complete recall. He/she would be more likely to phrase the search narrowly, aiming to obtain just a few relevant documents, without having to wade through a large number of nonrelevant ones.

Another medical measurement analogy from recall and precision has been defined by Bachmann et al. (2002): the *number needed to read* (NNR), which is the inverse of precision, i.e., 1/precision. The NNR defines the total number of articles that must be read to find each relevant one. This analogy can actually be carried back to the medical measurement realm, with the inverse of the positive predictive value (equivalent of precision) representing the number needed to test.

1.6.2.2   *F*-Measure

Another measure commonly used to combine recall and precision is the *F*-measure (van Rijsbergen, 1979). This measure is the harmonic mean of recall and precision, and uses a parameter α that gives added value to recall as it increases. When $\alpha = 1$, the measure is called F_1, and it represents the harmonic mean of recall and precision. For a search situation where precision was important, one would set α to a lower level, i.e., less than one:

$$F = \frac{(1 + \alpha)RP}{\alpha P + R} \tag{1.3}$$

1.6.2.3   Ranked Systems

Many IR systems use relevance ranking, whereby the output is sorted by means of measures that attempt to rank the importance of documents, usually based on factors related to frequency of occurrence of terms in both the query and the document. In general, systems that feature Boolean searching do not have relevance ranking, while those featuring natural language searching tend to incorporate it. Systems that use relevance ranking tend to have larger but sorted retrieval outputs, and users can decide how far down to look. Since the more relevant documents tend to be ranked higher, this approach gives users a chance to determine whether they want lower recall and higher precision (just look at the top of the list) or higher recall and lower precision (keep looking further down the list).

One problem that arises when one is comparing systems that use ranking vs. those that do not is that nonranking systems, typically using Boolean searching, tend to retrieve a fixed set of documents and as a result have fixed points of recall and precision. Systems with relevance ranking, on the other hand, have different values of recall and precision depending on the size of the retrieval set the system (or the user) has chosen to show. For this reason, many evaluators of systems featuring relevance ranking will create a recall–precision table (or graph) that identifies precision at various levels of recall. The "standard" approach to this was defined by Salton and McGill (1983), who pioneered both relevance ranking and this method of evaluating such systems.

To generate a recall–precision table for a single query, one first must determine the intervals of recall that will be used. A typical approach is to use intervals of 0.1 (or 10%), with a total of 11 intervals from a recall of 0.0 to 1.0. The table is built by determining the highest level of overall precision at any point in the output for a given interval of recall. Thus, for the recall interval 0.0, one would use the highest level of precision at which the recall is anywhere greater than or equal to zero and less than 0.1.

Since the ranked output list is scanned from the top, the number of relevant documents is always increasing. Thus, each time a new relevant document in the list is identified, it must first be determined whether it is in the current interval or the next one (representing higher recall). For the appropriate interval, the new overall precision is compared with the existing value. If it is higher, then the existing value is replaced.

When there are fewer relevant documents than there are intervals (e.g., ten intervals but fewer documents), one must interpolate back from the higher interval. For example, if there are only two relevant documents, then the first relevant one would fall at a recall level of 0.5 and would require interpolation of the current overall precision value back to the preceding levels of recall (i.e., 0.4, 0.3, 0.2, 0.1, and 0.0). Conversely, when there are more relevant documents than intervals, one must compare each level of precision within the recall interval to all the others to determine the highest one.

An example should make this clearer. Table 1.7 contains the ranked output from a query of 20 documents retrieved, and 7 are known to be relevant. Table 1.8 is a recall–precision table for the documents in Table 1.7 with recall intervals of 0.1. Note that there are fewer intervals than documents, so interpolation is needed.

The first document in Table 1.7 is relevant. Because there are seven relevant documents, the recall is 1/7 or 0.14. The overall precision at this point is 1/1 or 1.0, and its value is entered into the table for the recall level of 0.1. Since there are fewer than ten relevant documents, there will be separate precision for the recall level of 0.0, so the value from the recall level of 0.1 is interpolated back to the 0.0 level. The second document is not relevant, but the third document is. The overall level of recall is now 2/7 or 0.28, so the new level of precision, 2/3 or 0.67, is entered into

Table 1.7 Example ranked output of 20 documents with 7 known to be relevant

Rank	Relevance	Recall and precision[a]
1	Rel	$R = 1/7, P = 1/1$
2	NRel	
3	Rel	$R = 2/7, P = 2/3$
4	NRel	
5	Rel	$R = 3/7, P = 3/5$
6	Rel	$R = 4/7, P = 4/6$
7	NRel	
8	NRel	
9	Rel	$R = 5/7, P = 5/9$
10	NRel	
11	NRel	
12	NRel	
13	NRel	
14	Rel	$R = 6/7, P = 6/14$
15	NRel	
16	NRel	
17	NRel	
18	NRel	
19	NRel	
20	Rel	$R = 7/7, P = 7/20$

Rel relevant document, *NRel* nonrelevant one
[a] Each time a relevant document is encountered, recall (R) and precision (P) are calculated to be entered into the recall–precision table (see Table 1.8)

Table 1.8 Recall–precision table resulting from the data in Table 1.6

Recall	Precision
0.0	1.00
0.1	1.00
0.2	0.67
0.3	0.60
0.4	0.60
0.5	0.67
0.6	0.56
0.7	0.56
0.8	0.43
0.9	0.35
1.0	0.35

the recall level of 0.2 in Table 1.8. The following document is not relevant, but the fifth document is, moving the overall recall level up to 3/7 or 0.42. The new precision is 3/5 or 0.60, and it is entered into Table 1.8 at the recall level of 0.4. Notice that there was no value to enter into the recall level of 0.3, so the value at the

0.4 level is interpolated back to the 0.3 level. The rest of the results are shown in Table 1.8.

For a whole set of queries, the values at each recall level are averaged. In general, the values for precision over a set of queries will fall with increasing level of recall. To compare different systems, or changes made in a single system, three or more of the precision levels are typically averaged. When the recall interval is 0.1, one might average all 11 intervals or just average a few of them, such as 0.2, 0.5, and 0.8.

An approach that has been used more frequently in recent times has been MAP, which is similar to precision at points of recall but does not use fixed recall intervals or interpolation (Voorhees, 1998; Buckley and Voorhees, 2005). MAP is calculated from the mean of average precision (AP) for each topic. AP represents the average of precision at each point a relevant document is retrieved or, for relevant documents not retrieved, a value of 0. As such, it is a recall-oriented measure (despite having "precision" in its name), since it measures retrieval across the entire set of relevant documents for a topic.

Here is how AP would be calculated for the ranked output of Table 1.7:

$$\mathrm{AP} = \frac{\frac{1}{1} + \frac{2}{3} + \frac{3}{5} + \frac{4}{6} + \frac{5}{9} + \frac{6}{14} + \frac{7}{20}}{7} = \frac{4.27}{7} = 0.61. \tag{1.4}$$

If the retrieved documents in positions 14 and 20 in the output were not relevant, and those other relevant documents had not been retrieved at all, then AP would be calculated as follows:

$$\mathrm{AP} = \frac{\frac{1}{1} + \frac{2}{3} + \frac{3}{5} + \frac{4}{6} + \frac{5}{9} + 0 + 0}{7} = \frac{3.49}{7} = 0.501. \tag{1.5}$$

Another approach to aggregating recall and precision with ranked output has been proposed by Jarvelin and Kekalainen (2000), who have put forth two measures related to the value to the degree of relevance and rank of the document in the output list. The measure to add value based on relevance is called cumulative gain (CG). A cumulative score is kept, with additional score added based on the degree of relevance of the document:

$$\mathrm{CG}(i) = \mathrm{CG}(i - 1) + G(i), \tag{1.6}$$

where i is the document's rank in the output list (e.g., the top ranking document has $i = 1$) and $G(i)$ is the relevance value. The measure based on document rank is called the discounted cumulative gain (DCG):

$$\mathrm{DCG}(i) = \mathrm{DCG}(i - 1) + \frac{G(i)}{\log(i)}. \tag{1.7}$$

When $i = 1$, CG(1) is set to 1 if there is no relevant document and DCG(1) is set to 1 to avoid dividing by zero. The authors advocate that CG be plotted vs. DCG, with the performance of systems assessed based on the value of CG relative to DCG.

For all of the above measures, a system is evaluated by taking the mean or average of a given measure over a set of topics. For a recall–precision table, the average precision at each point of recall is calculated, while for AP, the MAP across all topics is calculated. We will explore these measures and their usage further in Chaps. 7–9, along with actual evaluation results of systems. We will also explore some of their limitations.

1.6.3   Challenge Evaluations

The field of computer science has a long history of *challenge evaluations*, where developers of different systems compare their efficacy with some sort of standardized task and/or data collection. The IR field is no exception. The largest and best-known IR challenge evaluation is the Text REtrieval Conference (TREC, http://trec.nist.gov), organized by the US National Institute of Standards and Technology (NIST, http://www.nist.gov/) (Voorhees and Harman, 2005). Started in 1992, TREC has provided a series of challenge evaluations and a forum for presentation of their results. TREC is organized as an annual event at which the tasks are specified and queries and documents are provided to participants. Figure 1.9 shows the usual steps in the annual cycle for each task organized in TREC. The original TREC events were numbered, e.g., TREC-1 (in 1992), TREC-2 (in 1993), etc., to TREC-9 (in 2000). Thereafter, each year's TREC was named with the year, e.g., TREC 2001.

Challenge evaluations are usually based on test collections, which have three basic components:

1. Documents: used very generically here, documents can be articles, Web pages, bibliographic records, images, or any other item that is a unit of retrieval.
2. Topics: statements of information need, ideally derived from real-world situations. It should be noted that the statements themselves are usually described as topics whereas the search statements entered into actual systems are typically called queries.
3. Relevance judgments: judgments of relevance of documents to the topics. This is typically done via the pooling method where a certain number of top ranking documents from each system participating in the challenge evaluation are included in a pool for relevance judging for each topic.

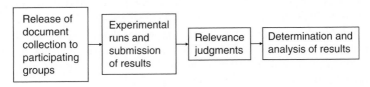

Fig. 1.9 Annual cycle of most TREC tracks and tasks

One of the motivations for starting TREC was the observation that much IR evaluation research (prior to the early 1990s) was done on small test collections that were not representative of real-world databases. Furthermore, some companies had developed their own large databases for evaluation but were unwilling to share them with other researchers. TREC was therefore designed to serve as a means to increase communication among academic, industrial, and governmental IR researchers. Although the results were presented in a way that allowed comparison of different systems, conference organizers advocated that the forum not be a "competition" but instead a means to share ideas and techniques for successful IR. In fact, participants are required to sign an agreement not to use results of the conference in advertisements and other public materials (Voorhees and Harman, 2005).

The original TREC conference featured two common tasks for all participants. An ad hoc *retrieval task* simulated an IR system, where a static set of documents was searched using new topics, similar to the way a user might search a database or Web search engine with an information need for the first time. A *routing task*, on the other hand, simulated a standing query against an oncoming new stream of documents, similar to a topic expert's attempt to extract new information about his or her area of interest. The original tasks used newswire and government documents, with queries created by US government information analysts. System performance was measured by a variety of measures similar to those described previously. Relevance judgments have been performed by the same information analysts who create the queries (Voorhees, 1998).

By the third TREC conference (TREC-3), interest was developing in other IR areas besides ad hoc tasks and routing. At that time, the conference began to introduce *tracks* geared to specific interests, each of which developed one or more tasks in each annual cycle. In an overview of TREC, Voorhees recently categorized the tasks and the names of the tracks associated with them (Voorhees and Harman, 2005):

- Static text: ad hoc
- Streamed text: routing, filtering
- Human in the loop: interactive
- Beyond English (cross-lingual): Spanish, Chinese, and others
- Beyond text: OCR, speech, video
- Web searching: very large corpus, Web
- Answers, not documents: question answering
- Domain-specific: genomics, legal

TREC has, for the most part, focused on newswire and/or government documents. With the exception of the Genomics Track, led by this author (Hersh, Bhupatiraju et al., 2006b), TREC has not focused on biomedical content. The TREC Genomics Track (http://ir.ohsu.edu/genomics/) was one of the largest and longest running challenge evaluations in biomedicine. The tasks of each year are listed in Table 1.9 and described in more detail later in the book. Instructions for obtaining the test collections for research use are available on the track's Web site.

Table 1.9 Tasks of the TREC Genomics Track (http://ir.ohsu.edu/genomics/)

Year	Task description	Document collection	Topics
2003 (Hersh and Bhupatiraju, 2003)	Ad hoc retrieval	A 1-year subset (4/2002–4/2003) of 525,938 MEDLINE records	Gene names, with the goal of finding all MEDLINE references that focus on the basic biology of the gene or its protein products from the designated organism
2003 (Hersh and Bhupatiraju, 2003)	GeneRIF (Mitchell, Aronson et al., 2003) annotation from article titles and abstract	139 articles that had been assigned GeneRIFs, derived from all articles appearing in five journals during the latter half of 2002	Assigned GeneRIFs
2004 (Hersh, Bhuptiraju et al., 2004)	Ad hoc retrieval	A 10-year subset (1994–2003) of 4,591,008 MEDLINE records	50 information needs statements with title, information need, and context (background)
2004 (Hersh, Bhuptiraju et al., 2004)	Categorization of documents containing data about gene function suitable for "triage" to annotators assigning Gene Ontology (GO) codes for Mouse Genome Informatics database	A 3-year set of 11,880 full-text articles for three journals obtained from Highwire Press	N/A
2005 (Hersh, Cohen et al., 2005)	Ad hoc retrieval	A 10-year subset (1994–2003) of 4,591,008 MEDLINE records	50 information needs statements similar to 2004 but classified into one of five Generic Topic Types (GTTs)

(continued)

Table 1.9 (continued)

2005 (Hersh, Cohen et al., 2005)	Categorization of documents containing data about gene function suitable for "triage" to annotators assigning GO codes or identifying for inclusion into databases about tumor biology, embryologic gene expression, or alleles of mutant phenotypes for Mouse Genome Informatics	A 3-year set of 11,880 full-text articles for three journals obtained from Highwire Press	N/A
2006 (Hersh, Cohen et al., 2006)	Retrieval of passages (from part of sentence to paragraph in length) with linkage to five entities (e.g., genes, proteins) and the source article	Collection of 162,259 full-text HTML documents from 49 journals that publish electronically via Highwire Press	28 question statements based on GTTs
2007 (Hersh, Cohen et al., 2007)	Entity-based question answering based on retrieval of passages linked to 14 entities and the source article	Collection of 162,259 full-text HTML documents from 49 journals that publish electronically via Highwire Press	36 question statements based on the 14 entities

The TREC experiments have led to research about evaluation itself. Voorhees (1998), for example, has assessed the impact of different relevance judgments on results in the TREC ad hoc task. In the TREC-6 ad hoc task, over 13,000 documents among the 50 queries had duplicate judgments. Substituting one set of judgments for the other was found to cause minor changes in the MAP for different systems but not their order relative to other systems. In other words, different judgments changed the MAP number but not the relative performance among different systems. Zobel (1998) has demonstrated that the number of relevant documents in the ad hoc track is likely underestimated, hence recall may be overstated.

TREC has also had its share of critics. Those who have argued that system assessments based solely on topical relevance assessments and not employing real users are implicitly criticizing the TREC model (Swanson, 1977; Harter, 1992; Hersh, 1994). Blair (2002) noted the problems in calculating recall that have been put forth by others and further argued that the TREC ad hoc experiments overemphasized the importance of recall in the operational searching environment. He did not, however, acknowledge the TREC Interactive Track, which addressed some of his concerns (Hersh, 2001).

Some TREC tracks have been so successful that they have spawned their own separate organizational structures. The first of these was the Cross-Language Track, which spawned two TREC-like initiatives:

1. Cross-Language Evaluation Forum (CLEF, http://www.clef-campaign.org/): focused on European languages, CLEF features a number of tracks that mimic those in TREC, such as ad hoc and Web searching. CLEF also includes an image retrieval task, ImageCLEF, which itself includes a medical image retrieval task whose organizers include this author (http://ir.ohsu.edu/image/) (Hersh, Müller et al., 2006). In the ImageCLEF medical task, the "documents" of the test collection are comprised of images and their annotations.
2. NTCIR (http://research.nii.ac.jp/ntcir/index-en.html): focused on East Asian languages (predominantly Japanese and Chinese), this forum also provides a full spectrum of IR tasks, including retrieval, question answering, Web searching, and text summarization.

Another track that spawned its own initiative is the Video Track, which has evolved into the separate TRECVID (http://www-nlpir.nist.gov/projects/trecvid/) (Smeaton, 2005). Another IR evaluation forum focusing on retrieval from XML documents, the INitiative for the Evaluation of XML Retrieval (INEX, http://inex.is.informatik.uni-duisburg.de/) (Lalmas and Tombros, 2007).

Other collections made available for research have included query logs. Such logs from major Web engines have provided a snapshot of the information people are looking for (or at least type into search engines). This research lets us know, for example, that most users enter very short queries and rarely look at results beyond the first page of ten results (Jansen, Spink et al., 1998; Spink, Jansen et al., 2002). America Online created a stir in 2006 when it released, with great fanfare, a collection of 20,000 user queries from its system. After it was quickly discovered that the queries contained some personally identifiable information, the data set was withdrawn and never posted again (Hafner, 2006).

Chapter 2
Health and Biomedical Information

Chapter 1 defined the basic terminology of information retrieval (IR) and presented some models of the use of IR systems. Before proceeding with the details of IR systems, however, it is worthwhile to step back and consider the more fundamental aspects of information, especially as it is used in the health and biomedical domain. In this chapter, the topic of information itself will be explored by looking at what it consists of and how it is produced and used. Consideration of this topic allows a better understanding of the roles as well as the limitations of IR systems.

2.1 What Is Information?

The notion of *information* is viewed differently by different people. The American Heritage Dictionary offers a number of different definitions that include the following:

- Knowledge derived from study, experience, or instruction.
- Knowledge of specific events or situations that has been gathered or received by communication; intelligence or news. See synonyms at knowledge.
- A collection of facts or data: statistical information.
- The act of informing or the condition of being informed; communication of knowledge: Safety instructions are provided for the information of our passengers.
- Computer Science: processed, stored, or transmitted data.
- A numerical measure of the uncertainty of an experimental outcome.
- Law: A formal accusation of a crime made by a public officer rather than by grand jury indictment.

Others have attempted to define information by comparing it on a spectrum containing data, information, and knowledge (Blum, 1984). *Data* consists of the observations and measurements made about the world. *Information*, on the other hand, is data brought together in aggregate to demonstrate facts. *Knowledge* is what is learned from the data and information, and what can be applied in new situations to understand the world.

Whatever the definition of information, its importance cannot be overemphasized. This is truly the information age, where information (or access to it) is an indispensable resource, as important as human or capital resources. Most corporations have a chief information officer who wields great power and responsibility. Some of the best-known very wealthy Americans (e.g., Bill Gates, Paul Allen, Larry Ellison, and Ross Perot) each made their fortunes in the information industry. Information is important not only to managers, but to workers as well, particularly those who are professionals. Many health-care professionals spend a significant proportion of their time acquiring, managing, and utilizing information.

2.2   Theories of Information

One way of understanding a complex concept such as information is to develop theories about it. In particular, one can develop models for the generation, transmission, and use of information. This section will explore some of the different theories of information, which provide different ways to view information. More details in all the theoretical aspects of information can be found in the books by Losee (1990) and Cover and Thomas (2006).

The scientists generally credited with the origin of information theory are Shannon and Weaver (1949). Shannon was an engineer, most concerned with the transmission of information over telephone lines. His theory, therefore, viewed information as a signal transmitting across a channel. His major concerns were with coding and decoding the information as well as minimizing transmission noise. Weaver, on the other hand, was more focused on the meaning of information, and how that meaning was communicated.

Figure 2.1 depicts Shannon and Weaver's model of communication. In information communication, the goal is to transfer information from the source to the destination. For the information to be transmitted, it must be encoded and sent by the transmitter to a channel, which is the medium that transmits the message to the destination. Before arriving, however, it must be captured and decoded by the receiver. In electronic means of communication, the signal is composed of either

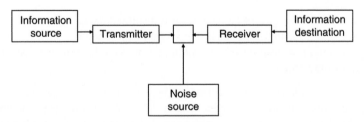

Fig. 2.1 Shannon and Weaver's model of communication (adapted from Shannon and Weaver, 1949)

waves (i.e., the analog signals of telephone or radio waves) or binary bits (i.e., in a digital computer).

From the standpoint of the sender, the goal is to deliver information as efficiently as possible. Therefore, information is a measure of *uncertainty* or *entropy*. Shannon actually defines this quantitatively. The simplest form of this expression is

$$I = \log_2\left(\frac{1}{p}\right) = -\log_2(p) \tag{2.1}$$

where p is the probability of a message occurring. If base two is used for the logarithm, then information can be measured in terms of bits. An alternative view is that the quantity of information is measured by q, the logarithm of the number of different forms that a message can possibly take. In this case, the measurement of information is expressed as

$$I = \log_2(q) \tag{2.2}$$

Obviously messages of greater length have a higher number of possible forms.

As an example of the measure of information, consider the transfer of a single letter. If each letter has an equal probability of occurring, then the chance of any one letter occurring is 1/26. The information contained in one of these letters, therefore, is $-\log_2(1/26) = 4.7$ bits. This can be alternatively expressed as having 26 different forms, with the information contained in a letter as $\log_2(26) = 4.7$ bits. Similarly, the information in a coin flip is $-\log_2(1/2) = \log_2(2) = 1$ bit. Therefore, there is more information in a single letter than in a coin flip. These examples indicate that the more likely a message is to occur, the less information it contains. Shannon's measure is clearly valuable in the myriad of engineering problems in transmitting messages across electronic media.

Weaver, as mentioned earlier, was more concerned with the transmission of meaning (Shannon and Weaver, 1949). He noted that Shannon's view of communication was only one of three levels of the communication problem, and that the other two levels also must be considered in the communication of information. These levels were as follows:

1. The technical level – issues of engineering, such as how to efficiently encode information and move it across a channel with a minimum of noise.
2. The semantic level – issues of conveying meaning, such as whether the destination understands what the source is communicating.
3. The effectiveness level – issues of whether information has the desired effect at the destination level. A well-engineered communication system may have good semantic representation, but if it does not provide proper behavioral outcomes at the other end, then the system is not effective.

Others have attempted to refine and extend Shannon and Weaver's model. Bar-Hillel and Carnap (1953) added a layer of semantics to the measurement of information. They noted that information does not consist just of isolated bits; it actually contains objects with relationships (or predicates) between them. These objects and relationships can be encoded in logical forms, and therefore, information can be defined as the set of all statements that can be logically excluded from a message. In other words, information increases as statements become more precise. Belis and Guiasi (1968) worked at Weaver's effectiveness level by adding values of utility of messages for both the sender and receiver. Certainly a message over a paramedic's radio that a patient in cardiac arrest is on the way to the Emergency Department has a great deal more utility for sender and receiver than one announcing that someone with a fractured wrist is coming. Belis and Guiasi added factors based on utilities of these types to Shannon's original equations.

Although information science is concerned with these theoretical notions of information and communication, most work has a more practical basis. In particular, information scientists are most concerned with written communication, which plays an important role in the dissemination of historical events as well as scholarly ideas. Information scientists focus on written information, from both archival and retrieval perspectives. Written information has been viewed not only from theoretical perspectives, such as the measuring of the "productivity" of scientists, but also from practical standpoints, such as deciding what books and journals to put in libraries and, more recently, how to build and disseminate IR systems.

2.3   Properties of Scientific Information

As just noted, information scientists study many facets of information but are usually most concerned with the written form. In the course of this work, they have identified many properties of information. Since the focus of information science is also usually based on scholarly and scientific information, most of these properties turn out to be quite pertinent to health information. This section will explore the growth, obsolescence, fragmentation, and linkage of scientific information.

2.3.1   Growth

Scientific information has been growing at an exponential level for several centuries and shows no signs of abating. Price (1963) found that from the first known scientific journals in the 1600s, the doubling time of the scientific literature was about 15 years. Pao (1989) noted that Price's model predicted an accumulation of 2.3 million scientific papers by 1977 (based on an initial paper in 1660), which was very close to the 2.2 million documents that were indexed by members of the National Federation of Abstracting and Indexing Services in that year (Molyneux, 1989). Durack (1978) and Madlon-Kay (1989) followed the weight growth of the (no longer produced) *Index Medicus* books of the medical literature, noting that they also followed Price's doubling time. They lamented practically that this might exceed the shelving space of libraries, though did not foresee the replacement of *Index Medicus* by the electronic MEDLINE database, whose 56 GB can be stored on a small number of lightweight DVD disks.

Will the exponential growth in scientific information continue? There are some practical issues, such as whether there will be enough trees to produce the paper to print the increasing numbers of journals on, although as trees become more scarce and electronic media more developed and affordable, there could just be a shift from print to electronic publication. Another factor that may slow the growth of scientific information is the slowing rate of growth of funding of science by government agencies (Loscalzo, 2006). With fewer scientists, especially those funded by public means, who are more likely to publish in the scientific literature, there could be a leveling off of the growth of scientific literature. But even if the rate of information growth slows, there will still be plenty of new information for scientists and professionals to assimilate.

2.3.2 Obsolescence

Despite its exponential growth in size, another property of scientific information is that it becomes obsolete, sometimes rather quickly. Newer literature not only reports on more recent experiments, but is also more likely to provide a more up-to-date list of citations to recent work. Furthermore, new experimental findings often cause underlying views of a topic change over time. As new results are obtained, older experiments may be viewed in a different light.

A classic example of how views change over time because of new experimental results is seen with respect to the role of serum cholesterol in heart disease (Littenberg, 1992). When the link between serum cholesterol and coronary artery disease was first discovered, there was no evidence that lowering the cholesterol level was beneficial. But as experimental studies began to demonstrate that benefits could occur, the earlier beliefs were displaced (though such assertions remained in the literature in the form of outdated papers). Even more recently, however, it has become clear that not everyone benefits from lowering serum cholesterol. In particular, for primary prevention of heart disease, many individuals must be treated to obtain benefit in a relatively few, and those likely to benefit cannot be predicted.

Some phenomena, such as medical diseases, change over time. For example, the presentation of many infectious diseases has changed drastically since the beginning of the antibiotic era, while the incidence of coronary artery disease continues to decline. Even phenomena from chemistry and physics, which themselves do not change, are seen in a different light when methods of measuring and detecting them are refined.

These changes over time indicate that more recent literature is clearly advantageous and that some information becomes obsolete. The actual rate of information obsolescence varies by field. Price (1963) found that half of all references cited in chemistry papers were less than 8 years old, while half of those in physics papers were less than 5 years old. This type of observation is not just theoretical; it has practical implications for those designing libraries and IR systems. For the former, there are issues of shelves to build and librarians to hire, while for the latter there are issues of how much data to store and maintain.

Fortunately, knowledge itself becomes obsolete less quickly than citations. This was demonstrated in a study of the "truth survival" of conclusions in the domain of cirrhosis and hepatitis (Poynard, Munteanu et al., 2002). The goal of the study was to determine whether information generated by the best evidence-based means had a longer survival when obtained in studies of higher methodological quality. The authors identified 474 conclusions in the published literature from 1945 to 1999 and found that 285 (60%) were still true in 2000, 91 (19%) were obsolete, and 98 (21%) were false. The half-life of truth in this domain was 45 years (in stark contrast to the half-life figures for citations presented earlier for chemistry and physics). The survival of conclusions was not higher in studies of better methodological quality than those of lesser quality, and that the 20-year survival of conclusions derived from systematic reviews (a type of summarization of the literature described in Sect. 2.5.4) was lower (57%) than those from nonrandomized studies (87%) or randomized controlled trials (RCTs; 85%).

Another study on information obsolescence assessed only systematic reviews, determining how quickly "signals" for their updating became known (Shojania, Sampson et al., 2007). These signals could be quantitative or qualitative. The former were defined as changes in statistical significance or 50% or more relative change in effect magnitude of one of the primary outcomes or of any mortality measure. The latter were defined as "substantial" changes with new information about harms or concerns about previously described findings. On the basis of this approach applied to 100 systematic reviews, the authors discovered a signal for updating 57% of all reviews, with a median duration of "survival-free" signal for updating of 5.5 years. The signal for updating occurred within 2 years for 23% of systematic reviews and by the publication date for 7% of them.

Of course, just because literature is old does not mean it is obsolete. When a healthy volunteer died after being given the compound hexamethonium in a recent clinical trial, it was noted that the toxicity of this compound had been documented in earlier literature (McLellan, 2001). Since, however, the pertinent literature was published before the advent of MEDLINE in 1966, it was not included in the MEDLINE database. This case led to the call for more systematic searching of older literature by researchers.

Related to information obsolescence is the long lead time for the dissemination of information. A common dictum in health care is that textbooks are out of date the moment they are published. As it turns out, they may be out of date before the authors even sit down to write them. Antman et al. (1992) showed that the information of experts as disseminated in the medical textbooks, review articles, and practice recommendations they produce often lagged far behind the edge of accumulated knowledge. As a result, important advances go unmentioned and/or ineffective treatments are still advocated. Extending the analysis of Antman et al., Balas and Boren (2000) estimated that the average medical treatment advance takes 17 years to go from original discovery and studies into routine clinical practice. Other research notes that the early stoppage of large-scale RCTs due to adverse outcomes and their publication results in incomplete changes in clinical practice, i.e., clinicians are still prescribing disproven therapies for some time after publication and widespread publicity of these findings (Hersh, Stefanick et al., 2004; Stafford, Furberg et al., 2004).

2.3.3   Fragmentation

Ziman (1969) noted another property of the scientific literature, namely, that a single paper typically reports only on one experiment that is just a small part of overall picture. Ziman observed that the scientific literature is mainly written for scientists to communicate with their peers and thus presumes a basic understanding of the concepts in the field. Ziman also maintained that the literature is not only fragmented, but also derivative, in that it relies heavily on past work and is edited, which provides a quality control mechanism.

Part of the reason for the fragmentation of the scientific literature is the scientist's desire to "seed" his or her work in many different journals, where it may be seen by a larger diversity of readers. In addition, the academic promotion and tenure process encourages scientists in academic settings to "publish or perish." A common quip among academicians is to slice results into "least publishable units" (or "minimal publishable units") so that the maximum number of publications can be obtained for a body of work (Refinetti, 1991). The extent to which this is done is not clear, but to the extent that the practice exists, more fragmentation of the scientific literature is a result.

2.3.4   Linkage and Citations

Another property of scientific information is linkage, which occurs via citation. The study of citations in scientific writing is a field unto itself called *bibliometrics*. This field is important in a number of ways, such as measuring the importance of individual contributions in science, indicating the likely places to find information on a given topic and, as is known to Google users and we will discuss in Chap. 5, offering potential ways to enhance IR systems (i.e., the Google PageRank algorithm).

The bibliography is an important part of a scientific paper. It provides background information, showing the work that has come before and indicating what research has motivated the current work. It also shows that the author is aware of others working in the field. Authors also use citations to substantiate claims. Thus, a scientific paper on a new treatment for a disease will usually cite papers describing the disease, its human toll, and the success of existing therapies. An author arguing for a certain experimental approach or a new type of therapy, for example, may cite evidence from basic science or other work to provide rationale for the novel approach.

Citations can be viewed as a network, or as a directed acyclic graph. Although reasons for citation can often be obtuse (i.e., a medical paper may cite a statistical paper for a description of an uncommon method being used), networks can give a general indication of subject relationship. One of the early workers in bibliometrics was Garfield (1964), who originated the *Science Citation Index* (Institute for Scientific Information, Philadelphia, PA), a publication that lists all citations of every scientific paper in journals.

Being cited is important for scientists. Academic promotion and tenure committees look at, among other things, how widely cited an individual's work is, as do those who review the work of candidates for grant funding. In a study of several different fields, Price (1965) found that in certain fields, half of all citations formed a core of a small number of papers representing authors and publications with major influence on a given subject. Some advocate using citation patterns to judge the quality of the work of scientists but others have warned against it (Adam, 2002).

What factors are associated with increased likelihood of a paper being cited? One important factor in the modern era is the easy electronic availability of the paper. Lawrence (2001) found that computer science papers freely available on the Web had a higher likelihood of being cited than those that were not. Antelman (2004) recently verified this for four other fields: philosophy, political science, mathematics, and electrical engineering. Likewise, Eysenbach (2006) found that for articles published in *Proceedings of the National Academy of Sciences*, which offers both open-access (a more open approach to publishing described in Sects. 2.6.1 and 6.4.3) and non-open-access publishing to authors, those published under the former approach were 2–3 times more likely to be cited. Of course, these articles were not "randomized," and so there may have been confounders leading to the different citation rate. It has also been found that sharing detailed research data in biomedicine is also associated with a higher rate of citation (Piwowar, Day et al., 2007).

Others, however, have questioned whether open-access publishing and other forms of making articles freely available may not lead to increased citation. In reviewing more recent studies on this question, Craig et al. (2007) note other possible explanations for their higher citation impact, such as selection bias, where more prominent authors are likely to post their articles online, and early-view bias, where the earlier availability of articles leads to more citations. In other words, more widespread availability of articles may lead to quicker citation of articles, especially of those by more prominent researchers.

What other factors lead to higher rates of citations? A pair of studies has looked at Norwegian scientists, most of whom publish in international journals and are cited by international authors. The first study compared highly cited with "ordinary" cited papers (Aksnes, 2003). It found that while most papers were regular articles (81%), review articles (12%) were overrepresented relative to their regular rate of appearance. Highly cited papers followed the usual pattern of initial rise and then decline of citation frequency over time. They received citations from many different journals and from both close and remote fields, which was also true of ordinary papers, although their high rate of citation made them appear in higher absolute numbers in different journals and fields. The second study found that, in general, the rate of citation of papers correlated well with scientists' perceived importance of the research (Aksnes, 2006). However, because of individual variance, it was difficult to apply this at the single-paper level.

As mentioned, the field of bibliometrics is concerned with measuring the individual contributions in science as well as the distribution of publications on topics. This field has also generated two well-known laws that deal with author productivity and subject dispersion in journals: Lotka's law and Bradford's law respectively. It has also developed the impact factor (IF), which attempts to measure the importance of journals. Two other aspects of note with regard to citations are cocitation analysis and the Erdös Number Project.

2.3.4.1 Author Productivity: Lotka's Law

Most readers who work in scientific fields know that there is a small core of authors who produce a large number of publications. A mathematical relationship describing this has been described by Lotka and verified experimentally by Pao (1986). Lotka's law states that if x is the number of publications by a scientist in a field and y is the number of authors who produce x publications each, then

$$x^n \times y = C \tag{2.3}$$

where C is a constant. For scientific fields, the value for n is usually near 2.0. Thus in scientific fields, the square of the number of papers published by a given author is inversely proportional to the number of authors who produce that number of papers.

Lotka's law is also known as the *inverse square law of scientific productivity* (Pao, 1986). If the number of single paper authors is 100, then number of authors producing 2 papers is $100/2^2 = 25$ and the number of authors producing 3 papers is $100/3^2 = 11$, etc. In general, 10% of the authors in a field produce half the literature in a field, while 75% produce less than 25% of the literature.

2.3.4.2 Subject Dispersion: Bradford's Law

Bradford (1948) observed, and several others have verified (Urquhart and Bunn, 1959; Trueswell, 1969; Self, Filardo et al., 1989), a phenomenon that occurs when the names of journals with articles on a topic are arranged by how many articles on that topic each publication contains. The journals tend to divide into a nucleus of a small number of journals followed by zones containing n, n^2, n^3, etc., journals with approximately the same number of articles. This observation is known as *Bradford's law of scattering*. Its implication is that as a scientific field grows, its literature becomes increasingly scattered and difficult to organize. But Bradford's law also indicates that most articles on a given topic are found in a core of journals. This fact is of importance to libraries, which must balance the goal of comprehensiveness with space and monetary constraints. Bradford's law has been found to apply to other phenomena in IR, such as distribution of query topics to a database (Bates, 2002).

This phenomenon has been demonstrated in the medical literature in the area of the acquired immunodeficiency syndrome (AIDS) (Self, Filardo et al., 1989). In 1982, shortly after the disease was identified, only 14 journals had literature on AIDS. By 1987, this had grown to over 1,200. The authors plotted the cumulative percent of journal titles vs. journal articles for AIDS (Fig. 2.2), and found a Bradford distribution, with the first third of articles in 15 journals, the second third in 123 journals (=15 × 8.2), and the final third in 1,023 journals ($\approx 15 \times 8.2^2$).

Other data support the notion of scattering. Wilczynski et al. (2007) have found in the area of nephrology that 2,779 articles cited in systematic reviews were concentrated in 466 journals and that 90% of the titles were in a set of 217. Another medical demonstration of Bradford's law has been in Web site citation analysis. Cui (1999) analyzed the Web citations (links) from library sites of 19 of the top 25 ranked medical schools in the USA. The distribution of top-level domain (e.g., .com or .edu), first-level domain (e.g., the part of the URL up to the first slash), and whole URLs was analyzed. When the total number of first-level domains were segregated

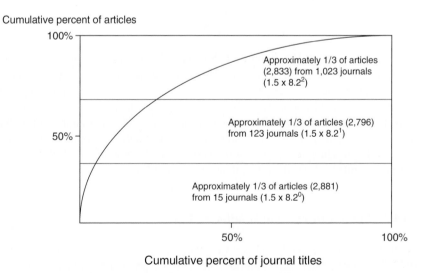

Fig. 2.2 The Bradford distribution for articles on AIDS (adapted from Self, Filardo et al., 1989)

into three groups based on total frequency (1,731), their absolute counts came close to obeying the $1:n:n^2$ distribution (78:452:1,201 or 1:4:42). This study also found that 90% of the top-level domains were for the US-based top-level domains (.com, .edu, .gov, .org).

One implication of both Lotka's law and Bradford's law is that scientists and journals that are already successful in writing and attracting articles are likely to continue to be so in the future. In Sect. 2.5.2 on peer review, aspects of the scientific publishing process that indicate why successful scientists in a field continue their good fortune are explored.

2.3.4.3 Journal Importance: Impact Factor

Linkage information can also be used to measure the importance of journals, based on the IF, which was introduced by Garfield (1994). The assumption underlying the IF is that the quantity of citations of a journal's papers is associated with that journal's importance. As with other linkage measures, IF can be used to make decisions about the journals to which a library should subscribe.

IF is usually measured with a formula that is the ratio of the number of citations in a given time period to the number of articles published. The formula also has a variant that adjusts for self-citations within a journal. The IF for current year citations of articles published over the last 2 years would thus be

$$IF = \frac{\text{Citations in current year to articles published in prior two years}}{\text{Number of articles published in prior two years}} \qquad (2.4)$$

Table 2.1 shows the IF for the top journals in general medicine, medical informatics, biotechnology, and information systems.

Not everyone agrees that IF is the best determinant of journal quality. West (1996) pointed out that the importance of scientific articles is influenced by other factors, such as the nature of the underlying research, variations in the number of references different publications include, journal editorial policies that limit the number of references per article, different-sized readerships, (which may lead to differences related to audience size) scientists' conformity in often citing papers that are currently cited, authors' tendencies to cite their own work, and referees' tendencies to recommend inclusion of references to their work.

However, a number of studies have found positive association between IF and other measures of journal quality. Lee et al. (2002) have found that IF and other measures of journal quality (e.g., citation rate, acceptance rate, listing in MED-LINE, circulation) are associated with higher methodological quality of a given publication. Likewise, Callaham et al. (2002) have found IF to be more important in the subsequent citing of a scientific paper than even the quality of the study methodology. Saha et al. (2003) asked 113 physicians who were predominantly practitioners and 151 physicians who were graduates of advanced training

Table 2.1 Impact factors of journals from selected fields for 2006

Journal title	Impact factor
General medical	
New England Journal of Medicine	51.296
Lancet	25.8
Journal of the American Medical Association	23.175
Annals of Internal Medicine	14.78
PLoS Medicine	13.75
Annual Review of Medicine	13.237
British Medical Journal	9.245
Archives of Internal Medicine	7.92
Canadian Medical Association Journal	6.862
Medicine	5.167
Medical informatics	
Journal of the American Medical Informatics Association	3.979
Journal of Medical Internet Research	2.888
Journal of Biomedical Informatics	2.346
Statistics in Medicine	1.737
Medical Decision Making	1.736
International Journal of Medical Informatics	1.726
Methods of Information in Medicine	1.684
Artificial Intelligence in Medicine	1.634
IEEE Transactions on Information Technology in Biomedicine	1.542
Statistical Methods in Medical Research	1.377
Biotechnology	
Briefings in Bioinformatics	24.37
Nature Biotechnology	22.672
Nature Reviews Drug Discovery	20.97
Genome Research	10.256
Stem Cells	7.924
Trends in Biotechnology	7.843
Mutation Research – Reviews in Mutation Research	7.579
Pharmacogenetics	7.221
Genome Biology	7.172
Current Opinion in Biotechnology	6.949
. . .	
Bioinformatics	4.894
. . .	
BMC Bioinformatics	3.617
Computer Science, Information Systems	
ACM Transactions on Information Systems	5.059
MIS Quarterly	4.731
Journal of the American Medical Informatics Association	3.979
Journal of Chemical Information and Modeling	3.423
Very Large Database Journal	3.289
Journal of the ACM	2.917
IEEE Wireless Communications	2.577
IEEE Transactions on Mobile Computing	2.55

(continued)

Table 2.1 (continued)	
Data Mining and Knowledge Discovery	2.295
IEEE Network	2.211
...	
Information Retrieval	1.744
International Journal of Medical Informatics	1.726
Methods of Information in Medicine	1.684
Journal of The American Society for Information Science and Technology	1.555
Information Processing and Management	1.546

Adapted from *Journal Citation Reports* (Institute for Scientific Information, http://www.isi.com/)

programs in clinical and health services research to rate the quality of nine general medical journals. The correlation of IF with physicians' ratings of journal quality was high overall, and somewhat higher for the group of researchers than for the practitioners. McKibbon et al. (2004) also found an association between IF and the quantity of high-quality (i.e., evidence-based) studies published by medical journals.

Nakayama et al. (2003) assessed the IFs of the citations included in the US government's *Guide to Clinical Preventive Services*, second edition, which reflects the best evidence for clinical preventive services. Not surprisingly, the largest number of citations came from journals with high IFs. Of the 1,740 citations in the 25 chapters of the report, the most commonly represented journals were *Journal of the American Medical Association* (135), *American Journal of Preventive Medicine* (102), *British Medical Journal* (77), and *Lancet* (70). The IFs of the 56 journals having five or more citations in the report were widely distributed, however. Six (11%) journals had an IF > 10, but half of the journals (28, or 50%) had an IF < 3, and the median IF was 2.76. There was a correlation between IFs and number of times cited in these guidelines. However, this analysis showed that many articles having high-quality clinical evidence were published in low-IF journals. An editorial in *British Medical Journal* (BMJ) assessed some of the other social aspects of IFs, such as academic promotion, in light of these findings and advocated avoiding the use of IFs for these purposes (Abbasi, 2004). Still, many journal editors consider them important, and the tongue-in-cheek dialogue by two editors of a dermatology journal is representative of how journals strive to increase their IF (verified personally by this author's participation in several editorial boards of other journals) (Goldsmith and Hall, 2006).

The inventor of the IF, Garfield, recently defended it in a JAMA commentary (Garfield, 2006). He noted the value of quantitative measurement of a journal's importance for decision-making concerning the value of journals as well as decisions for library subscriptions. He did, however, warn against its use for evaluating the contributions of individual scientists. Dong et al. (2005) also recently reviewed the IF. They provided a list of how the measure can be biased, including the following:

- Incomplete journal coverage by the Science Citation Index, with an overrepresentation of English-language journals
- Different citation patterns across research fields and subject areas
- Differences among journals that increase IF but have nothing to do with quality, such as citations to "noncitable" items (i.e., items not counted in the IF denominator), availability of the abstract and/or full text online, and presence of longer articles
- Inaccuracy of data
- IF calculated for whole journals whereas citations are to single articles
- Journals manipulating IF, such as by requesting authors to cite papers in their journal

They noted that while IF was effective in measuring the quality of a journal, it had little value in assessing individual articles, whether for their scientific contribution or how evidence-based they were (e.g., the Nakayama paper mentioned earlier).

Just as scientific literature is linked, so is information on the Web. Indeed, Ingwersen (1998) has proposed a Web impact factor (WIF), which is defined as the proportion of pages that link to a site from some defined area of the Web, such as a site or a group of sites devoted to a specific topic. It is defined mathematically as follows:

$$\text{WIF} = \frac{\text{number of pages linking to a site}}{\text{total number of pages in site}} \tag{2.5}$$

Two kinds of pages contribute to the denominator, external-link pages from outside the site and internal-link pages from within the site. Most analyses have used the "external WIF" to omit internal links within a Web site. As an example, consider a Web site of an academic medical informatics program. The external WIF would be calculated by all pages that point to that site (e.g., 10) divided by some universe of pages considered to be in the realm of medical informatics (e.g., 1,000). The external WIF would be 10/1000 = 0.01. It can be calculated from Web search engines (limited insofar as the engines do not completely cover the entire Web). For example, the Google query +link:<domain>-url:<domain> will return all Web pages that point to a specific Web domain except those within the domain. The number of such pages divided by the number of pages in a site gives the external WIF.

Almind and Ingwersen (1998) used the WIF to determine that Denmark was less visible on the Web than were other Nordic countries. Smith (1999) found no correlation between research output (measured in numbers of papers published) and the external WIF for Australasian universities, while Thelwall (2000) did find a positive trend between the WIF and a measure of general rating for 25 British research universities. However, Thomas and Willett (2000) found such an association when they narrowed the view to British library and information science departments. Smith also considered whether the WIF could serve as a sort of journal IF for Web-based journals and found it to be unreliable.

A more recent analysis found that while higher rated scholars produce more Web content, the impact as measured by in-links to those pages is not increased for those scholars (Thelwall and Harries, 2004). In other words, more productive researchers produce more Web-based content but the rate of links to their sites is not increased over those who are less productive. Thelwall (2003) also attempted to categorize links between academic Web sites and found four general categories of links:

- General navigation – allowing browsing to nonspecific information
- Ownership – allow navigation to co-owners or coauthors of a project
- Social – recognition that the site being linked to is important in the social context of a field
- Gratuitous – links acknowledging institutions or other entities

2.3.4.4   Cocitation Analysis

Another type of analysis done in bibliometrics is *cocitation analysis*, which measures the number of times that pairs of authors are cited together by another paper. Cocitation analysis can help show authors whose work is similar in scope. Andrews (2003) performed such an analysis for the field of medical informatics, with a particular focus on members of the American College of Medical Informatics (http://www.amia.org/acmi/acmi.html), a body of elected fellows who have made significant and sustained contributions to the field. This article showed that the work of this author is closest to that of Keith Campbell, Betsy Humpreys, Mark Tuttle, and Christopher Chute. In addition, he is the 21st most highly cited individual in this group of leaders of the field.

Another analysis of publication and citation in the medical informatics field was recently carried out by Eggers et al. (2005). They analyzed 10 years of publications and citations in 22 journals in the field. In addition to measuring numbers of publications, they calculated an "authority score," based on frequency of citation by other highly frequent publishers. This author ranked tenth in the list of authority scores. They also mapped closeness of authors, which converged into five topic areas of the field. This analysis placed this author close to Homer Warner, Steve Johnson, Arthur Elstein, and Patricia Brennan, which seems less logical than Andrews' analysis.

Related to cocitation analysis is the recognition of the importance of research collaboration, especially with the emergence of "team science" and the large teams that take part in large, cutting-edge research projects. Indeed, a motivation of the National Institutes of Health (NIH) Roadmap initiative is to encourage collaboration of multidisciplinary teams of scientists to accelerate research findings into benefit for human health (Zerhouni, 2003). Guimera et al. (2005) have found that research team size increases as scientific fields (as well as production of Broadway plays) increase and as the complexity and required creativity for advancement increase.

2.3.4.5   Erdös Number Project

Another large-scale project of bibliographic linkage is the Erdös Number Project. This project is, according to its Web site (http://www.oakland.edu/enp/), part of the "folklore of mathematicians," who measure their distance in coauthorship from the prolific Hungarian mathematician, Paul Erdös. Erdös published over 1,400 scientific papers and had over 500 coauthor collaborators. The mathematical community has undertaken building a collaboration graph for its community with ~337,000 authors of 1.6 million authored items in the Math Review database. Erdös is at the center of that graph. An "Erdös number" is thus the smallest number of coauthorship links between an individual and Erdös. Therefore, someone who coauthored with Erdös has an Erdös number of 1. Anyone who coauthored with any one of those coauthors has an Erdös number of 2. This author has a relatively low Erdös number of 4, thanks to his former postdoc Andrew Turpin (http://goanna.cs.rmit.edu.au/~aht/), who was a graduate student of Alistair Moffat (http://www.cs.mu.oz.au/~alistair/), who has one of the lowest Erdös numbers (2) in the IR community.

2.3.5   Propagation

A final property of information is propagation. Interest in this area has been revived with the growth of the Internet and Web, which provide a vast new medium for information spread. The notion of the propagation of information can be traced back to Dawkins (1976), whose book laid out the ideas of *memes*, which are information patterns that are held in a person's memory but can be copied to another. The field that studies the replication and evolution of memes is called memetics. There are many Web sites devoted to memetics, e.g., http://pespmc1.vub.ac.be/TOC.html.

Dawkins gives examples of memes as "tunes, ideas, [and] catch-phrases," that propagate from "brain to brain." Memes have been likened to genes, but may be more appropriately compared to viruses, which cannot replicate themselves but take over a cell's DNA to cause it to make millions of copies of itself. According to Dawkins, memes can affect the mind like a parasite, causing an individual to change his or her behavior and/or pass the idea on to others. Memes are selected or, in genetic terms, have fitness by a variety of properties such as novelty, coherence, and self-reinforcement. If they do not have the capability to survive, then they may die out.

The Internet is a (relatively) new medium for the wide spread of memes. The frequent forwarding of e-mails as well as visiting of Web sites are common means for memes to propagate. One consequence of such easy spread of information is the propagation of misinformation, which are sometimes called "urban legends" (e.g., http://www.urbanlegends.com, http://www.snopes.com).

2.4   Classification of Health Information

Now that some basic theories and properties of information have been described, attention can be turned to the type of information that is the focus of most of this book, textual health information. It is useful to classify it, since not only are varying types used differently, but alternative procedures are applied to its organization and retrieval.

Table 2.2 lists a classification of textual health information. *Patient-specific* information applies to individual patients. Its purpose is to tell health-care providers, administrators, and researchers about the health and disease of a patient. This information comprises the patient's medical record. Patient-specific data can be either *structured*, as in a laboratory value or vital sign measurement, or in the form of *free (narrative) text*. Of course, many notes and reports in the medical record contain both structured and narrative text, such as the history and physical report, which contains the vital signs and laboratory values. For the most part, this book does not address patient-specific information, although Chap. 9 discusses the processing of clinical narrative text. As will be seen, the goals and procedures in the processing of such text are often different from other types of medical text.

The second major category of health information is *knowledge-based* information. This is information that has been derived and organized from observational or experimental research. In the case of clinical research, this information provides clinicians, administrators, and researchers with knowledge derived from experiments and observations, which can then be applied to individual patients. This information is most commonly provided in books and journals but can take a wide variety of other forms, including computerized media. Of course, some patient-specific information does make it into knowledge-based information sources, but with a different purpose. For example, a case report in a medical journal does not assist the patient being reported on, but rather serves as a vehicle for sharing the knowledge gained from the case with other practitioners.

Knowledge-based information can be subdivided into two categories. *Primary* knowledge-based information (also called primary literature) is original research that appears in journals, books, reports, and other sources. This type of information reports the initial discovery of health knowledge, usually with original data. Revisiting the earlier serum cholesterol and heart disease example, an instance of primary literature could include a discovery of the pathophysiological process by

Table 2.2   A classification of textual health information

1. Patient-specific information
a. Structured – laboratory results, vital signs
b. Narrative – history and physical, progress note, radiology report
2. Knowledge-based information
a. Primary – original research (in journals, books, reports, etc.)
b. Secondary – summaries of research (in review articles, books, practice guidelines, etc.)

which cholesterol is implicated in heart disease, a clinical trial showing a certain therapy to be of benefit in lowering it, a cost-benefit analysis that shows which portion of the population is likely to best benefit from treatment, or a systematic review that uses meta-analysis to combine all the original studies evaluating one or more therapies.

Secondary knowledge-based information consists of the writing that reviews, condenses, and/or synthesizes the primary literature. The most common examples of this type of literature are books, monographs, and review articles in journals and other publications. Secondary literature also includes opinion-based writing such as editorials and position or policy papers. It also encompasses clinical practice guidelines, systematic reviews, and health information on Web pages. In addition, it includes the plethora of pocket-sized manuals that are a staple for practitioners in many professional fields. As will be seen later, secondary literature is the most common type of literature used by physicians.

Another approach to classifying knowledge-based information comes from Haynes (2001), taking the perspective of evidence-based medicine (EBM) (Straus, Richardson et al., 2005), which we will discuss at greater length in Sect. 2.8. As depicted in Fig. 2.3, Haynes defines a hierarchy of evidence, with the original *studies* forming the foundation of knowledge. These studies are in turn aggregated into *syntheses*, often called *systematic reviews* or *evidence reports*, which systematically identify and synthesize all the evidence on a given topic. Where appropriate in systematic reviews, meta-analysis is performed, in which the results of multiple appropriately homogenous studies are combined to achieve an aggregate result, which usually also has larger statistical power. Systematic reviews are distinct from *narrative reviews*, which just provide a general overview of a topic that is usually broader but less exhaustive in coverage. A further distillation of knowledge occurs with *synopses*, which provide a summary (ideally derived from an evidence-based synthesis) on a topic. The ultimate level of the hierarchy is *systems*, which consist of actionable knowledge structured in a way that can be used by information systems, such as a clinical decision support module of an electronic health record.

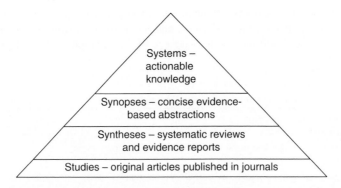

Fig. 2.3 The "4S model" of hierarchy of evidence (adapted from Haynes, 2001)

2.5 Production of Health Information

Since the main focus of this book is on indexing and retrieval of knowledge-based information, the remainder of this chapter will focus on that type of information (except for Chap. 9, where patient-specific information is discussed, but only in the context of processing the text-based variety). This section covers the production of health information, from the original studies and their peer review for publication to their summarization in the secondary literature.

2.5.1 The Generation of Scientific Information

How is scientific information generated? Figure 2.4 depicts the "life cycle" of scientific information. The process begins with scientists themselves, who make and record observations, whether in the laboratory or in the real world. These observations are then written up and submitted for publication in the primary literature, where they undergo peer review. If the paper passes the test of peer review, it is published, usually in a scientific journal. If the paper does not pass muster in peer review, the author usually revises it and resubmits it to the same or a different journal. Other steps that may occur if the paper is published is that the author may be required to relinquish the copyright, usually to the publisher of the journal, and/or the information in the paper may make its way into secondary publications, such as a textbook. The research will also likely feed back to motivate new research that may then follow a new cycle through the process.

One of the most widely cited descriptions of the scientific process is Thomas Kuhn's *The Structure of Scientific Revolutions* (Kuhn, 1962). Kuhn noted that science proceeds in evolutions and revolutions. In the evolutionary phase of a science, there is a stable, accepted paradigm. In fact, Kuhn argued, a field cannot be a science until there is such a paradigm that lends itself to common interpretation

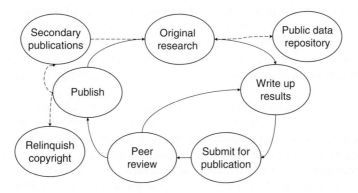

Fig. 2.4 The "life cycle" of scientific information

and agreement on certain facts. A science evolves as experiments and other observations are performed and interpreted under the accepted paradigm. This science is advanced by publication in peer-reviewed journals. In the revolutionary phase, however, evidence in conflict with the accepted paradigm mounts until it overwhelmingly go against the paradigm, overturning it. The classic example of this described by Kuhn came from the work of Copernicus, who contributed little actual data to astronomy but showed how the astronomical observations of others fit so much better under a new paradigm in which the planets revolved around the sun rather than around the earth.

Just about all research undergoes peer review by scientist colleagues, who decide whether the paper describing the research is worthy of publication. The goal of this process is to ensure that the appropriate experimental methods were used, that the findings represent a new and informative contribution to the field, and that the conclusions are justified by the results. Of course, what is acceptable for publication varies with the scope of the journal. Journals covering basic biomedical science (e.g., *Cell*) tend to publish papers focusing on laboratory-based research that is likely to focus on mechanisms of diseases and treatments, whereas clinical journals (e.g., *Journal of the American Medical Association*) tend to publish reports of large clinical trials and other studies pertinent to providing clinical care. Specialized journals are more likely to publish preliminary or exploratory studies. Bourne (2005) has provided some simple rules to those aspiring to achieve scientific publication in the field of computational biology, but these easily apply to other fields.

Peer-reviewed journals are not the only vehicle for publication of original science. Other forums for publication include the following:

- Conference proceedings – usually peer-reviewed, publishing either full papers or just abstracts
- Technical reports – may be peer reviewed, frequently providing more detail than journal papers do
- Books – may be peer-reviewed

In general, however, nonjournal primary literature does not carry the scientific esteem accorded to journal literature. These varying sources of nonjournal primary literature are sometimes called "grey literature," and their identification can be important, as they may impact the results of systematic reviews and meta-analyses. In particular, they are less likely to show a treatment effect and thus may lead to exaggeration of meta-analysis results when not included (McAuley, Pham et al., 2000).

Many authors, such as Ziman (1969), have noted that the scientific method is the best method humans have devised for discerning the truth about their world. Although a number of limitations with the peer-review process and the scientific literature itself will be seen in ensuing sections, the present author agrees that there is no better method for understanding and manipulating the phenomena of the world than the scientific method. Flaws in science are usually due more to flaws in scientists and the experiments they devise than to the scientific method itself.

To standardize the publishing process, the editors of the major medical journals have formed a committee (International Committee of Medical Journal Editors, ICMJE, http://www.icjme.org/) to provide general recommendations on the submission of manuscripts to journals. They have defined the so-called Vancouver format for publication style, which journals will agree to accept upon submission even if their own formats vary and will require editing later. Equally important, however, they have defined a number of additional requirements and other statements for biomedical publishing (Anonymous, 2006i):

- Redundant or duplicate publication occurs when there is substantial overlap with an item already published. One form of redundant publication that is generally acceptable is the publication of a paper whose preliminary report was presented as a poster or abstract at a scientific meeting. Acceptable instances of secondary publication of a paper include publication in a different language or in a journal aimed at different readers. In general, editors of the original journals must consent to such publication and the prior appearance of the material should be acknowledged in the secondary paper.
- Authorship should be given only to those who make substantial contribution to study conception or design and data acquisition, analysis, or interpretation; drafting of the article or revising it critically for important intellectual content; and giving final approval for publication.
- A peer-reviewed journal is one that has most of its articles reviewed by experts who are not part of the editorial staff.
- While journal owners have the right to hire and fire editors, the latter must have complete freedom to exercise their editorial judgment.
- All conflicts of interest from authors, reviewers, and editors must be disclosed. Financial support from a commercial source is not a reason for disqualification from publishing, but it must be properly attributed.
- Advertising must be kept distinguishable from editorial content and must not be allowed to influence it.
- Competing manuscripts based on the same study should generally be discouraged, and this requires careful intervention by editors to determine an appropriate course of action.

Another publication from the IJCME (Davidoff, DeAngelis et al., 2001) elucidated further the issue of conflicts of interest and authorship.

Scientific information would not be generated at all were it not for research funding. The process to determine research funding is also done via peer review. The largest grantor of funding in the world is the NIH. Of its $28 billion annual budget, 80% supports research and training outside NIH. Each of the 20+ institutes of the NIH allocates funds for research in a competitive process. (The major institute for biomedical informatics research is the NLM, which also receives substantial funding for its library operations.) The NIH receives about 80,000 grant proposals per year, recruiting more than 15,000 experts to review them. Proposals are usually grouped by subject and/or grant type, with a group of reviewers recruited to form a *study section*. The general process is to assign a *priority score*, from 100 (*best*) to 500 (*worst*), and then funding proposals by priority until funds are exhausted. The institutes have some leeway to adjust scores and prioritize funding. The director of the NIH Center for Scientific Review recently provided an overview of the system and areas of concern (Scarpa, 2006). There is growing concern that the leveling off of NIH funding growth is difficult not only for individual scientists, but also for the institutions who depend on them to get funding to cover salaries of the time spent doing research. There are also concerns at the long lead time required for funding decisions, on average about 9 months. This not only delays research but also creates funding uncertainties for researchers and the institutions that employ them. A related concern is that basic research is not being "translated" quickly enough into benefits for human health, with the NIH now funding centers for translational research under the Clinical and Translational Science Award (CTSA) initiative (Zerhouni, 2007).

There are some additional concerns about the generation of knowledge. One is that some knowledge is never obtained because it is "forbidden" to be studied (Kempner, Perlis et al., 2005). Knowledge may be forbidden because it can only be obtained through unethical means, e.g., human experiments conducted by Nazi scientists. But other research is prohibited by what Kempner et al. call "informal constraints." This may involve fear from results being attacked by political groups across the spectrum, from religious groups to animal rights activists. Clearly there must be some ethical constraints on the conduct of science, but not merely if they offend the political agenda of a particular group.

Related to forbidden knowledge is the focus of scientific literature on diseases and their treatments pertinent to developed countries. Raja and Singer (2004) note that much content in the major journals is not relevant to developing countries, although their research found that British journals do a better job than their American counterparts in this regard.

Another concern about the production of biomedical literature is that the clinical trials carried out do not meet the needs of "decision-makers," in particular, those who develop policy, practice guidelines, and so forth. Tunis et al. (2003) have called for more effort on pragmatic or practical clinical trials. The characteristics of practical clinical trials they deem most important include the selection of clinically relevant interventions for comparison, diverse populations of study participants, recruitment from heterogeneous practice settings, and data collection from a broad range of clinical outcomes. They lament that the major funders of clinical research, namely the NIH and the medical products industry, do not focus on supporting these types of clinical trials.

2.5.2   Peer Review

Although peer review had its origins in the nineteenth century, it did not achieve widespread use until the midtwentieth century (Burnham, 1990). As noted earlier, the goal of peer review is to serve as a quality filter to the scientific literature.

Theoretically, only research based on sound scientific methodology will be published. In reality, of course, the picture is more complicated. Awareness that what constitutes acceptable research may vary based on the quality or scope of the journal has led to the realization by some that the peer-review process does not so much determine whether a paper will be published as where it will be published.

Most journals have a two-phase review process. The manuscript is usually reviewed initially by the editor or an associate editor to determine whether it fits the scope of the journal and whether there are any obvious flaws in the work. If the manuscript passes this process, it is sent out for formal peer review. The results of the peer-review process vary widely. The BMJ states on its author submission page (http://resources.bmj.com/bmj/authors) that only 7% of submitted papers are accepted. Among smaller journals, the rate of acceptance varies widely, from 13 to 91% (Hargens, 1990). The recommendations of acceptance or rejection by reviewers vary equally widely.

The peer-review process serves other purposes besides assessing the quality of science. For example, review of papers by peers also leads to improvement in the reporting of results and conclusions. Purcell et al. (1998) found that peer review identified five types of problem with papers: too much information, too little information, inaccurate information, misplaced information, and structural problems. These can be corrected during the editorial process. Even if the paper is not accepted, peer review can be beneficial to authors who are likely to implement suggested changes before submitting their material to a different journal (Garfunkel, Lawson et al., 1990).

Why do papers get rejected by peer review? One study of papers in the field of medical education research found that the top reasons for rejection included statistical problems, overinterpretation of results, problems with instrumentation, inadequate or biased sample size, writing that was difficult to follow, insufficiently detailed statement of the research problem, inaccurate or inconsistent data reported, inadequate review of the literature, insufficient data presented, and problems with tables or figures (Bordage, 2001). The main strengths identified in the accepted manuscripts were the importance or timeliness of the problem studies, excellence of writing, and soundness of study design. The author concluded that while some of the problems (e.g., overstating the results and applying the wrong statistics) could be fixed, others (e.g., ignoring past literature, poor study design, use of inappropriate instruments, poor writing) were likely to be fatal flaws that warranted rejection.

2.5.2.1 Is Peer Review Effective?

Has peer review been shown to improve the quality of publications or, better yet, the advancement of human health or scientific knowledge? In one systematic review, Jefferson et al. (2002) found that all studies to date have focused on surrogate and intermediate measures and none have compared peer review with other methods. Twenty-one studies of the process were found and led to a variety of conclusions (number supporting each conclusion in parentheses):

- Concealing identities of peer reviewers or authors does not appear to affect quality of reviews (9)
- Checklists and other attempts at standardizing the process do not appear to help (2)
- Training of referees does not improve the quality of reviews (2)
- Electronic media do not improve quality (2)
- Peer review does not detect bias against unconventional drugs (1)
- The process may improve readability and general quality of papers (2)

Some believe that the peer review system tends to serve to keep control of science in the hands of those who already have it. Readings (1994) argues that peer reviewers "take exciting, innovative, and challenging work by younger scholars and reject it." Because those who do peer reviewing have already passed into the inner circle, they have incentive to keep others out. Agger (1990) states that there is not enough room for everybody in the prestigious journals, and so those on the inside are likely to want to minimize the number of new entrants. Given the growing competitiveness for research grants, those who have already achieved success in science do have incentives to minimize new competition. Roberts (1999) advocates a more moderate view, arguing that peer review is beneficial and that the Internet opens up a new means to make it more open and efficient.

Is peer review necessary in this era of widespread access to the Internet and World Wide Web? Some have suggested that posting submitted papers online and allowing public comment and update could substitute for it. To this end, the journal *Nature* carried out an experiment of one approach to open peer review (Anonymous, 2006f). For a 4-month period, they gave authors the option of having their submissions posted for public comment in addition to the usual peer-review process. Only 71 (5%) of the 1,369 authors submitting papers during the 4 months of the period agreed to take part. For these papers, comments were posted on only 38 (54%) of them. A total of 92 technical comments were posted (i.e., about 2.5 per paper commented upon). The number of comments varied widely by subject domain. The authors were asked about the utility of the comments, and most were found to be not helpful, though some editorial comments were found to be of value. The editors of *Nature* concluded that this approach would not be pursued further for now.

Is the peer-review process "broken?" McCook (2006) notes that the growing number of submissions and the pressures for scientists to publish, especially in prestigious journals, and to obtain promotion and/or continued grant funding, are taxing the system. This also leads to hyping the conclusions and downplaying the limitations of studies. McCook lists three specific complaints with the current peer-review system and quotes editors and others with suggestions for change:

1. Editors at commercial (e.g., *Nature*, *Cell*) are in general younger than those at society or nonprofit journals and thus less experienced. It is unclear, however, that the age of an editor matters, as they may have more experience but also formed stronger opinions and networks of colleagues.

2. Journals with sister publications steer papers into them to increase their profiles. A deputy editor of JAMA is quoted as denying this.
3. Peer reviewers delay or otherwise sabotage reviews of competing scientists. The editor-in-chief is quoted as noting this is an "extreme exception."

The article discusses advantages for and against open peer review (i.e., the reviewer is identified to the authors), which is done at BMJ and *Biomed Central*. Even though the evidence is unclear that the process works better, many editors believe that it leads to more constructive reviews. Others caution that reviewers may lose objectivity and fear repercussions, especially from senior leaders in the field.

Many scientists would no doubt agree with the information scientist Tefko Saracevic, who has said (personal communication) that the peer-review process determines more where an article is published than whether it is published. Perhaps a lesson can be learned from observations about professional basketball, which is that those who are already successful tend to continue achieving success. In the book *The Jordan Rules* (Smith, 1994) an analysis of NBA referees found a tendency to give this superstar (and probably others) the benefit of the doubt in foul calls.

2.5.2.2   How Can Peer Review Be Improved?

There is a fairly substantial body of disparate literature on what works in peer review and how it can be improved. One simple suggestion for improving peer review has been the separation of improving writing from judgment of scientific merit (Kaplan, 2005). A variety of other studies have looked at who makes good reviewers, how they are best helped, and where the process falls down. Similar to their simple rules for getting published, Bourne and Korngreen (2006) have also provided simple rules for individuals being good reviewers.

Some research has attempted to identify the characteristics of good peer reviewers. The only consistent factor associated with high-quality reviewing has been younger age, in particular advanced enough to know the field but not too senior so as to be too busy or cynical. One researcher (Stossel, 1985) found that the best reviews came from faculty of junior academic status, while another (Evans, McNutt et al., 1993) showed that the best reviews came from younger faculty working at top academic institutions or who were known to the editors. Nylenna et al. (1994) found that younger referees with more experience refereeing had a better chance at detecting flaws in problematic papers. Black et al. (1998) also showed that younger reviewers and those who had training in epidemiology or statistics produced better reviews, though their study found in general that reviewer characteristics could explain only 8% of the variation in review quality. Callaham et al. (1998) found that subjective ratings of reviewers correlated with the ability to detect flaws in manuscripts.

Another question relating to peer review is whether the process is biased by institutional prestige or geographic location of the reviewers. Garfunkel et al. (1994) observed that institutional prestige did not influence acceptance of major manuscripts at the journal *Pediatrics*, though it was found to correlate positively with brief reports. Link (1998) noted that US-based and non-US-based reviewers had comparable rates of recommendation of acceptance when reviewing for the journal *Gastroenterology*.

Other research has addressed ways of improving the process so that peer reviewers can do their job more effectively. One intervention that has been shown to be effective is to provide reviewers with abstracts and preprints of related papers (Hatch and Goodman, 1998). Another intervention has been to blind reviewers to the identity of the authors of the paper being reviewed. It is presumed that this reduces bias in reviews. Of course, complete blinding of reviewers can be difficult. Even if author identities are stripped from manuscripts, references to past work, location of the study, funding source, or other aspects may reveal their identity. Indeed, one study of masking found that it was successful only 68% of the time, and less often for well-known authors (Justice, Cho et al., 1998). One study has shown that blinding produced better reviews (McNutt, Evans et al., 1990), while several more recent studies have provided evidence that it does not (Godlee, Gale et al., 1998; Justice, Cho et al., 1998; vanRooyen, Godlee et al., 1998). Two of these studies also assessed whether unmasking the identity of reviewers to authors led to higher quality reviews, with both showing that it did not (Godlee, Gale et al., 1998; vanRooyen, Godlee et al., 1998). These studies have led BMJ to adopt an "open review" policy, where the names of peer reviewers are disclosed to authors. A recent study of reviews of conference proceedings abstracts found a bias in favor of authors from the USA, other English-speaking countries, and prestigious institutions, which was eliminated when this information was blinded (Ross, Gross et al., 2006).

One common practice in peer review, especially outside medicine, is to ask authors for suggested reviewers. Does this make a difference? One analysis of 329 manuscripts from ten leading journals found that the quality of the reviews was judged similar but that author-suggested reviewers tended to make more favorable recommendations concerning publication (Schroter, Tite et al., 2006). Similar findings were found in another analysis (Wager, Parkin et al., 2006).

Most editors of peer-reviewed journals are not trained in editorial practices, tending to come from the ranks of accomplished academicians and clinicians. Most of these individuals are likely to have had prior experience with publishing and/or peer reviewing, however. The editors of the major journals devote full-time effort to editing, while editors of specialty journals usually devote part-time effort. Most specialist clinical medical journals tend to be edited by practicing clinicians who are self-taught, part-time editors (Garrow, Butterfield et al., 1998).

Of course, the peer-review process is not without imperfections. Even the relatively sterile world of science is susceptible to human tendencies toward competitiveness, arrogance, and even dishonesty. The ensuing discussion of the problems should inform the reader of the limitations of the process, rather than leading to rejection of its merits.

It was seen that Lotka's law indicates that current success in a scientific field is a good predictor of future success. Certainly those who have already produced good work are likely to continue to do so. However, there may also be an unfair bias toward those who are already successful. Evidence for this was shown most strikingly in an experiment by two psychologists Peters and Ceci (1982), who took 12 psychology articles that were already published in prestigious psychology journals and resubmitted them with different author names and slight rewording of titles. These articles were eventually disseminated to 38 reviewers, only three (8%) of whom detected that the article was a resubmission. For the remaining nine articles where a resubmission was not detected 16 of 18 reviewers recommended against acceptance, and all but one of the articles were rejected for publication. The most common reason for rejection of these previously accepted papers was "serious methodologic flaw."

Peters and Ceci's paper was published with a large number of rebuttals from various psychology journal editors and other psychologists. A variety of limitations of the study were proposed, including its small sample size and possibility that the results represented a regression toward the mean. Peters and Ceci acknowledged the small sample size but refuted the assertion that the results were due to chance or some other statistical anomaly. Clearly, the rejection of findings previously deemed suitable for publication but now described by unknown authors indicated that already esteemed authors have a better chance of publication.

A more recent variant of this type of study was done in the social work literature (Epstein, 2004). In this study, two "stimulus" articles, written with both a positive and negative interpretation, were submitted to 31 social work journals. The acceptance rates between the positive and negative versions were statically significantly different for one of the articles but not the other. The timeliness and quality of the peer reviews were considered inadequate in 73.5% of the reviews.

Other findings raise some concerns about the peer-review process. Ingelfinger (1974), a former editor of the *New England Journal of Medicine*, noted that for nearly 500 consecutive papers submitted to that journal, the concordance between the two reviewers for each article was only slightly better than chance. Among the problems he cited in the peer-review process were reviewers wrongly assumed to be knowledgeable on a particular topic based on their stature in the field as a whole, reviewers not skilled in detecting poor writing that obscured the quality of an underlying message, and reviewer bias toward or against others in the individual's field. A more recent study showed that in secondary review of accepted manuscripts, although there was high concordance among reviewers for accepting or rejecting the paper, there was a wide divergence in the identification of problems deemed to warrant further revision (Garfunkel, Ulshen et al., 1990).

The peer-review process of grant proposals has been less studied than peer review of journal articles. The most investigated aspect concerns funding rates of basic vs. clinical research. Two recent analyses show that applications for clinical research on average receive worse priority scores (Kotchen, Lindquist et al., 2004, 2006). Other findings include that smaller study sections result in worse priority scores for clinical but not basic science research.

Commenting on inadequacies in the peer-review process for grant proposals, Stumpf (1980) noted a number of problems, which also occur with journal peer review:

- For scientific pioneers, there are often few peers who are knowledgeable enough to adequately review their work.
- For all scientists, the closest peer is a competitor, who may not be appropriate as a reviewer.
- While reviewers have the opportunity to criticize every aspect of the submitter's work, there is little, if any, chance for rebuttal.
- Reviewers are anonymous, hence are shielded from their own deficiencies and bias.

Stumpf also called into question the value of anonymous peer review.

2.5.3   Primary Literature

As already noted, the primary literature consists of reports of original research. Key features of primary literature are that it reports on new discoveries and observations, describes earlier work to acknowledge it and place the new findings in the proper perspective, and draws only conclusions that can be justified by the results. Another feature of most primary literature is that it has not been published elsewhere, especially in non-peer-reviewed forums. Indeed, most journals adhere to the "Ingelfinger rule," which states that a manuscript will be accepted for publication only if it has not been published elsewhere (Ingelfinger, 1969). Exceptions are made for articles that have been presented at scientific meetings, situations in which early publication would have a major impact on public health, and cases in which findings have been released for government deliberations (Angell and Kassirer, 1991). The ease of posting research results on the Web has challenged the Ingelfinger rule, but most medical journals still adhere to it (Altman, 1996).

The highest quality (i.e., most evidence-based) studies tend to be published in a small number of journals. McKibbon et al. (2004) looked at publications that provide summaries of "clinically important" articles (e.g., *ACP Journal Club* and *Evidence-Based Medicine*), assessing 60,352 articles in 170 journals. They found the following results by field:

- In internal medicine (*ACP Journal Club*), four titles provide 56.5% of articles, while 27 supply the rest.
- In general/family medicine (*Evidence-Based Medicine*), five titles provide 50.7% of articles, while 40 supply the rest.
- In nursing (*Evidence-Based Nursing*), seven titles provide 51.0% of the articles, while 34 supply the rest.
- In mental health (*Evidence-Based Mental Health*), nine titles provide 53.2% of the articles, while 34 supply the rest.

The discussion on peer review indicates that good science sometimes does not make it through the peer-review process because of reasons not having to do with its quality. The converse occurs as well, with poor or even invalid science sometimes getting published. Furthermore, medical journals, online databases, and libraries are not well equipped to handle fraudulent science. The remainder of this section addresses these issues.

2.5.3.1   Methodological Issues in Primary Literature

Problems in the methodology used in clinical studies have been a problem for decades. Fletcher and Fletcher (1979) lamented that weak methods were quite prevalent in the literature, such as studies using nonrandomized designs or very small sample sizes. Even now, studies of case series or case reports, with no experimental or observational control, still manage to get published. While such studies can have value in generating hypotheses for further research, their appearance in the literature (and literature databases, such as MEDLINE) gives them an aura of value that may not be warranted. Even large-scale observational studies can be problematic, as demonstrated by the Women's Health Initiative study. Previous observational reports from case-control studies had shown a clear association between postmenopausal hormone replacement therapy (and positive clinical outcomes. A large-scale RCT, however, showed the opposite (Anonymous, 2002e), and later analysis found that the observational studies had been confounded by the fact that women who had used hormone replacement therapy were of higher socioeconomic status, and their better health hid the negative effects of the therapy (Humphrey, Chan et al., 2002).

It has also been found that lower-quality studies are more likely to be later "overturned" (Ioannidis, 2005a). This is probably due to their relatively small sample sizes, which prevent complete knowledge of all effects, especially relatively uncommon adverse ones. Ioannidis (2005b) has further generalized this observation to assert that "most published research findings are false." He makes this claim based on the observations that most studies and the effects they discover are small, and that the proper range of hypotheses is not tested. He also expresses concern about research groups "vigorously chasing" statistical significance such that research findings may just be a result of "prevailing bias."

There are also a number of practical issues in the conduct of biomedical research that raise concerns – for example, some studies that are stopped early because a strong and statistically significant treatment effect has occurred (Montori, Devereaux et al., 2005). These studies are usually published in the major five medical journals and funded by industry. However, despite this happening more commonly, they often fail to fully document their reasons for stopping early. Mueller et al. (2007) have reviewed the ethical issues in this setting and advocate continuing recruitment and monitoring of patients randomized to the favorable group to minimize the risk of overestimate of its benefit.

Another common problem in methodology is inappropriate use of statistics. Glantz (1980) found that nearly half of all studies in medical journals utilized statistics incorrectly, with the most common error being the inappropriate use of the t test in comparing more than two groups of means. Freiman et al. noted that many studies inadequately reported the statistical power of the methods used to discern a difference when one exists (Freiman, Chalmers et al., 1978). An analysis by Garcia-Berthou and Alcaraz (2004) found that one or more incongruence occurred with statistical reporting in the prestigious journals *Nature* and BMJ in 38% and 25% of papers respectively. In 12% of these instances, the significance levels (p value) could be incorrect by an order of magnitude or more. Most errors were presumed to be due to rounding, transcription, or type-setting problems.

A related issue is inadequate statistical power, where an inadequate sample size may fail to discern a statistically significant difference that may actually exist. Moher et al. (1994) found that many published clinical trials do not have a large enough sample size to be able to detect clinically meaningful relative differences. Halpern et al. (2002) have deemed the continued performing and reporting of underpowered clinical trials as an ethical dilemma. There have been some efforts to improve statistical reporting. In an assessment of an attempt to improve statistical reporting at the BMJ, it was found that the rate of papers considered statistically acceptable improved from 11% at submission to 84% by publication (Gardner and Bond, 1990).

It should be noted that even if statistical methods and results are reported correctly, readers will not necessarily understand them. A number of studies have found that professionals who read scientific journals tend to understand natural frequencies much better than probabilities (Hoffrage, Lindsey et al., 2000). Thus, these readers can calculate the risk of a disease better by using natural frequencies (e.g., 10 of 100) than probabilities (e.g., 10%).

Also a problem in the literature is the manipulation of study design to achieve a beneficial outcome. Smith (2005) has catalogued the ways that pharmaceutical companies and others have "gamed" studies to get good results. He also provides "advice" on how to perform this process:

- Conduct a trial against a drug known to be inferior instead of the best current treatment
- Conduct a trial against a competitor by using too low (to get a better result) or too high (to have less toxicity) a dose
- Conduct trials with samples too small to show a difference from competitor
- Use multiple endpoints and select those that show best benefit
- Do multicenter trials but only report results from centers that are favorable
- Conduct subgroup analysis and report only those that are favorable
- Report results most likely to impress, i.e., report relative rather than absolute risk reduction

Smith has also noted that the publication of a positive study can be lucrative, i.e., worth billions, for a drug that treats a common condition. Actual scientific papers look more "professional" than advertisements, and paper reprints of them passed out by sales representatives are a large source of revenue for journals, up to 70% profit margin. This has led Smith to call the medical journals and pharmaceutical companies "uneasy bedfellows" (Smith, 2003) and advocate that medical journals not publish such studies, but instead serve as a forum to review their findings and limitations.

Does pharmaceutical company funding compromise clinical studies? About 66–75% of all trials published in major medical journals are funded by industry (Egger, Bartlett et al., 2001). In a systematic review of studies comparing research sponsored by the pharmaceutical industry with that sponsored by others, Lexchin et al. (2003) analyzed 30 studies and found that the latter were more likely to have a positive outcome and less likely to be published. Their analysis did not, however, find that these studies were of poorer quality. The better outcomes were explained by inappropriate comparator products and publication bias. Perlis et al. (2005) has documented similar problems in the psychiatry literature.

One series of methodological manipulations gave critical mass to a major change by journals, namely the requirement of clinical trial registration to prevent changes after the trial was started and ensure complete reporting (Dickersin and Rennie, 2003). These manipulations were of studies on COX-2 inhibitors, touted as a "better" nonsteroidal anti-inflammatory drug for pain control that would reduce the known gastrointestinal complications of older drugs in this category (e.g., ibuprofen). In one study (Silverstein, Faich et al., 2000), the researchers (from the manufacturer) omitted 6 months of data because they believed it was invalid (Silverstein, Simon et al., 2001). These data were published on the Web site of the US Food and Drug Administration (FDA) and discovered by a number of researchers (Hrachovec and Mora, 2001; Wright, Perry et al., 2001), and when added to the data reported in the paper, the original conclusions of safety were no longer warranted (Jüni, Rutjes et al., 2002). The latter authors also noted that the paper had been cited by 169 other papers and 30,000 reprints had been ordered before these problems came to light. In another study on a different COX-2 inhibitor (Bombardier, Laine et al., 2000), three patients suffering myocardial infarctions were excluded from the study despite the authors knowing about them, and their inclusion would have changed the conclusion of the paper to the agent being harmful (Curfman, Morrissey et al., 2005).

Another example of failure to publish negative studies was documented for trials of antidepressants (Turner, Matthews et al., 2008). These authors identified 74 RCTs performed on 12 antidepressants that were registered by the FDA to obtain approval to market the drug. While nearly all of the studies with positive results were published (37 of 38), a majority of the studies with negative results were either not published (22 of 36) or published in a way that the authors believed conveyed a positive outcome (11 of 36). As a result, although 94% of trials appeared to be positive, only 51% were actually so. A meta-analysis done on patient-level data from these trials showed that the nonpublication created an apparent 32% better (11–69% for individual drugs) effect size for the drugs than was warranted by all the data.

The outrage over the changes in the nonsteroidal anti-inflammatory drug trials being made after their inception increased the long-standing calls for pretrial registration. Long advocated by many EBM advocates to protect integrity of RCT conduct and reporting, registration requires those conducting RCTs to register them with details of hypotheses, methods, etc. (Dickersin and Rennie, 2003). Therefore, any changes that are made must be documented and scrutinized. After the COX-2 and related (e.g., SSRI inhibitors and suicide, (Anonymous, 2004c)) debacles, the ICMJE adopted a policy of requiring it at the inception of study (DeAngelis, Drazen et al., 2004). Now, RCTs must be registered in ClinicalTrials.gov (Zarin, Tse et al., 2005) or other comparable databases (Haug, Gotzsche et al., 2005), and acceptance has been high (Laine, Horton et al., 2007). In addition, the new Ottawa Statement has been adopted that reflects principles of data to be entered into such registration databases (Krleza-Jeric, Chan et al., 2005). The process of registering trials has had the usual challenges in any large-scale informatics project, i.e., minimizing inadvertent duplicate entries, standardizing intervention names, and providing robust searching (Zarin, Ide et al., 2007).

Is Smith right that journals not publish RCTs? He instead advocates that there should be more public funding of RCTs, especially large head-to-head ones, and RCT protocols and results should be made available on Web sites, with the role of journals being instead to critically critique them. If RCTs were to be published elsewhere, where would that be? A number of clinical trials results databases have been developed, none of which has comprehensive coverage and for which concerns about lack of peer review have been expressed (Fisher, 2006). Some have suggested increased use of the FDA Dockets Management system (http://www.fda.gov/ohrms/dockets/default.htm), which contains information required of pharmaceutical companies for FDA approval of their drugs. Many researchers find it to be a source of clinical trials data beyond that which is reported in articles. However, the site is extremely user-unfriendly, which is thought to be deliberate by some. Another possibility would be the use of the new drug application database of the FDA (Turner, 2004). A different proposal is to develop a Global Trial Bank (Sim and Detmer, 2005), which has been promoted by the American Medical Informatics Association (http://www.amia.org/gtb/) and is based on capturing all the elements believed necessary to allow others to analyze all data of trial.

2.5.3.2 Reporting Issues in Primary Literature

Another problem with the primary literature has been inadequate reporting of methods and results. DerSimonian et al. (1982) identified 11 factors deemed important in the design and analysis of studies, such as eligibility criteria for admission to the trial, method of randomization used, and blinding, and found that only slightly over half of all studies in four major medical journals reported them adequately. Others also have found that randomization methods were poorly described in the obstetrics and gynecology literature (Schulz, Chalmers et al., 1994). Bailar (1986) has lamented that some scientific practices border on the deceptive, such as the selective reporting of results in some experiments, which is sometimes done to improve chances for publication.

Reporting of methods and results has been found to be particularly problematic in the area of the RCT. As will be further described in Sect. 2.8, the RCT is considered to be the best type of evidence for the effectiveness of a health-care intervention, whether in the treatment of a disease or its prevention. Furthermore, the data in RCTs are used in *meta-analysis*, which is the aggregation of the results of many similar trials to obtain a more statistically powerful result (see Sect. 2.5.4). It is therefore imperative that RCTs report their data in a way that can be understood by readers and used by other researchers. Authors and journals, however, appear to be falling short. For example, one review of the use of selective serotonin-reuptake inhibitors for depression found that only 1 of 122 RCTs described the randomization process unequivocally (Hotopf, Lewis et al., 1997). This is important, since one of the most important predictive factors of the quality of an RCT is whether the randomization process is concealed from those involved in care of the patient (Schulz, Chalmers et al., 1995).

The problems in the reporting of methods and results in RCTs has led to the formation of the *Con*solidated *S*tandards *o*f *R*eporting *T*rials (CONSORT) statement, which provides a checklist of 22 items to include when reporting an RCT (Moher, Schulz et al., 2001). Most of these elements are included because it has been found that their omission is associated with biased evidence favoring the treatment being studied. For example, studies not using masked assessments of the outcome (i.e., the person judging whether a patient got better did not know whether the patient had received the experimental or control intervention), studies rated as low quality, and studies not concealing the allocation of the patients to the experimental or control intervention all have been found to have a higher average treatment effect than do studies of better quality (Moher, Pham et al., 1998). This finding was also observed in studies of selective digestive decontamination, where there was an inverse relationship between methodological quality score of RCTs and the benefit of treatment (vanNieuwenhoven, Buskens et al., 2001). A more recent analysis, however, found that quality measures do not always correlate with treatment effects (Balk, Bonis et al., 2002). Use of the CONSORT statement has been shown to result in improvements in the quality of RCT reports (Moher, Jones et al., 2001), although others (Huwiler-Muntener, Juni et al., 2002) have found that good reporting is not strictly correlated with good quality of the study itself. The success of the CONSORT statement generally has led to the development of a similar approach for observational studies, the *St*rengthening the *R*eporting of *Ob*servational Studies in *E*pidemiology (STROBE) statement (von Elm, Altman et al., 2007).

Another problem with articles about RCTs is inadequate reporting of adverse events. Chan et al. (2004) assessed 102 clinical trials and their clinical outcome measures that were approved by ethics committees in Denmark during 1994–1995. They found that 50% of the efficacy outcomes and 65% of the harm outcomes were incompletely reported. About 62% of the trials had at least one clinical outcome that had been changed, introduced, or omitted from the original study protocol. A survey of trial authors denied the existence of unreported outcomes despite their existence identified by Chan et al. Related to this problem is that RCTs in general tend to underreport adverse effects or not to have text words or indexing terms that enable their retrieval (Derry, Loke et al., 2001; Fromme, Eilers et al., 2004; Golder, McIntosh et al., 2006). This makes it vitally important that postmarketing surveillance of approved drugs occur (Fontanarosa, Rennie et al., 2004).

Also a limitation of RCTs is that some clinical interventions require training or skill that is not always taken into account. One way to address this has been proposed is "expertise"-based trials, where only those with enough training and skill to carry out the intervention do so (Devereaux, Bhandari et al., 2005). Related to this is a problem of rapidly changing technologies, which includes informatics applications, such that the intervention becomes different due to improvements or other changes in the technology. For this reason, "tracker trials" that maintain the intervention but track its change have been advocated (Lilford, Braunholtz et al., 2000).

RCTs are not the only type of study considered to be problematic in the medical literature. The reporting of diagnostic test research studies has also been criticized (Reid, Lachs et al., 1995). Similar to RCTs, it has been found that inadequate methodology used in evaluating diagnostic tests tends to overestimate their accuracy (Lijmer, Mol et al., 1999). Likewise, Udvarhelyi et al. (1992) found that studies on cost-effectiveness and cost-benefit similarly have reporting problems.

Another reporting-related issue is the understandability of benefits and risks of medical interventions by clinicians, other professionals such as policymakers, and patients. In an overview of what is known, Politi et al. (2007) have noted that our understanding is incomplete not only with regard to the meaning of various adjectives that are commonly used to quantify the level of risk (e.g., severe, minimal, etc.) but also concerning the uncertainty of our knowledge. One challenge is a tendency for authors to report relative over absolute risks, which may make an intervention seem more effective than is warranted, especially when a condition is uncommon. For example, the relative risk reduction of a treatment that lowers mortality from 2/100 patients to 1/100 patients is 50%, whereas the absolute risk reduction is only 1%. This has led to calls for more standardized reporting of benefits and harms in the literature and communication of both relative risk and frequencies (Sawaya, Guirguis-Blake et al., 2007; Sedrakyan and Shih, 2007).

With the growing access to medical information by patients, some have assessed the best ways to report scientific literature to nonprofessionals. One study compared various methods for presenting results to patients and found that relative and absolute risk reduction were more readily understood than number needed to treat, a common approach used to convey the magnitude of treatment benefit to clinicians (Sheridan, Pignone et al., 2003). However, in another study, number needed to treat was found to yield a higher consent rate for a treatment of known benefit than presenting the benefit as how long the treatment would postpone an adverse outcome.

Also found to be a problem in journal articles is incomplete reporting of past studies. Gotzsche and Olsen (2001) found that subsequent references to seven RCTs of mammography screening tended to omit important limitations of the trials. They advocated that study protocols remain available on the Web after the results have been published. Clarke et al. (2002) noted that only 2 of 25 RCTs where prior trials existed described the new results in the proper context of prior trials. Similarly, Tatsioni et al. (2007) have documented the persistence of citing observational studies in the literature where results of large-scale clinical trials have superceded their conclusions. A related problem is weaknesses identified in follow-up correspondence. Horton (2002) found that half of the criticisms in postpublication correspondence of the three RCTs went unanswered. In addition, criticisms of the studies raised in such correspondence were not noted in subsequent practice guidelines.

Authorship is another area that can be problematic in reporting. Although it probably does not affect the quality of the information being reported, authorship is important nonetheless in terms of academic promotion and funding. As many as 19% of articles in major journals may have authors who do not meet the ICMJE criteria for authorship, that is, are "honorary" authors (Flanagin, Carey et al., 1998). Conversely, up to 11% show evidence of having "ghost" authors. Laine et al. (2001) have found that 93% of first authors of papers in *Annals of Internal Medicine* and *Radiology* satisfy the ICMJE criteria, while fewer authors in other positions do so (72% of second authors, 51% of third authors, 54% of last authors, and 33% of authors in other positions). Van Rooyen et al. (2001) found that only 17% of papers in the BMJ adhere to the reporting standards of the ICMJE criteria.

A related concern to authorship is conflict of interest. ICMJE guidelines do not prevent authors with a financial interest from publishing, requiring only that they disclose such interests. While the explicit financial interest that authors have is not well reported (Gupta, Gross et al., 2001), studies having such interests have actually been found to be associated with higher quality of methodological reporting (Olson, Rennie et al., 2001). There is also no association between trial quality or outcome, although the authors of this study noted that their analysis was limited because the reporting of these interests was voluntary (Clifford, Moher et al., 2001).

Even when the methods and results are adequately described, the writing may be problematic. As mentioned earlier, scientists who serve as peer reviewers may not be skilled at ensuring that a paper will describe its findings and conclusions as clearly and succinctly as possible (Ingelfinger, 1974). Even when the body of a paper is written soundly, the abstract may not accurately convey the nature of the results. One study of six major medical journals found that 18–68% of abstracts contained data that either were inconsistent or were not found in the body of the article (Pitkin, Branagan et al., 1999). This problem is of increased gravity when practitioners access bibliographic databases (such as MEDLINE) that have only titles and abstracts. They may not have the time or motivation to seek the primary reference and thus may be misled by an inaccurate abstract. These problems have motivated the use in virtually all major medical journals of *structured abstracts*, which require information about the objective, design, setting, participants, intervention, main outcome, results, and conclusions from a study (Haynes, Mulrow et al., 1990). The *Annals of Internal Medicine* added a new item to structured abstracts starting in 2004, limitations (Anonymous, 2004a).

Journal articles may also have inaccuracies in citations and quotations. Unless noted by peer reviewers, these errors usually pass through the editorial process. In a study of three surgical journals, Evans et al. (1990) found that almost half of all references had errors such as misspelling of author names or partial omissions of titles and authors, although most of the errors were deemed to be minor. A more serious problem was the number of major errors in quotation, such as an article being referenced that did not substantiate, was unrelated to, or contradicted the authors' assertions. Each journal issue had over ten major quotational errors.

A decade later, citation errors are still found in 7–60% of journal articles, with 1–24% being so significant that the articles cannot be located based on the information given (Riesenberg and Dontineni, 2001; Wager and Middleton, 2001). Even recently, Aronsky et al. (2005) found this problem in the biomedical informatics literature. These authors assessed the five biomedical informatics journals with the highest IFs for each journal's first issue of 2004. They found 311 errors in 225 of the 656 references (34.3%) in 37 articles. The percentage of articles with errors varied by journal, from 22.1% for *Journal of the American Medical Informatics Association* to 40.7% for *International Journal of Medical Informatics*. The most common element with an error was the author name (31%), followed by the title (17%), page (7.4%), and year (3.5%).

A new wrinkle to the problem of inadequate citations is Web references provided in scientific papers that are inaccessible or incorrect. Crichlow et al. (2004) assessed URLs in the references of all original research papers in five major medical journals that were published in January 2004. In 91 articles analyzed, there were 68 URLs in the references, 8.6% of which were inaccessible. These authors noted that de Lacey et al. (1985) had found a similar 8% overall rate of errors in citations in the paper-based journal literature in 1985. A related problem is availability of URLs to supplementary data. A recent analysis found that about one quarter of such links become invalid, with a particular problem when the URL links to a site off that of the journal of publication (Anderson et al., 2006).

2.5.3.3 Publication Bias

An additional problem with the primary literature is the phenomenon of *publication bias*. Given studies of equal methodological rigor, those with "positive" results are more likely to be published (Dickersin, 1990). Publication bias tends to result because scientists want to report positive results and journal editors (and presumably their readers) want to read them. As will be seen in the next section, publication bias is particularly problematic with the growing use of meta-analysis, where the aggregation of studies presumes that individual studies represent the full spectrum of results.

There is strong evidence for publication bias. Sterling (1959) noted several decades ago that studies yielding statistically significant results were more likely to be published than those that did not, raising the possibility that studies with significant results may never be further verified. Rosenthal (1979) labeled this the "file drawer" problem, in that researchers would let languish negative results from their research in their file drawers. Dickersin and Min (1993) noted this problem with clinical trials, observing that studies approved by various institutional review boards and/or NIH funding agencies were more likely to be published if statistically significant results were achieved. Others have looked at a cohort of studies approved by a hospital review board and found that those with positive results were 2.3 times more likely to be published than those with negative results (Stern and Simes, 1997). The likelihood of publication for clinical trials was even higher (3.1 times more likely). Studies with indeterminate results were even less likely to be published, while those measuring qualitative outcomes did not seem to reflect the influence of publication bias.

There are other manifestations of publication bias. Some studies with positive outcomes tend to be published sooner than those with negative or equivocal outcomes. An additional finding from Stern and Simes (1997) was that the median time to publication for studies with positive results was significantly shorter (4.7–4.8 vs. 8.0 years). Likewise, Ioannidis (1998) found that clinical trials not achieving statistical significance of the results in the treatment of human immunodeficiency virus (HIV) were likely to be published later than those that did. A contrary result was found at JAMA, where studies with positive results were not found to be published more quickly than those with negative results (Olson, Rennie et al., 2002). Another facet of publication bias is that researchers from non-English-speaking countries tend to publish their positive results more in English-language journals (Egger, Zellweger-Zahner et al., 1997).

A related issue is conference proceedings abstracts that do not get published as full papers. A systematic review assessing the fate of biomedical meeting abstracts found that only about 46% of abstracts presented at such meetings achieved publication of the full paper in a journal (von Elm, Costanza et al., 2003). These authors also reviewed the fate of abstracts originally rejected, finding 27% were eventually published as full papers. Studies in basic science and those having a positive outcome were more likely to eventually be published as papers. Abstracts were more likely to be published if they were presented orally, at a small meeting, or a US meeting.

Negative results or the inability to obtain statistical significance are not reasons not to publish, since in the case of clinical trials, for example, it is just as important to know when a therapy is not more effective than the current standard or none at all. This is even more crucial with the current widespread use of meta-analysis, since data that should be part of a meta-analysis might not be used because it had never been published. Indeed, Chalmers (1990) has called failure to publish a clinical trial a form of "scientific misconduct." In recognition of this problem, more than 100 journals announced an "amnesty for unpublished trials" in September 1997, and authors of clinical trials not yet published were invited to report their register and report their results over the Web (Smith and Roberts, 1997). Friedman and Wyatt (2001) also raise concern about publication bias in fields such as medical informatics, where system developers often perform evaluations and are less likely to publish unfavorable results about their systems, especially when such data may detract from future grant funding.

2.5.3.4   Fraud in Primary Literature

A final issue associated with primary literature is the handling of invalid or fraudulent science. While the NLM has the means to retract incorrect or fraudulent literature from its databases (Colaianni, 1992), removing it from library shelves and the Web is considerably more difficult. A survey of 129 academic medical libraries in North America found that 59% have no policy or practices for calling retracted publications to the attention of their patrons (Hughes, 1998). Another 9% have no formal policies but attempt to notify users by one means or another. Among the means for identifying such research include tagging articles on the first page of the issue in which each one occurs or keeping lists of such articles at reference or circulation desks. Friedman (1990) has found that journals are inconsistent in how they identify retracted publications.

Specific instances of identified research fraud have been well publicized. In an analysis of the work of John Darsee, a Harvard researcher who was later found to have fabricated experimental results, two researchers found that the other publications of Darsee, whose validity may never be known, are still cited by other researchers in a positive light (Kochen and Budd, 1992). Others (Whitely, Rennie et al., 1994) did a similar analysis of the publications of Robert Slutsky, another scientist guilty of fraud, and found a similar phenomenon, though the rate of citation diminished as the case was publicized in the press. Likewise, another scientist known to publish fraudulent work, Stephen Breuning, was also found to have positive citations of his work long after he had pleaded guilty to deception (Garfield and Welljams-Dorof, 1990).

A more recent case was that of stem cell researcher Woo Suk Hwang of South Korea. He was viewed as a national hero after having made reported breakthroughs in the use of stem cells, which show promise in many human diseases but are controversial because of the only method for obtaining them being from the umbilical cords of aborted fetuses. Two papers published in *Science* were viewed as particularly seminal breakthroughs (Hwang, Ryu et al., 2004; Hwang, Roh et al., 2005). However, a Korean investigative news show was tipped off by some of Hwang's collaborators (Chong and Normile, 2006). Ultimately, all of his work was declared to be fraudulent, and *Science* retracted the two seminal papers (Kennedy, 2006). A retrospective analysis found a number of problems in the *Science* papers that were not detected by the peer-review process (Couzin, 2006).

Other documented cases of fraud abound (Couzin and Unger, 2006; Unger and Couzin, 2006). The NIH releases notices of scientific misconduct when fraud by researchers funded by its grants is uncovered. *Science* has raised the question of scientific misconduct in other areas, including "bubble fusion" (Service, 2006b) and chemical catalyzation (Service, 2006a). *Annals of Internal Medicine* reports a number of lessons learned, including the unwillingness of journals and academic institutions to take the necessary steps to ensure "cleansing" of the literature from the case of fraudulent research by Eric Poehlman (Sox and Rennie, 2006).

One case where fraud has not been documented but serious concerns remain about the research is in a study that assessed the value of distant prayer (from the USA and Australia) to facilitate in vitro fertilization in Korea (Cha and Wirth, 2001). One of the authors was a department chairman at Columbia University, and has since removed his name from the paper. However, the paper is still indexed in MEDLINE and present on the *Journal of Reproductive Medicine* Web site without any hints about these concerns. Flamm (2002, 2004) has documented significant problems with this research and the way concerns about it have been handled. It should be noted that an RCT of cardiac bypass patients receiving prayer found that it offered no benefit (Benson, Dusek et al., 2006).

There are additional concerns about compromised validity of information in journals short of outright fraud. One oft-cited culprit is the pharmaceutical industry, both through its influence on the content as well as advertising in journals. In an editorial, Fletcher (2003) noted that advertisements are a major source of revenue for journals and provide resources to support the journal or the organization (often a professional society) that publishes it. However, he notes that although physicians claim not to have their practices influenced by advertisements, the advertisers would unlikely spend thousands of dollars per physician per year that they do if they had no effect.

Advertisements themselves, which readers encounter alongside the scientific papers in journals, can be misleading in their content. Wilkes et al. (1992) found that 44% of advertising would lead to improper prescribing if the physician had no other information. They also noted that 92% of advertisements included at least one area that did not comply with regulations of the FDA. Villanueva et al. (2003) looked at all advertisements for blood-pressure-lowering and lipid-lowering medications in six Spanish medical journals during 1997. In a sample of references cited in the advertisements, they found that 18% of the references could not be retrieved. In addition, 44% of the claims made were not completely supported by the reference, usually because of the drug being recommended in a patient group other than in which it was studied.

Also problematic in advertisements may be the graphics. Cooper et al. (2003) analyzed all advertisements in ten US medical journals in 1999. Half of the advertisement area consisted of nonscientific figures and images. About 1.6% of the area contained scientific graphs. Over a third had some numerical distortion that led to overestimation or underestimation of the quantity being graphed, which is specifically prohibited by FDA regulations.

Another area of concern described in the text is conflict of interest. A recent episode led to the partial retraction of a paper by *Lancet*, when it was discovered that the primary author did not disclose funding by a group of lawyers representing alleged victims of autism due to the measles, mumps, and rubella vaccine (Horton,

2004). This demonstrates that conflicts of interests are not necessarily limited to those who stand to gain from sale of products.

A related problem is that of plagiarism. A group of case studies from the *Bulletin of Environmental Contamination and Toxicology* identified instances of self-plagiarism (title, coauthors, and data were changed), a paper published in Spanish that was translated into English and submitted, and the copying of figures without acknowledgment (Nigg and Radulsecu, 1994). Plagiarism may now be even easier with the growth of electronic publication on the Web. Kock (1999) reported a case of a paper of his that was copied from the Web and then submitted for publication to a journal. A case of a medical journal paper being assembled by plagiarism from a number of Web-based sources has also been identified (Eysenbach, 2000b).

2.5.4   Systematic Reviews and Meta-analysis

As noted earlier in the chapter, the scientific literature is fragmented, perhaps purposefully (Ziman, 1969). As will be seen in subsequent chapters, even experienced searchers have difficulty identifying all the relevant articles on a given topic. The proliferation of clinical trials, particularly when they assess the same diseases and treatments, has led to the production of systematic reviews, which have been described in Sect. 2.4. Systematic reviews are distinguished from traditional review articles, described in the next section, by their focused questions, exhaustive review of the literature, and use of evidence-based techniques (Petticrew, 2001). They are a major aspect of EBM, to be discussed in Sect. 2.8. When appropriate, systematic reviews involve the use of *meta-analysis*, where the results of appropriately similar trials are pooled to obtain a more comprehensive picture with greater statistical power. The term meta-analysis was coined by Glass (1976), and the technique is used increasingly in assessing the results of clinical trials. Meta-analyses are not limited to RCTs and have been used with diagnostic test studies (Glasziou and Irwig, 1998) and observational studies (Stroup, Berlin et al., 2000).

Several references describe the methods for producing systematic reviews in great detail: the *Cochrane Reviewers' Handbook* (Higgins, Green et al., 2006), an article (Pai, McCulloch et al., 2004), and a couple of books (Altman, Chalmers et al., 2001; Glasziou, Irwig et al., 2001). The *Annals of Internal Medicine* recently published a supplement describing the challenges of summarizing information (i.e., producing systematic reviews or evidence reports), with a focus on work done by the Evidence-Based Practice Center (EPC) program of the Agency for Healthcare Research and Quality (AHRQ) (Helfand, Morton et al., 2005). The supplement includes an overview of the EPC program and articles about challenges in various areas, such as efficacy of drugs (Santaguida, Helfand et al., 2005), use of nonrandomized studies (Norris and Atkins, 2005), and dissemination of reports (Matchar, Westermann-Clark et al., 2005).

What are the characteristics of systematic reviews published in the medical literature? Montori et al. (2004) assessed 170 well-known clinical journals for the year 2000, counting 60,330 articles. Of these articles, 26,694 were original research reports and 3,193 were review articles. Of the review articles, 768 (24%) were systematic reviews, defined as articles that clearly stated a clinical topic, how the evidence was retrieved, what sources the evidence was retrieved from, and what the inclusion and exclusion criteria were. The majority of systematic reviews were about therapy (63%), followed by causation and safety (29%), diagnosis (4.4%), and prognosis (2.1%). About 80% of all the systematic reviews were published in 11% of the journals. The IF of these journals was weakly but significantly associated with the publication of systematic reviews. Systematic reviews were more likely to be cited by other papers in these journals than narrative reviews.

One aspect that characterizes systematic reviews is their reporting of explicit search strategies and assessment of their effectiveness. Patrick et al. (2004) found that although the majority of meta-analyses (71%) reported a search strategy, only a small number (6.7%) reported evidence of the strategy's effectiveness. Despite the prevalence of IR systems, handsearching of the literature is still required to identify all trials to include in meta-analyses. Thirty-four assessments in a variety of topical areas have demonstrated that handsearching yields 92–100% of all reports of RCTs, whereas searching of MEDLINE and other databases reveals only 49–67% (Hopewell, Clarke et al., 2003).

The most common use of meta-analysis in health care is to combine the results of RCTs. The most common approach is to express the data as adverse event rates and compare the odds ratio (OR) between the control and experimental groups (Bland and Altman, 2000). In addition to knowing the point estimate of the treatment effect, one must know the precision of the value. That is, how likely is it that the point estimate from the patient sample represents the true value for the entire population? To determine the precision, the confidence interval (CI) is calculated (Bland and Altman, 2000). The 95% CI represents the range of values in which the true value of the population has a 95% likelihood of falling.

The OR and CI are usually displayed graphically. When the OR point falls to the left of the OR = 1 line, then the treatment is beneficial; and if the 95% CI does not touch the OR = 1 line, the difference is statistically significant. Usually the individual studies are displayed in rows, with the meta-analysis summary statistic in the last row. Sometimes the studies are displayed chronologically in a cumulative meta-analysis, where the treatment effect value and CI are shown cumulatively as each new study is added. This type of display allows investigators to determine when the result has achieved statistical significance. This approach has been used to show that many clinical interventions show statistically significant evidence of benefit long before experts begin to recommend them in textbooks and review articles (Antman, Lau et al., 1992). A *sensitivity analysis* can also be applied to meta-analysis, where the studies are sorted by those of highest quality and as the lower-quality studies are added to the analysis it becomes possible to state whether the aggregate result holds.

These concepts and the value of the meta-analysis are best demonstrated in the logo of the Cochrane Collaboration (see Fig. 2.5), a group devoted to production of systematic reviews of interventions in health care (Volmink, Siegfried et al., 2004).

Fig. 2.5 Logo of the Cochrane
Collaboration showing result of
meta-analysis demonstrating
benefit for use of corticosteroids in
preterm labor (courtesy of the
Cochrane Collaboration)

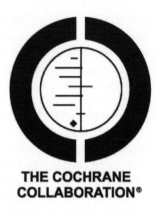

**THE COCHRANE
COLLABORATION®**

Fig. 2.5 Logo of the Cochrane Collaboration showing result of meta-analysis demonstrating benefit for use of corticosteroids in preterm labor (courtesy of the Cochrane Collaboration)

The logo demonstrates a meta-analysis done to assess whether steroids are beneficial to the fetus in premature labor. Of the seven trials identified at the time the logo was created, five showed statistically insignificant benefit (i.e., their CI crossed the OR = 1 line). However, when all seven trials were included in a meta-analysis, the results unequivocally demonstrated benefit, with the CI well to the left of the OR = 1 line. The Cochrane Collaboration has given inspiration to a similar effort in the social sciences, the Campbell Collaboration (http://campbell.gse.upenn.edu/).

Not everyone accepts the value of meta-analysis. Feinstein has called it "statistical alchemy" and warns that relying on it too heavily ignores such other factors in clinical decision-making as physiological reasoning and clinical judgment (Feinstein, 1995; Feinstein and Horwitz, 1997). (Although as is seen in Fig. 1.4, even in the context of EBM, evidence is not the sole criteria for making clinical decisions.) Hopayian (2001) is less critical, but does note that meta-analyses on the same topic do often reach different conclusions, usually because important clinical details are overlooked by those researchers focused purely on methodology. He recommends that they be conducted from the clinical as well as methodological viewpoint.

Even those who perform meta-analyses have noted pitfalls in the approach. As already described, RCTs of lower quality (Moher, Pham et al., 1998) and of smaller size (Kjaergard, Villumsen et al., 2001) tend to show a larger benefit for the treatment studied. In addition, at least 1 of 36 meta-analyses produced different results when non-English-language studies were added to an original English-only analysis (Gregoire, Derderian et al., 1995). One particular challenge in performing meta-analyses is identifying all the appropriate RCTs to include. As will be seen in Chap. 7, the literature-searching process requires assessing many articles to find the few that should be included. A possible source of additional studies beyond conventional database searching is the Internet (Eysenbach, Tuische et al., 2001).

The problem of publication bias described earlier is likely to be amplified in meta-analysis, since the analysis relies on the full spectrum of results for a given research question to be published. One approach to detecting publication bias is through the use of *funnel plots*, which are scatter plots of the treatment effect on the horizontal axis against a measure of the sample size on the vertical axis (Copas and

Shi, 2000). In general, an unbiased meta-analysis should show studies with small sample sizes having more scattered effect sizes than those with larger samples; that is, a funnel plot would appear as a symmetrical inverted funnel. Biased meta-analyses, however, are more likely to show asymmetrical funnel plots. This approach has been shown to explain why subsequent large RCTs contradict meta-analyses (i.e., the new large study added to the meta-analysis shows an asymmetrical funnel plot) and to demonstrate publication bias in meta-analyses (Egger, Smith et al., 1997). Two hypothetical funnel plots are shown in Fig. 2.6. Others have attempted to develop more mathematical approaches to detect publication bias (Iyengar and Greenhouse, 1988; Scargle, 2000), which have been shown to be useful though imperfect (Pham, Platt et al., 2001).

Another limitation of systematic reviews is that some studies may not be published in the journal literature. One analysis found that the exclusion of grey literature from meta-analyses was likely to exaggerate the benefit of interventions (McAuley, Pham et al., 2000), although another found that published trials demon-

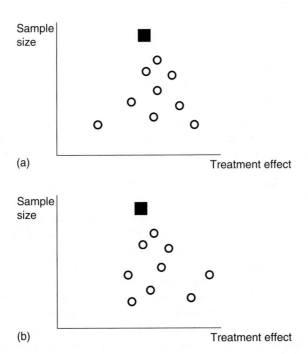

Fig. 2.6 Hypothetical funnel plots showing potentially (**a**) unbiased and (**b**) biased meta-analyses (courtesy of the Cochrane Collaboration)

strated an overall larger treatment effect (Hopewell, McDonald et al., 2003). The latter analysis also found that published trials were likely to be larger and of higher methodological quality. Grey literature most commonly consisted of either abstracts (49%) or unpublished data (33%). In addition, some meta-analyses are reported better than others. Jadad et al. (1998) have found that systematic reviews from the Cochrane Collaboration tend to use better methodologic rigor and are updated more frequently than those published in traditional medical journals.

An additional challenge for meta-analysis is duplicate publication (which is actually a problem beyond meta-analysis), since it results in single individuals being counted more than once, potentially affecting the results of the analysis. How prevalent is the problem of duplicate publication? von Elm et al. (2004) analyzed 141 systematic reviews published in anesthesiology and available on the Internet. Of these reviews, the authors of 56 acknowledged identification of duplicate articles (excluding abstracts, letters, and book chapters), leading them to identify 103 duplicates of 78 articles (60 were published twice and the remainder more than twice). The duplicates were not mere reproductions, but fell into more complex (one might say covert) patterns (number of article pairs in parentheses):

- Study samples identical

  – Outcomes identical – one report (21) or more than one report (16)
  – Outcomes different (24)

- Study samples different
  – Outcomes identical – increasing sample (11) or decreasing sample (11)
  – Outcomes different (20)

All but 5.3% of the papers referenced the earlier duplicates. Two thirds differed in authorship partially or completely. The annual citation rate was about equal for each in the pair. The median appearance of the duplicate was at about 1 year.

An earlier analysis looked at studies assessing the effect of the drug odansetron in postoperative emesis (Tramer, Reynolds et al., 1997). The authors identified a total of 84 RCTs that included 11,980 patients receiving odanseteron published from 1991 to 1996. Data from nine RCTs were published in 14 further reports (17% of trials) representing 3,335 (28%) patients. The overall efficacy of the drug in these trials was positive, but studies that were duplicated tended to show more positive results, with a 23% overestimation of efficacy of the drug.

A final concern of note is that most systematic reviews tend to focus on the "best" evidence, and this approach may be problematic for decision-makers, from policymakers to clinicians and patients, who need to make decisions based on all evidence. Mant (1999) has noted that while RCTs may be the best method for assessing an intervention, it is more difficult to know to whom the results apply, since most trials exclude precisely the patients with complications (i.e., with other comorbid conditions) who will receive the treatment in the real world. As such, Atkins (2007) has called on those who synthesize evidence to develop means to take into account other forms of evidence.

2.5.5 Secondary Literature

Because the primary literature is fragmented, its use is prohibitively difficult, and there is strong impetus to present the information in different formats. Another problem is that in many professional fields, health care included, practitioners apply scientific information but do not necessarily generate it and are therefore less likely to understand the scientific esoterica described by researchers. This is especially so for nonexpert professionals, such as clinicians, who must make decisions that are, however, based on specialized scientific information.

The need for overviews of primary literature is one of the motivations for the secondary literature. This literature consists of review articles (which are often published in the same journals that contain primary literature), books, editorials, practice guidelines, and other forms of publication in which original research information is reviewed. There are other motivations for generating this literature besides clinical use, such as for policy-making and administration.

The secondary literature, in the form of textbooks and review articles, has always been the major source of literature used by clinicians. Some of the review articles occur in the voluminous literature of the "throw-away" journals. These journals often serve as vehicles for pharmaceutical or other advertising, but nonetheless often feature well-written and concise articles on clinically pertinent topics. In fact, one study found that although such publications are of lower methodological quality from a research perspective, they communicate their message better via use of tables, pictures, larger fonts, and easier readability (Rochon, Bero et al., 2002). Of course, these publications are often justly criticized because it is unknown how the vested interests of the advertisers influence the editorial content.

Unfortunately, there are as many problems stemming from poor methodology and writing making it into secondary literature as there are for primary literature. It has also been found, for example, that the rigor of review articles, even in esteemed medical journals, can be lacking. Mulrow (1987) looked for eight criteria (purpose, data identification, data selection, validity assessment, qualitative synthesis, quantitative synthesis, summary, and future directives) in 50 review articles in major medical journals. For the categories of data identification, data selection, validity assessment, and quantitative synthesis, virtually all papers were inadequate. Mulrow argued that review papers were not complete without the details of the literature search as well as a quantitative synthesis such as a meta-analysis. A recent follow-up study, which added the criteria of addressing heterogeneity and addressing generalizability of data, showed that most review articles still were not measuring up (McAlister, Clark et al., 1999). This study found that less than one fourth of the articles assessed described how evidence was identified, evaluated, or integrated. It also noted that articles in journals with higher IF did not meet the criteria any better than those in journals with lower IF did.

The problem of inadequate literature identification in review articles has been further addressed by others. As will be described in more detail in Chap. 7, Dickersin et al. (1994) have found that even exhaustive searching in large literature databases such as MEDLINE does not yield all the studies pertinent to a review. Joyce et al. (1998) found that for 89 review articles on chronic fatigue syndrome, only three (3.4%) described the search strategy. Furthermore, authors from specific fields (in this case laboratory medicine and psychiatry) preferentially cited references from their own disciplines. Likewise, authors had a higher likelihood of citing from their own countries (i.e., the United States and the United Kingdom).

Another limitation of secondary literature is its potential to be incorrect. As noted earlier, Antman et al. (1992) and Balas and Boren (2000) have found that medical textbooks, review articles, and practice recommendations often lag behind the edge of accumulated knowledge. Sometimes secondary references do not provide the most accurate information. For example, Cohen (2001) has found that the *Physicians' Desk Reference* (Medical Economics, http://www.pdr.net/), a venerable information resource for clinicians and their patients, does not contain the full range of dosages for commonly prescribed drugs. Noting that the *Physicians' Desk Reference* contains the information in drug package inserts, he found that lower doses of 48 drugs discovered effective in clinical trials were not included in the recommendations for use.

Another problem in textbooks concerns the promulgation of information not very well investigated in the first place. One area where this has been found to be problematic concerns findings on physical examination in diseases. Richardson and Wilson (2002) have noted, for example, that frequencies of findings in diseases are often not described in popular internal medicine textbooks. A related issue concerns the description of eponymous physical findings, which are commonplace in medical textbooks and which often are used by veteran attending physicians to demonstrate their knowledge. Most of these findings, however, have been less subject to the modern scrutiny of diagnostic test evaluation. Babu et al. (2003) looked at 12 eponymous signs of aortic regurgitation, the condition where the aortic valve does not close completely and allows blood to "leak" back into the heart. This can lead to congestive heart failure and other complications. While these signs are described in major textbooks, the actual evidence supporting them is for the most part minimal. The authors call for physical findings to be evaluated using the more modern techniques of EBM (see Sect. 2.8).

Another type of secondary literature gaining increased interest as efforts to standardize health care evolve consists of clinical practice guidelines. These are, "systematically developed statements to assist practitioners and patient decisions about appropriate health care for specific clinical circumstances" (Field and Lohr, 1990). These guidelines are used as more than just documents for reading, for they also serve to guide documentation and provide decision logic for the provision of medical care (Shiffman, Brandt et al., 1999). As with other literature, guidelines become outdated quickly. A recent analysis, which found that a group of guidelines from AHRQ had a half-life of 5.8 years, recommended that all guidelines be updated at least every 3 years (Shekelle, Ortiz et al., 2001).

One concern with practice guidelines is their sheer number. A study of British general medical practices found that 855 different guidelines had been sent to physicians in 65 different practices, which could be stacked nearly 70-cm tall (Hibble, Kanka et al., 1998). Another concern with guidelines is that clinicians do not use them. Cabana et al. (1999) performed a systematic review assessing the reasons for lack of adherence to guidelines, finding a variety of factors often dependent on the unique characteristics of the locations where they were studied. The major categories of barriers include awareness of guidelines, agreement with them, altered expectations of patient outcomes, inability to overcome the inertia of previous practice, and barriers to carry them out.

Another concern with guidelines is the conflict of interest between those who perform studies for the industry as well and also develop clinical practice guidelines. Henry et al. (2005) found that Australian clinicians who performed research for pharmaceutical companies were more likely to receive gifts and/or obtain support for travel to international conferences. Likewise, Taylor and Giles (2005) found that 35% of 685 authors of guidelines reported a conflict of interest and that half of all guidelines published do not even have any declaration of conflict of interest. Related to this, pharmaceutical sales representatives are trained to downplay the risks of drugs when promoting their use (Waxman, 2005). Researchers may also be bound by gag clauses that limit their ability to publish or report certain adverse events (Steinbrook, 2005). All of these findings have led for leaders in medicine to call for more stringent policies limiting industry support, especially in academic medical centers (Brennan, Rothman et al., 2006).

2.6 Electronic Publishing

In the first edition of this book, IR systems were still viewed as a means to get to paper-based scientific journals. Although it was noted that online full-text journals had been in existence since the 1980s, high cost, low-resolution displays, and bandwidth-limited networks precluded their routine access. In the second edition, we noted that many journals and other resources were increasingly available electronically. With this third edition, we see that electronic publishing, at least for journals, is nearly ubiquitous. Even if not readily available to customers and/or planned for mostly paper-based distribution, most journals and other resources are at least produced electronically and probably available in some fashion through electronic means. This does not mean that anyone can get access at any time, an issue we will explore in greater depth in Chap. 6. In this section, we will raise the major issues for electronic publishing that set the context for the state-of-the-art of IR systems that follow in the ensuing chapters, which then leads into their coverage more deeply when discussing digital libraries.

Another phenomenon of electronic publishing has been the growth of the Web as a means to disseminate not only traditionally published health information but all sorts of other health information. The Web has been used to publish new forms of content not only for health-care professionals but also for their patients. This has given rise to a new concern about the quality of health information on the Web, especially as it related to consumer health information, which will also be discussed in this section.

The ease of replicating, deleting, and altering information on the Web has led the American Association for the Advancement of Science (AAAS) to define a "definitive publication" in science, especially in the context of the electronic environment (Frankel, Elliot et al., 2000). Such a publication should be peer-reviewed; the following statements apply as well:

- The publication must be publicly available.
- The relevant community must be made aware of its existence.
- A system for long-term access and retrieval must be in place.
- The publication must not be changed (technical protection and/or certification are desirable).
- It must not be removed (unless legally unavoidable).
- It must be unambiguously identified (e.g., by some sort of identifier).
- It must have a bibliographic record (metadata) containing certain minimal information.
- There must be a plan for archiving and long-term preservation.

2.6.1   Electronic Scholarly Publication

As noted above, electronic publishing of scientific journals and other publications is nearly ubiquitous. In addition to available content, the Internet and Web environment make possible all kinds of new capabilities, such as the ability to link directly to the full text of an article from its bibliographic record, and the linkage of sources that cite or make use of content in the resource. Another change is that journals can alter the form and quantity of what they publish, since editorial space, always at a premium in paper journals, is less constrained in electronic environments.

Some journals, most notably BMJ, have adopted an electronic-long/paper-short approach (Delamothe, Mullner et al., 1999). This provides the more casual reader with a shorter version of the paper, while researchers or others wanting more detail can read the long one. A sample of authors and readers were given three versions of articles to assess for their formatting preference: conventional scientific version, enhanced-abstract version, and journalistic version (Mullner, Waechter et al., 2005). The latter was essentially a narrative of the article that described why the research was done, how it was carried out, and what the results showed. Authors expressed a strong preference for conventional version (56%), followed by the journalistic version (34%) and the enhanced-abstract version (27%) (all differences statistically significant). Although readers still preferred the conventional version (42%), they did so with less strength (though still statistically significant), and they were nearly equally divided between the journalistic version (28%) and the enhanced-abstract version.

This new electronic environment may offer wonders to users, but it is not without new issues and challenges. In particular, the technical challenges to electronic scholarly publication have been replaced by economic and political ones

(Hersh and Rindfleisch, 2000; Anonymous, 2001c). Printing and mailing, tasks no longer needed in electronic publishing, comprised a significant part of the "added value" from publishers of journals. Since the intellectual portion of the peer-review process is carried out by scientists, the role of the publisher can be reduced or perhaps eliminated with electronic submission of manuscripts and their electronic distribution to peer reviewers. There is, however, still some value added by publishers, such as copyediting and production. Even if publishing companies as they are known were to vanish, there would still be some cost to the production of journals. Thus, although the cost of producing journals electronically is likely to be less, it is not zero, and even if journal content is distributed "free," someone has to pay the production costs.

The ease of distribution on the Web has given rise to a new publishing model called *open access* (Albert, 2006; MacCallum, 2007b). This model is sometimes called "author pays" based on the notion that publishing should be a cost incurred in research, which is usually funded by grants or contracts. In open-access publishing, after the article is accepted and the publishing cost paid, the article is then made freely available on the Web. We will describe the economics and related issues of publishing, including open access, in more detail in Chap. 6.

2.6.2   Consumer Health Information

Another phenomenon of the Internet and Web is the ability of nonprofessionals to seek and access information written not only for professionals but also for "lay" audiences. Indeed, as was noted in the last chapter, over 80% of Web users have searched for personal health information (Fox, 2006). As with electronic scholarly publication, this has led to new opportunities as well as challenges, the most serious of the latter being concern about the quality of information, i.e., whether it is correct or may mislead people, not only imperiling their health but also costing them money.

The Web is inherently democratic, allowing virtually anyone to post information. This is no doubt an asset in a democratic society such as the USA. However, it is potentially at odds with the operation of a professional field, particularly one such as health care, where practitioners are ethically bound and legally required to adhere to the highest standard of care. To the extent that misleading or incorrect information is posted on the Web, this standard is challenged.

A major concern with health information on the Web is the presence of inaccurate or out-of-date information. A systematic review of studies assessing the quality of health information through 2001 found that 55 of 79 studies concluded that quality of information was a problem (Eysenbach, Powell et al., 2002). In many of these studies, the sites evaluated were from academic medical centers or other prestigious medical institutions. Since academic sites are usually managed in a decentralized manner (i.e., individual departments and often individual faculty maintain their own pages), one cannot assume that quality-checking persists down to each department and faculty member with a Web page as it does on highly controlled corporate Web sites.

More recent studies show that this continues to be an issue. A study by Consumers International (Anonymous, 2002b) evaluated more than 460 sites for factors related to their credibility. Quoting from their results:

- 49% of health and financial sites failed to give warnings about the appropriate use of their information. For example, they did not warn consumers searching for health or financial advice that they should consult a professional before acting on advice given.
- At least 50% of sites giving advice on medical and financial matters failed to provide full information about the authority and credentials of the people behind that advice.
- Only 57% of general advice sites gave sources for that advice.
- 39% of sites that collected personal information did not have a privacy policy.
- 62% of sites contained claims that were vague and unspecific.
- 55% of sites said nothing about how up-to-date their content was.
- 30% of sites provided no address or telephone number.
- Only 41% of the sites that recommended products gave sources for their prices.
- 26% of sites gave no clear information about who owned them.
- 60% of sites provided no information that indicated whether or not their content was influenced by commercial interests (e.g., partners, sponsors, or advertisers).

Walji et al. (2004) assessed 150 sites for information related to three complementary and alternative medicine treatments: ginseng, gingko, and St. John's Wort. They found that one quarter of the sites contained statements that could lead to physical harm. Almost all sites had omitted information about potential harm of the treatments. There was no association between common measures of technical quality and potentially harmful information.

Another concern about health information Web sites is readability. It has been found that most patients (Overland, Hoskins et al., 1993; Foltz and Sullivan, 1996; Williams, Counselman et al., 1996) and parents of child patients (Murphy, 1994) read at an average of a fifth to sixth grade level. Reading ability also declines with age (Gazmararian, Baker et al., 1999). Those who deliver consumer health information must therefore take readability into account. The standard measure of assessing readability is the Flesch-Kinkaid score (Flesch, 1948). This measure calculates reading grade level (RGL) based on average sentence length (ASL, the number of words divided by the number of sentences) and average number of syllables per word (ASW, the number of syllables divided by the number of words):

$$RGL = (0.39 \times ASL) + (11.8 \times ASW) - 15.59 \tag{2.6}$$

Graber et al. (1999) found that a sample of patient education material from the Web was written at a tenth-grade level. O'Mahony (1999) reviewed a sample of Web sites in Ireland and also found that the average reading level was about tenth grade. Berland et al. (2001), who used the Fry Readability Graph (Fry, 1977), which is also validated in Spanish, determined that no English-language site they evaluated had readability below the tenth grade level, while over half were written at a college level and 11% at a graduate school level. Over 86% of Spanish sites were also written at the high school level or above.

Eysenbach and Diepgen (1998) note that the problem of poor-quality and hard-to-read information on the Web is exacerbated by a "context deficit" that makes poor-quality information more difficult to distinguish. These authors note that there are fewer less clear "markers" of the type of document (e.g., professional textbook vs. patient handout) and that the reader of a specific page may not be aware of the "context" of a Web site that includes disclaimers, warnings, and so forth. Furthermore, information may be correct in one context but incorrect in another, and this difference may not be detectable on a random page within a Web site (e.g. the differences in treatment in children vs. adults or across different ethnic groups).

New information resources raise new issues. One such resource is Wikipedia, a mass collaborative attempt to build a distributed online encyclopedia http://www.wikipedia.org/). One person has quipped, "If you don't like the facts in Wikipedia, you can change them" (source unknown), while another laments it is a "faith-based encyclopedia" (McHenry, 2004). However, research shows that Wikipedia is no less inaccurate that other comparable encyclopedias. The journal *Nature* compared 42 topics in Wikipedia and *Encyclopedia Britannica*, removing the text to obfuscate its source and sending it to experts in the respective fields (Giles, 2005; Anonymous, 2006f). A total of eight serious errors were found, four with each topic. However, there were more "factual errors, omissions, or misleading statements" in *Encyclopedia Britannica* (162) than in Wikipedia (123). Not surprisingly, *Encyclopedia Britannica* took great exception to the study, calling it "fatally flawed" (Anonymous, 2006c). *Nature* apparently has confidence in Wikipedia, because it uses the online encyclopedia, as many do, for definitions to words that appear on its Web site (Blackman, 2006). Another study showed that although Wikipedia was not comprehensive for four medical topics, the information present was highly accurate and comparable to another commercial consumer health product (Nicholson, 2006).

Another new and growing source of content on the Web is video, immensely popularized by the site YouTube. One recent analysis identified 153 videos covering immunizations (Keelan, Pavri-Garcia et al., 2007), a topic of much information of questionable validity on the textual Web (Chatterjee, 2003). The study on videos on the topic found that one half contradicted known scientific consensus on immunizations.

The impact of this poor-quality information is unclear. One systematic review of whether harm has resulted from information obtained on the Internet found 15 case reports (Crocco, Villasis-Keever et al., 2002). The review noted that larger studies of whether Internet information has caused general harm to patients have not been done. A dissenting view has been provided by Ferguson (2002), who argues that patients and consumers actually are savvy enough to understand the limits of quality of information on the Web and that they should be trusted to discern quality using their own abilities to consult different sources of information and communicate with health-care practitioners and others who share their condition(s). Indeed, the ideal situation may be a partnership among patients and their health-care practitioners, as it has been shown that patients desire that their practitioners be the primary source of recommendations for online information (Tang, Newcomb et al., 1997).

This lack of quality information has led a number of individuals and organizations to develop guidelines for assessing the quality of health information. These guidelines usually have explicit criteria for a Web page that a reader can apply to determine whether a potential source of information has attributes consistent with high quality. One of the earliest and most widely quoted set of criteria was published in JAMA (Silberg, Lundberg et al., 1997). These criteria stated that Web pages should contain the following:

- The name, affiliation, and credentials of the author – readers may differ on the value of an individual's credentials, but the information should be listed to be assessed by all.
- References to the claims made – if health claims are made, they should contain references to legitimate scientific research documenting the claim.
- Explicit listing of any perceived or real conflict of interest – a conflict of interest does not disqualify someone from posting information, but all perceived or real conflict of interests must be disclosed, as is required of those who teach continuing education courses.
- Date of most recent update – even though the Web is relatively new, health information becomes outdated quickly, and the date on which a page was most recently updated should be listed.

Another early set of criteria was the Health on the Net (HON) codes (http://www.hon.ch/), a set of voluntary codes of conduct for health-related Web sites. Sites that adhere to the HON codes can display the HON logo. These codes state the following:

1. Any medical or health advice provided and hosted on this site will only be given by medically or health trained and qualified professionals unless a clear statement is made that a piece of advice offered is from a nonmedically or health qualified individual or organization.
2. The information provided on this site is designed to support, not replace, the relationship that exists between a patient or site visitor and his or her existing physician.
3. Confidentiality of data relating to individual patients and visitors to a medical or health Web site, including their identity, is respected by this Web site. The Web site owners undertake to honor or exceed the legal requirements of medical or health information privacy that apply in the country and state where the Web site and mirror sites are located.
4. Where appropriate, information contained on this site will be supported by clear references to source data and, where possible, will have specific HTML links to these data. The date when a clinical page was last modified will be clearly displayed (e.g., at the bottom of the page).
5. Any claims relating to the benefits or performance of a specific treatment, commercial product, or service will be supported by appropriate, balanced evidence in the manner outlined here in Principle 4.

6. The designers of this Web site will seek to provide information in the clearest possible manner and provide contact addresses for visitors who seek further information or support. The Webmaster will display his or her e-mail address clearly throughout the Web site.
7. Support for this Web site will be clearly identified, including the identities of commercial and noncommercial organizations that have contributed funding, services, or material for the site.
8. If advertising is a source of funding it will be clearly stated. A brief description of the advertising policy adopted by the Web site owners will be displayed on the site. Advertising and other promotional material will be presented to viewers in a manner and context that facilitates differentiation between it and the original material created by the institution operating the site.

A number of other criteria for Web page quality have been put forth, often associated with checklists or other instruments that can be used to rate actual sites and their pages. These were reviewed by Kim et al. (1999), who found that there was fairly high agreement on the different criteria. These authors determined that most of the criteria could be grouped under 12 specific categories dealing with site content, design, disclosure, currency, authority, ease of use, accessibility, links, attribution, intended audience, contact or feedback, and user support.

In another review of quality criteria instruments, Gagliardi and Jadad (2002) took a less favorable view. These authors noted that most individual instruments were incomplete or inconsistent. They also pointed out that few such instruments have been validated. A case in point comes from the study on the quality of information concerning childhood cough described earlier (Pandolfini, Impiccatore et al., 2000); this study found no relationship between adherence to common indicators of quality and the amount of correct or incorrect information on a page.

More recently, Bernstam et al. (2005) identified 273 distinct tools purporting to help consumers assess the quality of health information on the Web, yet only seven met the usability criteria of having evaluation criteria publicly available, having ten or few items, and having elements that could be objectively evaluated. In another study, Bernstam et al. (2005) found that a set of 22 of these measures, when used in their original form, led to widely divergent reviews. However, when they were more precisely defined, 18 could be assigned reliably by medical experts.

Do Web sites actually adhere to quality standards? A study by Hersh et al. (1998) attempted to look at pages retrieved by a medical librarian attempting to answer questions generated in the course of clinical practice. They found that only 30% had a listed author, 12% had sources for claims made, and 18% showed the date of most recent update. Virtually no sites indicated any conflict of interest, regardless of whether one was present or not. Shon and Musen (1999) found a similar low rate of quality indicators on pages about breast cancer. The systematic review of Eysenbach et al. (2002) found similar rates of not having author names on pages, not providing references for claims made, not showing date of most recent update, and not indicating the presence or absence of conflict of interest.

Might it be possible for Web "robots" to automatically detect these criteria? Price and Hersh (1999) have looked into this possibility. While the results were too preliminary to be definitive, early indications were that some of these criteria can be detected and the output from a search can be reordered to give more prominent ranking of higher quality pages. One observation from the small data set used to evaluate the system was that the quality criteria listed earlier may not truly be associated with the actual quality of pages. These investigators noted, for example, that the low-quality pages were more easily identifiable from their exclamation points and "1–800" telephone prefixes to call to order products. A larger and more recent application of this approach found that a number of quality indicators could be detected with high accuracy (Wang and Liu, 2007).

Fallis and Fricke (2002) investigated the predictive nature of Web page attributes more comprehensively, aiming to ascertain which ones might be associated with quality. They assessed pages providing advice on treating childhood fever at home, an area in which wide consensus exists among experts. Pages were rated for accuracy by two independent observers. Those above the median accuracy scores were deemed "more accurate" and those below were deemed "less accurate." The authors found the following indicators to be most predictive of more accurate pages: organizational domain (i.e., a.*org* domain as opposed to a.*com* or.*edu* domain), display of the HON code logo, and claim of copyright.

Among the indicators not predictive of quality were those related to the criteria of Silberg et al. (1997), such as listing of authorship, currency, or references. Other nonpredictive indicators were the presence of spelling errors, exclamation points, advertising, and a high number of in-links to the page. A similar study by Kunst et al. (2002) similarly showed that source, currency, and evidence hierarchy had only moderate correlation with accuracy of information for five common health topics on well-known health-related Web sites. These authors concluded that apparently credible Web sites may not provide more accurate health information. Of course, one downside to publishing data such as these and using them to judge quality of output algorithmically is that those who seek to deceive may be motivated to "game" the system to make their pages to appear to be of higher quality.

Of course, misleading and inaccurate health information is not limited to consumer Web sites. Even resources one might normally consider to be of high repute have been found to have misinformation. Biermann et al. (1999), for example, found inaccurate information on the *Encyclopedia Britannica* Web site (http://www.britannica.com/). As noted earlier, even the *Physicians' Desk Reference* has been found to have incomplete information on drug dosages (Cohen, 2001).

Another source of sometimes inaccurate information is the news media, whose objective can often be to create sensational news stories and/or maintain the attention of their audience rather than go into the nuances of complex health-related information. Shuchman and Wilkes (1997) assessed the problems of health news reporting in the general press, noting four problem areas:

1. Sensationalism – there are a variety of reasons for sensationalism, from the desire of media executives to sell newspapers or increase television viewing to

the efforts of scientists or their institutions to garner publicity for prestige or funding, or both.

2. Biases and conflicts of interest – reporters may be misled by incomplete presentation of information or undisclosed conflict of interest by scientists, institutions, or the pharmaceutical industry.

3. Lack of follow-up – the press often has a short attention span and does not continue its coverage on stories that are initially sensationalized.

4. Stories that are not covered – health-related stories compete with other stories for coverage in the press. There are also instances of scientists who have, sometimes unwittingly, signed agreements forbidding publication of research not approved by the sponsor. One well-known case involved a study showing that generic versions of a thyroid medication were comparable to a brand-name drug (Rennie, 1997).

Other data support these observations. One particular problem is news media reporting of findings, usually preliminary, presented at scientific research meetings. Schwartz et al. (2002) found that of 149 such presentations receiving substantial attention in the news media, 76% were nonrandomized, 25% had fewer than 30 subjects, and 15% were nonhuman studies. Furthermore, half were not subsequently published in MEDLINE-indexed journals. A related concern is lack of news media coverage of retraction of studies. In one analysis of 50 retractions identified in the MEDLINE database, only three were reported in newspaper articles (Rada, 2007). This led Schwartz and Woloshin (2004) to recommend the following principles to journalists:

- In general, do not report preliminary findings.
- Communicate absolute (not relative) magnitudes of differences.
- Include caveats, i.e., limitations of studies.

They also advocated that the medical community also act responsibly by stopping courting of coverage of preliminary work and writing press releases to communicate the science and not generate press coverage. The latter should apply to biomedical journals, who also jockey for coverage in the general media.

What can be done to guide individuals to be good consumers of health information? The Federal Trade Commission has provided a set of guidelines to detect "virtual" treatments with a higher likelihood of being unproven (Anonymous, 2001e). Such content is likely to contain the following:

- Phrases like "scientific breakthrough," "miraculous cure," "exclusive product," "secret formula," and "ancient ingredient."
- Use of "medicalese" – impressive-sounding terminology to disguise a lack of good science.
- Case histories from "cured" consumers claiming amazing results. Such testimonials also imply that the experience recounted is typical for all consumers using the product or service. A Web page visitor who sees such a testimonial is well advised to ask for proof that the term "typical" has been properly used.
- A laundry list of symptoms the product cures or treats.

- The latest trendy ingredient touted in the headlines.
- A claim that the product is available from only one source, for a limited time.
- Testimonials from "famous" medical experts.
- A claim that the government, the medical profession, or research scientists have conspired to suppress the product.

When the information is less flagrantly invalid, the options are less clear. One might surmise that the prestige of the institution could be an indicator of quality. This is unfortunately not the case: several of the studies documenting incorrect information found some of their poor-quality information on the sites of prestigious medical institutions or highly reputable publishers.

Could governments play a role in regulating the quality of health information? Most believe that their role is likely to be limited. Hodge et al. (1999), for example, note that although the Federal Trade Commission has a mandate to regulate false or deceptive commercial information and the FDA is charged with regulating information about drugs and medical products, neither is likely to be able to comprehensively monitor all commercial health information on the Internet. And of course, an increasing fraction of that information is likely to arise outside the country, where US governmental entities have no jurisdiction at all. These authors conclude that self-regulation and education are likely to be the best approach. Such regulation may take the form of principles such as those maintained by the American Medical Association for its Web site (Winker, Flanagin et al., 2000). These guidelines cover not only issues related to quality, but also advertising, sponsorship, privacy, and electronic commerce.

One approach that has been advocated to ensure Web site quality may be approval or accreditation by a third party. One site with a well-documented ratings process is HealthRatings.org (http://www.healthratings.org/), which is a project of Consumer Reports and the Health Improvement Institute and for which a description of its methodology (Anonymous, 2007a) and the instrument used (Anonymous, 2007k) are available. A program for accreditation of Web sites is administrated by the American Accreditation HealthCare Commission (called URAC; http://www.urac.org/programs/prog_accred_HWS_po.aspx). This program requires 49 standards in eight categories to attain accreditation (Anonymous, 2007j). Uptake of the process, however, has been modest, with about two dozen sites accredited.

2.7   Use of Knowledge-Based Health Information

Information sources, print or computer, are approached for two reasons: the need to locate a particular item of information, such as a document or book, or the need to obtain information on a particular subject. Lancaster and Warner (1993) have defined *subject needs*, which may in modern parlance be called *use cases* (Cockburn, 2001) and fall into three categories:

- The need for help in solving a certain problem or making a decision
- The need for background information on a topic
- The need to keep up with information in a given subject area

The first two subject needs are called retrospective information needs, in that documents already published are sought, while the latter need is called a current awareness need, which is met by filtering new documents to identify those on a certain topic. Retrospective needs may also be classified by the amount of information needed (Lancaster and Warner, 1993):

- A single fact.
- One or more documents but less than the entire literature on the topic.
- A comprehensive search of the literature.
- It will be seen later that the interaction with an information system varies based on these different needs.

Wilkinson and Fuller (1996) describe four types of information needs for document collections:

- Fact-finding – locating a specific item of information
- Learning – developing an understanding of a topic
- Gathering – finding material relevant to a new problem not explicitly stated
- Exploring – browsing material with a partially specified information need that can be modified as the content is viewed

Another perspective on the use of information classifies the kinds of information needs characteristic of users of health information. Gorman (1995) defines four states of information need:

- Unrecognized need – clinician aware of information need or knowledge deficit
- Recognized need – clinician aware of need but may or may not pursue it
- Pursued need – information-seeking occurs but may or may not be successful
- Satisfied need – information-seeking successful

This section focuses on the information needs and uses of health-care practitioners and biomedical researchers. An overview of information-seeking in general has been published by Case (2006). This discussion begins with an overview of models of physician-thinking, followed by descriptions of what information they need and the sources they actually use, as well as comments on the usage of information by nurses, other health-care practitioners and biomedical researchers.

2.7.1 Models of Physician Thinking

Most work assessing the mental process of health care has focused on physicians. The traditional view of physician thinking is based upon the *hypotheticodeductive model* (Elstein, Shulman et al., 1978). In this model, the physician begins forming hypotheses based upon the initial information obtained, usually the patient's chief complaint. The skilled physician already begins to focus on data-driven hypotheses, which subsequently lead to hypothesis-driven selection of the next data to be collected. The process is iterated until one or more diagnoses can account for all the observations (or at least the observations deemed necessary to explain).

An alternative model, which is not necessarily at odds with the hypotheticode-ductive view, has been proposed by Schmidt et al. (1990). These authors note that one implication of the hypotheticodeductive model is that diagnostic failures arise from taking shortcuts or giving insufficient attention to details. However, they have observed that experienced clinicians actually gather smaller amounts of data and are able to arrive at correct diagnoses with fewer hypotheses.

Schmidt et al. theorize that medical knowledge is contained in "illness scripts," which are based not only on learned medical knowledge, but also past (and especially recent) experience. These scripts are based on causal networks that represent objects and their relationships in the world. These networks tell physi-cians, for example, that fluid in the lungs causes shortness of breath and that one of the causes of fluid in the lungs is heart failure. Medical education consists of building these causal networks in the mind. As the student progresses through medical education and attains clinical experience, the networks become compiled into higher level, simplified models that explain patient signs and symptoms under diagnostic labels.

There is considerable evidence for this model. First, the hypotheticodeductive model might imply that those with the best problem-solving skills should consis-tently be the best diagnosticians. Yet studies in which physicians and medical students were given patient management problems, which simulate the clinical setting, find that there is wide variation in performance on different problems by the same practitioners (Elstein, Shulman et al., 1978). Additional supporting evidence is that experienced physicians are much better able than students to recall details of patient encounters when the findings are randomly reordered (Schmidt, Norman et al., 1990). This is because more experienced practitioners attach specific patients to instances of the scripts. Another finding in support of this model is from Patel et al. (1989), who noted that experienced physicians tend to make minimal use of basic science in their diagnostic efforts; rather, they match patients to patterns of clinical presentations for various diseases. This is consistent with advanced training leading to building high-level scripts based on clinical findings.

Florance (1992) also looked at aspects of clinical decision-making and noted that it involves both declarative knowledge (i.e., facts) and procedural knowledge (i.e., how to apply those facts). She noted that the latter tends to be more useful for diagnosis, while the former is usually more beneficial for therapy. Since there tends to be more declarative knowledge in the literature, she calls for more procedural knowledge to be added to the literature. Of course computer applications, such as decision support systems, may be able to fill this void.

Some researchers express concern that clinicians rely too much on personal knowledge and experience and not enough on aggregated experience and/or pub-lished literature. Sox et al. (1988) note an *availability heuristic*, where clinicians inflate the diagnostic probability of a disease based on recent or otherwise well-remembered cases. Tanenbaum (1994) carried out an ethnographic study of physicians being exposed to outcomes and research data, finding that they often continued to rely on personal experience despite contrary data from outcomes research or the medical literature. Some medical editors have lamented that the journal literature is underused (Huth, 1989; Kassirer, 1992), yet others point out that this resource is too fragmented and time-consuming to use (Shaughnessy, Slawson et al., 1994; Hersh, 1999). McDonald (1996) has noted that there is often not enough evidence to inform clinical decisions and that clinicians rely on heuristics to guide their decision-making, advocating that such heuristics be improved when the robustness of evidence is sparse.

2.7.2   Physician Information Needs

As noted by Gorman (1995), physicians may have information needs that they do not immediately recognize. Some of these needs may become recognized, pursued, or satisfied. Understanding these needs is important to building health-care IR systems. Dawes and Sampson (2003) have done a systematic review summarizing the research in this area that we will describe in the coming sections.

2.7.2.1   Unrecognized needs

One of the difficulties in characterizing unrecognized information needs derives from the physicians' lack of direct awareness of their existence. As such, these needs can be identified only indirectly through the measurement of knowledge dissemination, knowledge stores, and outcomes of clinical practice that reflect application of knowledge.

Several older studies have demonstrated that medical knowledge is disseminated only slowly to the practitioner. Stross and Harlan (1979) looked at the dissemination of information on the use of photocoagulation in diabetic retinopathy, an important advance against the blindness that can complicate diabetes. Over 2 years after initial publication of the benefit of this therapy, less than half of primary care physicians were aware of the results. A similar finding was reported when physicians were asked about their knowledge of the Hypertension Detection and Follow-Up Study, which demonstrated the benefit of antihypertensive therapy: only half the physicians queried were aware of the findings 2–6 months after publication (Stross and Harlan, 1981). Williamson et al. (1989) performed a similar study, looking at six important then-recent medical advances and finding that anywhere from 20 to 50% of physicians were unaware of them. It is likely that the general increase of mass media coverage to medical topics has increased the dissemination of medical advances, especially in the Internet age, but no recent studies have ascertained quantitatively whether this is the case.

Another line of evidence demonstrating lack of information comes from physicians who take recertification examinations. The scores of family practitioners, who are required to recertify every 6 years, tend to decline with each recertification examination (Leigh, Young et al., 1993). Likewise, when internists with various levels of experience were given an 81-question subset of the American Board of Internal Medicine examination, a direct correlation was found between score and years out of residency training (Ramsey, Carline et al., 1991). Both of these studies were limited in two ways. First, it is unknown how examinations of these types correlate with practice skill. It has already been seen that experience is an important variable in addition to knowledge for physicians (recall the model of Schmidt, Norman et al. 1990). Second, physicians do use during their practice information resources that were not available during the test-taking situations. Thus some physicians who perform poorly at regurgitating knowledge might be quite effective at finding the required information and applying it.

Does this lack of information have a significant impact on patient care? This is a complex question, which is difficult to answer owing to the many variables present in a clinical encounter. There is evidence, however, that clinicians could be making better decisions. A report by the President's Advisory Commission on Consumer Protection and Quality in the Health Care Industry noted that significant problems in health care include medical error, overuse of services, underuse of services, and unexplained variation in use of services (Anonymous, 1998). A widely cited report by the Institute of Medicine has noted that twenty-first century health care must be quality-focused, patient-centered, and evidence-based (Anonymous, 2001b). Specific studies have shown, for example, that the antibiotics continue to be prescribed inappropriately 25–50% of the time, according to infectious disease experts (Kunin, Tupasi et al., 1973; Bernstein, Barriere et al., 1982; Gonzales, Bartlett et al., 2001). Likewise, adherence to published practice guidelines continues to be low: only 45–84% of recommended routine screening examinations are performed for diabetic patients (Weiner, Parente et al., 1995) and only one quarter of elderly patients are treated for hypertension in a way consistent with guidelines (Knight, Glynn et al., 2000). Similar lack of use of proven effective therapies for acute myocardial infarction has been demonstrated as well (Ellerbeck, Jencks et al., 1995). Of course the problems concerning the quality of health care, patient safety, and medical errors go well beyond access to IR systems, though the use of such systems will play a solution.

2.7.2.2 Recognized Needs

Physicians and other health-care practitioners do recognize they have unmet information needs. A number of studies described in this section have attempted to gain insight into the quantity and nature of questions asked in clinical practice. Many investigators have attempted to measure such needs, although their results differ as a result of variations in practice settings, types of physician studied, and how information need itself was defined (Gorman, 1995). Even though the results are not entirely consistent, they do reveal that physicians have significant unmet information needs.

The first study of this type, performed by Covell et al. (1985), found that although physicians thought they had an unmet information need for about 1 of every 77 patients, they actually had an average of two unmet needs for every three patients (0.62 unanswered questions per patient). Using a similar methodology with different physicians, Gorman and Helfand (1995) found a nearly identical frequency (0.60 per patient) of unmet information needs. The former study assessed urban internists and specialists in Los Angeles, while the latter focused on urban and rural primary care physicians in Oregon.

Other studies using different methodologies have obtained varying results, though they all demonstrate that physicians have significant unmet information needs in practice. Timpka and Arborelius (1990) studied "dilemmas" in a simulated environment with general practitioners in Sweden. While the most common dilemma type was social and organizational, there was an average of 1.84 medical knowledge dilemmas per patient. Osheroff et al. (1991), who used ethnographic techniques to assess information needs in teaching hospital rounds, found an average of 1.4 questions per patient (excluding those asked in the course of teaching). Dee and Blazek (1993) measured unmet needs in after hours interviews and found an average of 0.33 questions per patient. Ely et al. (1999) observed family physicians in Iowa, who were found to have 0.32 questions per patient.

Most of the foregoing studies attempted to identify the nature of the information needs observed. All found that they were highly specific to patient problems. Ely et al. (1999) developed a taxonomy of generic questions, finding 69 different types, the top 10 of which are listed in Table 2.3. This table also gives the percentage of

Table 2.3 Questions most commonly asked, pursued, and answered by physicians

Generic question	How many asked? (%)	How many asked were pursued? (%)	How many pursued were answered? (%)
What is the cause of symptom X?	9	9	50
What is the dose of drug X?	8	85	97
How should I manage disease or finding X?	7	29	83
How should I treat finding or disease X?	7	33	72
What is the cause of physical finding X?	7	18	46
What is the cause of test finding X?	4	40	72
Could this patient have disease or condition X?	4	14	67
Is test X indicated in situation Y?	4	29	83
What is the drug of choice for condition X?	3	47	76
Is drug X indicated in situation Y?	3	25	78

Adapted from Ely, Osheroff et al. (1999)

asked questions that were pursued as well as pursued questions that were answered, showing in general that treatment questions were more likely to be pursued and answered than diagnostic ones. This taxonomy was refined and validated with questions from Oregon primary care practitioners, and question types were found to be assignable with moderate reliability ($\kappa = 0.53$) (Ely, Osheroff et al., 2000).

Another study of questions generated in practices comes from New Zealand, where a group of 50 family physicians was observed (Arroll, Pandit et al., 2002). These physicians generated questions at a slightly lower rate than found by Covell et al. (1985), Gorman and Helfand (1995) and Ely et al. (1999) with an average of one question for every 3.4 patients. The types of questions and their proportions were comparable to the other studies.

Bryant (2004) recently published a quantitative and qualitative analysis of information needs of family physicians in one region of the United Kingdom. The most commonly perceived information needs were for clinical care, keeping up to date, and providing information for patients. The most commonly used resource was the physician's personal collection, followed by electronic resources. Medical library use was found to be small and declining. Physicians in practices that had medical trainees were somewhat more likely to use electronic resources as well as the library.

2.7.2.3   Pursued needs

One consistent finding in the studies on unmet information needs was that physicians decided against pursuing answers for a majority of the questions. Covell et al. (1985), Gorman and Helfand (1995), and Ely et al. (1999) found that answers were pursued only 30–36% of the time, indicating that 64–70% of information needs remained unmet. These studies also consistently found that when information was pursued, the most common sources were other humans, followed closely by textbooks and drug compendia. Use of journal articles as well as computer sources was low.

Gorman and Helfand (1995) attempted to define those factors that were most likely to be associated with the decision to pursue an answer to a question. They defined 11 attributes of clinical questions and used multiple logistic regression in an attempt to identify those most likely to correlate with an answer being sought, as shown in Table 2.4. The most likely factors to cause answer-seeking were as follows: the question required an urgent answer, it was likely to be answerable, and it would help manage other patients besides the one who had generated the question. The potential for a question to benefit a physician's general knowledge or to reduce his or her liability risk was not associated with pursuit of an answer.

Covell et al. (1985), who also attempted to identify the impediments to answer-seeking, found that physicians either were too busy or did not have immediate access to an answer. Another significant impediment to information-seeking was the disarray of the typical practitioner's library, consisting of out-of-date textbooks and inadequately indexed journal collections.

Table 2.4 Factors influencing a physician's decision to seek an answer to a question

Factors most associated with pursuit of an answer
Urgency – the question had to be answered soon
Answerability – the physician felt an answer was likely to exist
Generalizability – an answer would help manage other patients
Factors not associated with answer-seeking
Knowledge – how much was previously known about the problem?
Uneasiness – how uneasy did the physician feel about the problem?
Potential help – an answer could help the patient
Potential harm – not having an answer could hurt the patient
Edification – an answer would benefit the practitioner's general knowledge
Liability – the problem involved liability risk
Knowledge of peers – peers of the practitioner know the answer
Difficulty – how difficult would it be to find the answer?

Adapted from Gorman and Helfand (1995)

A number of survey studies have attempted to delineate the information resources used by physicians more precisely. One limitation in all these studies is that the information milieu has changed substantially in recent years. Indeed, as noted in the survey of physician computer use by the American Medical Association described in Chap. 1, the number of physicians using the Internet nearly doubled between 1999 and 2000 (Anonymous, 2001a). As such, the use of knowledge resource by physicians has likely changed substantially since many of the studies described throughout this section were performed. Nonetheless, some insight can be gained from looking at the resources used, which indicate the types of information physicians are wishing to pursue.

Ely et al. (1999) looked at information resources available in the offices of 103 family physicians. Among the resources owned were books (100%), reprint files (68%), posted (i.e., on wall or door) information (76%), computers (26% in the office but 45% having one at home), and "peripheral brains" (i.e., personal notebooks of clinical information) (29%). All physicians owned a drug-prescribing reference and all but one owned a general medical textbook. Other books likely to be owned covered adult infectious disease (89%), general pediatrics (83%), orthopedics (82%), dermatology (79%), and adult cardiology (77%).

The Arroll et al. (2002) study described earlier had a finding similar to that of other studies in that computers were infrequently used to pursue answers. Only 5% of questions were answered using a computer. One difference from earlier studies was that 78% of these physicians had computers in their offices, and most could access well-known clinical information resources. Thus, even though computer-based information resources were available in these physicians' offices, their use was still modest.

Ely and colleagues (2002) have also assessed obstacles to obtaining answers to clinical questions. They identified a total of 59 obstacles to accessing information. These were organized into five steps in asking and answering questions: recognizing a gap in knowledge, formulating a question, searching for relevant information, formulating an answer, and using the answer to direct patient care. They noted six obstacles that were particularly prominent to themselves and the clinicians they observed, quoted as follows:

- The excessive time required to find information
- Difficulty modifying the original question, which could be vague and open to interpretation
- Difficulty selecting an optimal strategy to search for information
- Failure of a seemingly appropriate resource to cover the topic
- Uncertainty about how to know when all the relevant evidence has been found so that the search can stop
- Inadequate synthesis of multiple bits of evidence into a clinically useful statement

Ely et al. (2005) recently continued their work assessing barriers to information for physicians. They followed 48 primary care physicians from small towns in Iowa, prompting them for information needs after they saw each patient during a half day. They later interviewed these physicians to ask them what recommendations they would have to improve knowledge resources. The 48 physicians generated 1,062 questions, an average of 5.5 per half day. Of these questions, 441 arose during the observation period (with the remainder arising before then). Of the 1,062 questions, 55% were pursued. Of those pursued, 41% were answered without difficulty, 31% were answered with difficulty, and 28% were not answered. The most common categories of resources used to answer questions were as follows:

- Single textbook – 31%
- Another human (informal consultation) – 18%
- Desktop computer application – 12%
- Multiple textbooks – 8%
- Human plus textbook – 6%
- Single journal article – 4%
- Handheld computer – 4%

No nonhuman resource was used for more than 7% of the answers, with the most common being a computer database (7%), a textbook (6%), and a handheld drug reference (4%).

The reasons for not pursuing an answer were identified for 212 questions (the physicians were too rushed or otherwise busy to provide reasons for the remainder). The most common reasons for not pursuing an answer were as follows:

- Doubted existence of relevant information – 25%
- Readily available consultation leading to referral rather than pursuit – 22%
- Lack of time to pursue – 19%
- Not important enough to pursue answer – 15%
- Uncertain where to look for answer – 8%

After the observation period, each of the 48 physicians was interviewed to provide recommendations for the knowledge resource developers. A qualitative analysis broke the recommendations down into content and access issues. The key content issues recommended were for comprehensive and trustworthy information. The important access issues were user-friendly and intuitive search function, rapid access to information, concise operation, and available anywhere all the time.

The researchers themselves then followed up on the 237 questions from the 585 that these physicians pursued but were unable to answer (Ely, Osheroff et al., 2007). They grouped the questions into 19 generic types but found that three of the types accounted for slightly more than half of the questions:

1. Questions about undiagnosed abnormal clinical findings
2. Questions containing subquestions qualifying otherwise simple questions, such as how to manage one disease given the presence of another
3. Questions about the association between two highly specific findings or diseases

Most studies of information needs and use have focused on primary care physicians. Shelstad and Clevenger (1996), however, assessed general surgeons in New Mexico and found that their needs were for the most part met with traditional paper resources. Significant impediments to the use of newer electronic resources existed for this group of surgeons. The most common reasons for seeking information among the New Mexico surgeons were patient care (98%) and continuing education (83%). The most common sources of information were professional meetings (97%), medical literature (96%), and colleagues (93%). Those who found it difficult to access information resource most often listed time demands of practice (71%), isolation from medical schools (30%), and computer illiteracy (28%).

2.7.2.4 Satisfied Needs

What information resources are most likely to satisfy an information need? In a study of knowledge resource preferences of family physicians, Curley et al. (1990) found that "cost" variables (e.g., availability, searchability, understandability, clinical applicability) were more closely associated with the decision to use a resource than "benefit" variables, such as its extensiveness and credibility. As with the studies described earlier, the family physicians in this study were more likely to use textbooks, compendia, and colleagues for information-seeking than journal literature and bibliographic resources (Connelly, Rich et al., 1990).

These observations led Shaughnessy et al. (1994) to propose a formula for the usefulness of information:

$$\text{Usefulness} = \frac{\text{Relevance} \times \text{Validity}}{\text{Work}} \tag{2.7}$$

That is, the value of information is proportional to its relevance and validity to the clinical situation and inversely proportional to how difficult it is to find and apply.

Some studies have also attempted to measure the use of computerized information sources. A number of these will be described in greater detail in Chap. 7, where the focus will be on how often and how successfully they are used. Not surprisingly, most of the early studies on pursued information needs found very little use of computers for seeking information. Covell et al. (1985), Williamson et al. (1989), Gorman and Helfand (1995), and Curley et al. (1990) found that fewer than 10% of physicians regularly use online literature searching. Even when use of online searching is prevalent, the frequency of its use pales with the frequency of information needs. In both inpatient (Haynes, McKibbon et al., 1990) and outpatient (Hersh and Hickam, 1994) settings, observed usage is never more than a few times per month among medical residents and faculty, which is far below the unmet information need frequency in the studies described.

Gorman et al. (1994) addressed the issue of whether physicians can meet their information needs through computer-based information sources. They chose a random sample of 50 questions that arose in clinical care where physicians chose not to pursue an answer. These questions were then given to librarians, who performed a literature search and returned three articles that might be relevant to the physicians. In 28 instances (56%), the physicians indicated that at least one of the articles was relevant to the question. They also stated that for 22 questions (46%), a clear answer to the question was provided, and for 19 questions (40%), the information would have had an impact on care of the patient. The limitation of this approach to obtaining information for physicians, they noted, was the time (averaging 43 min per search per librarian) and cost of searching (averaging $27 per search). Gorman (1993) also found in a subsequent study that only a third of the studies contained "high-quality" evidence, such as RCTs of therapeutic interventions.

A similar study was performed by Giuse et al. (1994), who looked at the answerability of questions about AIDS. Even though the study was simulated (i.e., questions were generated via chart review of patients already seen), the general categories of questions and their likelihood of being answered were comparable to those from field studies. About 92% of the questions were answerable: four fifths during a first phase that utilized information resources commonly available to general internists (paper-based general textbooks and MEDLINE) and the remainder during a more intensive second phase undertaken in an academic medical library. The most useful resources for the latter phase were specialty textbooks. This study showed that a variety of resources were needed to answer clinical questions in this domain.

Although few studies have addressed these questions in light of the massive growth of physician use of computers and the Internet, it is likely that with the growth of the Web, along with increasing use of handheld and other portable devices, physicians are using information resources during practice more frequently. There are still, however, impediments, which are due to a variety of factors, such as the need to find a computer to use, and the amount of time required to log on to the appropriate resource and search. Chueh and Barnett (1997) have argued that a new model is needed for delivery of information to clinicians, based on "just in time" principles of inventory management from the manufacturing industry. The model requires not only that information be readily (i.e., quickly) available, but also that it be specific to the context of the patient. One approach to doing this involves attempting to link from the context of the electronic medical record (e.g., diagnoses, medications, and conditions detected, such as rapid decrease in hemoglobin level) directly to appropriate information (Cimino, 1996). Studies remain to be done to determine whether direct linking based on information in the record or providing a pop-up query box is faster.

2.7.3 *Information Needs of Other Health-Care Professionals*

The information needs and usage of nonphysician health-care providers have been much less studied. In many ways, however, the data on nurses, the next-most studied group, show a picture similar to that for physicians. One limitation of these studies, however, is that almost all data are derived from surveys, without direct observation. Although this does not necessarily invalidate the results, one of the studies cited earlier showed considerable divergence between reported and observed needs (Covell, Uman et al., 1985), while another research group found a wide disparity when they measured pursued (Ely, Burch et al., 1992) vs. unmet needs (Ely, Osheroff et al., 1999).

The survey studies across different nursing professionals do show, however, fairly consistent results. Like physicians, nurses tend to rely on their own collections of textbooks and journals as well as on colleagues. A British study found that the most common sources of information used for nursing problems were books (22%), followed by nursing colleagues (21%), journals (14%), and medical colleagues (11%) (Williamson, 1990). An American study found an even larger percentage of nurses consulting other people for information needs as well as a lack of awareness of library resources (Bunyan and Lutz, 1991). On the latter point, it was noted that nurses comprised 34% of the hospital staff, yet only 6% of the hospital's library patrons.

Spath and Buttlar (1996) studied acute-care nurses in Ohio, most of whom were staff nurses with an RN degree. The most common information resources used were professional journals (79.4%), other nurses (64.7%), and the library card catalog (51.0%). Use of online or CD-ROM materials was minimal. More than half the respondents used the library for personal interest in a subject (68.6%) or to obtain information about a diagnosis (59.8%). Half reported that they read no or one professional journal regularly and another 42% reported reading two or three. A total of 9% spent 0 h per month reading professional literature, while 45% spent 1–3 h, 26% spent 4–6 h, and the remainder spent more.

The one study of observed needs was an ethnographic study of general medical and oncology nurses in Canada (Blythe and Royle, 1993). It was found that nurses sought information in two general areas, individual patient care and broader nursing issues. Most information-seeking was related to patient care. Information-seeking not related to patient care was generally done during quiet periods on a shift, while professional developmental reading tended to be done at home.

Urquhart and Crane (1994) attempted to assess nurses' information skills by using a simulated vignette in the library. They predefined "evidence of an information-seeking strategy" as behavior tending to support a belief that certain activity would yield a particular type of information or indicate that a particular sequence of steps was followed in gaining information. Slightly under half of all subjects displayed an information-seeking strategy, with those displaying such a strategy much more likely to consult more than two information sources. Both groups were equally likely to consult colleagues for information, and while those with an information-seeking strategy were more likely to use the library, they were no more likely to use literature-searching.

Corcoran-Perry and Graves (1990) performed a study on information-seeking by cardiovascular nurses that went beyond use of knowledge-based resources and included seeking of patient-specific information as well. They found that the most common reason for using "supplemental" (not available in personal memory) information was for patient-specific data (49%), such as general information about the patient, medications, or laboratory reports. The next most common type of information sought was institution-specific information (27%), such as tracking equipment, medications, reports, or people. The seeking of domain knowledge represented only 21% of supplemental information sought, most commonly related to medications or cardiovascular conditions. The most common sources of supplemental information were other people (nurses 26% of the time and other personnel 19% of the time), patient records (25%), references (15%), and a computer terminal (10%).

Beyond nursing, there are few information needs studies of other health-care professionals. Dental hygienists (Gravois, Fisher et al., 1995) and physical therapists (Bohannon, 1990), like physicians and nurses, have been found to rely on professional journals, colleagues, and continuing education, with little use of bibliographic databases. Among rural health-care practitioners in Hawaii, allied health professionals, social workers, and administrators tended to use journal articles less and newsletters, videos, and resource directories more commonly than physicians used them (Lundeen, Tenopir et al., 1994). They consulted colleagues at a rate comparable to that of physicians and rarely made use of the university library's online databases.

One recent study looked at information needs and seeking of nurse practitioners (Cogdill, 2003). The findings were not much different than those noted for physicians. The most frequent information needs reported were somewhat more focused than those of physicians and were on two specific areas: drug therapy (43%) and diagnosis (41%). Most commonly used information sources were supervising physicians, drug reference manuals, textbooks, journal articles, and other nurse practitioners. The generalness of a need was found to be a negative predictor of information-seeking.

2.7.4   Information Needs of Biomedical Researchers

Another group in the health-care field whose information needs have been minimally assessed is biomedical researchers. This is particularly pertinent in light of the recent growth of bioinformatics tools that they increasingly rely on to perform their work (MacMullen and Denn, 2005). Most work has focused on the information needs of genomics researchers. This group would presumably have great information needs because of the rapid growth of new "high throughput" biotechnologies that generate vast amounts of data, which in turn require researchers to need information about new genes, proteins, etc., involved in the biological systems they study. A prototype biotechnology is the gene microarray, which tests the expression of tens of thousands of genes (via their messenger RNA) in a given biological sample (Mobasheri, Airley et al., 2004). A researcher using a microarray might find dozens or more genes differentially expressed and now have the need to find out information about those genes or their protein products rapidly.

Roberts and Hayes (2008) collected and classified information requests to a library of a large pharmaceutical company. A total of 1,131 search requests were classified by the biological entity being searched (e.g., drug, disease, gene, etc.) and, when specified, type of document sought (e.g., scientific literature, business intelligence, patent record). The most common entities for which information was sought were drugs (31.3%), diseases (27.4%), genes (26.3%), companies (17.0%), methods (10.6%), authors (7.9%), geographic regions (5.7%), and drug sales (5.0%). About 36% of queries sought information on more than one of these entities, with the most common pairwise combinations being drug–disease, drug–company, and drug–sales. The type of document sought varied by search entity, with queries on genes most commonly seeking patent information, queries on diseases seeking journal articles, and queries on drugs seeking business intelligence. Of course, the searching in a pharmaceutical company is likely to have different characteristics than the searching in other sites for biomedical research.

Very little attention has been paid to the information tasks of biomedical researchers generally. Stevens, Goble et al. (2001) were the first to assess the information tasks in bioinformatics. Most tasks involved sequence similarity searching, with literature-searching representing a tiny fraction of their work. Tran et al. (2004) carried out a task analysis on a smaller sample of researchers but in more detail. There were too few researchers to generate reliable quantitative assessment of IR tasks, but several themes emerged from the analysis, including that laboratories lack procedural documentation of their information-related work, and that researchers use and stick to "home-grown" strategies and are unaware of many tools that are available. In a proprietary report, Strouse (2004) notes that biomedical researchers spend about 9 h (18%) of their work week gathering and reviewing information.

2.8   Evidence-Based Medicine

As noted already in this chapter, there has been considerable effort devoted to organizing scientific literature and teaching clinicians to use it to find the best evidence for making clinical decisions. The philosophy of this approach, EBM, is that clinical care should be guided by the best scientific evidence. As was seen in Fig.1.4, while factors in addition to evidence influence medical decision-making, when evidence is used in a decision, it should be of the highest quality. In fact, EBM is really just a set of tools to inform clinical decision-making. It allows clinical experience (art) to be integrated with best clinical science. Also, EBM makes the medical literature more clinically applicable and relevant. In addition, it requires the user to be facile with computers and IR systems.

There are many well-known resources for EBM. The original textbook in the field was first-authored by Sackett but now is in it third edition and led by Straus et al. (2005). A series of articles originally published in JAMA were assembled into a handbook (Guyatt and Rennie, 2001) and reference book format (Guyatt, Rennie et al., 2001). There are a number of comprehensive Web sites, including the Oxford University Centre for Evidence-Based Medicine (http://www.cebm.net) and the Canadian Centres for Health Evidence (http://www.cche.net).

The process of EBM involves three general steps:

- Phrasing a clinical question that is pertinent and answerable
- Identifying evidence (studies in articles) that address the question
- Critically appraising the evidence to determine whether it applies to the patient

The phrasing of the clinical question is an often-overlooked portion of the EBM process. There are two general types of clinical question: background questions and foreground questions (Sackett, Richardson et al., 2000). *Background* questions ask for general knowledge about a disorder, whereas *foreground* questions ask for knowledge about managing patients with a disorder. Background questions are generally best answered with textbooks and classical review articles, whereas foreground questions are answered using EBM techniques. Background questions contain two essential components: a question root with a verb (e.g., what, when, how) and a disorder or aspect of a disorder. Examples of background questions include, What causes pneumonia? and When do complications of diabetes usually occur?

Foreground questions have four essential components, based on the PICO mnemonic: the *p*atient and/or *p*roblem, the *i*ntervention, the *c*omparison intervention (if applicable), and the clinical *o*utcome(s). Some expand the mnemonic with two additional letters, PICOTS, adding the *t*ime duration of treatment or follow-up and the *s*etting (e.g., inpatient, outpatient, etc.). There are four major categories of foreground questions:

- Therapy (or intervention) – benefit of treatment or prevention
- Diagnosis – test diagnosing disease
- Harm – etiology of disease
- Prognosis – outcome of disease course

EBM has evolved since its inception. The original approach to EBM, called "first-generation" EBM by Hersh (1999), focused on finding original studies in the primary literature and applying critical appraisal. As already seen, accessing the primary literature is challenging and time-consuming for clinicians for a variety of reasons. This led to what Hersh (1999) called "next-generation" EBM and was focused on the use of syntheses, where the literature-searching, critical appraisal, and extraction of statistics operations were performed ahead of time. This approach put EBM resources in the context of more usable information resources as advocated in the InfoMastery concept of Shaughnessy et al. (1994) and JIT (just in time) information model of Chueh and Barnett (1997).

One statement was recently published by a group of experts who defined *evidence-based practice* (EBP) as medical practice requiring that health-care decisions be based on the "best available, current, valid, and relevant evidence" (Dawes, Summerskill et al., 2005). They defined a five-step model of EBP that included the following:

1. Translation of uncertainty to an answerable question
2. Systematic retrieval of the best evidence
3. Critical appraisal of the evidence for validity, clinical relevance, and applicability
4. Application of results in practice
5. Evaluation of performance

They also advocated that EBP practitioners need to be able to distinguish "evidence from propaganda (advertisement), probability from certainty, data from assertions, rational belief from superstitions, and science from folklore." Of course, in light of the manipulation of evidence by the manufacturers of COX-2 inhibitors and other treatments described earlier in the chapter, additional help may be needed to truly sort out fact from fiction.

Slawson and Shaughnessy (2005) argue that teaching clinicians to find evidence, such as that in synopses, is a much more important skill than critical appraisal. They advocate for three skills to be taught in medical training that are essential to applying evidence: foraging – keeping up with new knowledge, hunting – finding important information just in time, and the ability to make the best decisions based on applying evidence in specific scenarios of care. Ogrinc et al. (2003) have developed learning objectives for teaching EBM and related topics in the larger framework of improving health-care quality.

Haynes, one of the founders of the concept of EBM, wrote a historical perspective on EBM in 2002 (Haynes, 2002). He noted in retrospect that the originators of EBM should probably not have touted it as an alternative paradigm for medical practice, but instead should have promoted it to augment (rather than replace) individual clinical experience and understanding of basic disease mechanisms. He advocated that EBM must evolve not only to respond to theoretical and moral challenges in its use but also to address practical concerns such as dissemination and generalizability. More recently, Haynes (2004) noted that despite the progress, much remains to get the best evidence to clinicians and allow them to apply it in their practices. Gray (2004) argues that we also need to be more evidence-based in health-care policy.

2.8.1   Studies

When first developed, EBM focused on identifying the appropriate foreground question, finding evidence in the primary literature (usually individual studies), and critically appraising it. Table 2.5 gives an overview of the major question types,

Table 2.5 Overview of major question types, best studies for evidence, and most important questions to ask for study design in evidence-based medicine

Category of question	Best type of study for evidence	Most important questions to ask of study design
Therapy	Randomized controlled trial	Was the assignment of patients to treatments randomized?
		Were all the patients who entered the trial properly accounted for and attributed at its conclusion?
Diagnosis	Blinded comparison with gold standard	Was there an independent, blind comparison with a reference standard?
		Did the patient sample choice include an appropriate spectrum of patients similar to that to which the test would be applied in clinical practice?
Harm	Randomized controlled trial (if possible) or case-control study	Were there clearly identified comparison groups that were similar with respect to important determinants of outcome (other than the one of interest)?
		Were outcomes and exposures measured in the same way in groups being compared?
Prognosis	Follow-up of representative and well-defined group with a disease or condition	Was there a representative patient sample at a well-defined point in the course of the disease?
		Was follow-up sufficiently long and complete?

the best studies for evidence, and the most important questions to ask for study design. Discussed later are the best sources of information for these studies (Chap. 3) and how well various strategies work in finding them (Chaps. 5 and 7). After studies with evidence have been identified, they need to be critically appraised by three questions:

- Are the results valid?
- What are the results?
- Will they help in caring for the patient?

RCTs are considered to be the best evidence for therapy or interventions because their basic design minimizes bias by ideally keeping everything the same except for the intervention being studied, which is then randomized. For example, while many individuals tout the value of vitamin C for the prevention of the common cold, a meta-analysis of numerous RCTs has shown the vitamin to be ineffective for this purpose (Hemila, 1997). Also, RCTs tend to emphasize clinical end points and patient-oriented outcomes. It has been observed that minor cardiac arrhythmias, such as premature ventricular contractions after an acute myocardial infarction, are associated with more serious arrhythmias, such as ventricular fibrillation, which is fatal without defibrillation. As a number of new drugs were discovered that reduced the frequency of these minor arrhythmias, it was assumed that this would result in a corresponding decrease of more serious arrhythmias. However, RCTs (strengthened by follow-up meta-analyses) have shown that while the drugs do suppress arrhythmias, they are associated with a higher mortality because of other problems arising from their use (Sadowski, Alexander et al., 1999).

All kinds of health interventions, from surgery to alternative medicine, can be assessed by means of RCTs. There is nothing inherently "biomedical" about them. There are other study designs that can be used to assess interventions, and it may be that their evidence yields results similar to those of RCTs. Both prospective cohort studies and retrospective case-control series have been found to lead to similar results in one analysis of five clinical topics (Concato, Shah et al., 2000) and in another analysis of 19 clinical topics (Benson and Hartz, 2000). It has also been argued that papers presenting evidence of lower quality, namely, case reports and case series, still have value in the medical literature (Vandenbroucke, 2001). They potentially allow recognition of new diseases, new manifestations of old diseases, and detection of adverse effects of treatment. Others have noted that RCTs have their limitations as well, such as the modification of the intended treatment (due to protocol error or lack of compliance) and the lack of outcome determination (due to difficulty in ascertaining outcomes or because the patient was not studied for long enough) (Rabenback, Viscoli et al., 1992).

The first RCT is usually ascribed to a study carried out by the Medical Research Council of the United Kingdom and published in the *British Medical Journal* in 1948 (Anonymous, 1948). However, the earliest trials may have been performed by James Lind, MD, in the mid-1700s, where he determined that lack of vitamin C was the cause of scurvy in sailors on British ships and they could be treated by carrying citrus fruit on ships. A Web site devoted to Lind's work has been developed (http://www.jameslindlibrary.org).

A number of limitations of studies-based EBM have been noted (Hersh, 1999):

1. Time – as mentioned earlier and described in more detail in Chap. 7, the process outlined in this section takes a great deal of time, which a busy clinician is unlikely to have.
2. Expertise – although this is changing, very few clinicians are skilled in applying EBM as described here.
3. Comprehensiveness – relying on single studies for EBM calculations is problematic because there are often numerous studies on a given topic.
4. Publication bias – as seen earlier, publication bias may result in the exclusion of some results from the literature.

Another concern about EBM is whether its skill set can be learned by clinicians. Most studies of instruction in EBM have focused on medical students and residents. A systematic review of earlier studies found that gains in knowledge were more likely to occur when the subjects instructed in its use were students rather than residents (Norman and Shannon, 1998). A more recent study of first-year internal medicine residents found that skills in question formulation, literature-searching, and understanding quantitative outcomes were significant and durable over time, although skills in critical appraisal were not (Smith, Ganschow et al., 2000).

2.8.2   Syntheses

The limitations of first-generation EBM led to the premise that not every clinician needed to do critical appraisal on each problem de novo. Instead, experts should create and maintain "synthesized" or "predigested" EBM content. This approach will likely assist in overcoming the first-generation problems of time (evidence is found more quickly), expertise (critical appraisal is done by experts), and comprehensiveness (techniques such as meta-analysis are a staple of this approach). Of course, the problem of publication bias will not be ameliorated with this approach and may actually be exacerbated, given the greater reliance on meta-analysis.

The best-known producer of systematic reviews is the Cochrane Collaboration (Levin, 2001). This collaboration is named after Archie Cochrane, who noted, "It is surely a great criticism of our profession that we have not organized a critical summary, by specialty or subspecialty, adapted periodically, of all relevant randomized controlled trials" (Cochrane, 1972). The Cochrane Collaboration is an international one with the aim of preparing and maintaining systematic reviews of the effects of health-care interventions. The *Cochrane Database of Systematic Reviews* has over a thousand reviews across medicine and will be described in greater detail in Chap. 3. Traditional journals are increasingly publishing systematic reviews. The Evidence-Based Practice Centers of AHRQ are also a source of systematic reviews (which the centers call evidence reports).

2.8.3   Synopses

Of course, systematic reviews and evidence reports can be quite long and detailed, and are still likely to be difficult for routine use by front-line clinicians. As such, there is increasing interest in more synoptic forms of information, especially for the busy clinical setting. Of course, clinicians have always used synoptic forms of information to help with clinical care, but as noted already, paper-based handbooks and compendia go out of date quickly and are not necessarily created based on evidence-based principles.

One form of synopsis is called *critically appraised topics* (CATS). These were originally defined to be "quick and dirty" systematic reviews of one or a few articles on a given topic, but their definition has been expanded for the purposes of this discussion to include any collection that summarizes the evidence less formally than systematic reviews. In fact, many CATS are summaries of systematic reviews. The original CATS adhered to a template that followed the critical appraisal approach of EBM and would be collected in databases. A number of Web sites provide access to a wide variety of CATS, such as the previously mentioned Oxford University Centre for Evidence-Based Medicine.

Additional CATS-like information resources have been developed. These resources are characterized by their relevance to clinical practice, use of exclusively patient-oriented outcomes (symptoms, mortality, cost, or quality of life as opposed to test results), and their ability to allow users to change their clinical practice. One approach has been *Patient-Oriented Evidence That Matters* (POEMS) (Shaughnessy, Slawson et al., 1994). POEMS are published by the *Journal of Family Practice* as well as on a Web site (http://www.infopoems.com/). Another publication that provides highly distilled evidence is *Clinical Evidence*. To the extent that they are built using evidence-based techniques, clinical practice guidelines can fall under this category of EBM information as well.

2.8.4 Systems

As noted in the clinical evidence hierarchy of Fig. 2.3, at the top sits systems or what may be described as knowledge that can be acted upon by decision support technology. Although the market for such content is currently tiny compared to that for medical journals and textbooks, it is likely to grow in the future as more health-care organizations adopt clinical decision support technology, whose benefit is increasingly documented (Choudhry, Fletcher et al., 2005; Garg, Adhikari et al., 2005). Although such content has historically been "home grown" by institutions developing clinical decision support systems and integrating them into their clinical environments, a number of medical publishers have begun to market content such as clinical decision rules and order sets. Among the early providers of such content are Thomson Publishing (http://clinical.thomsonhealthcare.com/) and Zynx Health (http://www.zynx.com/).

2.8.5 Limitations of EBM

The entire medical community has not unequivocally embraced EBM. Feinstein (1995), as already noted, expresses concern about the use of meta-analysis and the lack of judgment that may emanate from a strictly "by the numbers" approach (Feinstein and Horwitz, 1997). Miles et al. (1997) lament that EBM is so narrowly focused on sound methodology that it may lose the bigger clinical picture. Alderson (2004) has noted that "absence of evidence is not evidence of absence," i.e., there may be no evidence to support or refute the use of a test or treatment because no research (or sufficiently powered research) has been done.

Cohen et al. (2004) published a categorization of the major criticisms of EBM. In particular, they noted the following problems with EBM from a philosophical standpoint:

- It relies solely on empiricism and not other forms of scientific investigation and analysis, such as physiological processes and reasoning.
- Its definition of evidence is narrow and excludes other types of scientific studies, e.g., cohort studies.
- It is not evidence-based, i.e., the practice of EBM itself has not been demonstrated to lead to improved clinical outcomes.
- Its usefulness to individual patients is limited, e.g., studies of highest quality evidence are not necessarily applicable to individual patients and tend to be limited to the most common diseases.
- It may threaten the autonomy of the patient–physician relationship by limiting diagnostic and therapeutic options.

A tongue-in-cheek criticism (with many inside jokes) has also been published (Anonymous, 2002c).

Norman (1999) acknowledges these criticisms and argues that proponents of EBM must conduct research on its effectiveness, incorporate more holistic perspectives on evidence, move from teaching appraisal skills to practitioners toward expert reviews (as described in Sect. 2.8.2), develop better strategies for teaching its use in clinical practice, and acknowledge and address the concerns of its critics.

Part II
State of the Art

Chapter 3
Content

In the first edition of this book, describing the content available in information retrieval (IR) systems was relatively simple. The Web was in its infancy, so most content could be classified as either bibliographic or full text. The former consisted of databases that cataloged books or periodicals, while the latter contained the full text of a relatively small number of books, periodicals, and other resources available in electronic form. Most available full-text content was distributed via CD-ROM, with online content limited mainly to text-only displays of periodicals. By the second edition, the use of the Web was becoming widespread, although a substantial amount of material was still paper-based. With this third edition of the book, the knowledge world is almost completely electronic. This does not mean that paper is not still widely used, but most journal articles, textbooks, and other resources are available electronically, and an increasing amount of material is distributed only in electronic format.

This chapter begins our exploration of the "state of the art" of IR systems. We will begin with looking at content, i.e., what health and biomedical information resources are available. Our goal is not to be exhaustive, but rather representative, covering the diversity of content that is available. We will approach this via a classification scheme for content. This will be followed in subsequent chapters by coverage of indexing, retrieval, and digital libraries.

3.1 Classification of Health and Biomedical Information Content

The classification schema is shown in Table 3.1. It is not a pure schema, for some of the subcategories represent type of content (e.g., literature reference databases) while others describe its subject (e.g., the -omics databases). Nonetheless, the schema does cover the major types of health and biomedical information available electronically, even if the boundaries between the categories have some areas of fuzziness. The classification will be revisited again in Chap. 5 when we cover approaches to searching various resources.

W. Hersh, *Information Retrieval: A Health and Biomedical Perspective,*
doi: 10.1007/978-0-387-78703-9, © Springer Science + Business Media, LLC 2009

Table 3.1 Classification of health and biomedical information content

1. Bibliographic
   (a) Literature reference databases
   (b) Web catalogs and feeds
   (c) Specialized registries
2. Full text
   (a) Periodicals
   (b) Books and reports
   (c) Web collections
   (d) Evidence-based medicine resources
3. Annotated
   (a) Images
   (b) Videos
   (c) Citations
   (d) Molecular biology and -omics
   (e) Other
4. Aggregations
   (a) Consumer
   (b) Professional
   (c) Body of knowledge
   (d) Model organism databases

The first category consists of *bibliographic* content. It includes what was for decades the mainstay of IR systems: *literature reference databases*. Also called *bibliographic databases*, this content is still a key online health and biomedical information resource. Even with essentially the entire scientific publishing enterprising online, literature reference databases are still in widespread use as an entry point into the scientific literature (especially since many publishers want to direct people to their resources that require a fee to use). A second, more modern type of bibliographic content includes *Web catalogs and feeds*. There are many Web catalogs, which consist of Web pages that contain mainly links to other Web pages and sites. Web feeds are bibliographic-like streams of information that inform users of new content on Web sites and in other databases. The final type of bibliographic content is the *specialized registry*. This resource is very close to a literature reference database except that it indexes more diverse content than scientific literature.

The second category is *full-text* content. A large component of this content consists of the online versions of periodicals, books, and reports. As already noted, much of this content, from journals to textbooks, is now available electronically. The electronic versions may be enhanced by measures ranging from the provision of supplemental data in a journal article to Web linkages or multimedia content in a textbook. This category also includes the specialized textbook-like resources related to evidence-based medicine (EBM). The final component of this category is what we will call the Web collection. Admittedly, the diversity of information on Web collections is enormous, and they may include every other type of content described in this chapter. However, in the context of this category,

"Web collection" refers to the vast number of static and dynamic Web pages that reside at a discrete Web location.

The third category consists of *annotated* content. We make the subtle distinction between this content and bibliographic content by virtue of the annotation being tightly integrated with the content as opposed to being in a separate bibliographic database. Annotated content includes images, videos, citation databases, and bio-medical research data. The latter are particularly prevalent in molecular biology and the -omics (e.g., genomics, proteomics, etc.), which consist of nucleotide or protein sequences, chromosome maps, and biological pathways. All these types of content are usually annotated with some amount of text and searched with IR-like systems, although their make-up is predominantly nontextual or text that is nonnarrative.

The final category consists of *aggregations* of the first three categories. A number of Web sites consist of collections of different types of content, aggregated to form a coherent resource. We will look at examples in biomedical research, clinical content, and consumer content. In one sense, the entire Web can be viewed as one big aggregation, but as we will see, there are plenty of more confined aggregations that provide value within their (not always distinct) boundaries.

3.2 Bibliographic Content

Bibliographic content consists of references or citations to complete resources. It tends to be richer than other content in metadata. This is not surprising, since bibliographic databases in essence consist of metadata. The original IR databases from the 1960s were bibliographic databases that typically contained references to literature on library shelves. Library card catalogs are also a type of bibliographic database, with the electronic version usually called an *online public access catalog* (OPAC). Biblio-graphic data-bases were designed to steer the searcher to printed resources, not to provide the information itself. Most have fields not only for the subject matter, such as the title, abstract, and indexing terms, but also for other attributes, such as author name(s), publication date, publication type, and grant identification number.

In this section, we begin our discussion with literature reference databases, fol-lowed by descriptions of Web catalogs and feeds and then specialized registries. Although not typically thought of as bibliographic databases, many Web catalogs and feeds can be viewed as bibliographic in that they provide links to other informa-tion sources. Indeed, some modern bibliographic databases offer direct linkage to the literature they are referencing, hence are becoming similar to Web catalogs.

3.2.1 Literature Reference Databases

As already noted, the literature reference database MEDLINE may be the best-known IR application in all of health and biomedicine. Produced by the National Center for Biotechnology Information (NCBI, http://www.ncbi.nlm.nih.gov/)

within the National Library of Medicine (NLM, http://www.nlm.nih.gov/), MED-LINE was virtually synonymous with online searching for health-care topics for many years. There are actually a substantial number of additional bibliographic databases, which are produced by the NLM and other information providers. A technical resource for all NLM resources is the *NLM Technical Bulletin* (http://www.nlm.nih.gov/pubs/techbull/tb.html).

3.2.1.1   MEDLINE

MEDLINE contains bibliographic references to all the biomedical articles, editorials, letters to the editors, and other content in over 5,000 scientific journals (Anonymous, 2007g). The journals are chosen for inclusion by the Literature Selection Technical Review Committee of the National Institutes of Health (Anonymous, 2007h). At present, more than 600,000 references are added to MEDLINE yearly (Anonymous, 2006d). Dating back to its inception in 1966, MEDLINE now contains more than 16 million references. The language of origin of nearly 89% of the citations is English, although journals representing 29 other languages are indexed. About 76% of the records have abstracts, including some non-English articles, although an English translation is always provided. The database is updated daily.

The MEDLINE database is the electronic version of *Index Medicus*, the print publication that was the most common way to access medical literature for over a century. *Index Medicus* was founded in the nineteenth century by Dr. John Shaw Billings, who headed the forerunner of the NLM, the Library of the Surgeon General's Office, from 1865 to 1895 (DeBakey, 1991). Billings was the first to diligently catalog the literature of medicine, culminating in the first volume of *Index Medicus* published in 1879. In 2004, the NLM finally "retired" the print version of *Index Medicus* (Anonymous, 2004b). One enduring value of *Index Medicus* is that it allows searching of pre-1966 literature, although NLM also maintains a database OLDMEDLINE that contains citations from before the official 1966 "start date" of MEDLINE. OLDMEDLINE continues to grow and now has more than 1.7 million references dating back to 1950 (Anonymous, 2007n).

MEDLINE has evolved over the years. Beginning in 1975, the NLM began adding abstracts for all references that contained them. The Medical Subject Headings vocabulary, used to index MEDLINE and other NLM resources and covered in the next chapter, has expanded to over 23,000 terms. Additional attributes have been added to MEDLINE, such as the secondary source identifier, which provides a link to records in other databases, such as the GenBank database of gene sequences and the ClinicalTrials.gov database of clinical trials. Other attributes have been enhanced, such as publication type, which lists, for example, whether the article is a meta-analysis, practice guideline, review article, or randomized controlled trial. Another feature of MEDLINE that has been retired is the old MEDLINE Unique Identifier (UI), which has been replaced by the PMID as the unique identifier for MEDLINE and OLDMEDLINE citations (Tybaert and Rosov, 2004).

The current MEDLINE record contains more than 50 fields, the most important of which are listed in Table 3.2 (Anonymous, 2007l). Table 3.3 contains the special tags that NLM uses for comments and corrections, such as when an article has an editorial or letter to the editor or has a correction or retraction (Anonymous, 2007f).

Table 3.2 Most important fields in MEDLINE (Anonymous, 2007l)

Tag	Name	Description
AB	Abstract	Abstract
AD	Affiliation	Institutional affiliation and address of the first author, and grant numbers
AID	Article identifier	Values may include the pii (controlled publisher identifier) or doi (digital object identifier)
AU	Author	Authors' names
CI	Copyright information	Copyright statement
CN	Corporate author	Corporate author or group names with authorship responsibility
DEP	Date of electronic publication	Electronic publication date
DP	Date of publication	Date the article was published
EDAT	Entrez date	Date the citation was added to PubMed
FAU	Full author	Full names of authors
FPS	Full personal name as subject	Full name of the subject of the article
GR	Grant number	Grant number, acronym, and agency
GS	Gene symbol	Abbreviated gene names (used 1991–1996)
IP	Issue	Number of the issue, part, or supplement of the journal in which the article was published
IS	ISSN	International Standard Serial Number of the journal
JID	NLM unique ID	Unique journal ID in NLM's catalog of books, journals, and audiovisuals
JT	Journal title	Full title of journal
LA	Language	Language in which the article was published
LR	Date last revised	Date a change was made to the record during a maintenance procedure
MH	MeSH terms	Subject headings from NLM's controlled vocabulary
MHDA	MeSH date	Date MeSH terms were added to the citation
NM	Substance name	Name of substance that RN or EC number identifies
PG	Pagination	Full pagination of the article
PHST	Publication history status	History status date
PL	Place of publication	Journal's country of publication
PMID	PubMed unique identifier	Unique number assigned to each PubMed citation

(continued)

Table 3.2 (continued)

PS	Personal name as subject	Individual who is the subject of the article
PST	Publication status	Publication status
PT	Publication type	Type of material the article represents
PUBM	Publishing model	Medium/media in which the cited article is published (print or electronic)
RF	Number of references	Number of bibliographic references for review articles
RN	Registry number/ EC number	Number assigned by the Enzyme Commission to designate a particular enzyme or by the Chemical Abstracts Service for Registry Numbers
SB	Subset	Code for a specific set of journals
SI	Secondary source ID	Identifies a secondary source that supplies information (e.g., other data sources, databanks, and accession numbers of molecular sequences discussed in articles)
SO	Source	Composite field containing bibliographic information
STAT	Status	Status of record (e.g., in-process, MEDLINE, PubMed-not-MEDLINE, etc.)
TA	Journal title abbreviation	Standard journal title abbreviation
TI	Title	The title of the article
TT	Transliterated title	Nonroman alphabet language titles are transliterated
VI	Volume	Journal volume

Courtesy of the National Library of Medicine
MeSH Medical Subject Headings

A clinician may only be interested in just a handful of MEDLINE fields, such as the title, abstract, and indexing terms. But other fields contain specific information that may be of great importance to a more focused audience. For example, a genome researcher might be highly interested in the secondary source identifier field to link to genomic databases. Even the clinician may, however, derive benefit from some of the other fields. For example, the publication type field can help in the application of EBM, such as when one is searching for a practice guideline or a randomized controlled trial. The PubMed subset (SB) field allows searches to be limited to MEDLINE, in-process citations, publisher-supplied citations, and several subject subsets, all of which are listed in Table 3.4. A sample MEDLINE record is shown in Fig. 3.1.

The major way that most users access MEDLINE is via the PubMed system at the NLM (http://pubmed.gov/), which provides access to other NLM databases as well and is free of charge (Anonymous, 2006b). PubMed refers to both the software system used to access MEDLINE as well as the system plus content that includes some additional material beyond just MEDLINE, such as OLDMEDLINE, in-process citations that have not yet been indexed, and citations that precede the date a journal was selected for inclusion in MEDLINE (Anonymous, 2006j). There are other ways to access MEDLINE. Some information vendors, such as Ovid

Table 3.3 Comments and corrections in the MEDLINE database (Anonymous, 2007f)

Tag	Name	Description
CON	Comment on	Cites the reference upon which the article comments
CIN	Comment in	Cites the reference containing a commentary about the article (appears on citation for original article)
EIN	Erratum in	Cites a published erratum to the article (appears on citation for original article)
EFR	Erratum for	Cites the original article for which there is a published erratum
CRI	Corrected and Republished in	Cites the final, correct version of a corrected and republished article (appears on citation for original article)
CRF	Corrected and Republished from	Cites the original article subsequently corrected and republished
PRIN	Partial retraction in	Cites the reference containing a partial retraction of the article (appears on citation for original article)
PROF	Partial retraction of	Cites the article being partially retracted
RPI	Republished in	Cites the subsequent (and possibly abridged) version of a republished article (appears on citation for original article)
RPF	Republished from	Cites the first, originally published article
RIN	Retraction in	Cites the retraction of the article (appears on citation for original article)
ROF	Retraction of	Cites the article(s) being retracted
UIN	Update in	Cites an updated version of the article (appears on citation for original article)
UOF	Update of	Cites the article being updated
SPIN	Summary for patients in	Cites a patient summary article
ORI	Original report in	Cites a scientific article associated with the patient summary

Courtesy of the National Library of Medicine

Technologies (http://www.ovid.com/) and Aries Systems (http://www1.kfinder. com/), license the content for a fee and provide value-added services that can be accessed for a fee by individuals and institutions.

3.2.1.2 Other NLM Bibliographic Resources

MEDLINE is only one of many databases produced by the NLM. Not only are a number of more specialized databases also available, but they are also accessed from a variety of interfaces. Although most of these databases are bibliographic, some provide full text (described in Sect. 3.3). In general, the NLM's other databases have fields defined in ways similar or identical to MEDLINE.

In response to the growing number of databases and users' desires to mix and match them differently, the NLM reorganized its bibliographic databases in 2002 into three general categories (Anonymous, 2000):

Table 3.4 PubMed subsets (Anonymous, 2004d)

Subset	Description
AIDS	Journal citations in the area of AIDS and HIV
Abstracts	All journal citations containing abstracts
Ahead of print	Journal citations that appear on the Web in advance of the journal issue's release
Bioethics	Journal citations in the area of bioethics
Cancer	Journal citations in all areas of cancer
Complementary medicine	Journal citations in the area of complementary and alternative medicine
Consumer health	Journal citations in the area of consumer health
Core clinical journals	Journal citations within a list of 120 core clinical journals; formerly the *Abridged Index Medicus*
Dental journals	Journal citations in the area of dentistry
History of medicine	Journal citations in the area of the history of medicine
Index Medicus journals	Journal citations from over 5,000 journal titles found in the *Index Medicus*
MEDLINE	Over 16 million journal citations from 1966 to present
MEDLINE and OLDMEDLINE	Over 18 million journal citations from the 1950s to present
Nursing journals	Journal citations in the area of nursing
OLDMEDLINE	Journal citations before 1966
PubMed	Search all of PubMed without any filters or limits
PubMed Central	Digital archive of life sciences journal literature
Space Life Sciences	Journal citations in the area of space life sciences
Systematic Reviews	Journal citations identified as systematic reviews and evidence-based medicine
Toxicology	Journal citations in the area of toxicology

Courtesy of the National Library of Medicine

1. Citations to journal and other periodical articles from 1966 to the present
2. Citations to books, monographs, whole serials, and audiovisual material
3. Citations to selected journal articles published prior to 1966 and scientific meeting abstracts

The primary interface for journal citations is PubMed, which itself is part of the large Entrez system (http://www.ncbi.nlm.nih.gov/sites/entrez). The main interface for access to books, serials, and audiovisual materials is provided by LOCATOR-plus (http://locatorplus.gov), which is essentially the NLM's OPAC, though it also contains some materials that do not reside at the NLM, such as those owned by the regional libraries of the National Network of Libraries of Medicine or other organizations that have agreements with NLM. The Entrez system has also added the ability to search the "NLM Catalog," which has all the content present in LOCATORplus (Jacobs, 2004).

```
UI  - 88050247
PMID- 3675956
DA  - 19871231
DCOM- 19871231
LR  - 20001218
IS  - 0889-7190
VI  - 33
IP  - 3
DP  - 1987 Jul-Sep
TI  - Effects of 25(OH)-vitamin D3 in hypocalcemic patients on
chronic hemodialysis.
PG  - 289-92
AD  - Department of Medicine, College of Medicine, University of
Illinois, Chicago.
AU  - Kronfol NO
AU  - Hersh WR
AU  - Barakat MM
LA  - eng
PT  - Journal Article
CY  - UNITED STATES
TA  - ASAIO Trans
JC  - ASA
JID - 8611947
RN  - 0 (Parathyroid Hormones)
RN  - 32222-06-3 (Calcitriol)
RN  - 7440-70-2 (Calcium)
RN  - 7723-14-0 (Phosphorus)
RN  - EC 3.1.3.1 (Alkaline Phosphatase)
SB  - IM
MH  - Alkaline Phosphatase/blood
MH  - Calcitriol/*therapeutic use
MH  - Calcium/blood
MH  - Comparative Study
MH  - Human
MH  - Hypocalcemia/*drug therapy/etiology
MH  - Parathyroid Hormones/blood
MH  - Phosphorus/blood
MH  - Renal Dialysis/*adverse effects
EDAT- 1987/07/01
MHDA- 1987/07/01
PST - ppublish
SO  - ASAIO Trans 1987 Jul-Sep;33(3):289-92.
```

Fig. 3.1 Sample MEDLINE record (courtesy of the National Library of Medicine)

Historically, the NLM did not index scientific meeting abstracts except in a few specific subject areas and continues not to do so generally. This is because, in general, conference proceedings publications are thought to be less critically peer-reviewed than journal publications as well as of less interest to searchers outside the specialty from which they were generated. However, some conference proceedings abstracts are in MEDLINE, while others are available through the NLM Gateway described in Sect. 3.5.2.

3.2.1.3   Non-NLM Bibliographic Databases

The NLM is not the sole producer of bibliographic databases. A number of other entities, public and private, produce a wide variety of databases. Many of these databases used to be available from the two largest online information vendors, BRS (assets now owned by Ovid) and Dialog (Dialog Corp., http://www.dialog. com/). Now, however, many information producers provide access to their bibliographic databases directly on their own Web sites. In the discussion that follows, we consider non-NLM bibliographic databases that we group into those of large general coverage, subject-specific, and content-type specific.

There are other large general biomedical bibliographic databases besides MEDLINE. One of these is Scopus (http://www.scopus.com/), a product of Elsevier (http://www.elsevier.com/) that includes 29 million records covering 15,000 journals from 4,000 publishers, including 5,300 health science journals (Burnham, 2006). Scopus also includes links to the full text of articles as well as cited and citing documents. The database also contains patents and scientific Web pages. Elsevier also publishes a subset of these in another database called EMBASE (http://info.embase.com/), which is complementary to MEDLINE. EMBASE has a more international focus, including more non-English-language journals. These journals are often important for those carrying out systematic reviews and meta-analyses, who need access to all the studies done across the world.

Another bibliographic database of sorts, although perhaps an example of how the borders of our content classification schema can blur, is Google Scholar (http:// scholar.google.com/), which contains links to full-text scientific articles on the Web, even those that are protected by passwords (for subscribers) (Banks, 2005; Henderson, 2005). As will be noted in Chaps. 4 and 5, the interface to Google Scholar is similar to that of Google, with searching by words in articles and sorting of results by number of Web links to the article. Google Scholar has inspired other approaches, such as Microsoft's Windows Academic Live (http://academic.live. com/), which is currently limited to mostly computer science, electrical engineering, and physics journals, although some biomedical content has started to appear.

A variety of subject-specific bibliographic databases have existed for several decades, but have evolved in the modern era. Some come from other US government agencies. For example, the Department of Education produces the ERIC (*Educational Resources Information Center*) database (http://www.eric.ed.gov/), which has more than 1.2 million citations from education-related literature. Others come from private companies. For example, the major database for the nursing and allied health fields is CINAHL (*Cumulative Index to Nursing and Allied Health Literature*, CINAHL Information Systems, http://www.cinahl.com/), which covers nursing, physical therapy, occupational therapy, laboratory technology, health education, physician assistants, and other allied health fields. Another prominent subject-specific database is PsycINFO (http://www.apa.org/psycinfo/), which is produced by the American Psychological Association. PsycINFO is a bibliographic database with more than 2.3 million references from more than 2,150 journals dating back to 1887. A database of peer-reviewed journal literature for the complementary and alternative medicine field is the *Manual Alternative and Natural Therapy Index System* (MANTIS, http://www.healthindex.com/), which has more than 280,000 records and indexes from more than 1,000 journals in its database. In the bioinformatics/text mining community, a new bibliographic database is *Biomedical Literature (and text) Mining Publications* (BLIMP, http://blimp.cs. queensu.ca/).

A number of computer and information science bibliographic resources are valuable for the biomedical informatics field. One is CiteSeer (also at one point called ResearchIndex, http://citeseer.ist.psu.edu/), which maintains a database of computer-science-oriented (including biomedical informatics) scientific literature. Each record contains bibliographic data, links to the full text (if available), and links to other papers that it cites as well as those that cite it. Other bibliographic databases for computer science include the following:

- The Collection of Computer Science Bibliographies – http://liinwww.ira.uka.de/ bibliography/
- Digital Bibliography & Library Project – http://www.informatik.uni-trier.de/ ~ley/db/
- ACM Guide to Computing Literature – http://portal.acm.org/guide.cfm
- Computer Network Bibliography – http://www.cs.columbia.edu/~hgs/netbib/

Some bibliographic databases tend to be focused more on specific types of content. Two well-known databases that provide alternate access to the medical literature are *Current Contents* (Thomson Scientific, http://scientific.thomson.com/products/ ccc/) and *BIOSIS Previews* (BIOSIS, http://www.biosis.org/). The *Current Contents* series provides bibliographic indexes with abstracts for a variety of scientific fields, including biomedicine. The databases began as monthly diskette subscription products but now are all available on the Web. *BIOSIS Previews* offers access to a number of resources that are not available in the databases already mentioned, including citations to research and technical reports, conference proceedings, symposia, and other sources.

Other bibliographic databases provide access to online resources. For medical educators, the Association of American Medical Colleges has developed MedEd-PORTAL (http://www.aamc.org/mededportal/), a database of peer-reviewed medical education resources. Each record in the database contains metadata about the resource, such as its educational objectives and document type. Also of interest to medical educators and others is HEAL (*Health Education Assets Library*, http:// www.healcentral.org/), a repository of free, Web-based multimedia teaching materials in the health sciences. A more general database of learning objects is MERLOT (*Multimedia Educational Resource for Learning and Online Teaching*, http://www.merlot.org/). Likewise, for computer programmers, a bibliographic resource is Krugle (http://www.krugle.org/), which is a database of open source computer code as well as information about computer code.

A database of all available books is *Books in Print* (R.R. Bowker, http://www. booksinprint.com/). Of course, the major online booksellers such as Amazon.com (http://www.amazon.com/) and Barnes & Noble (http://www.bn.com/) also can be considered to maintain bibliographic databases of books (that they sell). Another important database is *Dissertation Abstracts* (ProQuest Information and Learning, http://wwwlib.umi.com/dissertations/), which provides a citation for virtually every dissertation submitted to North American universities since 1861. Abstracts of dissertations were added in 1980, and in 1988, citations from a number of European universities began to be included.

3.2.2   Web Catalogs and Feeds

Although some may not consider Web catalogs to be bibliographic content, they share many features with traditional bibliographic databases. This is especially true for Web catalogs that provide other content on their sites or more exhaustive descriptions of Web sites than a traditional bibliographic database might. One of the original Web catalogs was Medical Matrix (http://www.medmatrix.org/), which existed before the Web as a text file of medical resources on the Internet. It has since developed an exhaustive database of sites that are rated by its editorial board consisting of physicians and other health-care professionals. For each topic area, a variety of links are provided for different types of resources. Some other early medical Web catalogs, now defunct, include Cliniweb (Hersh, Brown et al., 1996) and HealthWeb (Redman, Kelly et al., 1997).

A variety of other health-oriented Web catalogs exist, each with unique features. Some are oriented to health professionals and include the following:

- Intute (http://www.intute.ac.uk/healthandlifesciences/medicine/) – formerly called OMNI, a Web catalog maintained by universities in the United Kingdom, with a medical portion listed at the above-mentioned link
- HON Select (http://www.hon.ch/HONselect/) – a European catalog of clinician-oriented Web content from the Health on the Net Foundation
- Translating Research into Practice (TRIP, http://www.tripdatabase.com/) – allows searching over the titles and/or full text of a wide variety of evidence-based online resources, including full-text journals, electronic textbooks, and EBM databases

Other Web catalogs are oriented to consumers. A number of the large general search engines have portions with catalogs of health content, such as Google (http:// www.google.com/Top/Health/), Yahoo (http://health.yahoo.com/), and Open

Directory (http://www.dmoz.org/Health/). Some specific consumer-oriented catalogs include the following:

- HealthFinder (http://www.healthfinder.gov/) – consumer-oriented health information maintained by the Office of Disease Prevention and Health Promotion of
  the US Department of Health and Human Services.
- MedStory (http://www.medstory.com/) – recently acquired by Microsoft, this
  site features health information filtered by specific "media partners" vetted for
  producing content of high quality.
- WebMD (http://www.webmd.com/) – a Web catalog is part of this much larger
  consumer health information site.

A growing bibliographic-type resource on the Web is RSS, which is claimed to
stand for either Really Simple Syndication or Rich Site Summary (Hammersley,
2005). RSS feeds provide short summaries, typically of news or other recent
postings on Web sites. Many news sites, such as CNN (http://www.cnn.com/) and
BBC (http://www.bbc.co.uk/), make extensive use of them. Users receive RSS
feeds by an RSS aggregator that can typically be configured for the site(s) desired
and to filter based on content.

There are unfortunately a number of different versions of RSS, although each
has the fundamental fields and most aggregators can handle all of the different
versions. The various versions can be grouped into two categories. One category
(version 1.0) builds on the Resource Description Framework and aims to allow rich
metadata, while the other category (version 2.0) uses plain XML and aims to be
simpler. The fundamental fields of RSS include the following:

- Title - name of item
- Link - URL of full page
- Description - brief description of page

Here is an example of XML code from an RSS item from the BBC:

```
<title>
Google maps give fresh perspective
</title>
<link>
http://news.bbc.co.uk/go/rss/-/2/hi/technology/4448807.stm
</link>
<description>
Search engine Google offers users the chance to see satellite photos of many
locations in North America.
</description>
```

RSS is not limited to news feeds. In fact, there are a growing number of innovative
uses for it in scientific fields (Hammond, Hannay et al., 2004). Certainly it can be
used for newly published scientific papers as an information notification application, similar to the electronic table of contents most journals already offer. This is
already being done by the Nature Publishing Group and Highwire Press. *Nature*

also circulates its job advertisements via RSS. More recently, NLM has made MEDLINE records available via RSS (Canese, 2005).

3.2.3   Specialized Registries

A specialized registry overlaps with literature reference databases and Web catalogs but can be considered to be distinct in that it points to more diverse information resources. An example of a specialized registry is the *Catalog of U.S. Government Publications*, which provides bibliographic links to all governmental publications whether in print, online, or both (http://www.access.gpo.gov/su_docs/locators/cgp/).

Another specialized registry of great importance for health care is the *National Guidelines Clearinghouse* (NGC, http://www.guideline.gov/). Produced by the Agency for Healthcare Research and Quality (AHRQ), it contains exhaustive information about clinical practice guidelines. Some of the guidelines produced are freely available, published electronically or on paper, or both. Others are proprietary, in which case a link is provided to a location at which the guideline can be ordered or purchased. The overall goal of the NGC is to make evidence-based clinical practice guidelines and related abstract, summary, and comparison materials widely available to health-care and other professionals. The fields provided in the NGC are listed in Table 3.5.

The criteria for a guideline being included in the NGC are as follows:

- Contains systematically developed statements that include recommendations, strategies, or information that assists physicians and/or other health-care practitioners and patients in making decisions about appropriate health care for specific clinical circumstances
- Produced under the auspices of medical specialty associations; relevant professional societies: public or private organizations: government agencies at the federal, state, or local level; or health-care organizations or plans
- Corroborating documentation can be produced and verified that a systematic literature search and review of existing scientific evidence published in peer-reviewed journals was performed during the guideline development
- Written in the English language, current, and the most recent version produced (i.e., documented evidence can be produced or verified that the guideline was developed, reviewed, or revised within the last 5 years)

3.3   Full Text Content

Full-text content contains the complete text of a resource as well as associated tables, figures, images, and other graphics. If a database has a corresponding print version, then the text portions of the electronic and print versions should be nearly

Table 3.5 Fields in National Guideline Clearinghouse

Attribute
Guideline title
Bibliographic source(s)
Number of references
Guideline availability
Availability of companion documents
Availability of related patient resources
Guideline status/Update information
Guideline length
Issuing organization(s)
Guideline developer(s)
Guideline developer comment
Guideline endorser(s)
Adaptation
Organization type
Source(s) of funding
Funding source ID
Guideline committee
Composition of group that authored the guideline
Date released
Guideline category
Clinical specialty
Disease/Condition(s)
Guideline objective(s)
Method of review of the guideline recommendations
Description of method of review of the guideline recommendations
Implementation plan developed? (Yes/No)
Description of implementation strategy
Intended users
Target population
Age of target population
Sex of target population
Interventions and practices considered
Major outcomes considered
Cost analysis
Methods used to collect the evidence
Description of methods used to collect the evidence
Number of source documents
Methods used to assess the quality and strength of the evidence
Rating scheme for the strength of the evidence
Methods used to analyze the evidence
Description of methods used to analyze the evidence
Qualifying statements
Major recommendations
Clinical algorithm(s)
Type of evidence supporting recommendations
Potential benefits
Subgroup(s) of patients most likely to benefit
Potential harms
Subgroup(s) of patients most likely to experience these harms

Courtesy of the Agency for Healthcare Research and Quality

identical. The original full-text databases were online versions of journals and thus tended to be either primary literature or mixtures of primary and secondary literature. As the price of computers and CD-ROM drives fell in the early 1990s, adaptation of nonjournal secondary sources such as textbooks increased. This trend has not only continued with the growth of the Internet but led to the development of vast Web sites with information aimed at a variety of audiences.

Full-text products usually do not have associated human-assigned indexing terms. Instead, the indexing terms are typically the words that appear in the text, as will be described in Chap. 5.

3.3.1 Periodicals

The technical impediments to electronic publishing of journals have long passed, and as was discussed in Chap. 2, the challenges now are mostly political and economic (Hersh and Rindfleisch, 2000). Just about all scientific journals, certainly those in health and biomedicine, are now published electronically. Commercial publishers such as Springer (http://www.springer.com/) and Elsevier (http://www.elsevier.com/) tend to sell vast collections of their journals to large customers, such as libraries, instead of individual subscribers. Many health and biomedical journals published by nonprofit publishers (typically scientific and medical societies) publish their journals though Highwire Press (http://www.highwire.org/), a spin-off of the Stanford University Library that provides a Web site, searching and browsing interfaces, and development tools for journals whose publishers have not moved directly into electronic publishing. Some well-known journals that utilize Highwire Press include the *British Medical Journal* (http://www.bmj.com/), the *New England Journal of Medicine* (http://content.nejm.org/), and *Journal of the American Medical Informatics Association* (http://www.jamia.org/).

Some journals have been developed exclusively in electronic format, such as the journals of Biomed Central (http://www.biomedcentral.com/) and *Journal of Medical Internet Research* (http://www.jmir.org/). Many of these journals follow the open-access publishing model introduced in Sect. 2.6.1 and described more fully in Sect. 6.4.3). Biomed Central features more than 180 peer-reviewed journals on a variety of biological and health topics, including medicine, cell biology, medical informatics, etc. The success of Biomed Central in the biomedical domain has spawned similar efforts in chemistry (http://www.chemistrycentral.com/) and physics, mathematics, and computer science (http://www.physmathcentral.com/). Another family of open-access journals, some of which are published in paper, is the Public Library of Science (PLoS, http://www.plos.org/). One recent innovation from PLoS is PLoS ONE, which aims to break down the disciplinary walls between journals and also provide an open and innovative form of postpublication peer review (after the initial traditional peer review to deem acceptance) (MacCallum, 2007a).

A number of government entities provide periodical information in full-text form. Among the best known of these are *Morbidity and Mortality Weekly Report* (MMWR, http://www.cdc.gov/mmwr/) from the Centers for Disease Control and Prevention and *AHRQ WebM&M: Morbidity and Mortality Rounds on the Web* (http://www.webmm.ahrq.gov/).

Electronic publication of journals allows additional features that were not possible in the print world. Journal editors often clash with authors over the length of published papers (editors want them short for readability whereas authors want them long to be able to present all ideas and results). To address this situation, *British Medical Journal* initiated an electronic-long, paper-short system that provided longer versions of papers on the Web site, which did not appear in the shorter print versions in the journal. Journal Web sites can provide additional description of experiments, results, images, and even raw data. A journal Web site also allows more dialogue about articles than could be published in a Letters to the Editor section of a print journal. Electronic publication also allows true bibliographic linkages, both to other full-text articles and to the MEDLINE record, typically from PubMed. These features are also facilitated by the Highwire software. Most journals provide access to PDF versions of articles that print in a more readable format than a Web page, usually in a layout identical to the printed version.

Another source for full-text journal articles is the repository PubMed Central (PMC, http://pubmedcentral.gov/), the rationale for which is explained in Chap. 6. PMC contains articles from several hundred journals that deposit them. It also includes manuscripts submitted by authors representing research done via funding from NIH grants, based on a policy adopted that encourages grantees to submit the final document submitted to the journal after peer review but before typesetting (Anonymous, 2005f). These are submitted by authors using the NIH Manuscript Submission System (NIHMS, http://www.nihms.nih.gov/).

NLM and PMC have attempted to bring more standardization to electronic journal publishing with the NLM Journal Archiving and Interchange Document Type Definition (http://dtd.nlm.nih.gov/). This provides a standard way to format content for NLM databases in XML. There are four specific tag sets for archiving and interchanging:

1. Archiving and Interchange Tag Set – enables an archive to capture as many of the structural and semantic components of existing printed and tagged journal material as conveniently as possible, with no effort made to model any particular sequence or textual format
2. Journal Publishing Tag Set – optimized for the archives that wish to regularize and control their content, not to accept the sequence and arrangement presented to them by any particular publisher
3. Article Authoring Tag Set – designed for authoring new journal articles, where regularization and control of content is important
4. NCBI Book Tag Set – written specifically to describe volumes for the NCBI online libraries

Another effort of PMC is the Back Issue Digitization Project, which aims to scan back issues of participating journals (http://www.pubmedcentral.gov/about/scanning.html). The scanned pages for each article are combined into a single PDF file. The text has optical character recognition (OCR) applied for searching, although OCR errors are not corrected.

3.3.2   Books and Reports

The most common secondary literature source is the traditional textbook, an increasing number of which are available in electronic form. One of the first textbooks available electronically was *Scientific American Medicine*, now *ACP Medicine* (http://www.acpmedicine.com/). Other venerable print textbooks now available electronically include the *Physician's Desk Reference* (Medical Economics, Inc., http://www.pdr.net/) and the *Merck Manual* (Merck & Co., http://www.merck.com/mmpe/). The latter is one of the few traditional medical textbooks available for free on the Web.

A common approach with textbooks is to bundle them, sometimes with linkages across the aggregated texts. An early bundler of textbooks was *Stat!-Ref* (Teton Data Systems, http://www.statref.com/), which like many began as a CD-ROM product and then moved to the Web. *Stat!-Ref* offers more than 30 textbooks. Another early product that implemented linking early was a combination of *Harrison's Principles of Internal Medicine* and the drug reference *U.S. Pharmacopeia*, which is now part of a large collection called *AccessMedicine* (http://www.access-medicine.com/). Some other well-known providers of multiple online textbooks are *MDConsult* (http://www.mdconsult.com/) and eMedicine (http://www.emedicine.com/).

Electronic textbooks offer additional features beyond text from the print version. Although many print textbooks do feature high-quality images, electronic versions offer the ability to have more pictures and illustrations. They also have the ability to use sound and video, although few do at this time. As with full-text journals, electronic textbooks can link to other resources, including journal references and the full articles. Many Web-based textbook sites also provide access to continuing education self-assessment questions and medical news. And finally, electronic textbooks let authors and publishers provide more frequent updates of the information than is allowed by the usual cycle of print editions, where new versions come out only every 2–5 years.

Making a textbook or other tertiary literature source usable as an electronic database requires some reorganization of the text. The approach used by most vendors is to break books down into "documents" along their hierarchical structure. Since the text of most books is divided into chapters, sections, subsections, and so forth, a typical approach will be to reduce the text to the lowest level in a subsection. Figure 3.2 demonstrates how this is done in the *Merck Manual*. The indexing and retrieval based on this approach are described in the next two chapters.

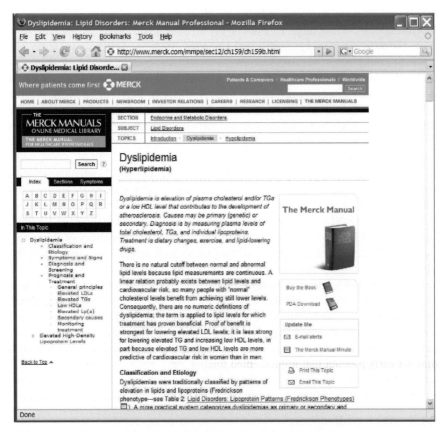

Fig. 3.2 A section from the textbook *Merck Manual* (courtesy of Merck)

Another type of publication long of interest to clinicians in print form is collected summaries of journal articles. Probably the best known among these are the Massachusetts Medical Society's *Journal Watch* (http://www.jwatch.org/) and, from the American College of Physicians (ACP), *Journal Club* (http://www.acpjc. org/). The latter is a supplement to ACP's journal *Annals of Internal Medicine* and uses a highly structured format designed to provide the reader all the important details of the study, including pertinent EBM statistics, such as patient population, intervention, and number needed to treat (McKibbon, Wilczynski et al., 1995).

A growing trend is to redesign full-text information for use on personal digital assistants (PDAs). The advantage of these devices for IR databases is their portability, though they are limited by constraints in screen size and memory capacity. They are often not connected to networks, though their synchronization capability allows information to be updated frequently, including over the Internet. In addition to many of the standard textbooks and references are those designed explicitly for

PDAs, probably the best-known being the drug reference ePocrates (http://www.epocrates.com/). Some large vendors of PDA-based medical content include Skyscape (http://www.skyscape.com/) and Unbound Medicine (http://www.unbound-medicine.com/).

Another large and growing collection of online textbooks is the NCBI Bookshelf (http://www.ncbi.nih.gov/entrez/query.fcgi?db=Books). Part of the NCBI Entrez system, this resource provides access to the full text of several dozen commercially published textbooks. Some of these books are also formatted for handheld devices and can be downloaded for loading on to them (http://www.ncbi.nlm.nih.gov/entrez/query/Books.live/Help/mobile.html).

One noteworthy title in this collection is *The NCBI Handbook*, which provides a great deal of information about NCBI databases and their searching (McEntyre and Ostell, 2005). Another important full-text resource, not part of NCBI Bookshelf but available through NLM Entrez, is *Online Mendelian Inheritance in Man* (OMIM, http://www.ncbi.nlm.nih.gov/sites/entrez?db=OMIM). A key feature of this reference is its linkage to references in MEDLINE as well as genomics databases, the latter of which are described in more detail in Sect. 3.4.4.

Consumer health information also has been an area of rapid growth in full-text information (Eysenbach, 2000a; Slack, Lewis et al., 2005). While traditional consumer-oriented books on health topics are still plentiful in bookstores, and some have migrated online (e.g., *The Merck Manual Home Edition*, http://www.merck.com/mmhe/), the real growth has occurred with consumer-oriented Web sites, which are described in the next section.

3.3.3   Web Collections

As noted at the beginning of the chapter, we use the term "Web collection" for the classification of discrete collections of Web pages providing full-text information. Health-oriented Web sites are produced by everyone from individuals to nonprofit entities to companies to governments. The Web has fundamentally altered the publishing of health information. To begin with, the bar of entry has been significantly lowered. Virtually anyone can have access to a Web server, and with that access, he or she can become a "publisher" of health or any other type of information. The ease of producing and disseminating has had ramifications; for example, the ease of copying content threatens protection of intellectual property, and the ease of pasting can lead to plagiarism. The Internet, through Web sites, news groups, e-mail lists, and chat rooms, also rapidly speeds the dissemination of information and misinformation. Nonetheless, there are a great many Web sites that empower the health-care provider and consumer alike.

Probably the most effective user of the Web to provide health information is the US government. The bibliographic databases of the NLM, NCI, AHRQ, and others have been described. These agencies have also been innovative in providing comprehensive full-text information for health-care providers and consumers as well. Some of these (in particular MedlinePlus) are described later as aggregations (Sect. 3.5), since they provide many different types of resources. Smaller yet still comprehensive Web sites include the following:

- The Diseases and Conditions (http://www.cdc.gov/DiseasesConditions/) and Traveler's Health (http://wwwn.cdc.gov/travel/) Web sites of the Centers for Disease Control and Prevention
- Health Information from other NIH institutes besides NLM, such as the National Cancer Institute (http://www.cancer.gov/), National Institute of Diabetes and Digestive and Kidney Diseases (http://www.niddk.nih.gov/), and the National Heart, Lung, and Blood Institute (http://www.nhlbi.nih.gov/)
- Drug use and regulatory information from the Food and Drug Administration (FDA) for professionals (http://dailymed.nlm.nih.gov/) and consumers (http://www.fda.gov/consumer/)

A large number of commercial consumer health Web sites have emerged in recent years. Of course they include not only just collections of text, but also interaction with experts, online stores, and catalogs of links to other sites. Sites with the largest amounts of full-text consumer health information include the following:

- Clinical Reference Systems – http://www.patienteducation.com/
- Healthgate – http://www.healthgate.com/
- Intelihealth – http://www.intelihealth.com/
- Netwellness – http://www.netwellness.com/
- WebMD – http://www.webmd.com/

Among the many entities that provide information for patients are the following:

- American Academy of Dermatology – http://www.skincarephysicians.com/
- American Academy of Family Physicians – http://familydoctor.org/online/fam-docen/home.html
- Federal Consumer Health Information Center – http://www.pueblo.gsa.gov/health.htm
- Oregon Health & Sciences University (OHSU) Health – http://www.ohsuhealth.com/
- RxMed – http://www.rxmed.com/

Some sites provide handouts in low-literacy formats and/or other languages, such as Spanish. These include the following:

- FDA – easily read handouts on drug topics (http://www.fda.gov/opacom/lowlit/englow.html)
- OHSU/Hood River Community Health Outreach Project – handouts in English and Spanish (http://www.ohsu.edu/library/hoodriver/pamphlets/pamphletindex.shtml)

A number of organizations have used the Web to publish the full text of their clinical practice guidelines, including the following:

- American College of Cardiology – http://www.acc.org/qualityandscience/clinical/statements.htm
- American College of Physicians – http://www.acponline.org/sci-policy/guidelines/
- American Academy of Pediatrics – http://www.aap.org/policy/paramtoc.html
- Institute for Clinical Systems Improvement – http://www.icsi.org/guidelines_and_more/
- International Diabetes Federation – http://www.d4pro.com/diabetesguidelines/
- University of California at San Francisco – http://medicine.ucsf.edu/resources/guidelines/

A number of new types of Web content have achieved prominence in recent years and found use in health and biomedicine (KamelBoulos, Maramba et al., 2006). One of these is the wiki, or free encyclopedia. Wikis allow any individual in a community to write or edit an entry. This allows massive distributed and collaborative work to be done. For example, the prototype wiki, Wikipedia (http://en.wikipedia.org/wiki/Main_Page), has millions of entries in a variety of languages. At least two wikis are devoted to general medical topics:

- Ask Dr. Wiki (http://askdrwiki.com/) – aims to be a wiki medical textbook for health-care professionals
- Clinfowiki (http://www.clinfowiki.org/) – devoted to clinical informatics

Another growing type of Web content is the weblog. Also know as a blog, it consists of running commentary on a topic and is usually maintained by a person or community. Although probably less widespread for health and biomedical topics, blogs are extremely popular in the political realm. They are also popular in virtual communities with an interest in a diversity of topics.

3.3.4 Evidence-Based Medicine Resources

Although in some ways textbooks and in other ways Web collections, evidence-based medicine (EBM) resources deserve special mention because of their unique resources as well as importance to health care. As noted in Chap. 2, there has been an evolution in EBM to make it more useful for busy clinicians with the emergence of the 4-H model of Haynes (2001) (see Fig. 2.3). This section organizes description of EBM content into the four levels of that model.

3.3.4.1 Studies

The ultimate collection of studies themselves, of course, is the full text of the articles describing those studies. Those are among the periodicals described in Sect. 3.3.1 and often accessed via the bibliographic databases discussed in Sect. 3.2.1.

Always popular among clinicians have been summaries of articles, from the abstracts as part of them to more comprehensive overviews. In the past, the latter consisted of summaries such as Current Contents and *Journal Watch*, although publications such as *ACP Journal Club* and *Evidence-Based Medicine* take a more systematic and evidence-based approach.

3.3.4.2 Syntheses

As noted in Sect. 2.8, there has been a growing tendency toward syntheses, usually in the form of systematic reviews, which may include meta-analysis when enough studies exist and are homogeneous enough to have their results combined. Many systematic reviews are published in medical journals, but once that is done, they tend to become static documents that are not updated when new studies become available. This shortcoming has led to the development of the *Cochrane Database of Systematic Reviews* (http://www.cochrane.org), which is the largest collection (though far from covering all of medicine) of systematic reviews of health and medical interventions. The Evidence-Based Practice Centers of AHRQ are also a source of systematic reviews (which they call evidence reports).

3.3.4.3 Synopses

Although some EBM purists argue that Up to Date (http://www.uptodate.com/) is not completely evidence-based, i.e. not all statements are tagged with levels of evidence or support from studies of the highest quality evidence, the resource is comprehensive and very popular among clinicians as well as those in training. Up to Date has about 4,500 topic reviews in adult and pediatric medicine, which are updated continually. Each topic has an outline that allows easy navigation. One of those outline headings is "Recommendations," which quickly gives the specific clinical recommendations for diagnosis and/or treatment of the problem. Topics are linked to both the MEDLINE references of articles cited as well as a drug compendium for specific prescribing information. Up to Date also provides a "What's New" area for each clinical topic, describing the latest clinical news in a given field. The system also has links to a drug reference, PubMed MEDLINE references, and patient education information.

Another resource growing in size and comprehensiveness is The Physicians' Information and Education Resource (PIER, http://pier.acponline.org/) from ACP. PIER is designed to be the comprehensive information resource for practitioners of adult primary care medicine. PIER is organized into modules that are categorized under seven topic types:

- Diseases
- Screening and Prevention
- Complementary/Alternative Medicine

- Ethical and Legal Issues
- Procedures
- Quality Measures
- Drug Resource

As of now, the largest category of modules is Diseases, with more than 500 developed. Figure 3.3 shows the front page of a sample disease module. The content for each disease is organized under the following headings:

- Prevention
- Screening
- Diagnosis
- Consultation for Diagnosis – when to consider obtaining subspecialty consultation for the diagnosis
- Hospitalization – important issues to address in the patient hospitalized with the disease
- Nondrug Therapy
- Drug Therapy
- Patient Education – pertinent issues to educate the patient about with the disease

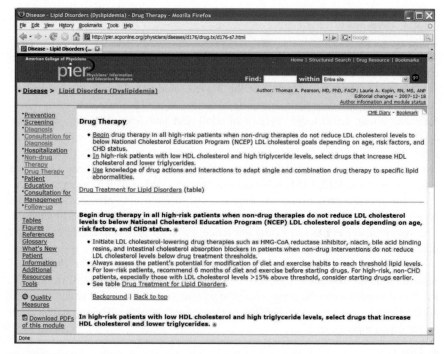

Fig. 3.3 A disease module from the Physicians' Information and Education Resource (courtesy of American College of Physicians)

- Consultation for Management – when to consider obtaining subspecialty consultation for management
- Follow-up

Modules also include references, patient information, additional references, and a PDF file of entire module for printing. A handheld version is also available (http://pier.acponline.org/pierpdajump.html), and the underlying system is constructed in a modular way to allow access via other applications, such as electronic health records. PIER has also been licensed, not only by some conventional publishers but also by some electronic health record vendors for context-aware linkage from the medical record. PIER has also completed the full circle back to paper, setting the foundation for a series in *Annals of Internal Medicine* devoted to providing evidence-based overviews of diseases, such as diabetes mellitus (Laine, Goldmann et al., 2007).

Every single guidance statement and recommendation in PIER is given a strength of recommendation rating to help the clinician assess its usefulness. The evidence criteria vary for the study type (e.g., randomized controlled trials for therapeutic or preventive interventions). References drawn from the medical literature are also given a level of evidence rating.

Another widely distributed and comprehensive resource is *Clinical Evidence* (http://www.clinicalevidence.com/). Billed as an "evidence formulary," *Clinical Evidence* classifies each intervention for a given medical condition into the following categories:

- Beneficial – interventions for which effectiveness has been demonstrated by clear evidence from RCTs, and for which expectation of harms is small compared with the benefits
- Likely to be beneficial – interventions for which effectiveness is less well established than for those listed under "beneficial"
- Trade off between benefits and harms – interventions for which clinicians and patients should weigh up the beneficial and harmful effects according to individual circumstances and priorities
- Unknown effectiveness – interventions for which there are currently insufficient data or data of inadequate quality
- Unlikely to be beneficial – interventions for which lack of effectiveness is less well established than for those listed under "likely to be ineffective or harmful"
- Likely to be ineffective or harmful – interventions for which ineffectiveness or harmfulness has been demonstrated by clear evidence

An additional comprehensive collection of EBM content consists of POEMS ("patient-oriented evidence that matters"), which are short evidence-based synopses. Topics are selected based on whether they address a question faced by physicians, measure outcomes that physicians and their patients care about (e.g., symptoms, morbidity, quality of life, and mortality), and have the potential to change the way medicine is practiced. The main component of InfoPOEMS (http://www.infopoems.com/) is InfoRetriever, a resource that includes a variety of evidence-based content and tools, including all POEMs, *Cochrane Database of Systematic Reviews* abstracts, decision support tools, diagnostic calculators supporting selection and interpretation of diagnostic tests and the history and physical examination, summaries of practice guidelines, and the reference *Five-Minute Clinical Consult*.

The Family Practice Inquiries Network (http://www.fpin.org/) is a project led by leading Departments of Family Medicine in the US. It features several resources:

- Clinical Inquiries (http://www.fpin.org/CI/) – The goal of this resource is to develop a resource that answers 80% of primary care clinical questions in 60 s. This is being done by collecting the most common clinical questions and providing specific answers to them. In some ways this is analogous to the "Frequently Asked Questions" (FAQs) seen on many Web sites.
- Evidence-Based Practice (http://www.ebponline.net/) – a newsletter that contains "help desk" answers to clinical questions.
- PEPID (http://www.pepid.com/) – a suite of information resources for various specialties of practicing physicians.

A number of commercial publishers have begun to offer "evidence-based" products, such as Thomson (http://www.micromedex.com/products/) and Elsevier (http://www.elsevier.com/wps/subject/cws_home/H03). Another evidence-based resource focused specifically on complementary and alternative medicine is Natural Standard (http://www.naturalstandard.com/).

3.3.4.4   Systems

As noted in Sect. 2.8.4, the market for systems content is still quite small. Some of the early providers of this content, such as order sets and clinical decision support rules, are Thomson Publishing (http://clinical.thomsonhealthcare.com/) and Zynx Health (http://www.zynx.com/).

3.4   Annotated Content

As noted earlier, annotated content has its metadata tightly integrated with the content (as opposed to being in a separate bibliographic database). It includes resources such as images, citation databases, and biomedical research data. Although these types of content are usually annotated with some amount of text, and searched with IR systems, their make-up is of predominantly nontextual material or nonnarrative text.

3.4.1   Images

Images have always been an important part of health-care practice, education, and research, and a variety of image collections have been made available on the Web. These collections tend to come and go, and often their Web addresses change over time. Table 3.6 provides a sampling of current image databases. Another listing of image sites is available at http://www.library.uthscsa.edu/internet/ImageDatabases. cfm.

Some image collections in Table 3.6 merit special mention. One is the *Visible Human Project* of the NLM, a collection of three-dimensional representations of normal male and female bodies (Spitzer, Ackerman et al., 1996). It consists of cross-sectional slices of cadavers, with sections of 1 mm thickness in the male and 0.3 mm thickness in the female. Also available from each cadaver are transverse computerized tomography and magnetic resonance images. The raw images themselves are very large: each of the 1,871 cross-sectional anatomic images is 2,048 × 1,216 pixels at 24-bit color, for a size of 7.5 MB per image. Compressed (e.g., JPEG) versions of the images have also been made available, which are more feasible for use in Web-based applications. A variety of searching and browsing interfaces have been created that can be accessed via the project Web site (http:// www.nlm.nih.gov/research/visible/visible_human.html).

There are some noteworthy aspects of some of the image databases listed in Table 3.6. The Digital Anatomist Project (http://sig.biostr.washington.edu/projects/ da/) models anatomical structures and the knowledge associated with them (Brinkley and Rosse, 1997). Its indexing approach is described in the next chapter. MyPACS allows clinicians to post and discuss cases. The Goldminer project provides access to images in a group of radiology journals (Kahn and Thao, 2007).

A number of commercial image collections are also available, such as Images. MD (Current Medicine, http://www.images.md/) and VisualDx (Logical Images, http://www.logicalimages.com/prodVDx.htm). A site of growing prominence for nonmedical images is Flickr (http://www.flickr.com/), which lets individuals upload their pictures and allows anyone to annotate them. Fickr was recently acquired by Yahoo.

3.4.2   Videos

The growth of broadband (high-speed) connections has made possible the delivery of videos over the Web. Although not nearly as prolific as the established image collections described in the previous section, there are a growing number of videos and sites that serve them. Two examples are the Medical Gross Anatomy Dissection Videos (University of Michigan, http://anatomy.med.umich.edu/courseinfo/video_index. html) and a collection of surgical procedure videos (NLM, http://www.nlm.nih.gov/ medlineplus/surgeryvideos.html).

Table 3.6 A sampling of medical image databases on the Web

Name	Organization	Web address
General purpose		
Visible Human	National Library of Medicine	http://www.nlm.nih.gov/ research/visible/ visible_human.html
Images from the History of Medicine	National Library of Medicine	http://wwwihm.nlm.nih.gov/
Mascagni	University of Iowa	http://www.lib.uiowa.edu/ hardin/mascagni/
HON Media	Health on the Net Foundation	http://www.hon.ch/ HONmedia/
Dermatology		
Atlas of Dermatology	Loyola University Medical Center	http://www.meddean.luc.edu/ Lumen/MedEd/medicine/ dermatology/melton/atlas.htm
Dermatology Imaging Bank	University of Utah	http://library.med.utah.edu/kw/ derm/
Dermatologic Image Database	University of Iowa	http://tray.dermatology.uiowa. edu/DermImag.htm
Dermatology Image Atlas	Johns Hopkins University	http://dermatlas.med.jhmi.edu/ derm/
Dermatologic On-Line Image Atlas	University of Heidelberg and University of Erlangen	http://www.dermis.net/
DermNet Skin Disease Image Atlas	Interactive Medical Media LLC	http://www.dermnet.com/
Pathology		
WebPath	University of Utah	http://www-medlib.med.utah.edu/ WebPath/webpath.html
Pathology Education Instruction Resource (PEIR)	University of Alabama at Birmingham	http://www.peir.net/
Pathology Atlas of Gross and Microscopic Images	Columbia University	http://cpmcnet.columbia.edu/dept/ curric-pathology/pathology/ pathology/pathoatlas/
Urbana Atlas of Pathology	University of Illinois	http://www-s.med.uiuc.edu/m2/ pathology/PathAtlasf/titlepage. html
Radiology		
BrighamRad	Brigham and Women's Hospital	http://brighamrad.harvard.edu/ education/online/tcd/tcd.html
Interactive Radiology Atlas	SUNY Downstate Medical Center	http://ect.downstate.edu/ courseware/rad-atlas/
MedPix Medical Image Database	Uniformed Services University	http://rad.usuhs.edu/medpix/
Cardiothoracic Imaging	Yale University	http://info.med.yale.edu/intmed/ cardio/imaging/
MyPACS	Vivalog Technologies	http://www.mypacs.net/
Goldminer	American Journal of Roentgenology	http://goldminer.arrs.org/

Of course, an increasingly well-known site for general videos is YouTube (recently acquired by Google, http://www.youtube.com/). A site that is both a repository for academic videos and an ongoing research project is the Open Video Digital Library (http://www.open-video.org/) (Marchionini, Wildemuth et al., 2006).

3.4.3 Citations

Chapter 2 described bibliometrics, the field concerned with linkage of the scientific literature. Bibliometric databases can be very useful in IR; that is, searchers may wish to find new articles by tracing references from those they have found. The *Science Citation Index* (SCI) and *Social Science Citation Index* (SSCI) are databases of citations in the scientific literature that are available in *Web of Science* (Thomson Scientific, http://scientific.thomson.com/products/wos/). Figure 3.4 shows a screen with citations to some of the author's works.

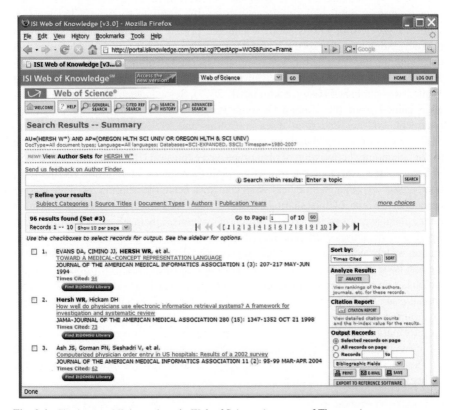

Fig. 3.4 Citations and links to them in *Web of Science* (courtesy of Thomson)

Another system for citation indexing is the Research Index (formerly called CiteSeer, citeseer.nj.nec.com) (Lawrence, Giles et al., 1999). This index uses a process called *autonomous citation indexing* that adds citations into its database by automatically processing the papers from the Web. It also attempts to identify the context of citations, showing words similar across citations such that the commonality of citing papers can be observed. The Research Index is not as complete or up-to-date as the Web of Science.

3.4.4   Molecular Biology and -Omics

In Sect. 3.3.4, we explored a variety of types of full-text content and then focused in on one specific domain, EBM. In this section we will do likewise, focusing further on annotated content from molecular biology and the various -omics (e.g., genomics, proteomics, metabolomics, etc.). The first -omics to gain prominent was genomics, the field studying genetic material in living organisms. A milestone in genomics was reached in 2001 with the publication of a "working draft" of the human genome published simultaneously by the publicly sponsored Human Genome Project (Anonymous, 2001d) and the private company Celera Genomics (Venter, Adams et al., 2001). The final sequence of the 3 billion nucleotides that constitute the human genome was completed in 2003 (Collins, Morgan et al., 2003). More recently, the complete publication of the founder of Celera Genomics, Craig Venter, was published (Levy, Sutton et al., 2007). Some have argued that the knowledge gained from the Human Genome Project will revolutionize the diagnosis, treatment, and prevention of disease (Collins and McKusick, 2001). Since then, other sources of -omics data have emerged and been shared publicly all the way up to the "phenome," consisting of phenotype data expressed (Butte and Kohane, 2006).

One unique aspect of the molecular biology research community (certainly in comparison to other biomedical sciences) has been the sharing of data among researchers. Some of this sharing has been made possible by the development of public databases from the NCBI. However, scientists themselves as well as those developing databases with genome-related content have in general made their information widely available. The myriad of genomics databases are reviewed annually in the first issue of the journal *Nucleic Acids Research* (http://nar.oxfordjournals.org/), which is now published as open access and is freely available on the Web. A related annual issue has emerged more recently devoted to Web services providing access to bioinformatics tools (Fox, McMillan et al., 2007). Another aggregation of bioinformatics resources has been developed by the University of Pittsburgh (http://www.hsls.pitt.edu/guides/genetics/obrc) (Chen, Chattopadhyay et al., 2007).

The NCBI organizes molecular biology databases into the following categories (Wheeler, Barrett et al., 2007):

- Database retrieval tools
- Sequence-similarity search programs (BLAST and related programs)
- Resources for gene-level sequences (including polymorphisms)

- Resources for genome-scale analysis (including chromosome maps)
- Resources for analysis of patterns of gene expression and phenotypes
- Resources for molecular structure and proteomics

All of these databases are linked to related resources among each other; for example, a nucleotide sequence is linked to a gene, its location on a chromosome, and its three-dimensional structure. The resources are also linked to PubMed and OMIM (Online Mendelian Inheritance in Man) in the NCBI's Entrez system (http:// www.ncbi.nlm.nih.gov/Entrez/).

The prototype nucleotide sequence database is GenBank (Benson, Karsch-Mizrachi et al., 2007). This resource contains millions of nucleotide sequences and billion base pairs for thousands of different living species. GenBank is continually updated as researchers add more data and as linkages to other databases become available. It can be searched at the NLM Web site or downloaded for loading into local databases.

One of the main purposes of genomes is to transcribe nucleotide sequences into proteins. As such, there are many protein-related resources, many of which are now under the umbrella of the Universal Protein Resource (UniProt) (Anonymous, 2007v). Since the function of proteins is highly dependent upon their three-dimensional structure, protein structure databases are of increasing importance. A database of protein structures is maintained in the Molecular Modeling Database (Wang, Addess et al., 2007). Likewise, there are growing collections of annotated information related to the gene microarrays of functional genomics (Barrett, Troup et al., 2007; Demeter, Beauheim et al., 2007), the metabolome (Wishart, Tzur et al., 2007), and the phenome (Bogue, Grubb et al., 2007). One resource that attempts to bring together the names, annotations, and linkages to data sets for genome-scale analysis is SOURCE (http:// source.stanford.edu/), developed at Stanford University (Diehn, Sherlock et al., 2003).

Some NCBI databases are aggregations of other databases. Entrez Gene brings together various information about single genes (Maglott, Ostell et al., 2007), including Gene Reference in Functions (GeneRIFs), which are short annotations about the function of a gene described in an article (Mitchell, Aronson et al., 2003). The Entrez Map Viewer gives a graphical depiction of the location of a specific gene on a given chromosome, as well as links to each gene's Entrez Gene record (see Fig. 3.5). MEDLINE records that contain information about a gene in Entrez Gene now allow linkage to it through the "Link Out" function. The NLM's approach to gene indexing was recently described by Ward (2005).

The NLM has also released some other innovative genomics-related resources. One is dbGAP, the database of Genotype and Phenotype (http://view.ncbi.nlm.nih. gov/dbgap) (Mailman, Feolo et al., 2007). This database is a repository of data from genomewide association studies that attempt to associate findings in genes (genotype) with features of living organisms (phenotype). Another recent genomics resource from NLM is the *Genetics Home Reference* (http://ghr.nlm.nih.gov/) (Mitchell, Fun et al., 2004). This resource draws on publicly available resources, most of which are written for professionals, but presents them with additional material to provide a view more understandable to the lay public (Fomous, Mitchell et al., 2006).

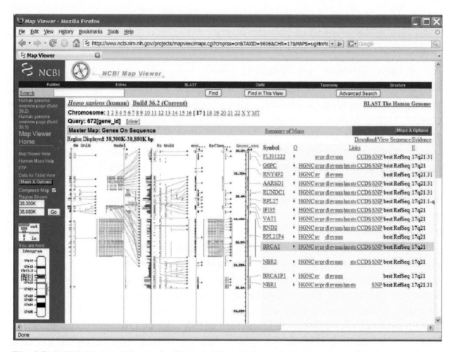

Fig. 3.5 NCBI (National Center for Biotechnology Information) map viewer for the *BRCA1* gene (courtesy of the National Library of Medicine)

Of course, the "central dogma" of molecular biology, where DNA is transcribed into RNA and translated into protein, is under increasing challenge. One project aiming to investigate other functions of DNA is the Encyclopedia of DNA Elements Project (ENCODE, http://www.genome.gov/10005107). A portal has been developed to provide access to all the data and tools for this project (Thomas, Rosenbloom et al., 2007).

3.4.5 Other Databases

There are a variety of other databases of annotated content:

- *Computer Retrieval of Information on Scientific Projects* (http://crisp.cit.nih. gov/) – a database of all of grants, contracts, and other projects conducted or funded by the NIH.
- PubChem – The growing amount of chemical information, particularly that which is relevant to biological activity, has led the NLM to create the PubChem database (http://pubchem.ncbi.nlm.nih.gov/) (Sayers, 2005). This resource shows chemical structures, related substances, biological activity, and linkages to the biomedical literature.
- HSRProj – a database of ongoing projects in health services research (http:// www.nlm.nih.gov/hsrproj/).

- Google Maps – This is not the first map application, but it provides Google's typical ease of use and links the drawn maps to satellite images (http://maps.google.com/).
- Google Earth – provides more detailed images and maps in an application that runs on a local machine (http://earth.google.com/).
- Search capabilities over the documents, e-mails, viewed Web pages, and so forth, on one's own computer. Both the Windows and Macintosh operating systems allow searching over information in files on their disks these days. In addition, Web search engine vendors such as Google offer "desktop searching" tools (http://desktop.google.com/). There is a growing concern that these tools may allow "leakage" of corporate and other (potentially medical) data outside protected networks, since the indexing data is stored remotely (i.e., on Google's desktop searching site) (Bednarz and Dubie, 2006).
- Cartograms – redrawing of maps of countries or states to represent other items of interest, such as economic status, prevalence of diseases, or voting patterns (http://www-personal.umich.edu/~mejn/cartograms/).
- MedWatch – Web site for reporting of, and published reports on, safety and adverse events from medical drugs and devices (http://www.fda.gov/medwatch/).

Another database specifically worthy of mention is ClinicalTrials.gov. Beginning as a database of clinical trials sponsored by NIH, ClinicalTrials.gov has taken on a new role with the requirement for registration of clinical trials. After problems were uncovered with postinception protocol changes in clinical trials, the International Committee of Medical Journal Editors adopted a policy of requiring registration at inception of study (DeAngelis, Drazen et al., 2005). This requires that clinical trials be registered in ClinicalTrials.gov (Zarin, Tse et al., 2005) or other comparable databases (Haug, Gotzsche et al., 2005) before they begin in order to be later published. The data elements required for registration in ClinicalTrials.gov have been published and are summarized in Table 3.7 (Anonymous, 2007d).

ClinicalTrials.gov does not contain results of clinical trials, although many advocate that it or other comparable resources provide results of clinical trials (Korn and Ehringhaus, 2006). Not only could readers get more details about the results of such trials, but those who carry out systematic reviews would have easier and better access to data. Indeed, Derry et al. (2001) have noted that articles of clinical trials in the medical literature are usually inadequate for reporting adverse events discovered in those trials. Some advocate even larger availability of raw data from clinical trials, although others have expressed caution that not only peer review but also patient privacy protection could be compromised (Fisher, 2006). One large-scale approach currently advocated is the Global Trial Bank, promoted by the American Medical Informatics Association (Sim and Detmer, 2005). A recent report commissioned by the NLM focused on clinical trials reporting and databases for the purpose of improving the efficiency of systematic reviews (Carson, Cohen et al., 2007). Table 3.8 lists other databases of clinical trials beyond ClinicalTrials.gov.

Table 3.7 Required elements to register a clinical trial in ClinicalTrials.gov

1. Unique trial number	The unique trial number will be established by the primary registering entity (the registry).
2. Trial registration date	The date of registration will be established by the primary registering entity.
3. Secondary IDs	May be assigned by sponsors or other interested parties (there may be none).
4. Funding source(s)	Name of the organization(s) that provided funding for the study.
5. Primary sponsor	The main entity responsible for performing the research.
6. Secondary sponsor(s)	The secondary entities, if any, responsible for performing the research.
7. Responsible contact person	Public contact person for the trial, for patients interested in participating.
8. Research contact person	Person to contact for scientific inquiries about the trial.
9. Title of the study	Brief title chosen by the research group (can be omitted if the researchers wish).
10. Official scientific title of the study	This title must include the name of the intervention, the condition being studied, and the outcome (e.g., The International Study of Digoxin and Death from Congestive Heart Failure).
11. Research ethics review	Has the study at the time of registration received appropriate ethics committee approval (yes/no)? (It is assumed that all registered trials will be approved by an ethics board before commencing.)
12. Condition	The medical condition being studied (e.g., asthma, myocardial infarction, depression).
13. Intervention(s)	A description of the study and comparison/control intervention (s). (For a drug or other product registered for public sale anywhere in the world, this is the generic name; for an unregistered drug the generic name or company serial number is acceptable.) The duration of the intervention(s) must be specified.
14. Key inclusion and exclusion criteria	Key patient characteristics that determine eligibility for participation in the study.
15. Study type	Database should provide drop-down lists for selection. This would include choices for randomized vs. nonrandomized, type of masking (e.g., double-blind, single-blind), type of controls (e.g., placebo, active), and group assignment, (e.g., parallel, crossover, factorial).
16. Anticipated trial start date	Estimated enrollment date of the first participant.
17. Target sample size	The total number of subjects the investigators plan to enroll before closing the trial to new participants.
18. Recruitment status	Is this information available? (yes/no) (If yes, link to information.)
19. Primary outcome	The primary outcome that the study was designed to evaluate description should include the time at which the outcome is measured (e.g., blood pressure at 12 months).
20. Key secondary outcomes	The secondary outcomes specified in the protocol. Description should include time of measurement (e.g., creatinine clearance at 6 months).

Adapted from DeAngelis, Drazen et al., 2005

3.5   Aggregations

The real value of the Web, of course, is its ability to aggregate completely disparate information resources. This chapter so far has focused for the most part on individual resources. This section provides some examples of highly aggregated resources oriented toward consumers and professionals. We will also look in detail at two specific types of aggregations, the body of knowledge and model organism database.

3.5.1   Consumer Health Aggregations

One of the largest aggregated consumer information resources is MedlinePlus (http://medlineplus.gov/) from the NLM (Miller, Lacroix et al., 2000). It includes representatives of the types of resources already described, aggregated so that they are easily accessed for a given topic. At the top level, MedlinePlus contains the following:

- Health Topics
- Drugs and Supplements
- Medical Encyclopedia
- Dictionary
- News
- Directories

The selection of MedlinePlus topics is based on analysis of those used by consumers to search for health information on the NLM Web site (Miller, Lacroix et al., 2000). Each topic contains links to health information from the NIH and other sources deemed credible by its editorial staff. There are also links to current health news, a medical encyclopedia, drug references, and directories, along with a preformed PubMed search, related to the topic. Figure 3.6 shows the top of the MedlinePlus page for cholesterol.

Some MedlinePlus oriented to the elderly has been repackaged into the NIH Senior Health Web site (http://nihseniorhealth.gov/). Some innovative additional features of this site for elderly people with poor vision and/or low reading ability include the capability to enlarge the font size of the text, increase the contrast by using a black background with white or yellow text, and have the content delivered in spoken format.

A number of consumer health Web collections mentioned in Sect. 3.3.3 are actually part of larger aggregations of content that also provide features that can be used to manage health and health care. WebMD offers a variety of tools, including a personal health record and tools for risk assessment. A new consumer-oriented site, Revolution Health (http://www.revolutionhealth.com/), offers similar features.

Table 3.8 Clinical trials results databases

Database	Internet address	Sponsor
Pharmaceutical-industry-sponsored		
ClinicalStudyResults.org	http://www.clinicalstudyresults.org/home/	PhRMA
AstraZeneca	http://www.astrazenecaclinicaltrials.com/	AstraZeneca
Bayer Healthcare	http://www.bayerhealthcare.com/index.php?id=224&L=2	Bayer Healthcare
Boehringer Ingelheim	http://trials.boehringer-ingelheim.com/Trial_Results/index.jsp	Boehringer Ingelheim
Bristol-Myers Squibb	http://ctr.bms.com/ctd/ResultProductAction.do?type=all	Bristol-Myers Squibb
Eli Lilly	http://lillytrials.com/results/results.html	Eli Lilly
Forest	http://www.forestclinicaltrials.com/CTR/CTRController/CTRWelcome	Forest
Glaxo SmithKline	http://ctr.gsk.co.uk/welcome.asp	Glaxo SmithKline
Novartis	http://www.novartisclinicaltrials.com/clinicaltrialrepository/public/main.jsp	Novartis
Organon	http://www.organon.com/clinical_trials/Clinical_Trial_Results/index.asp	Organon
Roche	http://www.roche-trials.com/	Roche
Sanofi-Aventis	http://www.sanofi-aventis.us/live/us/en/layout.jsp?scat=E7C27A86-08F4-4798-8241-710051CE000A#p4	Sanofi-Aventis
Government-sponsored		
Drugs@FDA	http://www.accessdata.fda.gov/scripts/cder/drugsatfda/	FDA
European Medicines Agency	http://www.emea.eu.int/index/indexh1.htm	EMA
National Cancer Institute Clinical Trials	http://www.cancer.gov/clinicaltrials/results/	National Cancer Institute
ReFeR (Research FindingsRegistry) Department of Health research findings directory	http://www.refer.nhs.uk/ViewWebPage.asp?Page=Home	UK Department of Health
Other funding		
RCT Bank (Global Trial Bank Project)	http://rctbank.ucsf.edu/Presenter/ also http://www.globaltrialbank.org/	NLM, AMIA

Adapted from Carson, Cohen et al., 2007

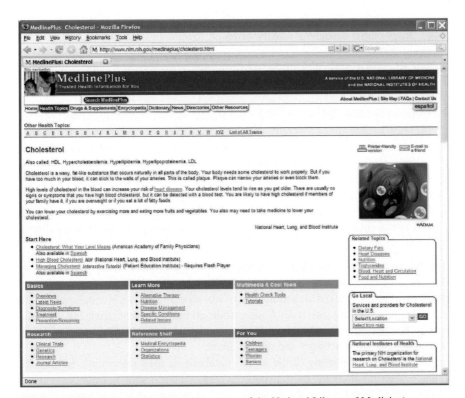

Fig. 3.6 MedlinePlus topic Cholesterol (courtesy of the National Library of Medicine)

3.5.2 Professionals' Content Aggregations

Consumers are not the only group for whom aggregated content has been developed. Some commercial efforts have also attempted to aggregate broad amounts of clinical content along with content about practice management, information technology, and other topics. These include the following:

- MDConsult (http://www.mdconsult.com/) – developed by several leading medical publishers.
- Unbound Medicine (http://www.unboundmedicine.com/) – another commercial resource for Web-based and PDA-based clinical content.
- Clineguide (http://www.clineguide.com/) – combines a summary of diseases and treatments with drug information, full-text resources from the SKOLAR system developed at Stanford, and the database access system Ovid into a single product.
- Merck Medicus (http://www.merckmedicus.com/) – developed by the well-known publisher and pharmaceutical house, available to all licensed US physicians, and including such well-known resources as *Harrison's Online*, MDConsult, and Dxplain.

- DrugBank (http://redpoll.pharmacy.ualberta.ca/drugbank/) – features a variety of drug-related resources mostly oriented toward researchers (Wishart, Knox et al., 2006).
- MICROMEDEX Healthcare Series (http://www.micromedex.com) – integrates a number of former standalone databases into a comprehensive clinical information resource.
- Partners in Information Access for the Public Health Workforce (http://phpartners.org/) – integrates a variety of information sources related to public health.
- United Kingdom National Library for Health (http://www.library.nhs.uk/) – A variety of free and commercial resources are available, including *Clinical Evidence*, the full text of over 800 journals, the Cochrane Library, and a variety of bibliographic databases.
- INFOMED – The Cuban National Health Care Telecommunications Network and Portal (http://www.sld.cu/) – from a more resource-limited country (Séror, 2006).

The NLM provides a number of aggregations. One is the Entrez system already described in several places in this chapter. Another is the NLM Gateway (http://gateway.nlm.nih.gov/), which aims to provide access to all NLM databases within via a single searching interface. A more focused but still comprehensive aggregation is ToxNet (http://toxnet.nlm.nih.gov/), which includes bibliographic and full-text resources on toxicology and related areas.

The innovation in many of the -omics databases is their integration. Indeed, the linkage of information and the way data are shared differ distinctly from conventions in the clinical world, where the databases, including many described in this chapter, exist as information islands or silos on the Web. Although most clinical databases are easy to reach and to navigate, there is no simple way to seamlessly move across them (e.g., link from a database of systematic reviews to the original studies comprising a review or a textbook description of the disease or treatment being reviewed). Likewise, a person cannot "mix and match" one's different favorite clinical resources into a unified digital library. Not surprisingly, the real barriers are economic, i.e., publishers do not want to link a user to the resources of a competitor.

3.5.3 Body of Knowledge

A growing approach to aggregation in a specific domain is the body of knowledge. One of the earliest and most comprehensive was the Software Engineering Body of Knowledge (SWEBOK, http://www.swebok.org/). The goal of this resource is to map all of the knowledge of the field of software engineering (Bourque et al., 1999). The paper by Bourque et al. summarized the challenges in creating such a resource. For example, where does one draw the line between the discipline of software engineering and related ones, such as computer science, cognitive science, management science, and systems engineering. Likewise, what should be the depth of the material presented? The project chose to adopt the approach of including "generally accepted" knowledge, which applies to most situations most of the time and has widespread consensus about its value and effectiveness. This type of knowledge was distinguished from "advanced and research" knowledge, which was not yet mature, and "specialized" knowledge, which was not yet generally applicable.

There is one body of knowledge project in biomedical informatics, the Health Information Management (HIM) Body of Knowledge managed by the American Health Information Management Association (AHIMA, http://library.ahima.org/). It includes the following:

- Most *Journal of AHIMA* articles published since January 1998
- Many *AHIMA Advantage* articles published since January 2002
- Various AHIMA practice briefs, position statements, reports, guidelines and white papers, job descriptions, and other AHIMA information
- Government publications such as parts of the Federal Register and Department of Health and Human Services documents
- Links to other useful HIM documents
- Practice guidance reports on current e-HIM topics

3.5.4 Model Organism Databases

A resource of growing importance in genomics is the model organism database, where all information (e.g., gene nomenclature, nucleotide and protein sequences, literature references, and other data) is brought together into a unified resource. What follows are among the most-developed model organism databases:

- Mouse Genome Informatics – *Mus musculus*, the house mouse (http://www.informatics.jax.org/)
- Ecocyc – genes and metabolism from the well-studied *Escherichia coli* bacterium (http://ecocyc.org/)
- Wormbase – the soil-dwelling worm, *Caenorhabditis elegans* (http://www.wormbase.org/)
- Saccharomyces Genome Database – the yeast *Saccharomyces*, which has importance for certain types of fermented beverages (http://www.yeastgenome.org/)
- FlyBase – the ubiquitous *Drosophila melanogaster* fruit fly (http://flybase.bio.indiana.edu/)

Naturally, the development of all these model organism databases has led to the development of a toolkit to facilitate their construction, the Generic Model Organism Database Construction Kit (http://www.gmod.org/) (Stein, Mungall et al., 2002).

3.5.5   Scientific Information

Some aggregations of science-oriented Web content go beyond health and biomedical science. The US government maintains a site called Science.gov that provides access by searching or browsing to the more than 50 million pages of scientific information produced by the various science-based agencies of the government. This is part of an even larger catalog of scientific information from around the world, WorldWideScience.org (http://worldwidescience.org/), which features a federated search engine that broadcasts search to each site's search engine.

Chapter 4
Indexing

In the first chapter, *indexing* was defined as the process of assigning metadata, consisting of terms and attributes, to documents. This process is also called *tagging*. There are two reasons to index document collections, one cognitive and one mechanical. The cognitive reason for indexing is to represent the content of individual documents so that searchers may retrieve them accurately. The mechanical reason for indexing is to enable computer programs to more rapidly determine which documents contain content described by specific terms and attributes.

In this chapter, we will explore the indexing process in more detail. After some introductory discussion, the two broad approaches to indexing, manual and automated, will be described. For manual indexing, approaches applied to bibliographic, full-text, and Web-based content will be presented. This will be followed by a description of automated approaches to indexing, with discussion limited to those used in operational retrieval systems. (Research approaches will be discussed in Chap. 8.) The problems associated with each type of indexing will also be explored. The final section will describe computer data structures used to maintain indexing information for efficient retrieval.

4.1 Types of Indexing

The indexing of documents for content long preceded the computer age. The most famous early cataloger of medical documents, John Shaw Billings, avidly pursued and catalogued medical reference works at the Library of the Surgeon General's Office (Miles, 1982). In 1879, Billings produced the first index to the medical literature, *Index Medicus*, which classified journal articles by topic. For over a century, *Index Medicus* was the predominant method for accessing the medical literature.

By the middle of the twentieth century, however, the chore of manually cataloging and indexing of the expanding base of medical literature was becoming overwhelming, but fortunately the beginning of the computer age was at hand. Although initial efforts at automation were geared toward improving the efficiency of the indexing and publishing process, the potential value of using computers for

W. Hersh, *Information Retrieval: A Health and Biomedical Perspective,*
doi: 10.1007/978-0-387-78703-9, © Springer Science + Business Media, LLC 2009

actual retrieval became apparent as well, with the birth of MEDLINE in the 1960s. By the 1990s, MEDLINE, the electronic version of *Index Medicus*, had made the paper version obsolete and the latter was retired in 2004 (Anonymous, 2004b).

Even though the medium has changed, the human side of indexing the medical literature for the most part has not. The main difference in the computer age is that a second type of indexing, automated indexing, has become available. Thus most modern commercial content is indexed in two ways:

1. Manual indexing – wherein human indexers, usually using standardized terminology, assign indexing terms and attributes to documents, often following a specific protocol
2. Automated indexing – wherein computers make the indexing assignments, usually limited to breaking out each word in the document (or part of the document) as an indexing term

Manual indexing has mostly been done with bibliographic databases. In the age of proliferating electronic databases, such as online textbooks, practice guidelines, and multimedia collections, manual indexing has become either too expensive or outright infeasible for the quantity and diversity of content now available. Thus there are increasing numbers of databases that are indexed only by automated means.

Recall from Chap. 1 that the indexing process uses one or more *indexing languages* to represent the content of documents and queries for retrieval of documents. In the human indexing process, the main indexing language is usually a controlled vocabulary of terminology from a field. When relationships among different terms are specified, this vocabulary is called a *thesaurus*. The indexing language for word indexing, however, consists of all the words that are used in the documents (often minus a small number of common function words, called a *stop list* or *negative dictionary*), with no control imposed.

Some authors classify indexing differently than the above-mentioned classification by distinguishing it as either *precoordinate* or *postcoordinate*. These distinctions are usually but not necessarily applied to human indexing, since they refer to whether the indexing terms are coordinated at indexing (precoordinate) or retrieval (postcoordinate) time. In precoordinate systems, the indexing terms are searchable only as a unit, thus they are "pre"-coordinated. Many early retrieval systems required precoordinated searching on full terms only, while most modern systems allow searching on the individual words of indexing terms, hence are "post"-coordinated.

4.2   Factors Influencing Indexing

A variety of factors influence indexing. Usually careful consideration must be given to selecting appropriate terms that lead to the most effective retrieval by users. Two measures reflect the depth and breadth of indexing, *specificity* and *exhaustivity*, respectively. These measures can also be used as criteria for evaluating the quality of indexing for any specific purpose. Another concern with the quality of indexing is inconsistency. While not an issue with automated systems whose computer algorithms produce the same results every time, manual indexing must be consistent for users who anticipate terms being assigned to documents they expect to retrieve. Of course, the ultimate measure of indexing quality is how well users can use the indexing to access the documents they need, which we will cover in Chap. 7.

The first measure of indexing, specificity, refers to the detail or precision of the indexing process and indicates its depth. The desired level of specificity is dependent upon both users and databases. Users with much knowledge of a subject area will likely want the highest level of specificity. Researchers, for example, may recognize distinct genes or clinical variations associated with a disease that are less known to clinicians. Thus a researcher might find indexing geared to the clinicians to be insufficiently specific, resulting in loss of precision when searching. Likewise, a clinician who found indexing geared to the researcher too specific might experience loss of recall owing to improper use of highly specific indexing terms. In general, more indexing specificity translates into better retrieval precision, assuming that searchers understand and apply the terms in their queries properly.

Exhaustivity indicates the completeness of indexing or its breadth. In the human indexing process, terms are generally assigned to documents when they are one of the focal subjects of a document. Increasing exhaustivity of indexing will tend to increase recall, since more possible indexing terms will increase the chance of retrieving relevant documents. On the other hand, excessive exhaustivity will result in diminished precision, especially if search terms are only loosely related to documents retrieved by the searcher.

The final measure of indexing quality is *consistency*. It has been shown that indexing consistency leads to improved retrieval effectiveness (Leonard, 1975). Hooper's measure has been used to indicate the percentage consistency of indexing (Funk and Reid, 1983):

$$\text{Consistency}(A, B) = \frac{i}{i + j + k} \qquad (4.1)$$

where A and B are the two indexers, i is number of terms A and B assign in agreement, j is the number of terms assigned by A but not B, and k is the number of terms assigned by B but not A. For example, if two indexers assigned 15 and 18 terms respectively, 11 of which were in agreement, their consistency would be $11 / [11 + (15-11) + (18-11)] = 0.5$ or 50%.

4.3 Controlled Vocabularies

Before discussing indexing processes in detail, it is important to describe controlled vocabularies. Although these vocabularies are most often used in manual indexing, numerous research projects have attempted to employ them for automated indexing, as described in later chapters. This section will first discuss some general principles in thesaurus construction, followed by a description of the controlled vocabulary used most often in medical IR systems, the *Medical Subject Headings* (or MeSH) vocabulary. This will be followed by a discussion of other controlled vocabularies and the Unified Medical Language System (UMLS) project.

4.3.1   General Principles of Controlled Vocabularies

Before discussing specific vocabularies, it is useful to define some terms, since different writers attach different definitions to the various components of thesauri. A *concept* is an idea or object that occurs in the world, such as the condition under which human blood pressure is elevated. A *term* is the actual string of one or more words that represent a concept, such as Hypertension or High Blood Pressure. One of these string forms is the preferred or *canonical* form, such as Hypertension in the present example. When one or more terms can represent a concept, the different terms are called *synonyms*.

A controlled vocabulary usually contains a list of certified terms that are the canonical representations of the concepts. Most thesauri also contain relationships between terms, which typically fall into three categories:

1. Hierarchical – terms that are broader or narrower. The hierarchical organization not only provides an overview of the structure of a thesaurus but also can be used to enhance searching (e.g., MeSH tree explosions described in Chap. 5).
2. Synonymous – terms that are synonyms, allowing the indexer or searcher to express a concept in different words.
3. Related – terms that are not synonymous or hierarchical but are somehow otherwise related. These usually remind the searcher of different but related terms that may enhance a search.

Another term that commonly comes up when discussing controlled vocabularies is *ontology*. There are many definitions of ontologies, and the word is sometimes used to describe any type of controlled vocabulary or terminology. A commonly cited definition and general overview of ontologies comes from Noy and McGuinness (2001). These authors describe an ontology as a "formal explicit description of concepts in a domain of discourse." Some commonly agreed upon components of an ontology are classes of general concepts, with specific instances or instantiations that represent concepts within them. Concepts have various attributes, usually connected via relationships. Concepts also have restrictions, sometimes called facets. In a pure sense, ontologies differ from terminologies in that the former richly represent a domain whereas the latter catalog its formal terms. Cimino and Zhu (2006) note that most major terminologies, while used successfully for many applications, have varying amounts to adherence to true ontological principles.

4.3.2 The Medical Subject Headings Vocabulary

Created by the NLM for indexing *Index Medicus*, the MeSH vocabulary was and is now used to index most of the databases produced by the NLM (Coletti and Bleich, 2001). MeSH now contains over 23,000 *headings* (the word MeSH uses for the canonical representation of its concepts and over 150,000 supplementary concept records in a separate chemical thesaurus (Anonymous, 2005c). In addition, MeSH contains the three types of relationships described at the end of Sect. 4.3.1:

1. Hierarchical – MeSH is organized hierarchically into 16 *trees*, which are listed in Table 4.1.
2. Synonymous – MeSH contains a vast number of *entry terms*, which are synonyms of the headings and consist mainly of variations of the headings and entry terms in plurality, word order, hyphenation, and apostrophes. These are also called *see references* because they point the indexer or searcher back to the canonical form of the term.
3. Related – terms that may be useful for searchers to add to their searches when appropriate are suggested for many headings.

The MeSH vocabulary files, their associated data, and their supporting documentation are available on the NLM's MeSH Web site (http://www.nlm.nih.gov/mesh/). There is also a Web site that provides a high-level overview (http://www.nlm.nih.gov/bsd/disted/mesh/) as well as a browser that facilitates exploration of the vocabulary (http://www.nlm.nih.gov/mesh/MBrowser.html). MeSH can also be searched via the PubMed interface (http://pubmed.gov/).

Table 4.1 The 16 trees in MeSH, under which all headings are classified

1. Anatomy [A]
2. Organisms [B]
3. Diseases [C]
4. Chemicals and Drugs [D]
5. Analytical, Diagnostic and Therapeutic Techniques and Equipment [E]
6. Psychiatry and Psychology [F]
7. Biological Sciences [G]
8. Natural Sciences [H]
9. Anthropology, Education, Sociology and Social Phenomena [I]
10. Technology, Industry, Agriculture [J]
11. Humanities [K]
12. Information Science [L]
13. Named Groups [M]
14. Health Care [N]
15. Publication Characteristics [V]
16. Geographicals [Z]
Courtesy of the National Library of Medicine

Figure 4.1 shows the screen image from the MeSH browser containing all the data in the vocabulary for the term `Hypertension`. The page displayed by the browser also displays the location of the term in the MeSH hierarchy. Figure 4.2 shows a partially pruned version of some of the terms in hierarchical proximity to `Hypertension`.

There are additional features of MeSH designed to assist indexers in making documents more retrievable. One of these is *subheadings*, which are qualifiers to headings that can be attached to narrow the focus of a term (Anonymous, 2006h). In the `Hypertension`, for example, the focus of an article may be on the diagnosis, epidemiology, or treatment of the condition. Assigning the appropriate subheading will designate the restricted focus of the article, potentially enhancing precision for the searcher. Table 4.2 lists the subheadings of MeSH and their hierarchical organization. There are also rules for each tree restricting the attachment of certain

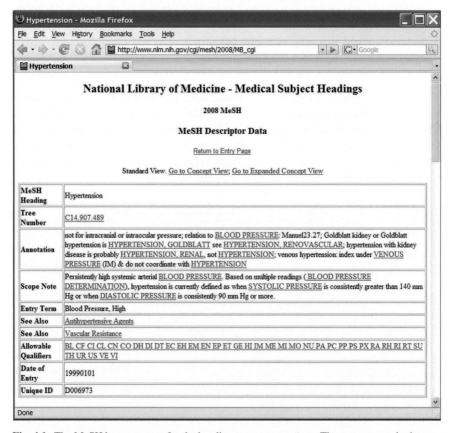

Fig. 4.1 The MeSH browser page for the heading `Hypertension`. The components in the note include the tree number, the text summarizing the term usage from the indexing manual, the scope note from the MeSH manual for searchers, an entry term (blood pressure, high), two related terms (antihypertensive agents and vascular resistance), the allowable subheadings, and other data (courtesy of the National Library of Medicine)

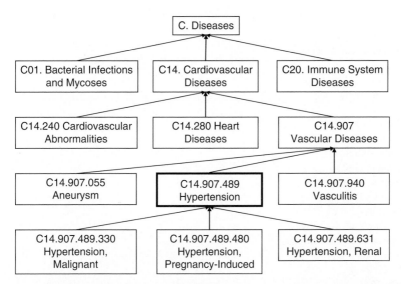

Fig. 4.2 The MeSH hierarchy for the heading `Hypertension`, which is denoted by the *heavy box*. Other (but not all) terms at each level are shown (courtesy of the National Library of Medicine)

subheadings. For example, the subheading `Drug Therapy` cannot be attached to an anatomic site, such as the femur. The allowed subheadings for a given term are shown as the *Allowable Qualifiers* in the browser (Fig. 4.1).

Another feature of MeSH that helps retrieval is *check tags*. These are MeSH terms that represent certain facets of medical studies, such as age, gender, human or nonhuman, and type of grant support. They are called check tags because the indexer is required to use them when they describe an attribute of the study. For example, all studies with human subjects must have the check tag `Human` assigned. Likewise, studies about pregnancy will require the check tags `Pregnancy` and `Female`. Related to check tags are the geographical locations in the Z tree. Indexers must also include these, like check tags, since the location of a study (e.g., Oregon) must be indicated.

Another important feature of MeSH is the *publication type*, which describes the type of publication or the type of study (Anonymous, 2006g). A searcher who wants a review of a topic will choose the publication type `Review`. Or, to find studies that provide the best evidence for a therapy, the publication type `Meta-Analysis`, `Randomized Controlled Trial`, or `Controlled Clinical Trial` would be used. MeSH features dozens of publication types (Anonymous, 2006g). (Unfortunately, `Systematic Review` is not a publication type but rather an entry term for the more general publication type `Review`. This belies the fact that systematic reviews are a special type of review, and that some systematic reviews are not amenable to meta-analysis.)

Although not necessarily helpful to a searcher using MeSH, the *tree address* is an important component of the MeSH record. The tree address shows the position

Table 4.2 MeSH subheadings

Analysis
  Blood
  Cerebrospinal fluid
  Isolation and purification
  Urine
Anatomy and histology
  Blood supply
  Cytology
  Pathology
  Ultrastructure
  Embryology
  Abnormalities
  Innervation
Chemistry
  Agonists
  Analogs and derivatives
  Antagonists and inhibitors
  Chemical synthesis
Classification
Drug effects
Diagnosis
  Pathology
  Radiography
  Radionuclide imaging
  Ultrasonography
Education
Ethics
Etiology
  Chemically induced
  Complications
  Secondary
  Congenital
  Embryology
  Genetics
  Immunology
  Microbiology
  Virology
  Parasitology
  Transmission
History
Injuries
Instrumentation
Methods
Organization and administration
  Economics
  Legislation and jurisprudence
  Manpower
  Standards
  Supply and distribution
  Trends
  Utilization
Pathogenicity

(*continued*)

Table 4.2 (continued)

Pharmacology
   Administration and dosage
   Adverse effects
   Poisoning
   Toxicity
   Agonists
   Antagonists and inhibitors
   Contraindications
   Diagnostic use
   Pharmacokinetics
Physiology
   Genetics
   Growth and development
   Immunology
   Metabolism
   Biosynthesis
   Blood
   Cerebrospinal fluid
   Deficiency
   Enzymology
   Pharmacokinetics
   Urine
   Physiopathology
   Secretion
Psychology
Radiation effects
Statistics and numerical data
   Epidemiology
   Ethnology
   Mortality
   Supply and distribution
   Utilization
Therapeutic use
   Administration and dosage
   Adverse effects
   Contraindications
   Poisoning
Therapy
   Diet therapy
   Drug therapy
   Nursing
   Prevention and control
   Radiotherapy
   Rehabilitation
   Surgery
   Transplantation
Veterinary

Indented terms are children terms hierarchically
Courtesy of the National Library of Medicine

of a MeSH term relative to others. At each level, a term is given a unique number that becomes part of the tree address. All children terms of a higher level term will have the same tree address up to the address of the parent. As seen in Fig. 4.2, the tree addresses for children terms for `Hypertension` have the same tree address up to the last number. It should be noted that a MeSH term can have more than one tree address. `Pneumonia`, for example, is a child term of both `Lung Diseases` (C08.381) and `Respiratory Tract Infections` (C08.730). It thus has two tree addresses, C08.381.677 and C08.730.610.

Another feature of MeSH is *related concepts*. Most well-designed thesauri used for IR have related terms, and MeSH is no exception. Related concepts are grouped into three types. The first is the *see related* references. These are used when one heading is reminded of another that may be more appropriate for a particular purpose. Some examples include the following:

- Between a disease and its cause, e.g., `Factor XIII Deficiency`, see related `Factor XIIIa`
- Between an organ and a physiological process, e.g., `Bone and Bones`, see related `Osteogenesis`
- Between an organ and a drug acting on it, e.g., `Bronchi`, see related `Bronchoconstrictor Agents`
- Between an organ and a procedure, e.g., `Bile Ducts`, see related `Cholangiography`

Another type of related concept is the *consider also* reference, which is usually used for anatomical terms and indicates terms that are related linguistically (e.g., by having a common word stem). For example, the record for the term `brain` suggests considering terms `cerebr-` and `encephal-`. A final category of related concepts consists of main heading/subheading combination notations. In these instances, unallowed heading/subheading combinations are referred to a preferred precoordinated heading. For example, instead of the combination `Accidents/Prevention and Control`, the heading `Accident Prevention` is suggested.

Figure 4.1 demonstrates two other features of MeSH terms. The first is the *Annotation*, which provides tips on the use of the term for searchers. For example, under `congestive heart failure`, the searcher is instructed not to confuse the term with `congestive cardiomyopathy`, a related but distinctly different clinical syndrome. Likewise, under `cryptococcus`, the searcher is reminded that this term represents the fungal organism, while the term `cryptococcosis` should be used to designate diseases caused by *Cryptococcus*. The second feature is the *Scope Note*, which gives a definition for the term.

4.3.3 Other Indexing Vocabularies

MeSH is not the only thesaurus used for indexing biomedical documents. A number of other thesauri are used to index non-NLM databases. CINAHL, for example, uses the CINAHL Subject Headings, which are based on MeSH but have additional domain-specific terms added (Brenner and McKinin, 1989). EMBASE, the so-called European MEDLINE that is part of *Excerpta Medica*, has a vocabulary called EMTREE, which has many features similar to those of MeSH (http://www.elsevier.com/wps/product/cws_home/707574). EMTREE is also hierarchically related, with all terms organized under 16 *facets*, which are similar but not identical to MeSH trees. Concepts can also be qualified by *link terms*, which are similar to MeSH subheadings. EMTREE includes synonyms for terms, which include the corresponding MeSH term.

As noted, a number of other entities use MeSH as part of the indexing process but add other attributes as well. For example, the NGC has a classification scheme that contains controlled terminology for attributes about guidelines in the following categories (http://www.guideline.gov/about/classification.aspx):

- Clinical specialty
- Disease/condition
- Guideline category
- Implementation tools
- Intended users
- IOM care need
- IOM domain
- Method of guideline validation
- Methods used to analyze the evidence
- Methods used to assess the quality and strength of the evidence
- Methods used to collect/select the evidence
- Methods used to formulate the recommendations
- Organization type
- Target population
- Treatment/intervention

The PsycINFO (http://www.apa.org/psycinfo/) database uses two indexing vocabularies. The first is the *Thesaurus of Psychological Index Terms*, containing over 8,000 terms and constructed like a typical thesaurus (Anonymous, 2007u). The second is a set of *Classification Categories and Codes*, a set of around 150 codes that classify references into broad categories of experimental psychology, treatment, education, and others (http://www.apa.org/psycinfo/about/classcodes.html).

Another vocabulary of increasing importance is the Gene Ontology (GO, http://www.geneontology.org), whose goal is to enable description of molecular biology aspects. GO covers three general areas:

- Molecular functions – the function of the gene product at the biochemical level
- Biological processes – the biological role of the gene product
- Cellular components – the part of the cell where a gene product is found

The primary use of GO is not in indexing content but rather structuring the knowledge of genes and their functions. Many of the model organism databases are devoting great resources to annotating the genes in their databases with GO codes. This work is usually done by curators who have advanced training in various fields of biology. There are more than 24,000 terms in GO, which is also now included in the UMLS Metathesaurus. An ongoing summary of the databases that use GO and the number of annotations within them are provided on the GO Web site (http://www.geneontology.org/GO.current.annotations.shtml).

GO also has *evidence codes* that indicate the level of evidence supporting the association of a term with a gene (http://www.geneontology.org/GO.evidence. html). The current evidence codes in use are shown in Table 4.3. Some of the evidence codes represent stronger levels of evidence. For example, the weakest forms of evidence are inferred from electronic annotation (IEA), where codes have been assigned based on genes identified in a sequence similarity search but have not been manually reviewed, and traceable author statement (TAS), where the author of a paper has made a statement about the function of a gene with a citation to a paper describing an experiment that has not been curated.

The Center for Bioinformatics of the National Cancer Institute (NCI, http:// ncicb.nci.nih.gov) has undertaken two vocabulary efforts, the NCI Thesaurus and the NCI Metathesaurus. The NCI Thesaurus (http://nciterms.nci.nih.gov/NCIBrowser/Dictionary.do) is focused on cancer science and covers basic, preclinical, and clinical research as well as administrative terminology associated with research management (Sioutos, deCoronado et al., 2007). Its goal is to provide a knowledge model that enabling cross-disciplinary workers to correctly interpret the meaning and relationships among entities from disciplines other than their own. The NCI Metathesaurus is described in the next section.

Table 4.3 Gene ontology evidence codes (http://www.geneontology.org/GO.evidence.html)

Curator-assigned evidence codes
Experimental evidence codes
IDA: inferred from direct assay
IPI: inferred from physical interaction
IMP: inferred from mutant phenotype
IGI: inferred from genetic interaction
IEP: inferred from expression pattern
Computational analysis evidence codes
ISS: inferred from sequence or structural similarity
IGC: inferred from genomic context
RCA: inferred from reviewed computational analysis
Author statement evidence codes
TAS: traceable author statement
NAS: nontraceable author statement
Curator statement evidence codes
IC: inferred by curator
ND: no biological data available
Automatically assigned evidence codes
IEA: inferred from electronic annotation

4.3.4   The Unified Medical Language System

One problem for the medical informatics field in general is the proliferation of different controlled vocabularies. Many of these vocabularies were developed for specific applications, such as epidemiological studies, coding for billing, and medical expert systems. It was recognized by the NLM and others as early as the 1980s that a significant impediment to the development of integrated and easy-to-use applications was the proliferation of disparate vocabularies, none of which was compatible with any other. Not only did this hamper individual applications, in that the user had to learn a new vocabulary for each application, but the integration of these applications was obstructed as well. The vision of a clinician seamlessly moving among the electronic health record, literature databases, and decision support systems could not be met if those applications could not communicate with each other by means of a common underlying vocabulary.

This is not necessarily surprising, since many vocabularies were created for different purposes. For example, MeSH is used for literature indexing while ICD-9 is used to code diagnoses for billing, SNOMED is used to represent patient-specific information, CPT-4 is used to code procedures, and so on. Many medical record systems as well as specialized decision support programs have their own vocabularies and cannot take data directly from sources other than user input. Applications designed to integrate or interact with other applications, however, cannot communicate because a common language is lacking. A number of analyses have shown that many vocabularies used in medicine for a variety of purposes do not provide comprehensive coverage of concepts (Cimino, 1998).

The UMLS Project was undertaken with the goal of providing a mechanism for linking diverse medical vocabularies as well as sources of information (Lindberg, Humphreys et al., 1993). When the project began, it was unclear what form the final products would take, and several years of work went into defining and building experimental versions of the UMLS resources (Barr, Komorowski et al., 1988; Evans, 1988; Masarie, Miller et al., 1991). There are now three components of the UMLS Knowledge Sources: the Metathesaurus, the Semantic Network, and the Specialist Lexicon (Humphreys, Lindberg et al., 1998; Bodenreider, 2004). This section focuses on the Metathesaurus, while the other components are described in connection with the research applications they are part of in later chapters. Documentation for the entire UMLS can be found at http://www.nlm.nih.gov/research/umls/documentation.html.

A major focus of the UMLS Metathesaurus has been to create linkages among these disparate vocabularies, not only assisting interprogram communication but also providing a richer vocabulary for IR and other applications. The Metathesaurus component of the UMLS links parts or all of more than 100 source vocabularies, including portions of those listed above. It is multilingual, in the sense that terms from non-English translations of its source vocabularies, mainly of MeSH, are "synonyms" of their English translations. The Metathesaurus is not a new, unified vocabulary, which some early workers advocated (Barr, Komorowski et al., 1988;

Evans, 1988; Masarie, Miller et al., 1991). Rather, it designates conceptual linkages across existing vocabularies. Another way to conceptualize the Metathesaurus is to think of it as a "repository" of vocabularies, with the source vocabularies kept unchanged and able to be extracted from the Metathesaurus.

In the Metathesaurus, all terms that are conceptually the same are linked together as a *concept*. Each concept may have one or more *terms*, each of which represents an expression of the concept from a source vocabulary that is not just a simple lexical variant (i.e., differs only in word ending or order). Each term may consist of one or more *strings*, which represent all the lexical variants that are represented for that term in the source vocabularies. Each string has an *atom* that represents the source vocabulary from which it came. One of each concept's strings is designated as the preferred form, and the preferred string of the preferred term is known as the *canonical* form of the concept. There are rules of precedence for the canonical form, the main one being that the MeSH heading is used if one of the source vocabularies for the concept is MeSH.

Each Metathesaurus concept has a single concept unique identifier. Each term has one term unique identifier (LUI), all of which are linked to the one (or more) concept unique identifier(s) with which they are associated. Likewise, each string has one string unique identifier, which in turn is linked to the LUIs in which it occurs. In 2004, a new Rich Release Format was introduced that added the atomic unit identifier (AUI), which provided a unique entry for each string in its original form from its source vocabulary, in essence allowing each string of a concept to be traced back to its source vocabulary.

Table 4.4 lists the concepts, terms, and strings for the concept `atrial fibrillation`. The English-language components are displayed graphically in Fig. 4.3. The canonical form of the concept and one of its terms is `atrial fibrillation`, with the other term being `auricular fibrillation`. Within both terms are several strings, which vary in word order and plurality.

The current Metathesaurus contains about 1.5 million concepts from more than 120 vocabularies. There are about 5 million terms, 5.5 million strings, and 7 million atoms. A total of 17 (and growing) different languages are represented. The Metathesaurus also contains a wealth of additional information. In addition to the synonym relationships between concepts, terms, and strings described earlier, there are also nonsynonym relationships between concepts. There are also a great many attributes for the concepts, terms, and strings, such as definitions, lexical types, and occurrence in various data sources. Also provided with the Metathesaurus is a word index that connects each word to all the strings it occurs in, along with its concept, term, and string identifiers.

Additional work with the Metathesaurus in the RxNorm project has aimed to improve its ability to represent clinical drugs, which may consist of more than one ingredient and have other attributes, such as brand names, strengths, and routes of administration (Nelson, Brown et al., 2002). This can be relevant to content from retrieval links that is linked to from applications such as electronic health records, e.g., an electronic prescribing application for which information about all the components of a multidrug formulation is to be displayed. The RxNav application

Table 4.4 Concept, terms, strings, and atoms for the Metathesaurus concept atrial fibrillation

Concept (CUI)	Term (LUI)	String (SUI)	Atom (AUI)
C0004238	**L0004238**	**S0016668**	**A0027665**
Atrial fibrillation (preferred)	Atrial fibrillation (preferred)	Atrial fibrillation (preferred)	Atrial fibrillation (from MSH)
Atrial fibrillations	Atrial fibrillations		**A0027667**
Auricular fibrillation			Atrial fibrillation (from PSY)
Auricular fibrillations			
		S0016669	**A0027668**
		Atrial fibrillations (plural variant)	Atrial fibrillations (from MSH)
	L0004327	**S0016899**	**A0027930**
	Auricular fibrillation	Auricular fibrillation (preferred)	Auricular fibrillation (from PSY)
	Auricular fibrillations (synonyms)		
		S0016900	**A0027932**
		Auricular fibrillations (plural variant)	Auricular fibrillations (from MSH)

CUI concept unique identifier, *LUI* term unique identifier, *SUI* string unique identifier, *AUI* atomic unit identifier
Courtesy of the National Library of Medicine

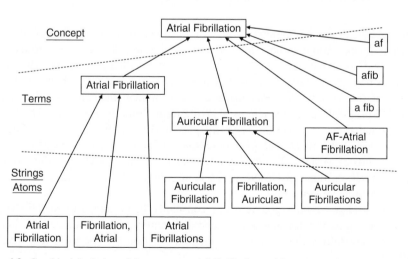

Fig. 4.3 Graphical depiction of the concept atrial fibrillation and its terms, strings, and atoms in the Unified Medical Language System Metathesaurus (courtesy of the National Library of Medicine)

has been developed that allows browsing of RxNorm (Bodenreider and Nelson, 2004).

The NCI Metathesaurus (http://ncimeta.nci.nih.gov/) is based on the UMLS Metathesaurus. Sources deemed not relevant to cancer are omitted from the UMLS Metathesaurus, while those believed to be valuable to cancer science have been added, such as Mitelman's terminology of chromosome aberrations in cancer and GO (although the latter is now in the UMLS Metathesaurus as well). The NCI Metathesaurus contains about 850,000 concepts mapped to 1.5 million terms. A public API is available for the NCI Metathesaurus server in the caCORE system (Komatsoulis, Warzel et al., 2007) (http://ncicb.nci.nih.gov/NCICB/infrastructure/cacore_overview/). The caCORE also contains a distribution of the NCI Thesaurus data.

4.4   Manual Indexing

As mentioned, manual indexing was the only type of indexing possible prior to the computer age. This circumstance may have influenced much of the early work in IR systems that focused only on this aspect of indexing (along with the fact that these early machines probably also lacked the power to build large indexes of words in databases). Virtually all human indexing systems utilize a controlled vocabulary.

4.4.1   Bibliographic Manual Indexing

Manual indexing of bibliographic content is the most common and developed use of such indexing. Bibliographic manual indexing is usually done by means of a controlled vocabulary of terms and attributes, often called a thesaurus. This function has been particularly developed by the NLM through MeSH, which will be the focus of this section. Most databases utilizing human indexing usually have a detailed protocol for assignment of indexing terms from the thesaurus. The MED-LINE database is no exception. The principles of MEDLINE indexing were laid out in the two-volume *MEDLARS Indexing Manual* (Charen, 1976, 1983). More recent descriptions of MEDLINE indexing are available on the NLM Web site (Anonymous, 2007i,o). Most MEDLINE indexers are trained in both biomedical sciences as well as manual indexing.

With a large volume of references constantly being added to MEDLINE, it would be impossible for indexers to read the entirety of every article they index. Rather, they follow the "read/scan" method outlined by Bachrach and Charen (1978):

1. Read and understand the title.
2. Read the introduction to the point at which the author states the purpose, and correlate it with the title.

3. Read chapter, section, and paragraph headings, noting italic and boldface copy; read charts, plates, and tables, laboratory methods, case reports.
4. Read the summary or conclusions.
5. Scan the bibliographic references.
6. Scan the abstract for hints about items missed in the text but confirm the existence of such items in the text.
7. Scan the author's own indexing if present.

After this process, the indexer assigns 5–12 headings, depending upon the complexity and length of the article (Bachrach and Charen, 1978). Terms are assigned if the concept is discussed and any of the following conditions is met:

- Occurs in the title, purpose, or summary
- Is significant in research generally or the results of this paper specifically
- Is a check tag
- Is covered by several sections or paragraphs
- Is in a table or figure

The major concepts of the article, usually from 2–5 headings, are designed as *central concept* headings, and designated in the MEDLINE record by an asterisk. (Noncentral concepts used to be called non-*Index Medicus* terms, since they were not represented in *Index Medicus*.) The indexer is also encouraged to assign the appropriate subheadings. Finally, the indexer must also assign check tags, geographical locations, and publication types.

The NLM also edits some of the other fields of the MEDLINE record. For example, author names are formatted with the last name followed by a space and then the initials of the first and middle (if present) names. The NLM policy on the number of authors included in the MEDLINE record has varied over the years. The current policy includes all author names, though in the past years it was limited to 10 (1984–1995) or 25 (1996–1999). When the policy changes, it applies only to new records added to the database (i.e., existing records are not changed). Author and institutional names are entered as they appear in the journal, which leads to much variation in authors' names and affiliations (e.g., some of this author's articles in MEDLINE have his name listed Hersh WR while others have `Hersh W`). Starting in 2002, the NLM added full author names to MEDLINE in the FAU field, with the previous abbreviated author name with last name and first and middle initials maintained in the old AU field (Nahin, 2003).

Another new addition to manual indexing is the indexing of gene function information in the Gene Reference into Function (GeneRIF) (Mitchell, Aronson et al., 2003). Assignment of GeneRIFs is now part of the MEDLINE indexing process, although others can nominate them to NCBI, and all GeneRIFs are added for a given gene to Entrez Gene (Maglott, Ostell et al., 2007). GeneRIFs describe the basic biology of the gene or its protein products from the designated organism, including the isolation, structure, genetics, and function of genes/proteins in normal and disease states.

McGregor (2003) has addressed the issues of indexing with MeSH outside the NLM, i.e., those who use it to index other resources. He notes that MeSH is well-tuned to indexing the biomedical literature and that the NLM devotes the resources to updating it with the terms it needs, a process that is likely to consume too much resources for most other organizations. Adding "enhanced" or "local" terminology to MeSH can be challenging. One problem is mapping terms into the proper location in the MeSH hierarchy. Another is maintaining those new terms when MeSH is revised or reorganized by the NLM. McGregor also notes that the addition of terms is sometimes political; for example, the developer of a new surgical procedure wants to be sure that the new procedure is in the index. A final problem he notes is the lack of use of the MeSH hierarchy. Non-NLM indexers usually do not follow the adage of indexing to the most specific level so searchers can take advantage of the explosion feature of retrieval (see Chap. 5), which leads to poorer search results.

4.4.2   Full-text Manual Indexing

Few full-text resources are manually indexed. One type of indexing that commonly takes place with full-text resources, especially in the print world, is that performed for the index at the back of the book. However, this information is rarely used in IR systems; instead, most online textbooks rely on automated indexing (see later). One exception to this is MDConsult (http://www.mdconsult.com/), which uses back-of-book indexes to point to specific sections in its online books.

4.4.3   Web Manual Indexing

The Web both is and is not a good place for manual indexing. On one hand, with tens of billions of pages, manual indexing of more than a fraction of it is not feasible. On the other hand, the lack of a coherent index makes searching much more difficult, especially when specific resource types are being sought. A simple form of manual indexing of the Web takes place in the development of Web catalogs and aggregations described in Chap. 3. These catalogs make not only explicit indexing about subjects and other attributes, but also implicit indexing about the quality of a given resource by the decision of whether to include it in the catalog. Some classifications are derived from well-formulated principles. The health topics selected for MedlinePlus, for example, were developed from analysis of consumers' searches on the NLM site (Miller, Lacroix et al., 2000).

This section focuses on more formal approaches to manual indexing of Web content. Several approaches to manual indexing have emerged on the Web, none of which are mutually incompatible. The first approach, that of applying metadata to Web pages and sites, is exemplified by the *Dublin Core Metadata Initiative* (DCMI, http://dublincore.org/). The second is to build directories of content, popularized initially by the Yahoo search engine (http://www.yahoo.com/). A more open approach to building directories followed with the Open Directory Project (http://www.dmoz.org/), which carries on the structuring of the directory and entry of content by volunteers across the world. Other approaches include user tagging, where individuals tag pages, and paid search, where bidders vie for having their results displayed for search terms entered by users.

4.4.3.1 Dublin Core Metadata Initiative

One of the first frameworks for metadata on the Web was the DCMI (Hillmann, 2005). The goal of the DCMI has been to develop a set of standard data elements that creators of Web resources can use to apply metadata to their content. The specification has defined 15 elements, as shown in Table 4.5 (Anonymous, 2007e). Each element is an attribute–value pair: for example, the attribute DC.Title contains the value of the name of the resource, and the attribute DC.Subject has values that list its subject domain. The elements in the DCMI do not differ greatly from metadata elements in conventional paper-based resources, such as the *Dewey decimal system* for library catalogs or the MEDLINE database for medical literature. A large number of projects have used the DCMI in a wide variety of topical areas (http://dublincore.org/projects/). The DCMI is also a standard of the National Information Standards Organization with the designation Z39.85 (Anonymous, 2007e).

The DCMI is more a semantic conceptualization than a definable syntax, and as such it does not completely identify how one is to represent the metadata. One simple approach, adopted by many organizations, is to put the metadata elements right in the Web page, using the HTML META tag. Figure 4.4 shows what metadata might be associated with this book if it were available on a Web site.

The original DCMI specification had a number of limitations. The most obvious was the lack of a standardized syntax, that is, no standard method for expressing the values of attributes. Dates are a well-known example. For example, the date 2008-2-5 is generally interpreted as February 5 in the United States and as May 2 in European countries. As any user of MEDLINE who is searching for articles by specific persons or their institutions knows, the lack of a standardized syntax, of course, is not unique to the DCMI. (Names and locations in MEDLINE are complicated by inconsistent usage in source articles.) The standardized syntax problem has been partially rectified with the development of Dublin Core Qualifiers, which recommend standards for elements such as DC.Format, DC.Language, and DC.Date (Anonymous, 2005g).

There have been several medical adaptations of the DCMI. The largest project applying the DCMI to healthcare resources is the *Catalogue et Index des Sites Médicaux Francophones* (CISMeF, http://www.cismef.org/) (Soualmia and Darmoni, 2005). A catalog of French-language health resources on the Web, CISMeF has used DCMI to catalog tens of thousands of Web pages, including information resources (e.g., practice guidelines, consensus development conferences),

Table 4.5 The Dublin core metadata element set (Anonymous, 2007e)

Dublin core element	Definition
DC.title	The name given to the resource
DC.creator	The person or organization primarily responsible for creating the intellectual content of the resource
DC.subject	The topic of the resource
DC.description	A textual description of the content of the resource
DC.publisher	The entity responsible for making the resource available in its present form
DC.date	A date associated with the creation or availability of the resource
DC.contributor	A person or organization not specified in a creator element who has made a significant intellectual contribution to the resource but whose contribution is secondary to any person or organization specified in a creator element
DC.type	The category of the resource
DC.format	The data format of the resource, used to identify the software and possibly hardware that might be needed to display or operate the resource
DC.identifier	A string or number used to uniquely identify the resource
DC.source	Information about a second resource from which the present resource is derived
DC.language	The language of the intellectual content of the resource
DC.relation	An identifier of a second resource and its relationship to the present one
DC.coverage	The spatial or temporal characteristics of the intellectual content of the resource
DC.rights	A rights management statement, an identifier that links to a rights management statement, or an identifier that links to a service providing information about rights management for the resource

```
<META NAME="DC.title" CONTENT="Information Retrieval: A Health and Biomedical
Perspective, Third Edition" >
<META NAME="DC.creator" CONTENT="William Hersh, M.D.">
<META NAME="DC.subject" CONTENT="Information storage and retrieval">
<META NAME="DC.subject" CONTENT="Biomedical Inforamtics">
<META NAME="DC.description" CONTENT="A book describing the use of information
retrieval systems in health and biomedicine.">
<META NAME="DC.publisher" CONTENT="Springer">
<META NAME="DC.date" CONTENT="2009-1-1">
<META NAME="DC.type" CONTENT="Book">
<META NAME="DC.identifier" CONTENT="http://www.irbook.info">
<META NAME="DC.language" CONTENT="en-US">
```

Fig. 4.4 Metadata for book Web site in *Dublin Core Metadata Initiative*

organizations (e.g., hospitals, medical schools, pharmaceutical companies), and databases. The Subject field uses the French translation of MeSH (http://ist. inserm.fr/basismesh/mesh.html) but also includes the English translations. For Type, a list of common Web resources has been enumerated, as given in Table 4.6 (Darmoni and Thirion, 2000).

Another large-scale Web content indexing initiative comes from Kaiser-Permanente, where a national effort aims to index all knowledge-based resources on the

Table 4.6 `DC.Type` enumeration from CISMeF

Advertisements (PT)
Architectural drawings (PT)
Commercial company
Community networks
Database (PT)
Database, bibliographic
Directory
Annual directory
Catalogs (PT)
Registry
Resource guides (PT)
Education
Teaching material
Educational courses
Instruction (PT)
Problems and exercises (PT)
Tutorial
Teaching structure
School
University
Training
Establishment, institution, organization
Foundation
Hospital
Hospital department
Image database
Library
Museum
Newsgroup and discussion list
Patient information
Periodicals (PT)
Publisher
Research structure
Scientific society
Search tools
Society
Software
Text
Bibliography (PT)
Congresses (PT)
Consensus development conference (PT)
Dictionary (PT)
Dissertation, memoir
Educational courses
Encyclopedias (PT)
Guide
Guidelines

(*continued*)

Table 4.6 (continued)

Practice guidelines
Journal article (PT)
Legislation (PT)
Medical thesis
Monograph (PT)
Problems and exercises (PT)
Technical report (PT)
Trade association, trade society

PT indicates MEDLINE publication type
Adapted from Darmoni and Thirion, 2000

health system's nationwide clinical intranet (Dolin, Boles et al., 2001). The Permanente Knowledge Connection uses a superset of the DCMI. Analysis of the indexing process found that metadata assignment for these mostly secondary literature resources was comparable to the time that human indexing is required for the primary literature in MEDLINE records by NLM indexers, which was about 15–30 min to initially catalog a resource and 5–10 min to update it when the content is revised.

The National Institute of Environmental Health Sciences (NIEHS, http://www.niehs.nih.gov/), an institute of the NIH, assessed the use of DCMI for resources on its Web site (Robertson, Leadem et al., 2001). An analysis of its use found that content authors were readily able to generate metadata and were able to do so with quality comparable to professional indexers (Greenberg, Pattuelli et al., 2002).

In addition to the problem of an underdeveloped syntax, early DCMI proposals suffered, perhaps unfairly, by being expressed in HTML. This tended to imply that the metadata would reside in Web pages. Metadata should not reside within a resource, however, particularly within Web pages. First, the practice encourages the author of the page to perform the indexing. However, the page author is not necessarily the best person to provide the metadata. He or she may be unskilled in indexing, may have an ulterior motive (such as using excess indexing terms in an attempt to increase page hits), or may not comply with the proper format of a given standard. Just as the NLM employs trained indexers to assign MEDLINE metadata, high-quality Web catalogs should employ standards of quality control and indexing expertise.

Another problem with the implication that DCMI should reside in Web pages is the assumption that all indexed resources should be at the granularity of the individual page. Like many information resources, print or electronic, many Web sites are not mere collections of HTML pages. Rather, they have organization and structure. A simple example is the online textbook in which the content is organized hierarchically. A more complex example is an aggregation Web site with pages providing not only information but also linkages across databases and applications.

The limitations in the DCMI and HTML-based metadata have been recognized, and solutions have been proposed. One emerging standard for cataloging metadata is the *Resource Description Framework* (RDF) (Manola and Miller, 2004).

A framework for describing and interchanging metadata, RDF is usually expressed in Extensible Mark-up Language (XML), a standard for data interchange on the Web. Key features of XML are its ability to express complex data, its readability, and the growing array of tools to parse and extract data from encoded documents. RDF consists of the following entities:

- A *resource* is anything that can have a unique resource identifier, which can be a Web page (identified by a URL) or an XML structure.
- A *property* is an attribute of a resource, such as an author or subject.
- A *statement* is the combination of a resource, a property, and a value for the property.

RDF is expressed in a subject–predicate–object format. An example of an RDF statement is a book (resource) authored (property) by William Hersh (value). The object can be a literal (string) or a resource. In this example, the author can be a name (literal) or structured resource, such as an XML structure with the author's name, address, phone, e-mail, and so on. RDF properties can be represented in XML. Figure 4.5 shows the metadata of Fig. 4.4 reformulated in RDF. An additional enhancement to RDF has been made. RDF does not provide mechanisms for describing properties or the relationships between them. For this reason, RDF Schema has been developed, which provides additional semantics for capturing this type of information (Brickley and Guha, 2004).

Using RDF to represent DCMI moves the metadata outside the Web page, thus decoupling metadata and content. As a result of this advantage, different metadata providers can maintain different sets of metadata. Much as the metadata of MEDLINE and EMBASE cover the same content (journal articles) but with varying overlap (higher representation of non-English journals in the latter) and different metadata schemas (e.g., MeSH vs. EMTREE), RDF allows different entities to maintain their own collections of metadata. This permits different "brands" of

```
<!DOCTYPE rdf:RDF SYSTEM "http://purl.org/dc/schemas/dcmes-xml-20000714.dtd">
<rdf:RDF xmlns:rdf="http://www.w3.org/1999/02/22-rdf-syntax-ns#"
     xmlns:dc="http://purl.org/dc/elements/1.1">
 <rdf:Description>
  <dc:title>Information Retrieval: A Health and Biomedical
          Perspective, Third Edition</dc:title >
  <dc:creator>William Hersh, M.D.</dc:creator>
  <dc:subject>Information storage and retrieval</dc:subject>
  <dc:subject>Biomedical Informatics</dc:subject>
  <dc:description>A book describing the use of information retrieval
          systems in health and biomedicine.</dc:description>
  <dc:publisher>Springer</dc:publisher>
  <dc:date>2009-1-1</dc:date>
  <dc:type>Book</dc:type>
  <dc:identifier>http://www.irbook.info<dc:identifier>
  <dc:language>en-US</dc:language>
 </rdf:Description>
</rdf:RDF>
```

Fig. 4.5 Metadata for book Web site in *Resource Description Framework*

indexing, which can compete with each other to provide the best metadata for their intended audiences. Put another way, RDF allows individuals or groups to define a common semantics expressed in a standardized syntax.

4.4.3.2 Open Directory

Another approach to cataloging content on the Web has been to create directories of content. The first major effort to create these was the Yahoo! search engine, which created a subject hierarchy and assigned Web sites to elements within it (http://www.yahoo.com/). When concern began to emerge that the Yahoo directory was proprietary and not necessarily representative of the Web community at large (Caruso, 2000), an alternative movement sprung up, the Open Directory Project (http://www.dmoz.org/). There are 15 top-level categories in the Open Directory Project, one of which is Health. Within the Health category are subcategories such as Aging, Conditions and Diseases, Insurance, Weight Loss, and Women's Health.

4.4.3.3 User Tagging

Another approach that has emerged to index various types of Web content is user tagging (Morrison, 2007). This approach has also been called "social bookmarking" (Hammond, Hannay et al., 2005) or "collaborative filtering," where a community of users (sometimes anyone on the Web) indexes and/or even rates content. The ensuing vocabularies have been called *folksonomies* (Neal, 2007). They differ from the vocabularies described earlier in that they are not controlled. Web sites that apply user tagging are the photograph sharing website Flickr (http://www.flickr.com/), the social bookmarking website del.icio.us (http://del.icio.us/), and the video sharing website YouTube (http://www.youtube.com/). Some commercial sites, such as Amazon.com (http://www.amazon.com/) and Netflix (http://www.netflix.com/), employ a form of collaborative filtering to rate books and video discs respectively.

One form of collaborative filtering has begun use for clinical sites. Haynes and Walker-Dilks (Haynes, 2005; Haynes and Walker-Dilks, 2005) have described the McMaster Online Rating of Evidence (MORE) system, where clinicians rate journal articles already filtered for scientific (i.e., evidence-based) merit using the criteria of ACP Journal Club, evidence-based medicine, evidence-based nursing, etc. These clinicians rate the articles on 7-point scales for relevance and newsworthiness. The ratings are averaged for specific medical disciplines so that users of MORE will see ratings that have been made by physicians and nurses in their own specialties. A study of physician users from around the world found that they rated systematic reviews higher for relevance to clinical practice and original studies higher for newsworthiness (Haynes, Cotoi et al., 2006).

4.4.3.4 Paid Search

Although we do not think of it as "indexing" in the traditional sense, the growing application of "paid search" is a form of indexing, albeit search terms paid to the highest bidder. Paid search is the assignment of indexing terms to content based on how much someone is willing to pay for them (Jansen, 2005). Some search engines do not distinguish between search results based on paid search, while Google has developed a tremendously successful business model by clearly demarcating *Sponsored Links* separate from its regular search results. Google's Adwords approach works by advertisers bidding on given words and phrases for how much they are willing to pay when a user sees the advertisement and clicks through to the advertiser's site (Davis, 2006). Whoever is willing to bid more for a word or phrase will rank higher in the output. Advertisers are charged only when users click through, and can set a daily maximum to not exceed a specific budget. Once the daily maximum is reached, the advertiser's advertisement will no longer appear in the Sponsored Links until the following day. Google's approach is not the only one, but is most common (Fail and Pedersen, 2005). One challenge with approaches such as Adwords is *click fraud*, where competitors or others with malicious intent can set up robots that click through advertisements just to run up the advertiser's cost to their daily maximum (Kitts, LeBlanc et al., 2005).

4.4.4 Limitations of Human Indexing

The human indexing process is imperfect. Some of its limitations stem from the use of a thesaurus, which may not contain all the important terminology in a field or may not word the terms in a way that allows nonexpert users to readily identify and apply them. One study of 75 MEDLINE queries generated in a clinical setting contained terms that could not be found in the UMLS Metathesaurus, which is a superset of the MeSH vocabulary (Hersh, Hickam et al., 1994). A thesaurus also may not be up to date. In the mid-1980s, for example, knowledge and terminology related to AIDS expanded and changed, with MeSH lagging several years behind.

Another problem with human indexing, described earlier, is inconsistency. Funk and Reid (1983) evaluated indexing inconsistency in MEDLINE by identifying 760 articles that had been indexed twice by the NLM. The most common reasons for duplicate indexing were the accidental resending of an already-indexed article to another indexer and instances of a paper being published in more than one journal. Using Hooper's equation, Funk and Reid generated the consistency percentages for each category of MeSH term shown in Table 4.7. As can be seen, the most consistent indexing occurred with check tags and central concept headings, although even these only ranged in the level of 61–75%. The least consistent indexing occurred with subheadings, especially those assigned to noncentral

Table 4.7 Consistency of MEDLINE indexing by category of *Medical Subject Headings* (MeSH) (Funk and Reid, 1983; Marcetich, Rappaport et al., 2004)

Category of MeSH	Consistency (%)	
	Funk and Reid	Marcetich et al.
Check tags	74.7	74.5
Central concept headings	61.1	48.6
Geographics	56.6	Not measured
Central concept subheadings	54.9	46.1
Subheadings	48.7	43.4
Headings	48.2	Not measured
Central concept heading/subheading combination	43.1	28.3
Heading/subheading combination	33.8	24.3

concept headings, which had a consistency of less than 35%. This study was recently replicated in the new modern indexing environment of the NLM. The results have not been formally published but were presented in a public forum and showed that human indexing consistency has not changed substantially, as seen in Table 4.7 (Marcetich, Rappaport et al., 2004).

Crain (1987) used protocol analysis in an attempt to determine the reasons for interindexer inconsistency. She observed indexers during the actual indexing process, prompting them to think aloud and explain their rationales for MeSH term assignment. Three reasons were identified as leading to inconsistencies:

1. Prior experience in assigning a concept to a MeSH term – some indexers were so used to terms appearing in articles of certain types that they automatically assigned them without a great deal of cognitive reflection.
2. Idiosyncratic rules for assigning concept importance – indexers were more likely to assign terms unfamiliar to them.
3. Differing interpretation of the instructions provided by NLM for indexers, resulting in their being applied differently among indexers.

4.5 Automated Indexing

In automated indexing, the second type of indexing that occurs in most commercial retrieval systems, the work is done by a computer. Although the mechanical running of the automated indexing process lacks cognitive input, considerable intellectual effort may have gone into development of the process, and so this form of indexing still qualifies as an intellectual process. This section will focus on the automated indexing used in operational IR systems, namely, the indexing of documents by the words they contain.

4.5.1 Word Indexing

People tend not to think of extracting all the words in a document as "indexing," but from the standpoint of an IR system, words are descriptors of documents, just like human-assigned indexing terms. Most retrieval systems actually use a hybrid of human and word indexing, in that the human-assigned indexing terms become part of the document, which can then be searched by using the whole controlled vocabulary term or individual words within it. As will be seen in the next chapter, most MEDLINE implementations have always allowed the combination of searching on human indexing terms and on words in the title and abstract of the reference. With the development of full-text resources in the 1980s and 1990s, systems that allowed word indexing only began to emerge. This trend increased with the advent of the Web.

Word indexing is typically done by taking all consecutive alphanumeric sequences between "white space," which consists of spaces, punctuation, carriage returns, and other nonalphanumeric characters. Systems must take particular care to apply the same process to documents and users' queries, especially with characters such as hyphens and apostrophes. The process usually generates an inverted file, as described in Sect. 4.7. These files can store the part of the document in which the word occurs. They may also store the word's position in the document, which can use proximity searching as described in the next chapter.

4.5.2 Limitations of Word Indexing

Simple word indexing has a number of obvious limitations, as is well known by anyone who has tried to search for information on the computer programming language Java and ended up with articles about coffee (or vice versa). The potential pitfalls include the following:

- Synonymy – different words may have the same meaning, such as `high` and `elevated`. This problem may extend to the level of phrases with no words in common, such as the synonyms `Hypertension` and `High Blood Pressure`.
- Polysemy – the same word may have different meanings or senses. For example, the word `lead` can refer to an element or to a part of an electrocardiogram machine.
- Content – words in a document may not reflect its focus. For example, an article describing `Hypertension` may make mention in passing to other concepts, such as `congestive heart failure`, that are not the focus of the article.
- Context – words take on meaning based on other words around them. For example, the relatively common words `high`, `blood`, and `pressure`, take on added meaning when occurring together in the phrase `High Blood Pressure`.
- Morphology – words can have suffixes that do not change the underlying meaning, such as indicators of plurals, various participles, adjectival forms of nouns, and nominalized forms of adjectives.

- Granularity – queries and documents may describe concepts at different levels of a hierarchy. For example, a user might query for `antibiotics` in the treatment of a specific infection, but the documents might describe specific antibiotics themselves, such as `penicillin`.

A number of approaches to these problems have been proposed, implemented, and evaluated. For example, natural language processing techniques have been tried for recognizing synonyms, eliminating the ambiguity from polysems, recognizing the context of phrases, and overcoming morphological variation. The limited successes with these approaches have been difficult to generalize and are research problems that will be described in Chap. 8. The MeSH vocabulary and associated features in MEDLINE (e.g., the explosion function described in the next chapter) have handled granularity well in the manual indexing approach, while automated approaches to recognizing hierarchical relationships have not lent themselves to generalization.

4.5.3   Word Weighting

One limitation of word indexing that has been addressed with some success is content, or the ability to give higher weight to more important words in a document that improve retrieval output. Based on an approach developed by Salton in the 1960s (Salton, 1991), this approach has proven effective particularly for inexperienced searchers, who of course comprise the majority of those using Web search engines. Sadly, Salton, a true pioneer in the IR field, passed away in 1995 just as the approach he created was starting to achieve use in large-scale operational retrieval systems.

Salton's approach goes by a variety of names, such as automated indexing, natural language retrieval, statistical retrieval, and the vector-space model. A key element, no matter what the name, has been the use of techniques that do not require manual activities. Despite widespread adoption of the weighting of indexing terms and their use in natural language retrieval with relevance ranking, other techniques innovated by Salton remain research lines of investigation and will be covered in Chap. 8. The remainder of this section will focus on Salton's basic approach, sometimes called the TF*IDF approach.

Salton's work in the 1960s was influenced by work done in the 1950s by Luhn (1957), an IBM researcher who asserted that the content of documents themselves could be used for indexing. The majority of researchers until that time had assumed that human selection of indexing terms was the most appropriate method for indexing. Luhn noted that words in English followed the *Law of Zipf*, where frequency of the word in a collection of text times rank of the word by frequency is a constant. He proposed, therefore, that words in a collection could be used to rate their importance as indexing terms. He asserted that words of medium frequency had the best "resolving power," that is, were best able to distinguish relevant from nonrelevant documents, and advocated that words with high and low frequency be removed as indexing terms.

Table **4.8** The 10 most common words in the million-word *Brown Corpus*, with rank and frequency

Term	Rank	Frequency	(Rank × frequency)/1,000
the	1	69,971	70.0
of	2	36,411	72.8
and	3	28,852	86.6
to	4	26,149	104.6
a	5	23,237	116.2
in	6	21,341	128.0
that	7	10,595	74.2
is	8	10,099	80.8
was	9	9,816	88.3
he	10	9,543	95.4
Adapted from Salton and McGill 1983			

The most well-known data to support the Zipfian distribution of the English language came from the *Brown Corpus*, a collection of word frequencies based on a variety of English language texts totaling a million words (Kucera and Francis, 1967). Table 4.8 shows the ten most common words in English, along with the Zipfian constant. The *Brown Corpus* also showed that 20% of words in English account for 70% of usage.

Salton and McGill (1983) extended Luhn's ideas and Salton was the first to implement them in a functioning system. Salton asserted that Luhn's proposals were probably too simplistic. One would not want to eliminate, for example, high-frequency words such as diagnosis and treatment, which might be necessary to distinguish documents about these subtopics of a disease. Likewise, one would not necessarily want to eliminate very-low-frequency words such as glucagonoma, since there might be few documents about this rare type of tumor in any medical database.

Salton introduced the notion of an indexing term's *discrimination value*, which is its ability to distinguish relevant from nonrelevant documents on a given topic. In practice, a term with a high discrimination value is one that occurs frequently in a small number of documents but infrequently elsewhere. The value of this approach can be shown with a hypothetical example. Consider two databases, one focused on the topic of AIDS and another covering general medicine. In the former, a word such as AIDS would be unlikely to be useful as an indexing term because it would occur in almost every document and, when it did, would be nonspecific. The words more likely to be useful in an AIDS database would be those associated with specific aspects of the disease, such as pneumocystis, carinii, and zidovudine. In a general medicine database, on the other hand, only a small portion of documents would cover the topic of AIDS and thus it would probably be a good indexing term.

The first step in word-weighted indexing is similar to all other word-based indexing approaches, which is to identify the appropriate portions of a research amenable to such indexing (e.g., the title and text of an article or its MEDLINE reference) and break out all individual words. These words are filtered to remove *stop words*, which are common words (e.g., those at the top of the *Brown Corpus* list) that always occur with high frequency and hence are always of low discrimination value. The stop word list, also called a *negative dictionary*, varies in size from the seven words of the original MEDLARS stop list (and, an, by, from, of, the, with) to the list of 250–500 words more typically used. Examples of the latter are the 250-word list of van Rijsbergen (1979) and the 471-word list of Fox (1992). The PubMed stop list is shown in Table 4.9.

It should be noted, of course, that stop words can sometimes be detrimental. For example, most stop word lists contain the word a, whose elimination would be problematic in the case of documents discussing Vitamin A or Hepatitis A. In general, however, the elimination of stop words is beneficial not only for term discrimination purposes, but also for making indexing and retrieval more computationally efficient. For example, their removal leads to a reduction in size of the inverted disk files that store indexing information, since stop words tend to have a large number of postings and thus consume disk space. Eliminating these words also allows faster query processing, since stop words tend to occur in many documents, adding to the computational requirement of building and ranking retrieval sets.

In the next step, words not on the stop list undergo *stemming* to reduce them to their root form. The purpose of stemming is to ensure words with plurals and common suffixes (e.g., -ed, -ing, -er, -al) are always indexed by their stem form

Table 4.9 The PubMed stop list (Anonymous, 2007t)

A	a, about, again, all, almost, also, although, always, among, an, and, another, any, are, as, at
B	be, because, been, before, being, between, both, but, by
C	can, could
D	did, do, does, done, due, during
E	each, either, enough, especially, etc.
F	for, found, from, further
H	had, has, have, having, here, how, however
I	i, if, in, into, is, it, its, itself
J	just
K	kg, km
M	made, mainly, make, may, mg, might, ml, mm, most, mostly, must
N	nearly, neither, no, nor
O	obtained, of, often, on, our, overall
P	perhaps
Q	quite
R	rather, really, regarding
S	seem, seen, several, should, show, showed, shown, shows, significantly, since, so, some, such
T	than, that, the, their, theirs, them, then, there, therefore, these, they, this, those, through, thus, to
U	upon, use, used, using
V	various, very
W	was, we, were, what, when, which, while, with, within, without, would

Table 4.10 A simple stemming algorithm

1. If word ends in "ies" but not "eies" or "aies" then replace "ies" with "y"
2. If word ends in "es" but not "aes", "ees," or "oes" then replace "es" with "e"
3. If word ends in "s" but not "us" or "ss" then delete "s"
Adapted from Harman, 1991

(Frakes, 1992). The benefit of stemming, however, is less clear (Harman, 1991). Not only are actual experimental results mixed, but simple algorithmic rules for stemming can be shown to lead to erroneous results (e.g., stemming `aids` to `aid`). Stemming does, however, tend to reduce the size of indexing files and also leads to more efficient query processing. A simple stemming algorithm to remove plurals is shown in Table 4.10.

The final step is to assign weights to document terms based on discrimination ability. A commonly used measure that typically achieves good results is TF*IDF weighting, which combines the inverse document frequency (IDF) and term frequency (TF). The IDF is the logarithm of the ratio of the total number of documents to the number of documents in which the term occurs. It is assigned once for each term in the database, and it correlates inversely with the frequency of the term in the entire database. The usual formula used is as follows:

$$\text{IDF}(\text{term}) = \log \frac{\text{number of documents in database}}{\text{number of documents with term}} + 1 \qquad (4.2)$$

The TF is a measure of the frequency with which a term occurs in a given document and is assigned to each term in each document, with the usual formula:

$$\text{TF}(\text{term}, \text{document}) = \text{frequency of term in document} \qquad (4.3)$$

In TF*IDF weighting, the two terms are combined to form the indexing weight, WEIGHT:

$$\text{WEIGHT}(\text{term}, \text{document}) = \text{TF}(\text{term}, \text{document}) \times \text{IDF}(\text{term}) \qquad (4.4)$$

With this weighting approach, the highest weight is accorded to terms that occur frequently in a document but infrequently elsewhere, which corresponds to Salton's notion of discrimination value.

4.5.4 Link-Based Indexing

Another automated indexing approach generating increased interest is the use of link-based methods, fueled no doubt by the success of the Google search engine. These methods have a lineage back to bibliometrics, introduced in Chap. 2, where the notion of citation gives some idea of the quality of a publication. Extended to the Web, the "Google approach" gives weight to pages based on how often they are cited by other pages. The full description of the Google retrieval engine will be presented in the next chapter, but the PageRank (PR) algorithm that values pages based on linkages is presented here.

In a simple description, PR can be viewed as giving more weight to a Web page based on the number of other pages that link to it. Thus, the home page of the NLM or JAMA is likely to have a very high PR, whereas a more obscure page will have a lower PR. The PR algorithm was developed by Brin and Page (1998). To calculate it for a given page A, it is assumed that there is a series of pages $T_1 \cdots T_n$ having links to A. There is another function $C(A)$ that is the count of the number links going out of page A. There is also a "damping factor" d that is set between 0 and 1, by default at 0.85. Then PR is calculated for A as follows:

$$PR(A) = (1 - d) + d\left(\frac{PR(T_1)}{C(T_1)} + \cdots + \frac{PR(T_n)}{C(T_n)}\right) \qquad (4.5)$$

The algorithm begins by assigning every page a baseline value (such as the damping factor) and then iterates on a periodic basis. When implemented efficiently on a moderately powered workstation, PR can be calculated for a large collection of Web pages.

Although the actual operations of Google are now highly guarded trade secrets, a number of researchers have developed and published enhancements to the original PR algorithm to make it more efficient. One approach focuses on improving input/output efficiency and also has an understandable description of the basic algorithm. An entire book has actually been written on the mathematics of PR (Langville and Meyer, 2006). PR and other forms of link-based indexing have been applied to biomedicine using data from the *Science Citation Index* (Bernstam, Herskovic et al., 2006). As will be noted later, this approach has been shown to improve the effectiveness of searching for articles deemed "important" in specialized bibliographies.

It is often stated simplistically that PR is a form of measuring the in-degree, or the number of links, that point to a page. In reality, PR is more complex, giving added weight to pages that are pointed to by those that themselves have higher PR. Fortunato et al. (2005) assessed how closely PR is approximated by simple in-degree, finding that the approximation was relatively accurate, allowing Web content creators to estimate the PR of their content by knowing the in-degree to their pages.

4.5.5   Web Crawling

The Web presents additional challenges for indexing. Unlike most fixed resources such as MEDLINE, online textbooks, or image collections, the Web has no central catalog that tracks all its pages and other content. The fluid and dynamic nature of the Web makes identifying pages to be indexed a challenge for search engines. While some Web site developers submit their site URLs, the search engines themselves must still identify all the pages within the sites. The usual approach to finding Web pages for indexing is to use "crawling" or "spidering." Essentially, the search engine finds a page, indexes all the words on the page, and then follows all links to additional pages. The process is repeated for all pages not already indexed. This process is important to search engines, as they compete with each other to be able to boast the largest size. Sites can prevent parts or all of their content from being indexed by the Robots Exclusion Protocol, whereby they place a file in their directory called robots.txt that follows a convention for allowing or disallowing crawling (Koster, 1996). (The process is voluntary, though all major search engines obey the protocol.)

Henzinger et al. (2002) have described a number of challenges for Web-crawling search engines:

- Spam – Web sites try to "game" search engines to have their pages appear at the top of the retrieval list. This is very important on the Web, where results are presented ten at a time and users may not look beyond one or two screens of output. As such, Web sites try very hard to have their sites rank as high as possible in the output. A variety of techniques are used, such as hidden text to add indexing terms that will get indexed but not appear on actual pages and increased numbers of links from other pages to influence algorithms such as PR.
- Content quality – There is no way for search engines to control the quality of pages, which is a major issue, as described in Chap. 2.
- Quality evaluation – One means for assessing quality is user feedback about pages, but it is difficult to get users to provide this consistently, and it is challenging to try to obtain by analyzing search logs.
- Web conventions – Although many Web page authors follow conventions, such as providing a brief description of what is being linked to in the anchor text of a link, this is not done in a consistent manner that automated search engines can exploit.
- Duplicate hosts – A good deal of Web content is mirrored on other Web sites, but there is no formal method for notifying search engines of this.
- Vaguely structured data – HTML pages have some structure to them, e.g., titles and META tags, but these are not used consistently and thus cannot be relied upon to provide information that automated search engines can use.

4.6   Indexing Annotated Content

As noted in Chap. 3, a growing category of information people seek to retrieve is either nontextual or text that is highly structured. As such, retrieval is usually done by searching for annotations. In this section, we describe the indexing of certain types of such data.

4.6.1   Index Imaging

The indexing of images has been described by many authors, in a general textbook (Del Bimbo, 1999), a general scientific paper (Rui, Huang et al., 1999), and more medically focused journal articles (Lehmann, Güld et al., 2004; Müller, Michoux et al., 2004). In essence, there are two basic approaches to index imaging. One is *semantic indexing*, also called textual indexing, which uses textual annotations of the image (or group of images). The other major approach to image indexing is called *content-based indexing* or *visual indexing* (Müller, Michoux et al., 2004). In somewhat of an analogy to document indexing, the semantic approach can be considered to be "manual" indexing, while the content-based approach could be called "automated" indexing.

The semantic indexing of images can be quite varied, from simple free-text descriptions (from a simple description to the detailed findings in a radiology report) to the use of more structured metadata, such as DCMI. One approach gaining increasing visibility is the Google Image search tool (http://images.google.com/), which "indexes" images by the text of the Web pages in which they appear. Another approach to radiology images in the medical literature uses the text in figure legends (Kahn and Thao, 2007). While most systems that use controlled vocabularies for indexing images apply such standard resources as MeSH, one system has been developed specifically for radiological images called RadLex (Langlotz, 2006). Although image retrieval will be discussed at greater length in the next chapter on retrieval, it should be noted here that content-based image retrieval tools typically build vectors of these features and aim to retrieve images with similar features.

A key aspect of semantic metadata for imaging systems is standardization of the image type, orientation, modality, and so forth. One approach is Digital Imaging and Communications in Medicine (DICOM) standard, which describes not only content but also a wealth of information related to the image(s) for patient care (Graham, Perriss et al., 2005). Another effort is the Image Retrieval in Medical Applications classification (Lehmann, Güld et al., 2004), which classifies images along four axes:

- Technical – image modality
- Directional – orientation
- Anatomical – body region
- Biological – organ system

Greenes et al. (1992) have noted that most clinical observations are represented along a *findings–diagnosis continuum*, where they may be expressed differently based on how much diagnostic interpretation the clinician is adding. For example, an abnormality in a chest X-ray may be described as an `increased density` by one interpreter and a `nodule` by another. The latter contains more interpretation of the finding than does the former. Thus the authors advocate a semantic network-based approach to represent findings that makes the differences along the findings–diagnosis continuum explicit. In addition to the expected slots for anatomic site, procedure type, evaluation technique, and organism observation, there are slots for the following:

1. Elemental findings – the simplest description of a finding (e.g., increased density)
2. Composite findings – a description with some deductive information added (e.g., nodule)
3. Etiologic diagnosis – a diagnosis based on inference from the finding, such as the apical infiltrations seen on a classic chest X-ray in tuberculosis
4. Inference procedure – the procedure used to infer composite findings or etiological diagnoses from elemental findings

In content-based, computer algorithms identify *features* in the image. These features include aspects of an image that a computer algorithm can recognize, such as the following:

- Color, including the intensity and sets of color
- Texture, such as coarseness, contrast, directionality, linelikeness, regularity, and roughness
- Shape, including what types are present
- Segmentation, the ability to recognize boundaries

It can be seen, however, that these features do not necessarily identify what is in the image, e.g., a chest X-ray with pneumonia or a microscopic slide of a cell. Unlike text indexing, the state of the art for visual indexing is still fairly primitive. While we can process text documents automatically and get a good sense of what they are about, we still cannot, for example, process a chest X-ray and determine that an infiltrate from pneumonia or an enlarged heart is present. Smeulders et al. (2000) have noted a *semantic gap* between the low-level features that the current state of the art for image processing can detect vs. the higher-level concepts that humans understand from looking at an image. Problematic to both types of image retrieval, they note, is a *sensory gap* between the object in the real world and as recorded in an image (Smeulders, Worring et al., 2000).

A developing standard for metadata about images is the Z39.87 Data Dictionary for Technical Metadata for Digital Still Images, which aims to define a standard set of metadata elements for digital images. Supporting the draft standard is an XML schema, called Metadata for Images in XLM (http://www.loc.gov/standards/mix/). An emerging standard for video metadata comes from the Video Development Initiative (http://www.vide.net/), which is adapting the DCMI (Agnew and Kniesner, 2001).

4.6.2 Indexing Learning Objects

Another type of content attracting a great deal of interest from an indexing standpoint is e-learning content. An emerging view in this area is that educational content should be developed as *learning objects*. Ideally, learning objects should be sharable, reusable, and able to be discovered by their metadata. An emerging standard for e-learning content is the IEEE 1484 Learning Object Metadata (IEEE LOM) standard (Ogbuji, 2003), the most recent version of which is available on the IEEE Web site (http://ltsc.ieee.org/wg12/). The IEEE LOM consists of nine general categories:

1. General
2. LifeCycle
3. Metametadata
4. Technical
5. Educational
6. Rights
7. Relation
8. Annotation
9. Classification

A number of these elements map to the DCMI (see http://www.ischool.washington.edu/sasutton/IEEE1484.html). A comparison between IEEE LOM and DCMI was carried out for the iLumina Digital Library Project, which covers science, technology, engineering, and mathematics content for college undergraduates (Heath, McArthur et al., 2005). The authors found that IEEE LOM was more comprehensive than DCMI (it has many more elements), but most of the elements deemed most important in IEEE LOM had correlates in DCMI.

A medical-specific version of IEEE LOM, Healthcare LOM, has been developed by the Medbiquitous Consortium (http://www.medbiq.org/) and integrated with learning competencies (Hersh, Bhupatiraju et al., 2006a). Healthcare LOM is also being used in the MedEdPORTAL project (http://www.aamc.org/mededportal), a database of medical educational content (Sheffield, 2006). Another approach to indexing learning objects in medicine comes from the Health Education Assets Library (HEAL, http://www.healcentral.org). The primary goal of HEAL is to develop a metadata standard for medical education content such as images, cases, quizzes, lecture slides, and so forth, so that they can be readily shared by other medical educations (Candler, Uijtdehaage et al., 2003). HEAL is part of the National SMETE Digital Library (NSDL) initiative to develop digital libraries (see Chap. 6).

4.6.3 Indexing Biological Data

With the growing quantity of biological data being generated and deposited into public repositories, there arise complementary challenges to annotate it. Birney and Clamp (2004) have described some of the challenges in the design and implementation of biological databases. The growth of data has been accompanied by the proliferation of terminology, much of it uncontrolled. This was demonstrated by

Chen et al. (2005), who analyzed ambiguity in gene naming and found that it occurred most substantially in names across species but still not infrequently with general English terms as well as medical terms. Even where there are name sets for genes or other biological entities for a given organism and/or biological entity, there is no "metathesaurus" to integrate them all. The BioThesaurus project is an effort to provide such integration of names of genes, proteins, and related entities (http://pir. georgetown.edu/pirwww/iprolink/biothesaurus.shtml) (Liu, Hu et al., 2006).

Another effort aiming to provide standard identifiers for life science is the Life Sciences Identifier (http://lsids.sourceforge.net/), which assigns a unique identifier to all biomedical research data (Clark, Martin et al., 2004). Although not widely adopted yet, the LSID uses the uniform resource name format and contains the following elements:

- LSID designator
- Authority ID – Internet domain owned by organization that assigns this LSID to a resource
- Namespace ID – name of resource chosen by organization
- Object ID – unique name of item in context of database
- Revision ID – optional parameter to keep track of different versions of same item

Salamone (2004) gives examples of how the LSID would be used. A PubMed article, for example, would have the following LSID:

```
urn:lsid:ncbi.nlm.nih.gov:pubmed:12571434
```

Likewise, a second version of the protein 1AFT in the Protein Data Bank would have the following LSID:

```
urn:lsid:pdb.org:1AFT:2
```

The Digital Anatomist Project (http://sig.biostr.washington.edu/projects/da/) has devoted great effort to modeling anatomical structures and the knowledge associated with them. An overview of the project described its motivation and challenges (Brinkley and Rosse, 1997). A recent review described the issues in modeling structural information such as anatomy (Brinkley and Rosse, 2002). The conceptual framework of the Digital Anatomist organizes structural information into the following categories:

- Spatial Database – spatial information about individual structural objects, e.g., 2-D images, 3-D volume datasets, and 3-D surface reconstructions.
- Symbolic Database – symbolic information about individual structural objects, often used to identify the spatial information, e.g., the name of the patient who had an imaging study, where images are represented as files in the spatial database, image resolution and date of acquisition, person who segmented the images, and names of the files containing the spatial data.
- Spatial Knowledge Base – spatial models describing the shape and range of variation of structural objects, such as all normal kidneys, or models describing the relationships among different objects.

- Symbolic Knowledge Base – nonspatial information about classes of structural objects. This kind of information is often studied in artificial intelligence, and forms the basis for expert systems, belief networks, decision models, and so forth.

4.7　Data Structures for Efficient Retrieval

As mentioned at the beginning of the chapter, the second purpose of indexing is to build structures so that computer programs can rapidly ascertain which documents use which indexing terms. Whether indexing is by terms in a thesaurus or words, IR systems are feasible only if they can rapidly process a user's query. A timely sequential search over an indexed text database is infeasible if not impossible for any large document collection.

A computer index usually consists of a group of *inverted files*, where the terms are "inverted" to point to all the documents in which they occur. The algorithms for building and maintaining these structures are described well by Frakes and Baeza-Yates (1992). An inverted file group for a sample document collection as it would be stored on a computer disk is shown in Fig. 4.6. The first file is the *dictionary* file,

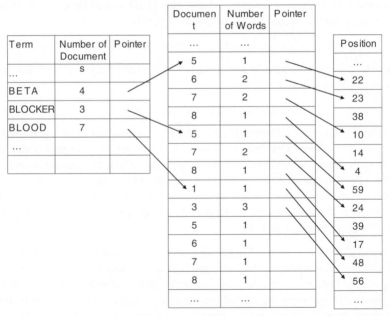

Fig. 4.6 Inverted file for a group of documents and their indexing terms BETA, BLOCKER, and BLOOD. The dictionary file contains the indexing terms, the number of documents in which they occur, and a pointer to the list of documents containing each term in the postings file. The postings file contains the document number for each indexing term, the number of words in the document, and a pointer to the list of word positions in the position file. The position file contains the word positions for the document. The pointers represent file addresses on the disk and are given by arrows rather than numbers to enhance readability

which contains each indexing term along with a number representing how many documents contain the term and a pointer to the *postings* file. The postings file consists of a sequential list of all the documents that contain the indexing term. If it is desired to keep positional information for the indexing term (to allow proximity searching), then the postings file will also contain a pointer to the *position* file, which sequentially lists the positions of each indexing term in the document. The structure of the position file depends on what positional information is actually kept. The simplest position file contains just the word position within the document, while more complex files may contain not only the word number but also the sentence and paragraph number within the document.

The final component of inverted files is a mechanism for rapid lookup of terms in the dictionary file. This is typically done with a B-tree, which is a disk-based method for minimizing the number of disk accesses required to find a term in an index, resulting in fast lookup. The B-tree is very commonly used for keys in a DBMS. Another method for fast term lookup is hashing (Wartik, Fox et al., 1992).

Of course, with the need to process millions of queries each minute, just having an efficient file and look-up structure are not enough. Systems must be distributed across many servers in disparate geographic locations. Although the details of its approach are proprietary, Google has published some on how it maintains its subsecond response time to queries from around the globe (Barroso, Dean et al., 2003; Dean and Ghemawat, 2008).

Chapter 5
Retrieval

Chapters 3 and 4 discussed the content and organization of textual databases. Chapter 3 covered the different types of databases available, while Chap. 4 showed how they are indexed for optimal retrieval. This chapter, which explores the interaction of the information retrieval (IR) system with the user, the person whom it is intended to serve, covers the entire retrieval process, from search formulation to system interaction to document access and/or delivery.

The relationship between the IR system and its users has changed considerably over the years. In the 1960s, users of the only database available, MEDLINE, had to undergo formal training at the National Library of Medicine (NLM) before being allowed access. Searching was done by filling out a form that had to be mailed to the NLM, with a "turnaround" time of 2–3 weeks for the results to be mailed back. In the 1970s, NLM databases could be directly accessed by trained searchers over time-sharing networks, though those wanting searches done still had to go through trained intermediaries, typically librarians. Of course, the user still had to make an appointment with the intermediary and wait for him or her to do the search and return the results, but this reduced the turnaround time to as low as 2–3 days. In the 1980s, online databases first became available to "early adopter" end users. Connecting to networks, then information providers, and then databases was still somewhat laborious. The 1990s saw the explosion of end user searching on the Web. The ease of use provided by powerful servers and graphical user interfaces as well as the general ubiquity of the Internet made searching a mainstream task performed by millions, with a turnaround time now down to two to three seconds. As we are in the first decade of twenty-first century, what advances will improve searching next?

We begin this chapter by discussing the search process. We then turn attention to the general principles of searching, including a description of exact-match and partial-match approaches. This is followed by discussion of specific searching interfaces. We then end with a discussion of document delivery and a specific type of retrieval known as information filtering.

W. Hersh, *Information Retrieval: A Health and Biomedical Perspective,*
doi: 10.1007/978-0-387-78703-9, © Springer Science + Business Media, LLC 2009

5.1   Search Process

Chapter 2 discussed the three general reasons for consulting IR systems (Lancaster and Warner, 1993): a need for help in solving a certain problem, a need for background information, and a need to keep up with a subject. Furthermore, for each information need, there was a spectrum of possible amounts of information needed, from a single fact to a few documents to an exhaustive collection of literature. The variation in these needs results in different strategies for interacting with the IR system.

Pao (1989) described four stages a searcher might go through before actually sitting down to an IR system:

1. Information problem – user determines that an information deficiency exists
2. Information need – user decides what must be known to solve the information problem
3. Question – user determines what motivates the interaction with the IR system
4. Request – user submits the search statement to the IR system

Based on the results of any stage, the user may return to earlier stages and modify them.

While any type of user can have any type of information need, the needs of certain groups of users are likely to differ from those of other groups. In the health and biomedicine field, one can readily discern the different needs of clinicians and researchers (Wallingford, Humphreys et al., 1990). Clinicians, including physicians, nurses, dentists, and other allied healthcare providers, are likely to have specific needs in solving problems (Gorman and Helfand, 1995). In general, they want a search to be more precise and to include the most relevant documents to their specific need. Researchers, on the other hand, are more likely to have broader needs on a given topic. For example, someone writing a paper will want a definitive overview of the topic, whereas a researcher exploring a new topic will want a great deal of background information. Researchers are likely to be more tolerant of retrieving nonrelevant references to make sure they find all the relevant ones and in fact may benefit from the "serendipity" of off-focus retrievals (Belkin and Vickery, 1985).

5.2   General Principles of Searching

Whereas each of the four stages identified by Pao (1989) is important in helping users to meet their information needs, the step of going from question to request is most important for IR system designers. After all, this is the step that will allow users to actually find documents that will meet their needs and ultimately solve their information problems. This section describes the general principles for retrieval in most currently available IR systems. It initially compares the two most common approaches to searching, exact-match (or Boolean or set-based) searching and partial-match (or natural language, ranked, or automated) searching. Then, the selection of search terms and attributes, to prepare for the description of specific searching interfaces, is discussed in Sect. 5.3.

5.2.1   Exact-Match Searching

In *exact-match searching*, the IR system gives the user all documents that exactly match the criteria specified in the search statement(s). Since the Boolean operators AND, OR, and NOT are usually required to create a manageable set of documents, this type of searching is often called *Boolean searching*. Furthermore, since the user typically builds sets of documents that are manipulated with the Boolean operators, this approach is also called *set-based searching*. Most of the early operational IR systems in the 1950s through 1970s used the exact-match approach, even though Salton was developing the partial-match approach in research systems during that time (Salton and Lesk, 1965). In modern times, exact-match searching tends to be associated with retrieval from bibliographic databases, while the partial-match approach tends to be used with full-text searching.

Typically, the first step in exact-match retrieval is to select terms to build sets. Other attributes, such as the author name, publication type, or gene identifier (in the secondary source identifier field of MEDLINE), may be selected to build sets as well. Since the user typically has an information need less broad than "all documents on a particular disease or treatment," the Boolean operators are used to focus the search output on all the elements in the information need. These operators also serve to create a document set that can be realistically analyzed. Blair (1980) spoke of the "futility point" of search results, the number of documents beyond which a searcher would stop looking at the results. He speculated that the value of this point was 50 documents, although modern search systems typically have 10 (Google) or 20 (PubMed) documents per screen of output.

Once the search term(s) and the attribute(s) have been selected, they are combined with the Boolean operators. The use of Boolean operators derives from *Boolean algebra*, which is based on *set theory*, the branch of mathematics dealing with sets and their algebraic manipulation. In set theory, a set is defined as a collection of elements. Examples of sets include all documents with the indexing term Hypertension or all students in a class. There are three common operations that are performed on sets, which correspond to the three common Boolean operators used in IR systems: intersection, union, and complement. These operations are depicted by Venn diagrams in Fig. 5.1.

The *intersection* of two sets is the set that contains only the elements that are common to both sets. This is equivalent to the Boolean AND operator. This operator is typically used to narrow a retrieval set to contain only documents about two or more concepts. For example, if one desired documents on the use of the drug propanolol in the disease Hypertension, a typical search statement might be propanolol AND Hypertension. Using the AND would most

AND – retrieve items only both

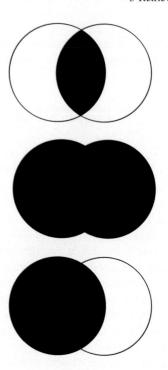

OR – retrieve items in either

NOT – retrieve items in one but not other

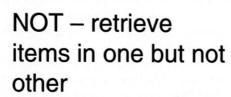

Fig. 5.1 The Boolean operators AND, OR, and NOT

likely eliminate articles, for example, on the use of `propanolol` in `migraine headaches` and the `diagnosis` of `hypertension`.

The *union* of two sets is the set that contains all the elements that occur in either set, equivalent to the Boolean OR operator. This operator is usually used when there is more than one way to express a concept. For example, the name of the virus that causes `AIDS` has carried a number of names and acronyms over the years. When simultaneously discovered by French and American scientists, it was assigned the names `Lymphadenopathy-Associated Virus` (LAV) and `Human T-Cell Leukemia Virus 3` (HTLV-3), respectively. It was later renamed `Human Immunodeciency Virus` (HIV). Likewise, one of the initial treatments for `AIDS` was originally called `azidothymidine` or `AZT`, but is now called `zidovudine`.

The *complement* of a set is the set with all the elements of some universal set that are not contained in the complemented set, equivalent to the Boolean NOT operator. However, for practical reasons, most IR systems use the NOT operator as a complement. In a large database such as MEDLINE, with its many millions of documents, the set of all documents that do not, for example, contain the term `Hypertension`, could be very large. As a result, most IR systems use NOT as a subtraction operator that must be applied to another set. Some systems more accurately call this the ANDNOT operator.

Boolean operations can be demonstrated by looking at Table 5.1, which shows a small five-document, five-term database. The query *A* AND *B* will only retrieve

Table 5.1 Five-document by five-term database

Terms	Documents						
	1	2	3	4	5	Documents with term	IDF
A	1	0	0	3	1	3	1.22
B	0	2	0	0	1	2	1.40
C	1	0	0	2	3	3	1.22
D	0	1	1	0	0	2	1.40
E	1	0	0	0	0	1	1.70

document 5, since that is the only term common to both documents. The query A OR B, on the other hand, will retrieve documents 1, 2, 4, and 5, since one of the query terms is present in these four documents. The query A NOT B will retrieve documents 1 and 4, since they contain term A but not B.

5.2.2 Partial-Match Searching

Although *partial-match searching* was conceptualized very early, it did not see widespread use in IR systems until the advent of Web search engines in the 1990s. This is most likely because exact-match searching tends to be preferred by "power users," whereas partial-match searching is preferred by novice searchers. Whereas exact-match searching requires an understanding of Boolean operators and (often) the underlying structure of databases (e.g., the many fields in MEDLINE), partial-match searching allows a user to simply enter a few terms and start retrieving documents. Despite the surface simplicity of partial-match searching, however, its effectiveness can be comparable to that of exact-match searching (see Chap. 7), and new research approaches using it (see Chap. 8) can be quite complex.

The development of partial-match searching is usually attributed to Salton (1991), who pioneered the approach in the 1960s. Although partial-match searching does not exclude the use of nonterm attributes of documents, and for that matter does not even exclude the use of Boolean operators (e.g., see Salton, Fox et al., 1983), the most common use of this type of searching is with a query of a small number of words, also known as a *natural language query*. Because Salton's approach was based on vector mathematics, it is also referred to as the *vector-space model* of IR. In the partial-match approach, documents are typically ranked by their closeness of fit to the query. That is, documents containing more query terms will likely be ranked higher, since those with more query terms will in general be more likely to be relevant to the user. As a result, this process is called *relevance ranking*. The entire approach has also been called *statistical retrieval*, *lexical–statistical retrieval*, and *ranked retrieval*.

The most common approach to document ranking in partial-match searching is to give each a score based on the sum of the weights of terms common to the document and query. Terms in documents typically derive their weight from the TF*IDF calculation described in Chap. 4. Terms in queries are typically given a weight of one if the term is present and zero if it is absent. The following formula can then be used to calculate the document weight across all query terms:

$$\text{Document weight} = \sum_{\text{all query terms}} \text{Weight of term in query}$$

$$\times \text{Weight of term in document.} \qquad (5.1)$$

This may be thought of as a giant OR of all query terms, with sorting of the matching documents by weight. The usual approach is for the system to then perform the same stop word removal and stemming of the query that was done in the indexing process. (The equivalent stemming operations must be performed on documents and queries so that complementary word stems will match.)

The sample database in Table 5.1 can demonstrate partial-match searching. To simplify calculations, Table 5.1 shows the IDF for each term and Table 5.2 shows the TF*IDF weighting for each term in each document. A query using the terms $A\ B\ C$ will retrieve four documents with the following ranking:

1. Document 5 (1.22 + 1.40 + 3.67 = 6.29)
2. Document 4 (3.67 + 2.44 = 6.11)
3. Document 2 (2.80)
4. Document 1 (1.22 + 1.22 = 2.44)

In general, documents that contain more of the query terms will be ranked higher. As seen in the sample query, document 5 contains three terms in the query, while document 4 contains two. However, document 2 only has one query term, while document 1 has two. But it achieves its higher ranking because the term present in document 2 has a higher weight than the two terms in document 1 combined. This result often occurs when a term has a higher IDF, which is consistent with the rationale of IDF in that terms which occur with less frequency across the entire database are more "discriminating" than those which are more common.

One problem with TF*IDF weighting is that longer documents accumulate more weight in queries simply because they have more words. As such, some approaches "normalize" the weight of a document. The most common approach is cosine normalization:

Table 5.2 TF*IDF weighting for the terms and documents in Table 5.1

Terms	Documents					
	1 (NR)	2 (R)	3	4 (R)	5 (NR)	Relevance feedback query
A	1.22	0	0	3.67	1.22	1.61
B	0	2.80	0	0	1.40	1.70
C	1.22	0	0	2.44	3.67	0.22
D	0	1.40	1.40	0	0	0.70
E	1.70	0	0	0	0	0

$$\text{Document weight} = \frac{\displaystyle\sum_{\text{all query terms}} \text{Weight of term in query} \times \text{Weight of term in document}}{\sqrt{\left(\displaystyle\sum_{\text{all query terms}} \text{Weight of term in query}^2\right)\left(\displaystyle\sum_{\text{all document terms}} \text{Weight of term in document}^2\right)}} \quad (5.2)$$

A variety of other variations to the basic partial-matching retrieval approach have been developed. All are considered to be research approaches and are covered in more detail in Chap. 8. Some apply different weighting than the simple TF*IDF, while others add more weight to certain parts of documents, such as the title or the anchor text in a Web link. Some apply different approaches to normalization.

Relevance feedback, a feature allowed by the partial-match approach, permits new documents to be added to the output based on their similarity to those deemed relevant by the user. This approach also allows reweighting of relevant documents already retrieved to higher positions on the output list. The most common approach is the modified Rocchio equation employed by Buckley et al. (1994a). In this equation, each term in the query is reweighted by adding value for the term occurring in relevant documents and subtracting value for the term occurring in nonrelevant documents. There are three parameters α, β, and γ, which add relative value to the original weight, the added weight from relevant documents, and the subtracted weight from nonrelevant documents, respectively. In this approach, the query is usually expanded by adding a specified number of query terms (from none to several thousand) from relevant documents to the query. Each query term takes on a new value based on the following formula:

$$\text{New query weight} = \alpha \times \text{Original query weight}$$

$$+\beta \times \frac{1}{\text{number of relevant documents}} \times \sum_{\text{all relevant documents}} \text{weight in document}$$

$$-\gamma \times \frac{1}{\text{number of nonrelevant documents}} \times \sum_{\text{all nonrelevant documents}} \text{weight in document.} \quad (5.3)$$

When the parameters α, β, and γ are set to one, this formula simplifies to

$$\text{New query weight} = \text{Original query weight}$$
$$+\text{Average term weight in relevant documents}$$
$$-\text{Average term weight in nonrelevant documents} \quad (5.4)$$

In its rightmost column, Table 5.2 shows the new weight for each query term when documents 2 and 4 are relevant, documents 1 and 5 are not relevant, and term D is added to the query (since it occurs in document 2, which is relevant). As can be seen, none of the query terms maintains its original weight of 1.0. The weights of terms in query are now:

1. $A = 1 + (3.67/2) - (2.44/2) = 1.61$
2. $B = 1 + (2.8/2) - (1.4/2) = 1.70$
3. $C = 1 + (2.44/2) - (4.89/2) = -0.22$
4. $D = 0 + (1.7/2) - 0 = 0.70$
5. $E = 0$ (no relevant docs, so none added)

By applying these new query weights to (5.1) above, the weight of terms in document can be recalculated, as shown in Table 5.3. These weights can then be used with (5.1) to reweight the documents after the relevance feedback process:

1. Document 2 = 4.75 + 0.98 = 7.72
2. Document 4 = 5.90 − 0.54 = 5.36
3. Document 5 = 1.97 + 2.38 − 0.81 = 3.53
4. Document 1 = 1.97 − 0.27 = 1.70
5. Document 3 = 0.98

As can be seen, document 2 has moved to the top of the list, while document 5 has fallen and document 3 has been added. These phenomena typically occur with relevance feedback, in general (but not always) achieving the goal of moving existing relevant documents higher in the output list, adding new relevant ones, and moving existing nonrelevant documents lower.

A number of IR systems offer a variant of relevance feedback that finds similar documents to a specified one. PubMed allows the user to obtain "related articles" from any given one in an approach similar to relevance feedback but which uses a different algorithm, which will be described in Chap. 8 (Wilbur and Yang, 1996). A number of Web search engines allow users to similarly obtain related articles from a specified Web page.

5.2.3   Term Selection

As noted already, search terms are generally either terms from a controlled vocabulary assigned by a manual indexing process or words extracted from the documents themselves by means of an automated process. While either type of term can

Table 5.3 Weighting of terms in documents after Rocchio relevance feedback process

Terms	Documents				
	1	2	3	4	5
A	1.97	0	0	5.90	1.97
B	0	4.75	0	0	2.38
C	−0.27	0	0	−0.54	−0.81
D	0	0.98	0.98	0	0
E	0	0	0	0	0

be used in either type of searching approach, controlled vocabulary terms are most commonly employed in exact-match systems. Typically in exact-match systems, when appropriate controlled terms are not available, document words are applied. Partial-match systems almost always use document words as indexing terms, though they may be qualified by where they occur, such as in the title or anchor text.

5.2.3.1 Term Lookup

Whereas early IR systems required users to enter search terms with minimal assistance (i.e., terms had to be found in telephone-book-sized catalogs and typed in exactly), most modern systems provide assistance with term lookup. PubMed, for example, provides a MeSH browser that allows users to type in one or more words from a term, select the appropriate term, and add it to the search. The Ovid system (http://www.ovid.com/) also allows user lookup of MeSH terms but uses a somewhat different approach, displaying a ranked list of MeSH terms that most commonly appear in MEDLINE references when the word(s) entered also occurs.

5.2.3.2 Term Expansion

Some systems allow terms in searches to be expanded by using the *wildcard character*, which adds all words to the search that begin with the letters up until the wildcard character. This approach is also called *truncation*. Unfortunately, there is no standard approach to using wildcard characters, so syntax for them varies from system to system. PubMed, for example, allows a single asterisk at the end of a word to signify a wildcard character. Thus, the query entry `can*` will lead to the words `cancer` and `Candida`, among others, being added to the search (although PubMed warns when more than 600 citations are retrieved). Ovid allows the use of four different wildcard characters. In its basic mode interface, the asterisk character can be used, and it functions similar to the asterisk in PubMed. In the advanced mode, however, there are three different wildcard characters:

- Limited truncation allows all terms with the root and the specified number of digits to be added to the query. It is specified by the dollar sign followed by a digit. For example, dog$1 retrieves documents containing `dog` and `dogs`, but not `dogma`.
- Mandated wildcard allows single characters to be substituted within or at the end of a word. It is specified by the pound sign (#). For example, `wom#n` will lead to retrieval of documents containing `woman` or `women`. There must be a character present, i.e., `dog#` will not retrieve `dog`.
- Optional wildcard allows zero or more characters to be substituted within or at the end of a word. It is specified by the question mark. For example, `colo?r` will lead to retrieval of documents containing `color` or `colour`. This character cannot be used after the first letter of a word.

5.2.3.3 Other Word-Related Operators

Some IR systems have operators that require more than just the term being present. The proximity operator, for example, specifies not only that two words be present but also that they occur within a certain distance of each other in the document. It is essentially an AND with the additional restriction that the words be within a specified proximity. These operators can help control for the context of words in a concept. For example, a user looking for documents on `colon cancer` might specify that the words `colon` and `cancer` appear within five words of each other. This would capture documents with phrases like `colon cancer` and `cancer of the colon` but would avoid documents that discuss `cancer` in one part and mention `colon` in another (e.g., description of the effect of a type of `cancer` that somehow affects `colon motility`).

As with other features, different systems implement and have varying syntax for proximity operators. PubMed does not provide proximity searching although it does, as will be described shortly, allow searching against a list of common multi-word phrases, such as `health planning`. Ovid, on the other hand, does provide this capability. Its ADJ operator requires words to be adjacent and in the order specified. For example, the query `blood ADJ pressure` will retrieve only documents that have the phrase `blood pressure`. The operator ADJ_n, where n is a digit, requires words to be within n characters of each other. For example, `colon ADJ₅ cancer` will retrieve documents with both `colon cancer` and `cancer of the colon`. The Web search engine AltaVista has a proximity operator NEAR, which requires target words to be within ten words of each other.

Another word-related term specification feature in Ovid is the FREQ command, which will not retrieve a document unless a word or a phrase is present a minimum number of times. One word-related feature no longer found in most systems is synonym specification. The now-retired STAIRS system from IBM has a SYN operator that allows a user to designate two words as synonymous. For example, entering `cancer SYN carcinoma` will cause the two words to be used interchangeably (i.e., connected to the other with OR whenever either is used).

5.2.3.4 Subheadings

Recall from Chap. 4 that some thesauri, including MeSH, contain *subheadings*, which are modifiers that can be attached to terms. For example, one can restrict the retrieval of documents on the subject of `Hypertension` to just those covering diagnosis or treatment. Many MEDLINE systems also allow searching with so-called *floating subheadings*, which allow the searcher to specify just the subheading itself, as if it were a solitary, unattached indexing term.

Subheadings have the effect of increasing the precision of a search, since documents on other aspects of the search term should be eliminated from the retrieval set. They should have no effect on recall, since the documents not retrieved should be focused on other aspects of the term. However, it is possible that the indexers may not assign a subheading where one is warranted; thus, the use of the subheading will preclude that document from being retrieved. Since subheading assignment is the least consistent area of indexing term assignment (see Chap. 4), most expert searchers advise care in the use of subheadings.

5.2.3.5 Explosions

Like the subheading, the *explosion* operation requires a controlled vocabulary. It further requires that the vocabulary have a hierarchical organization. The explosion operation is an OR of the term exploded with all the narrower terms below it in the hierarchy. It is typically used when a user wants to retrieve documents about a whole class of topics. For example, a user might want to obtain documents on all types of anemia. There are many types of anemia, due to nutrient deficiencies (iron, vitamin B12, folate), disease processes (hemolytic anemia, anemia of chronic disease), and genetic disorders (sickle cell anemia and other hemoglobinopathies). If a searcher wanted to obtain information on all those anemias in the MEDLINE database, the general MeSH term Anemia would be exploded, which would have the effect of combining the general and specific terms together with the OR operator. Another common reason for using explosions is to search on a category of drugs. For example, most drugs in the ACE Inhibitors category (e.g., captopril, enalapril, lisinopril) function similarly, so the user interested in the category would want to explode the general MeSH term ACE Inhibitors.

Most MEDLINE systems, including PubMed, automatically explode all terms that are not *terminal terms* or *leaf nodes* in the hierarchy (i.e., do not have a more specific term below them). While this approach is in general effective (especially for the examples just given), it can be detrimental when the MeSH hierarchy is not a true "is-a" or "part-of" hierarchy, i.e., the more general term is not a generalization of the more specific terms. This occurs with the MeSH term Hypertension, which is autoexploded. The terms underneath it in the hierarchy represent elevated blood pressure in specific body locations, such as the portal vein of the liver (Portal Hypertension) or the arteries of the lung (Pulmonary Hypertension). These terms are included in the autoexplosion, even though most searches on essential hypertension (designated by the MeSH term Hypertension) would not want to search on them.

As with subheadings, explosions require quality, consistent indexing. One of the principles taught to MEDLINE indexers to make explosions work well is that documents should be indexed to the "deepest" level of a hierarchy. Thus, if a document deals with a specific type of anemia, such as iron-deciency anemia, it will be indexed on that specific term. This allows searchers to home in on documents specifically about the disease with the MeSH term iron-deciency anemia, or still capture it more broadly by exploding the MeSH term, Anemia.

Explosions have the effect of increasing recall, since additional documents indexed on related but more specific terms are brought into the retrieval set. The effect on precision is variable, since the exploded topics may be relevant to the more general search term, or they may be too specific for the needs of the searcher.

5.2.3.6 Spelling Correction

A common feature of modern search engines, such as Google and PubMed, is detection of likely spelling errors and the offering of words for their correction. In PubMed, when a word entered in the search has few or no matches, the user is presented with an alternative spelling and the number of citations that would be retrieved if that option was selected (Canese, 2004; Wilbur, Kim et al., 2006). The spelling option is deactivated when the user enters a search tag, e.g., [mh]. An example of how the spelling correction of Google or PubMed works can be seen by entering `breast cancerr` into either, with orders of magnitude more documents made retrievable when the correct spelling is utilized.

5.2.4   Other Attribute Selection

As noted already, indexing not only consists of terms, but also entails other attributes about documents against which the user might desire to search. In MED-LINE, for example, the user might wish to search for papers by a specific author, in a specific journal, or representing a certain type of publication, such as a review article or a randomized controlled trial. On the Web, one might wish to search against only certain parts of Web pages, such as the text in a title or the anchor text in links. One might also wish to restrict Web searches to specific domains or hosts. The syntax for specifying these attributes is explained in the discussion of the different searching interfaces in the next section.

5.3   Searching Interfaces

In describing interfaces to various IR systems, the goal is not to exhaustively cover all features of all systems, but rather to demonstrate how features are implemented within various systems. Precedence is given to displaying systems of historical or market importance. The organization of this section follows the classification of content that was used described in Chap. 3.

Before we begin describing actual interfaces, let us make a few general comments. First, searching interfaces are constantly changing, so what is seen in this book reflects what they looked like when the book was written. Second, most systems do things somewhat differently, sometimes minimally and sometimes substantially. There is no standard approach to searching that has been adopted by all interfaces. Finally, many systems provide both "simple" and "advanced" interfaces, with the former allowing quick searches and the latter giving more control over refinement of the results.

5.3.1 Bibliographic

As noted in Chap. 4, bibliographic content includes literature reference databases, Web catalogs, and specialized registries. Literature reference databases, or bibliographic databases, continue to be the flagship IR application in healthcare. Even though most users want to obtain the full text of biomedical articles online, PubMed still provides an entry point to finding them.

5.3.1.1 Literature Reference Databases

Until the mid-1990s, MEDLINE was most commonly accessed using a command-line interface on a system called ELHILL over time-sharing networks accessed either by a dedicated line or a telephone modem connection. One early innovative system was PaperChase, which was the first MEDLINE system geared to clinicians (Horowitz, Jackson et al., 1983). It provided features taken for granted in modern systems, such as input of word fragments (instead of requiring the whole MeSH term), assistance with MeSH term lookup, intuitive description of the Boolean operators, and ability to handle American and British spelling variants.

Another innovative approach to MEDLINE came from the NLM in the 1980s. Grateful Med was the first MEDLINE system to run on a personal computer and feature a "full screen" interface that provided text boxes for specific fields (such as author, title, and subject), check boxes for tags such as English language and review articles, and expression of subject terms both as MeSH terms and text words (Haynes and McKibbon, 1987). Grateful Med eventually moved to the Web in Internet Grateful Med, sporting an expert assistant called COACH that helped users diagnose problematic searches (Kingsland, Syed et al., 1992), but was discontinued by NLM in favor of PubMed and the NLM Gateway.

PubMed is constantly being improved by NLM, both to respond to the needs of users and take advantage of new technology. It is also well documented. An overview of searching is provided in the NLM's help manual (Anonymous, 2007q). A variety of online training materials are available (http://www.nlm.nih.gov/pubs/web_based.html). Technical information about PubMed and other NLM services is available from the *NLM Technical Bulletin* (http://www.nlm.nih.gov/pubs/techbull/tb.html).

The initial searching screen for PubMed is shown in Fig. 5.2. Although presenting the user with a simple text box, PubMed does a great deal of processing of the user's input to identify MeSH and other subject terms, author names, and journal names, as described on the NLM Web site (Anonymous, 2007c). In automatic term mapping, the following steps are taken after removal of stop words:

1. *MeSH translation.* PubMed first tries to map input text to MeSH headings and entry terms. If this is unsuccessful, it then tries to map the text into subheadings, terms from publication types, phrases (from UMLS and elsewhere), pharmaceutical action terms, and supplementary concepts. When a term is found, it is

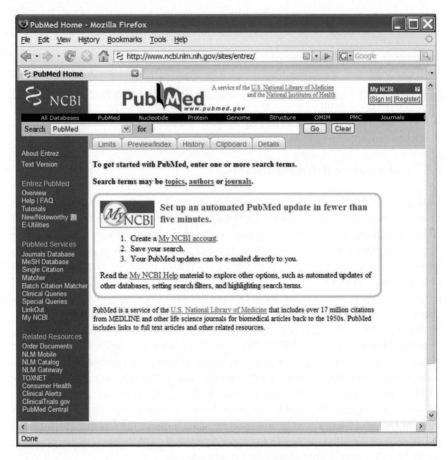

Fig. 5.2 PubMed search screen (courtesy of the National Library of Medicine)

searched as both the MeSH term and its text words. For example, the query `colon cancer treatment with radiation` is translated to the search `(("colonic neoplasms"[TIAB] NOT Medline[SB]) OR "co- lonic neoplasms"[MeSH Terms] OR colon cancer[Text Word]) AND ("therapy"[Subheading] OR ("therapeutic- s"[TIAB] NOT Medline[SB]) OR "therapeutics"[MeSH Terms] OR treatment[Text Word]) AND (("radiotherapy" [TIAB] NOT Medline[SB]) OR "radiotherapy"[MeSH Terms] OR "radiation"[MeSH Terms] OR radiation[Text Word])`.

2. *Journal name translation.* For all remaining words that do not map to MeSH (which could be all words if no MeSH terms are found), an attempt is made to map them to the journal abbreviation used in PubMed, although this is avoided for some journals whose names are common searches, such as `heart fail- ure` (McGhee, 2005). An example of journal name translation is the string `ann intern med` mapping to the journal `Annals of Internal Medicine`.

3. *Author mapping*. If the remaining words contain at least two words, one of which has only one or two letters, word pairs are matched against the MEDLINE full and abbreviated author fields. For example, the strings `William Hersh` or `hersh wr` map to an author search by this author.

The remaining text that PubMed cannot map is searched as text words (i.e., words that occur in any of the MEDLINE fields). As noted already, MEDLINE allows the use of wildcard characters. It also allows phrase searching in that two or more words can be enclosed in quotation marks to indicate they must occur adjacent to each other. If the specified phrase is in PubMed's phrase index, then it will be searched as a phrase. Otherwise, the individual words will be searched. Both wildcard characters and specification of phrases turn off the automatic term mapping.

PubMed allows specification of other indexing attributes by two means. First, the user may type the attribute and its value directly into the text box. (This can also be done to directly enter MeSH terms.) For example, a search of `asthma/ therapy [mh] AND review [pt]` will find review articles indexed on the MeSH term `Asthma` and its subheading `Therapy`. The use of field tags turns off automatic term mapping. Many attributes can also be specified via the PubMed "Limits" screen (see Fig. 5.3). These include publication types, subsets, age ranges, and publication date ranges (Canese, 2006).

As in most bibliographic systems, users search PubMed by building search sets and then combining them with Boolean operators to tailor the search. A "tabbed" interface allows stored searches to be displayed, with two default tabs being the search entered and that same search limited by `review [pt]`.

Consider a user searching for studies assessing the reduction of mortality in patients with `congestive heart failure` through the use of medications from the `angiotensin-converting (ACE) inhibitors` class of drugs. A simple approach to such a search might be to combine the terms `ACE Inhibitors` and `CHF` with an AND. The easiest way to do this is to enter the search string `ace inhibitors AND congestive heart failure`. (The operator AND must be capitalized because PubMed treats the lowercase and as a text word, since some MeSH terms, such as `Bites and Strings`, have the word `and` in them.)

A more advanced searcher might put `ACE Inhibitors` and `congestive heart failure` into separate sets for later manipulation in the searching process. Figure 5.4 shows the PubMed History screen we might develop. We see, for example, that there are 5,879 references about `ACE inhibitors` and `congestive heart failure`. If we are knowledgeable about evidence-based medicine (EBM), our next step is to try to limit the search to the best evidence. Since this question is about treatment of disease, we would likely use the Publication Type tag to limit retrieval to RCTs. This still yields 759 references. Additional knowledge of EBM, however, reminds us that if this many clinical trials have been done on this topic, someone has probably done a systematic review or meta-analysis. Employing the Publication Type tag `Meta-Analysis` reduces the output to 47 references,

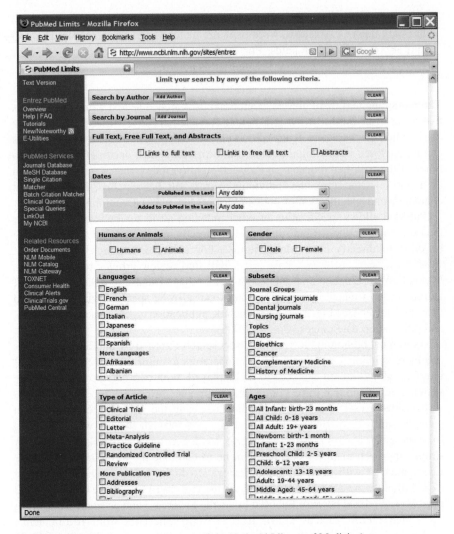

Fig. 5.3 PubMed limits screen (courtesy of the National Library of Medicine)

which is very manageable. We may also be interested in practice guidelines; this Publication Type tag can be used in a limit as well. PubMed also provides a Preview/Index screen that lets us build search sets directly without having to view intermediate results.

PubMed also features a variety of "special queries" designed to help users find specific types of information. This work first began with the development of "clinical queries," where the subject terms were limited by search statements designed to retrieve the best evidence based on principles of EBM for the four common types of clinical questions: therapy, diagnosis, harm, and prognosis

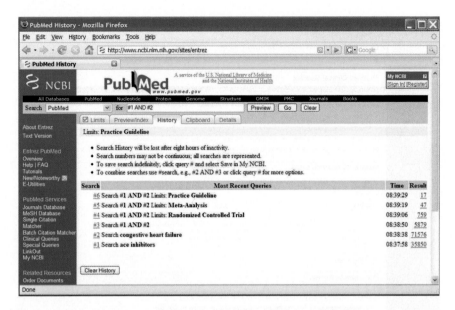

Fig. 5.4 PubMed history screen (courtesy of the National Library of Medicine)

(Haynes, Wilczynski et al., 1994). For each of the four question types, there were two strategies available, one emphasizing sensitivity (leading to higher recall, i.e., including as many relevant articles as possible) and the other emphasizing specificity (leading to higher precision, i.e., excluding as many nonrelevant articles as possible). Further "clinical queries" include the ability to find systematic reviews and perform genetics-related searches. When the clinical queries interface is used (see Fig. 5.5), the search statement is processed by the usual automatic term mapping and the resulting output limited (via AND) with the appropriate statement.

Clinical queries are actually part of a broader category of Special Queries (http://www.nlm.nih.gov/bsd/special_queries.html) that include:

- Queries – e.g., clinical, health service research, cancer
- Subjects – e.g., AIDS, complementary and alternative medicine, toxicology
- Interfaces – e.g., MedlinePlus, retracted publications
- Collections – e.g., core clinical journals, nursing journals

The Clinical Queries now feature three categories (http://www.ncbi.nlm.nih.gov/entrez/query/static/clinicalTable .html):

- Clinical studies – the original search strategies aiming for retrieval of best evidence for therapy, diagnosis, etiology, prognosis, and clinical prediction guides
- Systematic reviews – a strategy that limits retrieval to systematic reviews
- Medical genetics – strategies that limit retrieval to various aspects of genetics, including diagnosis, management, counseling, and testing

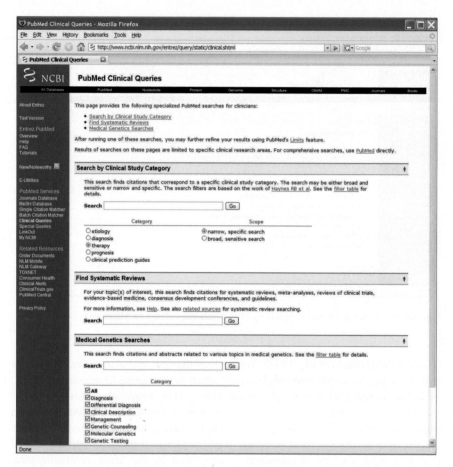

Fig. 5.5 PubMed clinical queries screen (courtesy of the National Library of Medicine)

Ongoing research has led to refinement of the search strategies for optimal retrieval of articles likely to contain scientifically strong studies (i.e., those likely to contain evidence for use in the practice of EBM; see (Table 5.4) (Wilczynski, Morgan et al., 2005). A list of publications describing updates of their strategies is available (http://www.nlm.nih.gov/pubs/techbull/jf04/cq_info.html). The search strategy for systematic reviews was based on work done by Shojania and Bero (2001) and improved by Montori et al. (2005). Recent research has also found that adding the word `randomised` to the specific/narrow strategy for therapy improves recall, mainly through the addition of recently published studies not yet indexed (Corrao, Colomba et al., 2006).

Additional effort has been devoted to making PubMed directly accessible to other Web-based applications that do not require its user interface. For example, an application may wish to send a query directly and receive results for its own formatting. One common application is the direct linkage to PubMed references,

Table 5.4 PubMed clinical queries (courtesy of the National Library of Medicine)

Category	Optimized for	Sensitivity (%)/specificity (%)	PubMed search
Therapy	Sensitive/ broad	99/70	((clinical[Title/Abstract] AND trial[Title/ Abstract]) OR clinical trials[MeSH Terms] OR clinical trial[Publication Type] OR random*[Title/Abstract] OR random allocation[MeSH Terms] OR therapeutic use[MeSH Subheading])
	Specific/ narrow	93/97	(randomized controlled trial[Publication Type] OR (randomized[Title/Abstract] AND controlled[Title/Abstract] AND trial[Title/Abstract]))
Diagnosis	Sensitive/ broad	98/74	(sensitiv*[Title/Abstract] OR sensitivity and specificity[MeSH Terms] OR diagnos*[Title/Abstract] OR diagnosis [MeSH:noexp] OR diagnostic*[MeSH: noexp] OR diagnosis,differential [MeSH:noexp] OR diagnosis [Subheading:noexp])
	Specific/ narrow	64/98	(specificity[Title/Abstract])
Harm	Sensitive/ broad	93/63	(risk*[Title/Abstract] OR risk*[MeSH: noexp] OR risk*[MeSH:noexp] OR cohort studies[MeSH Terms] OR group* [Text Word])
	Specific/ narrow	51/95	((relative[Title/Abstract] AND risk*[Title/ Abstract]) OR (relative risk[Text Word]) OR risks[Text Word] OR cohort studies [MeSH:noexp] OR (cohort[Title/ Abstract] AND stud*[Title/Abstract]))
Prognosis	Sensitive/ broad	90/80	(incidence[MeSH:noexp] OR mortality [MeSH Terms] OR follow up studies [MeSH:noexp] OR prognos*[Text Word] OR predict*[Text Word] OR course*[Text Word])
	Specific/ narrow	52/94	(prognos*[Title/Abstract] OR (first[Title/ Abstract] AND episode[Title/Abstract]) OR cohort[Title/Abstract])
Clinical prediction guide	Sensitive/ broad	96/79	(predict*[tiab] OR predictive value of tests [mh] OR scor*[tiab] OR observ*[tiab] OR observer variation[mh])
	Specific/ narrow	54/99	(validation[tiab] OR validate[tiab])

Source: http://www.ncbi.nlm.nih.gov/entrez/query/static/clinicalTable.html

e.g., as done by Highwire Press (http://www.highwire.org) and many medical textbooks. The Entrez Programming Utilities allow this functionality (Sayers and Wheeler, 2007).

PubMed has additional features available to the user once a MEDLINE record has been selected for viewing. As described earlier, a "related articles" command finds references similar to the current one by means of a relevance feedback process. As most journals are published electronically now, the user can also click on a button to be linked to the journal's Web site where the full text is available. The full text will appear if the article can be accessed without charge; if a subscription is required, the Web site can determine whether the user is eligible to view the article. From the MEDLINE record page, the user can also click on LinkOut, which will provide a page of links to other publishers that offer the article, general consumer information about the article's topic from MedlinePlus, and a library holdings feature. The latter allows libraries to restrict full-text linkages to the journals they subscribe to as well as link to other local resources, such as print-based holdings in special collections. Over 1,000 organizations take advantage of this feature, including the Oregon Health & Science University Library (http://www.ncbi.nlm.nih.gov/entrez/query.fcgi?holding=ohsulib). The PubMed interface also allows searching to be limited to various subsets of full-text literature with the following tags:

- PubMed Central – `pubmed pmc [sb]`
- Free full text – `free full text[sb]`
- Full text – `full text[sb]`

Another improvement to PubMed and other NLM databases has been the reformatting of Web pages to make them more friendly for display on the small screens of handheld devices, a growing number of which feature wireless connectivity to the Internet (Fontelo, Ackerman et al., 2003). Current applications, all of which are available at http://www.nlm.nih.gov/mobile/include:

- MD on Tap (http://mdot.nlm.nih.gov/proj/mdot/mdot.php): an application that runs on a Palm OS or PocketPC device that includes an interface that follows the PICO (patient/problem, intervention, comparison, outcome) framework and formats a search that takes advantage of PubMed's clinical queries (Fontelo, Nahin et al., 2005).
- PubMed for Handhelds (http://pubmedhh.nlm.nih.gov/): a variety of interfaces to PubMed and other NLM information resources, including an application called askMEDLINE that allows natural language queries to be entered (Fontelo, Liu et al., 2005).
- AIDSinfo's PDA Tools (http://aidsinfo.nih.gov/PDATools/): a variety of AIDS information resources available for a Palm OS or PocketPC device.
- Wireless Information System for Emergency Responders (WISER, http://wiser.nlm.nih.gov/): a system designed to assist first responders in hazardous material incidents, providing information on hazardous substances, including its identification, physical characteristics, human health information, and advice about containment and suppression.
- Several books from the NCBI Bookshelf that have been reformatted for smaller displays (http://www.ncbi.nlm.nih.gov/entrez/query/Books.live/Help/mobile.html)

Another major enhancement to PubMed is the MyNCBI system, which allows individuals to save searches and have them updated and sent via email on a periodic basis (Nahin, 2005). It also allows the designation of filters for limiting the output of all searches, such as to review articles, human studies, and/or various journal subsets. MyNCBI also lets the user specify properties associated with the LinkOut feature, such as automatic links to the holdings of specific libraries or to other databases, such as the NCBI Bookshelf or various genomics databases. The information filtering aspects of MyNCBI will be covered in Sect. 5.5.

PubMed is, of course, not the only interface for searching MEDLINE. Two well-known commercial interfaces used at many medical centers are produced by Ovid and Aries Systems (Knowledge Finder, http://www.kfinder.com/). The most notable features of Ovid are its different approach to mapping to MeSH, the availability of virtually all features via its "Limits" interface, and the direct linkage to full text of the articles also licensed by Ovid. Knowledge Finder is the only major MEDLINE interface to offer a partial-match approach to retrieval (though many exact-match features are available as well). It also provides linkages to EBM resources along with automated synonym mapping (e.g., `Advil` to `Ibuprofen`) and British/American spelling equivalents.

5.3.1.2 Web Catalogs

Web catalogs take a variety of approaches to searching. A number of them allow searching directly over their catalog and then provide links to the items referenced. For example, HealthFinder (http://healthfinder.gov/) offers a simple search interface that allows retrieval over titles and resource descriptions in the catalogs. All these systems also allow browsing of their subject classifications. The Open Directory project allows searching over the category names in its vast classification hierarchy. As seen in Fig. 5.6, topics might appear in a number of hierarchies, each with a different number of Web sites.

5.3.1.3 Specialized Registries

The National Guidelines Clearinghouse (NGC) offers a simple text-box searching interface and also provides a "detailed search" interface that allows all the attributes in the clearinghouse to be searched. These include the type of guideline, the type of organization that produces such guidelines, the intended users, and the clinical specialty (see Fig. 5.7) as well as limits on the content, target population, gender, and date of publication. The "results" interface allows not only viewing of the attributes for one guideline but also side-by-side comparison of the attributes of two or more guidelines. When the full text of the guideline is available on the Web, a link is provided directly to it.

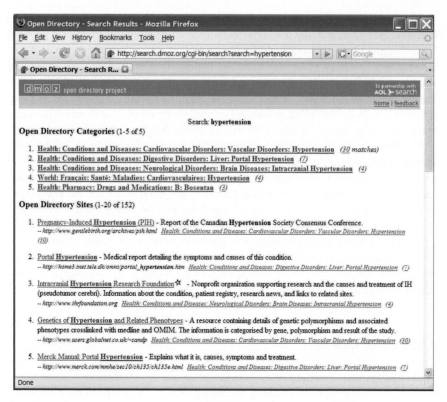

Fig. 5.6 Open Directory results of search on `hypertension` (courtesy of Open Directory)

5.3.2   Full Text

In general, full-text searching interfaces offer fewer features than their bibliographic counterparts. This is in part because the amount of metadata available for full-text resources is smaller. Unlike the rich metadata provided in bibliographic databases such as MEDLINE and the NGC, most full-text "documents" consist of just a title and body of text. One advantage of full text is its complete body of text, which provides more words to search against; but when those words do not represent the focus of the content of the document, this feature can be a disadvantage.

5.3.2.1   Periodicals

As noted in Chap. 4, many journals have become available in full text on the Web. A number of them use the facilities of Highwire Press. A number of high-profile journals are among the hundreds that deliver their full-text content via Highwire

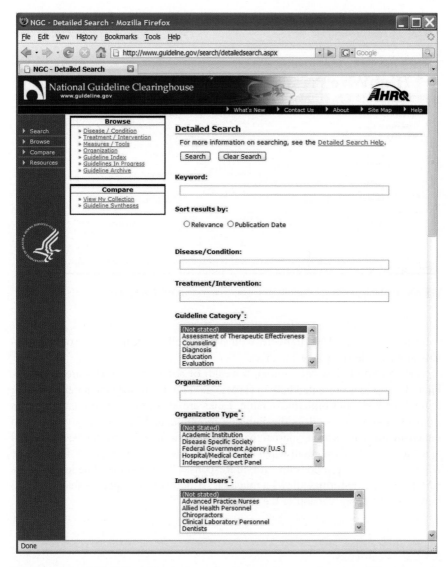

Fig. 5.7 National Guidelines Clearinghouse detailed search screen (courtesy of the Agency for Healthcare Research & Quality)

Press, as described in the last chapter. The Highwire system provides a retrieval interface that searches over the complete online contents for a given journal. Users can search for authors, words limited to the title and abstract, words in the entire article, and within a date range. The interface also allows searching by citation by entering volume number and page as well as searching over the entire collection of journals that use Highwire. Users can also browse through specific issues as well as

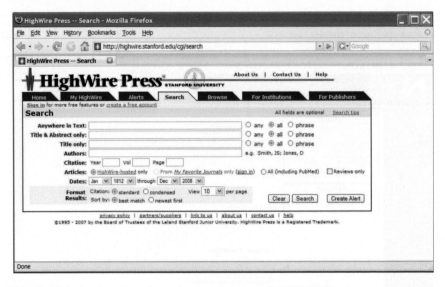

Fig. 5.8 Highwire Press journal search screen (courtesy of BMJ Publishing)

collected resources. The Highwire Web site also allows searching across all journals that they delivery (see Fig. 5.8).

Once an article has been found, a wealth of additional features are available. First, the article is presented both in HTML and PDF form, with the latter providing a more readable and printable version. Links are also provided to related articles from the journal as well as the PubMed reference and its related articles. Also linked are all articles in the journal that cited this one, and the site can be configured to set up a notification email when new articles cite the item selected. Finally, the Highwire software provides for "Rapid Responses," which are online letters to the editor. The online format allows a much larger number of responses than could be printed in the paper version of the journal.

5.3.2.2 Textbooks

Most electronic textbook searching interfaces offer variations on the basic theme of entering words to search against sections of the textbook organized along the book's organizational structure. One searching interface that offers somewhat more functionality is Stat!-Ref (http://www.statref.com/), which contains over 50 medical textbooks, from simple pocket guides to encyclopedic subspecialty tomes (Fig. 5.9). Its searching interface allows the user to select any number of textbooks. It also allows stemming or word synonym expansion to be optionally used. The results screen provides links that take the user right to the appropriate section of the textbook, from where he or she can navigate to other portions of the book.

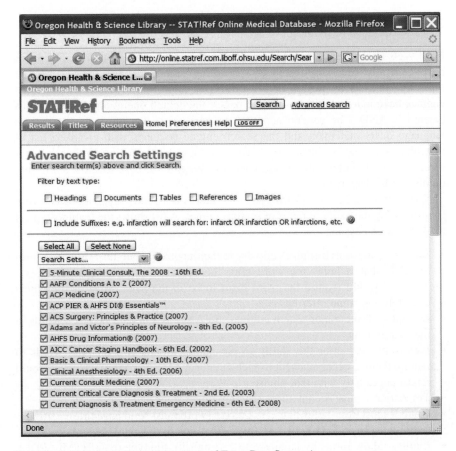

Fig. 5.9 Stat!-Ref search screen (courtesy of Teton Data Systems)

Up to Date (http://www.uptodate.com/) provides unique features for words in the query not found in the database. If a term is not found, it automatically removes one letter at a time from the end of the word until one is found. It also attempts to map nonfound words to common synonyms, abbreviations, and misspellings.

5.3.2.3 Web Search Engines

As noted in Chap. 1, Web search engines have become ubiquitous and economically important. Their features are constantly changing. SearchEngineShowdown is a frequently updated Web site that compares commercial search engines. Two pages cover their retrieval features:

1. A list of features by search engine – http://www.searchengineshowdown.com/features/

2. A list of search engines by feature – http://www.searchengineshowdown.com/
   features/byfeature.shtml

Most Web search engines use a basic variant of partial-match searching. The pages
have generally been discovered by "crawling" the Web, and their words are
typically indexed by means of a word-based approach. Because most search
engines have indexed billions of Web pages, the default operation between words
entered is AND. The general approach to retrieval is that users enter a natural
language query statement and the search engine responds with a ranked list of
matching Web pages. Most search engines show ten matching Web pages per
screen of output, but usually it is possible to configure the page to allow a different
number to be displayed.

The SearchEngineShowdown Table of features is a good organizing framework
for discussing the major features of search engines. A list shows the features typical
to Web search engines:

- Boolean – the search engines all vary in their approach, but most offer +, a form
  of AND that requires the word after the operator to be in the search, i.e.,
  +heart would require the word heart to be in the page. Most of the others
  offer OR and some offer NOT.
- Default – all the major search engines use AND as a default between words in
  the search input.
- Proximity – all offer the ability to put quotes around two or more words to
  require them to occur adjacent to each other, e.g., ''heart failure'' would
  return pages only with that phrase.
- Truncation – most do not allow searching over truncated words.
- Fields – most offer fields like intitle: (word must be in page title), inurl:
  (word must be in URL), link: (pages that link to this one), and others.
- Limits – allow limits by language (e.g., English), file type (e.g., HTML, PDF),
  date ranges (varies widely by engine, e.g., Google allows past 3, 6, or 12
  months), and Internet domain (e.g., http://www.billhersh.info/).
- Stop – most do stop word filtering, which can usually be overridden by use of the
  + operator.
- Sorting – all offer relevance ranking of some type, such as Google and its well-
  known PageRank algorithm and Microsoft Live Search using a combination of
  recency, popularity, and approximate vs. exact match.

Further review of Google demonstrates the power and complexity of its approach.
A description of its advanced features is at http://www.google.com/intl/en/help/
refinesearch.html. A list of the some of the limits it provides is shown in Table 5.5.
Google has a variety of other features, some of which are:

- Cached search – searches pages in Google's cache, especially useful when the
  retrieved page is unavailable.
- Calculator – typing in a mathematical expression returns the calculated result.
  It even does conversions such as 20 km in miles.

Table 5.5 Some of the field restrictions that can be applied in Google

Tag	Restriction	Example
intitle:	At least one word required to be in page title	`intitle: HIV AIDS` requires `HIV` or `AIDS` to appear in title
allintitle:	All words required to be in page title	`allintitle: HIV AIDS` requires both `HIV` and `AIDS` to appear in title
inurl:	At least one word required to be in page URL	`inurl: PDF Medical` requires `PDF` or `Medical` to appear in URL
allinURL:	All words required to be in page URL	`allinurl: PDF Medical` requires both `PDF` or `Medical` to appear in URL
site:	Page required to be in specified domain	`site: nlm.nih.gov` limits search to pages at NLM Web site
link:	Page required to have specified link	`link: pubmed.gov` limits search to pages that link to PubMed

- Definitions – preceding a word or phrase with `dene:` will provide a definition for that term, e.g., `dene: medical informatics`.
- Phone numbers – Google will also return the phone numbers for individuals whose name (last or first plus last) and location (city, state, zip, and/or area code) are entered. It will also provide a "reverse" lookup of giving the person when the phone number is entered.
- Q&A – attempts to answer simple questions.
- Search by number – a variety of tracking numbers, such as UPS, FedEx, and others.
- Similar – finds Web pages similar (based on having the same words) to one retrieved.
- Spell checker – checks query words for misspelling and suggests more common versions of their spelling if appropriate.
- Stock quotes – entering the stock ticker symbol gives a link for quotes on its current price, e.g., `INTC` (Intel).
- Street maps – typing an address or company name with an address provides a street map of the location through Google Maps.
- Synonyms – placing a tilde (~) in front of a word will cause Google to search for synonyms of that word in a process that has been well explained, e.g., `~informatics`.
- Travel information – entering the three-letter code for an airport followed by the word airport gives information about that airport, e.g., `pdx airport` (Portland International Airport). Typing the name of an airline plus a number gives the status of that flight, e.g., `united 250`.
- Translation – Google offers users to translate non-English pages from several languages into English. It also provides a variety of translation tools (http://www.google.com/language_tools?hl=en).
- Weather – provides weather forecasts for various locations, e.g., `weather portland, or`.

Google also provides an application programming interface (API) to its search engine, allowing others to build applications that access it using emerging Web Services standards (http://www.google.com/apis/). A book devoted to "Google hacks" demonstrates how to use this and other features (Calishain and Dornfest, 2004). With over hundreds of millions of queries per day, Google requires hardware and software that can handle this load. Papers have been published describing Google's system architecture (Hochmuth, 2003), file system (Ghemawat, Gobioff et al., 2003), and cluster architecture (Barroso, Dean et al., 2003).

A big challenge for search engines is how to make money for a service for which users do not pay. (Not only do they not pay, but also the results they find take them right off the search engine site.) Google has developed means to generate revenue streams without compromising its basic search results. While some other search engines feature sponsored links very prominently, Google continues to post them in a separate location clearly demarcated from the main results. In its Adwords program (http://adwords.google.com/select/), advertisers bid for their results to be placed in the sponsored links portion of the results, with those paying more ranking higher. A related program is AdSense (https://www.google.com/adsense/), which pays sites to put context-specific advertisements on their pages. Other search engines demarcate sponsored links less explicitly. One engine, Ask (http://www.ask.com/), only presents its results by paid placement.

5.3.3 Annotated

As noted in Chap. 3, a number of health resources on the Web consist of collections of annotated content. This section describes the searching approaches to these resources.

5.3.3.1 Images

The first group of annotated content is image databases. As explained in Chap. 4, image collections are generally indexed by textual descriptions of individual images. Most systems have relatively simple text-searching interfaces, usually consisting of simple word matching between query and image description terms. Few systems make use of visual retrieval techniques. One system that does is the GNU Image-Finding Tool (GIFT, http://www.gnu.org/software/gift/). As shown in Fig. 5.10, "searching" on one or more images tends to find others that "look like" it.

Most of the major Web search engines also feature some form of image retrieval. Their output usually displays images associated with the text of the Web pages on which they are located. Some of the features of Google are particularly useful in image retrieval, such as filetype (e.g., can limit to JPEG). When an image is retrieved, Google displays both a thumbnail of the image and the page from which it came. As with most of the major search engines, Google allows imaging

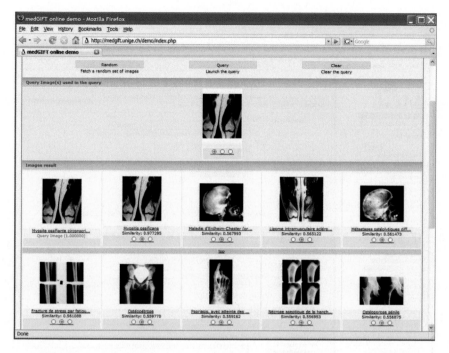

Fig. 5.10 GIFT image retrieval results screen (courtesy of VIPER Project)

from its main search page or has a separate image retrieval page (http://images.google.com/).

5.3.3.2 Citations

While the main use of citation databases is to identify linkages in the scientific literature, there is sometimes the need to search them in a conventional manner. If nothing else, the user needs to identify the specific works of an author or a particular citation. Or, a user who wishes to browse the database in a more exploratory manner might want to have the ability to search by author or title words. The Web of Science database has a relatively simple interface that allows such searching.

5.3.3.3 Molecular Biology and -omics

Another type of annotated content is molecular biology and -omics databases. Searching in these resources may involve text strings such as disease and drug names, and may also involve codes such as gene identifiers or numbers such as chromosome locations. All of these can be entered into the NLM Entrez interface. Both text strings and identifiers are treated similarly by Entrez, and they can be combined via Boolean sets and linked directly to them from the list of results.

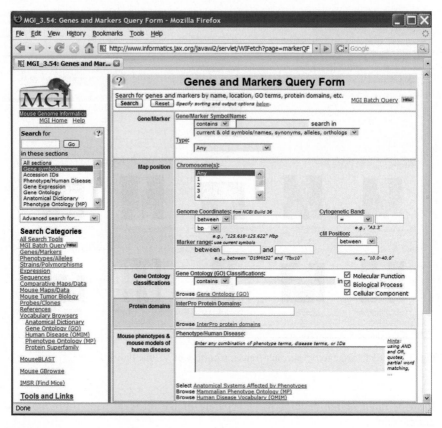

Fig. 5.11 Mouse Genomics Informatics search screen

Figure 5.11 shows the advanced search interface of the Mouse Genome Informatics system.

5.3.3.4   Other Databases

Chapter 3 listed a variety of annotated content in the "other" category. Most of these employ simple text-word searching. The ClinicalTrials.gov site has a simple text-box interface that searches over the text in the clinical trials records or an advanced search that provides an interface to search by disease, treatment, location, sponsor, etc. (see Fig. 5.12). The system attempts to map the simple search results into the categories of the advanced interface. For example, if the user enters the query `heart attack beta blockers portland`, the "Query Details" will map the phrase `heart attack` to `myocardial infarction`, recognize the phrase `beta blocker`, and find trials in cities named `Portland`.

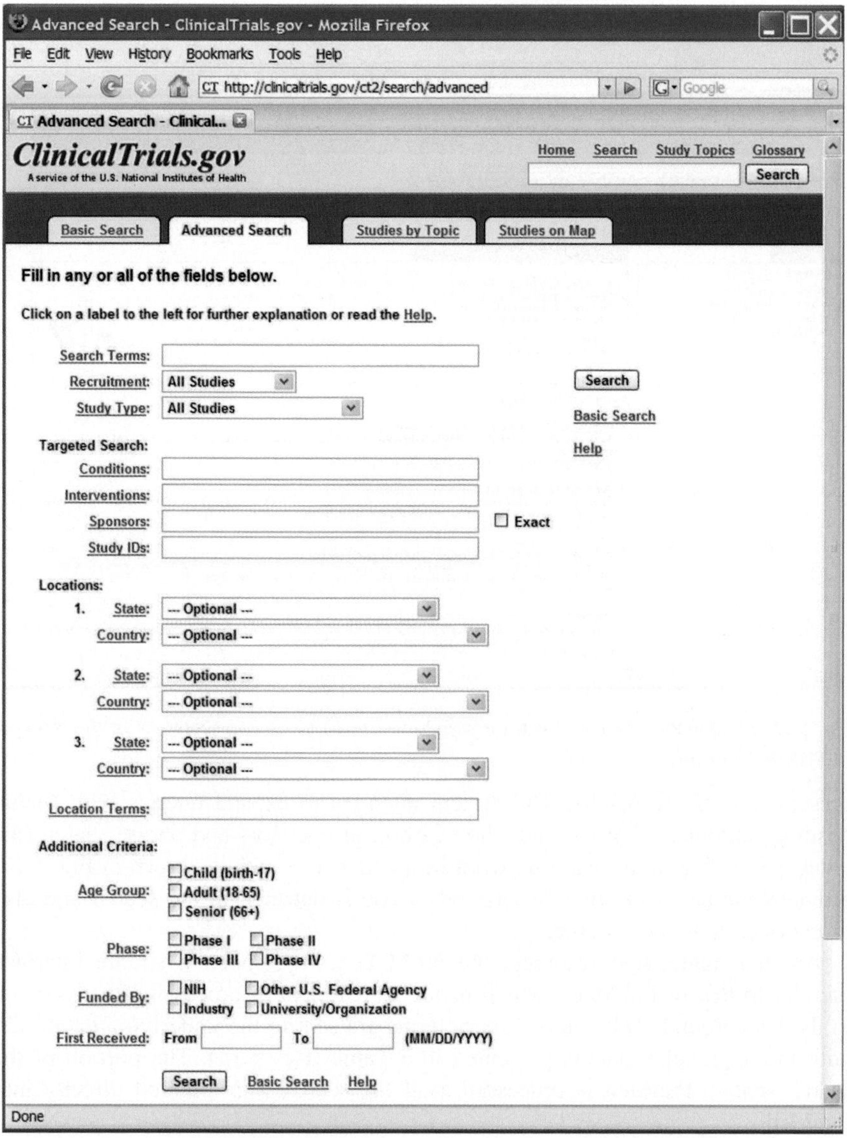

Fig. 5.12 ClinicalTrials.gov focused search screen (courtesy of the National Library of Medicine)

5.3.4 Aggregations

The final group of information resources described in Chap. 4 consisted of aggregations of content. The MedlinePlus system of aggregated consumer health resources provides a simple searching interface, but then offers more complexity with

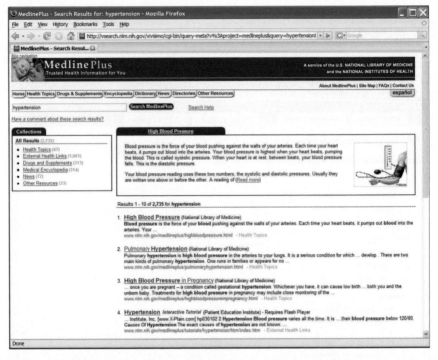

Fig. 5.13 MedlinePlus results screen for search on `hypertension` (courtesy of the National Library of Medicine)

presentation of the results. The system attempts to expand queries with MeSH headings automatically and also allows Boolean operators and phrase search (the latter via putting more than one word in quotes). The output, shown in Fig. 5.13, provides the definition of a disease when one is detected in the search and also categorizes results by source.

Another aggregated resource, the NLM Gateway, sports a simple interface (similar to that of PubMed), which belies a great deal of processing that goes on in the background. The entered query terms are sent to the underlying databases, with the aggregated results presented in a Table (Fig. 5.14). The portion of the search sent to PubMed is processed as if the search were entered directly into PubMed.

5.4 Document Delivery

Although there is much enthusiasm for access to online full-text journals, there is still demand for paper copies of journal articles to be delivered to individuals. Either the journal may not be available online or the user may not have a subscription permitting access to it. In these situations, paper documents must be

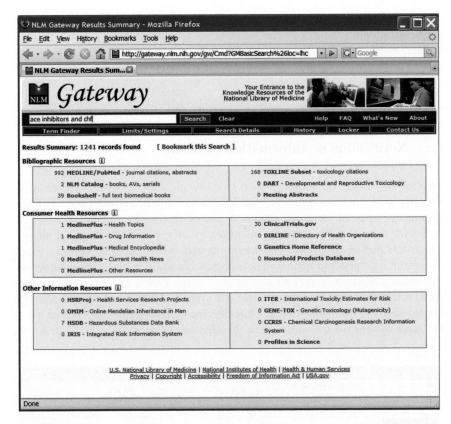

Fig. 5.14 NLM Gateway search screen (courtesy of the National Library of Medicine)

delivered by some means. In the traditional library searching setting, the user searches a bibliographic database, finds the appropriate references, and goes to the stacks to find the desired article. Because the particular reference may not be available in the library's collection, most libraries have an interlibrary loan department, which can obtain the reference or a copy from another library. With the increasing prevalence of IR system usage outside libraries, document delivery has become an important function of libraries. Many libraries have document delivery services, and some of the online services allow the user to order a copy of the document while viewing its reference online. NLM allows documents to be ordered through PubMed by means of its DOCLINE service (http://www.nlm.nih.gov/docline/newdocline.html). Requests are routed to regional libraries around the world, which provide the documents to users for a charge. Most commercial MEDLINE systems also provide the capability for users to order paper documents from institutions at which the systems are licensed.

The cost of document delivery is still rather high, averaging about $8–10 per article. In addition, there is a delay between the time a document is ordered and its delivery by surface mail. Some systems feature fax transmission of documents, but this is pricier still. Another option used increasingly is electronic mailing of a scanned version of the document.

5.5   Notification or Information Filtering

Another way of accessing information is via *notification, information filtering*, or *selective dissemination of information*. Information filtering is the retrieval of new documents from an incoming stream, a sort of electronic clipping system. It is suited for user who is perpetually interested in a topic, wanting to gather all new documents that are generated. The filtering system is used to set up a profile, which is a search statement run against all new documents added to one or more databases. Information filtering is very similar to IR, though Belkin and Croft (1992) note some distinct differences. For example, IR systems are oriented toward one-time use for distinct information needs, while filtering systems imply the repeated use of the same system for the same query. In addition, whereas IR systems deal with

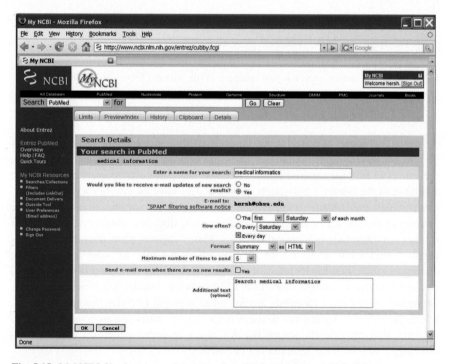

Fig. 5.15 MyNCBI filtering screen (courtesy of the National Library of Medicine)

relatively static databases, filtering systems are concerned with selection of information from dynamic streams of data. Finally, timeliness is more likely to be an important aspect of the functionality of filtering systems.

Information filtering has been around for decades, but some newer approaches make it easier and integrate it more effectively with other searching resources. Many systems make use of RSS feeds and allow users to receive them in a variety of ways, including directly through Web browsers such as Firefox. Most of the modern MEDLINE search systems offer some variant of information filtering. MyNCBI allows users to create a list of "saved searches" that can be run at specified intervals and delivered via email. The interface to set up a saved search is shown in Fig. 5.15.

Chapter 6
Digital Libraries

Our discussion of information retrieval (IR) systems thus far has focused on the provision of retrieval mechanisms to access online content. Even with the expansive coverage of some IR systems, such as Web search engines, they are often part of a larger collection of services or activities. An alternative perspective, especially when communities and/or proprietary collections are involved, is the *digital library* (DL). Sharing many characteristics with "brick and mortar" libraries, DLs provide some additional challenges.

Borgman (1999) notes that libraries of both types elicit different definitions of what they actually are, with researchers tending to view libraries as content collected for specific communities and practitioners alternatively viewing them as institutions or services. Weise (2004) reminds us that a library is still a physical place and that there is virtue to that place. She describes the value of the library, its mission, and the importance of professionalism in librarianship. Roush (2005) talks of the "infinite library," which extends its walls globally. Indeed, most who work in academic institutions take it for granted that the content from their library is available both at the library and over the Internet.

In this chapter, we will expand our perspective on IR systems and look at their role in the context of DLs. We will begin with overviews of libraries generally and then DLs specifically. Next, we will cover issues of access to DL content, copyright and intellectual property (IP) issues, and preservation of digital materials. We will end with a discussion of librarians and other professionals in the era of DLs.

6.1 Overview of Libraries

Libraries have traditionally performed a variety of functions, including the following:

- Acquisition and maintenance of collections
- Cataloging and classification of items in collections

W. Hersh, *Information Retrieval: A Health and Biomedical Perspective,*
doi: 10.1007/978-0-387-78703-9, © Springer Science + Business Media, LLC 2009

- Serving as a place where individuals can go to seek information with assistance, including information on computers
- Providing work or studying space (particularly in universities)

DLs provide some of these same services, but their focus tends to be on the digital aspects of their content.

There are a number of organizations concerned with libraries. The American Library Association (ALA, http://www.ala.org/) focuses on libraries in general, while the Special Library Association (SLA, http://www.sla.org/) takes a narrower view on scientific and technical libraries. As noted in Chap. 1, the Medical Library Association (MLA, http://www.mlanet.org/) addresses the issue of health science libraries.

Probably the main function of libraries is to maintain collections of published literature. They may also store nonpublished literature, such as letters, notes, and other documents, in archives. But the general focus on published literature has implications. One of these is that, for the most part, quality control can be taken for granted. At least until the recent past, most published literature came from commercial publishers and specialty societies that had processes such as peer review which, although imperfect, allowed the library to devote minimal resources to assessing their quality. While libraries can still cede the judgment of quality to these information providers in the Internet era, they cannot ignore the myriad of information published only on the Internet, for which the quality cannot be presumed.

The historical nature of paper-based traditional libraries also carries other implications. For example, items are produced in multiple copies. This frees the individual library from excessive worry that an item cannot be replaced. In addition, items are fairly static, simplifying their cataloging. With DLs, these implications are challenged. As noted in Chap. 2 and as described further shortly, there is a great deal of concern about archiving of content and managing its change when fewer "copies" of it exist on the file servers of publishers and other organizations. A related problem for DLs is that they do not own the "artifact" of the paper journal, book, or other item. This is exacerbated by the fact that when a subscription to an electronic journal is terminated, access to the entire journal is lost, i.e., the subscriber does not retain accumulated back issues, as is taken for granted with paper journals.

Another major function of libraries has been to provide access to their collections. The traditional means for accessing collections was the *card catalog*: users picked a subject or author name and flipped through cards representing items in the library. Card catalogs have largely been replaced by online public access catalogs (OPACs), which are similar to but have differences from document retrieval systems (Hildreth, 1989). The main difference emanates from the general differences between books and "documents." That books tend to be larger and to cover more subject material is exemplified by envisioning the difference between a medical journal article on a specific disease and its treatment and a book on internal medicine. As such, catalogers of books tend to use much broader indexing terms.

A major challenge for libraries is managing the physical size of their collections. Lesk (2005) notes that many aspects of libraries mimic the exponential growth curve documented in the growth of scientific literature by Price (1963), such as the number of volumes in libraries. Related to this challenge is the fact that libraries tend to be public or (even in private organizations) quasipublic entities that do not generate large revenue streams. Cummings et al. (1992) have documented that the costs of maintaining collections have exceeded the resources that libraries generally have available, resulting in a reduction of their purchasing power.

Because libraries are traditionally resource-poor, another major activity they undertake is sharing of collections. Few libraries can maintain complete collections, so most participate collaboratively with other libraries to attaining materials via *interlibrary loan* (ILL). This of course potentially sets up conflict, as the needs of publishers to maintain revenues to continue being in business must be weighed against the desire of libraries to reduce costs by sharing. Aspects of copyright and IP protection are covered in Sect. 6.4.

Another important goal of libraries is the preservation of library collections. In traditional libraries, the aim is for survival of the physical object. There are a number of impediments to preservation:

- Loss, theft, and general deterioration from use
- "Perfect binding" or the use of glue in binding instead of sewing, which reduces the longevity of books
- Acid paper, i.e., materials printed of paper produced by means of an acid process, used mainly between 1850 and 1950, which has led to an international resolution eschewing further use of such processes (Anonymous, 1989)

DLs have their own set of preservation issues, which are described in Sect. 6.5.

6.2 Definitions and Functions of DLs

A number of authors have attempted to define exactly what is meant by the term "digital library." Borgman (1999) reviewed all the definitions put forth by others and concluded that there were two competing views: a research-oriented view, with DLs defined to represent specific collections of content and/or technologies; and a service-oriented view, with DLs thought to represent a set of services provided to a specific community, such as a university or a company. Humphreys (2000) has examined DLs from the standpoint of being able to provide information in the context of the electronic health record (EHR), as described in Sect. 6.3.4.

A number of overviews of DLs have been written. These include books (Arms, 2001; Witten and Bainbridge, 2003; Lesk, 2005) and a journal, *Digital Library Magazine* (http://www.dlib.org/). A flurry of research in the area was funded by the National Science Foundation (NSF) Digital Libraries Initiative (http://dli2.nsf.gov/), which had participation by several other federal agencies, including the National Library of Medicine (NLM). A conference has emerged to address the scientific aspects of DLs, the Joint Conference on Digital Libraries (JCDL, http://www.jcdl.org/).

A number of authors have explored the larger issues in the transformation from paper-based libraries to DLs. Zhao and Resh (2001) have noted that the Internet transforms publishing, and thus DLs, with many effects:

- More efficient access to knowledge – e.g., via searching and access to full-text content
- New knowledge representations – access to hypertext, multimedia, and ultimately the Semantic Web
- Interdisciplinary integration – linkages across journals and other resources
- Transformation of production processes – streamlining of the peer review and editing processes
- Transformation of the consumption process – digital libraries bypassing conventional libraries and authors bypassing publishers

A large DL project in Europe, DELOS (http://www.delos.info/), has published a "manifesto" on DLs (Candela, Castelli et al., 2007). It presents a model with a three-tier framework containing the DL, the DL system, and the DL management system. Surrounding the framework is the DL *universe*, which addresses six core concepts: content, users, architecture, policy, quality, and functionality. This universe also features three roles of *actors*, consisting of end users, designers, system administrators, and application developers.

Another report has been published by the U.S. National Commission on Libraries and Information Science (NCLIS) (Anonymous, 2006e) and addressed information policy issues in the face of "mass digitization" of information. The report identified nine areas with potential impact on information policy:

1. Copyright – how should it be handled in digitization projects?
2. Quality – what is the quality of optical character recognition (OCR), content, and authentication?
3. Libraries – what are their roles and priorities for the digital age?
4. Ownership and preservation – who will assume long-term ownership of books, journals, and other media as well as preserve the public record?
5. Standardization and interoperability – how can systems and their content communicate with each other?
6. Publishers – what are the roles of publishers in this era?
7. Business models – what business models are needed and what will be the impact of the open-access movement?
8. Information literacy – what should be done about information illiteracy?
9. Assessment – what assessment is being undertaken? How will we know if content and systems are meeting people's needs?

One model of digital libraries (DLs) is the 5S model of Goncalves et al. (2004). These authors hypothesize that DLs can be modeled, or explained, according to these five elements:

1. Streams – sequences of elements of arbitrary types that can be static or dynamic

2. Structures – structures of the parts that comprise content in the digital library, usually defined via markup languages (e.g., XML, HTML)
3. Spaces – objects and operations on them that provide constraint yet meaning
4. Scenarios – the situation that describes how digital libraries are used by real people
5. Societies – the entities and their relationships, from the people to the technology systems

They also describe a taxonomy that defines the facets of a digital library based on these five elements:

1. Actors – who interacts with or within DLs?
2. Activities – what happens in DLs?
3. Components – what constitutes DLs?
4. Social, economic, and legal aspects – what surrounds DLs?
5. Environments – in what contexts are DLs embedded?

6.3   Access to Content

As noted earlier, the primary function of libraries is to provide content to its patrons. This process is usually aided by various forms of metadata. Earlier chapters focused on the importance of metadata in providing access to content. From the DL (and commercial publishing) perspective, the view of metadata is broader than what we have focused upon so far. This larger view incorporates the notion that content must be made available not only reliably, but also in a manner that allows use of IP to be appropriately tracked and expensed. In this section, we focus on access to individual items, collections of items, and the metadata that describes them.

6.3.1   Access to Individual Items

Probably every Web user is familiar with clicking on a Web link and receiving an error message that the page is not found. In the early days of the Web, this was the dreaded message: HTTP 404 – File not found. DLs and commercial publishing ventures need mechanisms to ensure that documents have persistent identifiers so that when the document itself physically moves, it is still obtainable. The original architecture for the Web envisioned by the Internet Engineering Task Force was to have every uniform resource locator (URL), the address entered into a Web browser or used in a Web hyperlink, linked to a uniform resource name (URN) that would be persistent (Sollins and Masinter, 1994). The combination of a URN and a URL, a uniform resource identifier (URI), would provide persistent access to digital objects. The resource for resolving URNs and URIs was never implemented on a large scale.

One approach that has achieved widespread adoption by publishers, especially scientific journal publishers, is the digital object identifier (DOI) (Paskin, 2006). A key aspect of the DOI initiative is the International DOI Foundation (IDF, http://www.doi.org/), a membership organization that assigns a portion of the DOI to make it unique. The DOI system consists of four components:

1. Enumeration – the location of the identifier, the DOI
2. Description – metadata of the entity association with the DOI
3. Resolution – the means to resolve the identifier to actually located the object
4. Policies – rules that govern the operation of the system

The DOI has attained the status of a standard by the National Information Standards Organization (NISO) with the designation Z39.84. The DOI itself is relatively simple, consisting of a prefix that is assigned by the IDF to the publishing entity and a suffix that is assigned and maintained by the entity. For example, the DOI for articles from the *Journal of the American Medical Informatics Association* has the prefix 10.1197 and the suffix jamia.M####, where #### is a number assigned by the journal editors. For example, a publication in JAMIA by this author on image retrieval (Hersh, Müller et al., 2006) has the DOI 10.1197/jamia.M2082.

The DOI can also be encoded into a URL and resolved by the DOI Web site in a standardized fashion. For example, the JAMIA article cited here (Hersh, Müller et al., 2006) is accessed by the URL http://dx.doi.org/10.1197/jamia.M2082, which is resolved to the URL on the JAMIA Web site http://www.jamia.org/cgi/content/abstract/13/5/488. In the long run, the DOI could become the identifier of the document, although in biomedicine, the PubMed Identifier (PMID) also vies for the title of universal content identifier.

An outgrowth of the standardization on the DOI is the CrossRef project, which aims to create an infrastructure for linking citations across publishers (http://www.crossref.org/01company/16fastfacts.html). Publishers who are members of Cross-Ref can insure that the DOIs for the content items they publish will resolve to a valid URL. They can also be assured that outbound links to other content adhering to the CrossRef standard will resolve to a valid URL. These resolutions will be maintained even if the actual URL of the content changes. CrossRef works hand in hand with OpenURL (Apps and MacIntyre, 2006), a standard for transporting metadata and identifiers within URLs. These URLs can have the transported information resolved when the object might exist in more than one place, but not have allowed access. For example, a library may not subscribe directly to a journal, but it may subscribe to an aggregation service that does. The library could then resolve the URL to point to the appropriate URL to access the object.

A related development for universal identification is that many publishers have agreed to make their proprietary content (i.e., that in the "invisible Web") for indexing by Google Scholar (http://scholar.google.com/) (Banks, 2005). This makes the content searchable via Google, although protected content still requires subscription or other means of paid access. In PageRank-like fashion, the content is ranked by the number of citations to it. Google Scholar has been compared to the Science Citation Index and URLs in the general Google search engine, with coverage and its overlap varying by discipline (Kousha and Thelwall, 2007). Both Google Scholar and the plain Google search engine have impacted searching for electronic publications. Many MEDLINE references as well as full-text articles are detected and indexed by the Google crawler. Analysis of journals published electronically by Highwire Press (Steinbrook, 2006) as well as just the *British Medical Journal* (Giustini, 2005) has found that over half of all accesses of their full-text articles come from links from Google or Google Scholar. A number of librarians have expressed concern about how the actions of Google challenge the functions and roles of academic libraries (Courant, 2006; MacColl, 2006).

Google is also undertaking additional activities with libraries and other producers of scholarly work. One such activity is its effort to digitize vast stores of books and other documents in a number of prominent university and other public libraries, including Oxford University, Harvard University, Stanford University, the University of Michigan, and the New York Public Library (Kousha and Thelwall, 2007). There are a number of challenges whose solutions are not clear, including how users will best interact with the content, how it will all be digitized, and how copyright issues will be resolved.

Some projects have arisen out of concern of the overly restrictive approach to the content being digitized by Google Books and related projects. One such project is the Open Content Alliance (OCA, http://www.opencontentalliance.org/participate.html), which aims to make cultural and other content as widely available as possible while respecting the rights of its owners and contributors. Another project, which is endorsed by the United Nations and the US Library of Congress, is the World Digital Library (WDL, http://www.worlddigitallibrary.org/). The goal of this project is to "make available on the Internet, free of charge and in multilingual format, significant primary materials from cultures around the world, including manuscripts, maps, rare books, musical scores, recordings, films, prints, photographs, architectural drawings, and other significant cultural materials."

Another effort to develop standards for metadata and interoperability in the medical community, not limited to knowledge-based applications, is the Medbiquitous Consortium (http://www.medbiq.org/). This consortium of medical specialty societies, universities, and publishers is aiming to develop Web Services-based standards that will facilitate interoperability of applications devoted to knowledge-based information, educational applications, and maintenance of certification in medical specialties. The current focus of work by Medbiquitous is on metadata for educational applications through enhancement of the Shareable Content Object Reference Model (SCORM, http://xml.coverpages.org/scorm.html), a set of 64 metadata elements that emanate from an expansion of the Dublin Core Metadata Initiative (DCMI) (http://www.lsal.cmu.edu/lsal/expertise/projects/developersguide/).

With the growing amount of digital scientific data on the Internet, there is also growing concern over how to make these data accessible and to preserve them. One workshop developed a series of recommendations that addressed the methods, costs, and terminology of archiving such data (Anonymous, 2003). More recently, Altman and King (2007) described the issues and proposed a standard for citing this data.

6.3.2 Access to Collections

With myriad resources online, there has always been a desire to provide seamless access to them. In the pre-Web era, a standard was developed to provide a standard means for IR clients and servers to interact with each other. Called Z39.50, it aimed to enable any server to allow searching on its collection (with appropriate restriction based on access rights) and at the same time to allow any client (with the proper access rights) to search on any server (Miller, 1999). This separation of the user interface from the back-end IR system allowed users on different platforms and with different clients to access the same collections. A limitation of this approach was that it limited the amount of retrieval capabilities, since each of the disparate components, client and server, needed to understand the functionality of the other. Early versions of the protocol, for example, did not provide for natural language searching capabilities. The momentum for Z39.50 was also hampered by the early search engines of the Web, which developed their own mechanisms for sending queries from Web page forms to IR servers.

Despite having lost momentum from its nonuse by Internet search engines, the Z39.50 effort has not been disbanded. The project is currently being led by the Library of Congress (http://www.loc.gov/z3950/agency/). The project has released specifications for Search/Retrieve for the Web (SRW, also called the Search/ Retrieve Web Service) and a Common Query Language (CQL). SRW has recently been enhanced to interoperate with the Open Archive Initiative (OAI) described in Sect. 6.3.3 (Sanderson, Young et al., 2005).

Another challenge for providing access to collections is the ability to link across disparate documents. In some fields, such as computer science, large amounts of scientific papers have been placed online by their authors and others. (This has generally not been the case for healthcare, where copyright restrictions have been adhered to with greater rigor.) Lawrence et al. (1999) have exploited the large amount of online content to build CiteSeer (http://citeseer.ist.psu.edu/), which uses a technique called autonomous citation indexing (ACI) to link the citations as well as the postings of the documents themselves to provide a comprehensive DL of scientific work in various areas of science.

6.3.3 Access to Metadata

As noted throughout this book, metadata are a key component for accessing content in IR systems. They take on additional value in the DL, where there is desire to allow access to diverse but not necessarily exhaustive resources. One key concern of DLs is *interoperability* (Besser, 2002). That is, how can resources from different producers and having heterogeneous metadata be accessed? One of the challenges with most current Web sites is that the content exists as a silo that can only be accessed through the terms of the Web site. As such, users must navigate to the

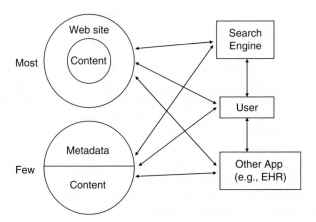

Fig. 6.1 Interoperability challenges in digital libraries. At present, most Web sites exist as silos without easy accessibility to their metadata

particular site to interact with the content and cannot easily cross "boundaries" to other sites. A notable exception to this is the NLM's Entrez Programming Utilities (eUtils) (Sayers and Wheeler, 2007). Nonetheless, most Web sites exist as silos that cannot be accessed in this manner, as shown in Fig. 6.1.

Arms et al. (2002) have noted that three levels of agreement must be achieved to attain the desired interoperability:

1. Technical agreements over formats, protocols, and security procedures
2. Content agreement over the data and the semantic interpretation of its metadata
3. Organizational agreements over ground rules for access, preservation, payment, authentication, and so forth

Probably the most widespread approach to interoperability has been the OAI (http://www.openarchives.org/) (Lagoze and Van de Sompel, 2001). This project had its origins in the E-Prints initiative, which aimed to provide persistent access to electronic archives of scientific publications (Van de Sompel and Lagoze, 1999). While the OAI effort is rooted in access to scholarly communications, its methods are applicable to a much broader range of content. Its fundamental activity is to promote the "exposure" of archives' metadata such that DL systems can learn what content is available and how it can be obtained. The OAI recognizes two classes of participants, both of whom agree to adhere to the OAI protocol that provides a low-cost, low-barrier approach to interoperability:

1. Data providers that expose metadata about their content
2. Service providers that harvest metadata to provide value-added services

Each record in the OAI system has an XML-encoded record. Each of these records contains three parts:

1. Header – a unique identifier and a date stamp indicating creation or latest modification

2. Metadata – a set of unqualified DCMI tags describing the resource
3. About – an optional container for information about the metadata, such as its schema

The DCMI tags are explicitly unqualified because the focus of the metadata is on discovery (i.e., providing systems with a description of what is there) as opposed to description (i.e., providing a mechanism for more detailed searching). The "about" container can be used to describe more about the metadata or, as suggested by Lagoze and Van de Sompel (2001), provide information about rights for access or terms and condition for usage. With this framework, the OAI protocol then allows selective harvesting of the metadata by systems. Such harvesting can be date based, such as items added or changed after a certain date, or set based, such as those belonging to a certain topic, journal, or institution. The harvesting protocol allows six different activities, as listed in Table 6.1.

The process of harvesting metadata in OAI is called the OAI Protocol for Metadata Harvesting (OAI-PMH) (Van de Sompel, Nelson et al., 2004). A number of open-source tools have been developed for the OAI-PMH, many of which can be accessed from http://www.openarchives.org/pmh/tools/. While straightforward for common metadata, challenges arise for the growing complex types of metadata, such as image thumbnails (Foulonneau, Habing et al., 2006) and learning objects (Richardson and Powell, 2004). A next step for OAI is the Open Archives Initiative Object Reuse and Exchange (OAI-ORE), which aims to define standards for the description and exchange of complex aggregations of Web resources.

Several medical publishers have been early adopters of OAI. Biomed Central has been very involved in promoting OAI for access to the metadata of its content (http://www.biomedcentral.com/info/libraries/oai/). Likewise, PubMed Central (PMC) provides OAI access to its content as well, using the PMC DTD at http://www.pubmedcentral.gov/about/oai.html.

There is emerging consensus not only that identifiers of digital content remain persistent but that metadata do so as well. A number of large-scale producers of metadata, including NLM, recently agreed to promote the use of URIs for this task (Baker and Dekker, 2003). A Web site has been developed to create a registry of

Table 6.1 Allowable actions in Open Archives Initiative Protocol for Metadata Harvesting (adapted from Lagoze and Van de Sompel, 2001)

Action	Description
GetRecord	Retrieve a single record
Identify	Retrieve information about a repository including, at a minimum, the name, base URL, version of OAI protocol, and e-mail address of the administrator of the resource
ListIdentifier	Retrieve list of identifiers that can be harvested from a repository
ListMetadataFormats	Retrieve metadata formats from a repository
ListRecords	Harvest records from a repository, with optional argument for filtering based on attributes of records, either date based or set based
ListSets	Retrieve set structure in a repository

such identifiers, http://info-uri.info/. A core concept behind their approach is that these URIs be nonreferenceable, meaning that they do not point to actual locations on the Internet or Web, but instead represent a persistent namespace for metadata elements. This is described in more detail on their Web site (http://info-uri.info/registry/docs/misc/faq.html).

As its use becomes more prolific, a growing concern about metadata is its quality (Bruce and Hillmann, 2004; Beall, 2006). A primer on metadata for science digital libraries is available from the National Science Digital Library (NSDL, http://nsdl.org/) (Dushay, 2006). A related challenge for metadata systems is the proliferation of different ones with different formats. Godby et al. (2004) have proposed a repository of crosswalks allowing translation among metadata elements. The lack of interoperability among knowledge-based resources on the Web means that current content is usually maintained in "silos" that dictate usage on their terms, e.g., their search engines, display format, etc. Linkage across resources from different publishers or across applications (e.g., EHR to IR systems) is difficult and nonstandardized.

6.3.4   Integration with Other Applications

Early DL researchers recognized the importance of linkage of information, even if the technology at the time did not permit optimal solutions. Work continues in the area of linking various aspects of content, some of which was described in state-of-the-art systems described earlier in the book. For example, the genomics databases described in Sect. 3.4.4 demonstrate how information from gene sequences (GenBank) to the scientific papers describing them (MEDLINE) to textbook descriptions of diseases they occur in (Online Mendelian Inheritance in Man) can be integrated. A glimpse of the same approach for clinical information has been hinted in some of the aggregated systems described in Sect. 3.5, but the barriers resulting from the proprietary status of the information have hindered integration of this kind of information. The remainder of this section will focus on two research areas that could serve as foci for integration of clinical information: linkage of knowledge-based content to the electronic medical record (EMR) and linkage of users to human knowledge.

6.3.4.1   Linkage to the Electronic Health Record

Most IR applications are stand-alone applications, i.e., the user explicitly launches an application or goes to a Web page. A number of researchers have hypothesized that the use of IR systems can be made more efficient in the clinical setting by embedding them in the EHR. Not only would this allow their quicker launching (i.e., the user would not have to "switch" applications), but the context of the patient could provide a starting point for a query. Cimino (1996) reviewed the literature on this topic and noted that embedding had been a desirable feature since the advent on the EHR. More recently, however, the ability to link systems and their resources via the Internet, particularly using Web browsers, has made such applications easier to develop and disseminate. Cimino noted that the process of linking patient information systems to IR resources consisted of three steps:

1. Identifying the user's question
2. Identifying the appropriate information resource
3. Composing the retrieval strategy

Humphreys (2000) notes that newer technologies enhance the prospects for linking the EMR to knowledge-based information systems. In particular, the Internet and the Web reduce the complexity of integrating disparate legacy systems, provide standards that facilitate development of applications, and allow users of all types to access resources from a variety of locations from the home to the clinical setting. She notes that three levels of integration are required to achieve this vision:

1. Technical connections – the gamut of pure technology-related issues that allow integration, such as hardware, software, telecommunications, access integration, and so on
2. Organizational connections – the means by which organizations license clinical applications and the information they access
3. Conceptual connections – the standardization of the structure of the information and the terminology to describe it

Most IR systems provide a simple mechanism for identifying the user's question: they provide a query box to enter it. Since, however, the EHR contains context about the patient, such as diagnoses, treatments, test results, and demographic data, it is conceivable this information could be leveraged to create a context-specific query. Some early approaches looked at extracting information from dictated reports (Powsner and Miller, 1989; Miller, Gieszczykiewicz et al., 1992) but were limited by the nonspecificity of much of the data in those reports. Cimino et al. (1993) developed *generic queries* that were based on analyses of real queries posed to medical librarians. They subsequently developed *infobuttons* that allowed the user to retrieve specific information. For example, an infobutton next to an ICD-9 code translated the code into a Medical Subject Headings (MeSH) term using the Unified Medical Language System (UMLS) Metathesaurus and sent a query to MEDLINE (Cimino, Johnson et al., 1992). Likewise, an infobutton next to a laboratory result generated a MEDLINE search with the appropriate term based on whether the result was abnormal or not (Cimino, Socratorus et al., 1995). Another approach to infobuttons was developed in the SmartQuery system by Price and Hersh et al. (2002) (see Fig. 6.2).

One challenge for linking clinical information to knowledge-based resources is determining what information to offer the user. This is especially so for clinical narratives which contain a wealth of words and concepts. Mendonça et al. (2001a) assessed narrative reports to determine how to promote the most important concepts on which a user is likely to search. They found that TF*IDF weighting of concepts

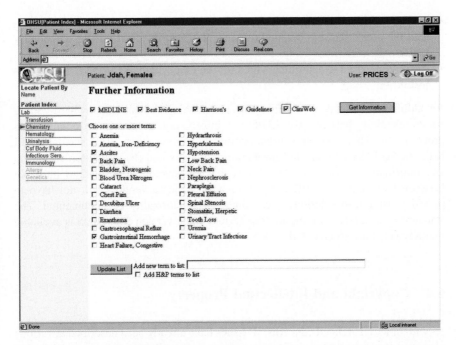

Fig. 6.2 Screen shot from SmartQuery, giving the user topics for searching based on the context of the electronic health record (Price, Hersh et al., 2002)

extracted by a natural language processing system was effective in promoting those of most interest to real human users. These authors also developed the means to formulate data extracted from other parts of the clinical record into the types of well-formed questions required in evidence-based medicine (Mendonça, Cimino et al., 2001b).

Additional work by Cimino and colleagues includes the development of an *Infobutton Manager*, which keeps track of the various information resources, generic questions that can be asked of them, and contexts in which those questions and resources might be used. The specific context of the patient is derived from the EHR or clinical information system (CIS), e.g., demographic information, diagnoses, test results, and so forth. The system then creates specific infobuttons that provide linkage to available resources with queries to find knowledge-based information appropriate to that context. The framework for this work was described by Cimino et al. (2002). The Infobutton Manager matches a group of context parameters to information needs and then matches those needs to actual resources. The context parameters include:

- User type – nurse, physician, patient
- Patient age – newborn, infant, child, adolescent, young adult, middle aged, and elderly
- Patient gender – male, female

- Concept of interest – datum (e.g., medication, test result, organism) that generated the user's request, mapped to concepts in the Medical Entities Dictionary (MED)
- Institution – used to determine which resources are available/preferred at a given institution

An additional challenge with infobuttons is that many of them work by hard-coding communications between the EHR and information resource. To address this problem, the HL7 standards organization has begun work on a standard API between (a) EHR systems and infobutton managers and (b) infobutton managers and information resources. The idea is that by developing a standard interface between these entities, EHR and information resource vendors will not have to provide customized solutions every time this functionality is implemented. The standard is currently evolving in draft format and a version from 2005 is available publicly (DelFiol, Rocha et al., 2005).

6.4 Copyright and Intellectual Property

As with other DL-related concerns, IP issues have already been described at various places in this book. IP is difficult to protect in the digital environment because although the cost of production is not insubstantial, the cost of replication is near nothing. Furthermore, in circumstances such as academic publishing, the desire for protection is situational. For example, individual researchers may want the widest dissemination of their research papers, but each one may want to protect revenues realized from synthesis works or educational products that are developed. The global reach of the Internet has required IP issues to be considered on a global scale. The World Intellectual Property Organization (WIPO, http://www.wipo.int/) is an agency of the United Nations attempting to develop worldwide policies, although understandably, there is considerable variation in opinion about what such policies should be.

6.4.1 Copyright and Fair Use

The right to protection of IP is enshrined in the U.S. Constitution (Article I, Sect. 8, Clause 8), which states that Congress has the power to "promote the progress of science and useful arts, by securing for limited times to authors and inventors the exclusive right to their respective writings and discoveries." Copyright law for the United States is detailed in Title 17 of the United States Code (http://www.copyright.gov/title17/). Within this law, however, is a provision for *fair use* (Sect. 107), which allows copyrighted work to be reproduced for purposes of "criticism, comment, news reporting, teaching (including multiple copies for classroom use), scholarship, or research." In particular, there are four factors to be considered whether an activity constitutes fair use:

1. Purpose of use – educational vs. commercial
2. Nature of work – photos and music more protected than text
3. Amount of copying – should be for use by individuals
4. Effect of copying – out-of-print materials easier to justify than in-print

Fair use guidelines vary among libraries. A Web site that provides pointers to a wide range of material on the topic has been developed by Stanford University Libraries (http://fairuse.stanford.edu/). The actual interpretation of fair use varies from library to library. Lesk (2005) lists some typical guidelines, e.g., copying guidelines might limit users to 1,000 words or 10% of book, a single journal article, or one illustration or image per book or journal. For libraries requesting materials from other libraries, the guidelines might limit copying to five articles from the most recent 5 years of a journal. Publishers have responded to fair use guidelines by creating the Copyright Clearance Center (CCC, http://www.copyright.com/), which attempts to standardize the process of royalty payments for use of journal articles that are reproduced. Royalty payments are usually listed at the bottom of the first page of journal articles. They apply to individual use and not reproduction in other published works. The CCC acts as a clearinghouse, with libraries and copy shops forwarding royalties to CCC, which distributes them to publishers.

Probably the ideal method for IP protection is to encode rules for it in the object's metadata. The schemes described earlier in the book (e.g., DCMI) do this at best in a rudimentary way. The DOI system attempts to encode metadata that includes the means by which objects are accessed and thus protected. The original metadata schema for the DOI system was the Interoperability of Data in e-Commerce System (INDECS). This system defined a small kernel of metadata as well as additional metadata that can be used. The kernel includes the following attributes:

- Identifier – the DOI
- Title – the name of the entity
- Type – the type of resource of the object
- Mode – the "sensory" mode by which the object is perceived (e.g., text, audio, video)
- Primary agent – the creator of the object
- Agent role – the role the primary agent played in creating the object

The concepts in INDECS have been operationalized by the ISO/IEC 21000-6 (MPEG-21 Rights Data Dictionary) initiative (http://www.iso21000-6.net/).

6.4.2 Digital Rights Management

The area of protecting online IP is most commonly called *digital rights management* (DRM) (Becker, Buhse et al., 2004). There are a number of ongoing open and proprietary efforts in this field, which are mired in political and economic struggles among commercial content producers (e.g., the Recording Industry Association of America, Microsoft Corp., etc.). There has been considerable effort focused at developing DRM standards in the more open research and education communities (Martin, Kuhlman et al., 2002), which are philosophically more akin to the health-care environment than, say, users of products from the entertainment industry. The DRM issue remains a thorny one, not only for protecting IP but also allowing fair use and respecting the privacy rights of users (Tyrväinen, 2005). Bailey (2006) argues that strong copyright and DRM in face of poor "network neutrality" are a recipe for "digital dystopia."

It is certainly understandable that publishers wish to protect their IP. The question is how to provide them the tools to protect that property while expanding the market for their content, which may in turn allow them to lower the unit price of access. A particular challenge is how to serve the single users or those in small groups. While those at academic and other large medical centers often have direct access to resources based on their Internet Protocol addresses, practitioners who do not reside at such centers usually do not. Even clinicians at large centers want to access resources that their institutions do not provide and are inconvenienced by the usual authentication schemes.

A comprehensive framework for an inventory of digital rights comes from Rosenblatt et al. (2002), who has defined categories of rights and user actions within them:

- Render rights – print, view, play
- Transport rights – copy, move, loan
- Derivative work rights – extract, edit, embed
- Utility rights – backup, cache, insure data integrity

As noted above, the approach of Martin et al. (2002) may work best for users in health and biomedical settings. Their solution aims at research and educational resources, where IP protection is important, but must be balanced by open and easy use. They describe their approach as "federated," in that administration of access controls is shared between the origin site and the resource provider. Their approach builds on open standards, such as the Shibboleth initiative from Internet2 (http://shibboleth.internet2.edu/) that keeps track of, among other things, access right of individuals and resources. Shibboleth in turn takes advantage of the Open Security Access Markup Language (OpenSAML, http://www.opensaml.org/), which defines rights for such resources and a single sign-on to access them. A guiding vision for DRM efforts should be a mechanism whereby individuals can gain access to resources with a single sign-on to all resources for which they and their institution have access rights. In addition, the DRM framework should allow easy and rapid access to resources for which they do not have subscription-style access. For example, if a user wants access to a systematic review from an online journal to which he or she does not subscribe, there should be a single dialog box asking if he or she would like to pay a certain amount from his or her online digital wallet and then get instant access after the one click required to accept making the payment. Coyle (2005) has described a metadata approach for copyright status.

Another approach to IP protection has been the Creative Commons License (http://creativecommons.org/). This approach is based on the premise that some people do not necessarily want full copyright protection (which is the default under law) to apply to their works, but instead desire to attach certain restrictions to its use. In essence, the Creative Commons License allows a creator of IP to retain some rights short of completely released the content into the public domain. The Creative Commons licensing process begins by completing a form on their Web site (http://creativecommons.org/license/). The licensee chooses four options for the license, as described in Table 6.2 and shown by the icons in Fig. 6.3.

For example, a person creating IP who desired to allow others to use his or her work unmodified and for noncommercial purposes would select a license that included all the above options. Someone giving permission for the work to be modified but not used commercially or with any restrictions would choose a license with the latter two options. In addition to these basic four options, there are some additional special ones, such as allowing royalty-free uses in developing nations while retaining full copyright in the developed world or allowing specified amounts of sampling. Once the appropriate license is chosen, the Creative Commons Web site generates three types of data:

Table 6.2 Options for Creative Commons licensing (http://creativecommons.org/)

Option	Condition
Attribution	Others may copy, distribute, and display the copyrighted work – and derivates of it – but must give credit.
Noncommercial	Others may copy, distribute, and display the copyrighted work, but only for noncommercial purposes.
No derivative works	Others may copy, distribute, and display only unmodified versions of the copyrighted work.
Share alike	Others can distribute derivative works only under a license identical to the one governing the original work.

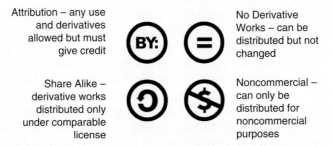

Fig. 6.3 The attributes of the Creative Commons licensing and their respective icons (http://creativecommons.org/)

1. Commons Deed – license in simple and plain language with appropriate icons
2. Legal Code – legal language designed to stand up in court
3. Digital Code – metadata to be included on Web sites and pages that enable search engines and other applications to know terms of use

The process also generates a logo with the Creative Commons logo and the statement, "Some Rights Reserved." The details of the licenses are described on the Creative Commons Web site (http://creativecommons.org/about/licenses/). Another project of the Creative Commons is the Science Commons (http://science-commons.org/), which aims to bring a comparable approach to the world of scientific data and publications. The Creative Commons Web site also has a search engine (http://creativecommons.org/find/) that allows searching over materials based on the options mentioned here (e.g., a search to find images that may be used for noncommercial purposes and may be modified).

6.4.3   Open-Access Publishing

A growing effort devoted to unimpeded access to scientific information has taken on the name *open-access* publishing. It is guided by the philosophy that access to scientific archives should be free and unimpeded, with other means used to finance the cost of scientific publishing. Another motivating factor is that most biomedical research is publicly funded (e.g., through the National Institutes of Health in the US), and the public should have the right to freely access its results. There is considerable debate over the merits of open-access publishing, including discussion of its financial feasibility as well as the issue of who controls scientific literature. The typical solution proposed for financing is that the author pays, based on the notion that most research is funded by grants, and a small additional charge for publishing should not adversely affect their budgets. (In fact, most researchers with grants consider the time they spend writing papers about the research to be part of their salary time that is funded.) Most open-access journals usually have provisions for those who cannot afford the page charges, especially scientists from developing countries. A bibliography of open-access publishing is maintained by Bailey (http://www.digital-scholarship.com/oab/oab.htm/).

The original open-access publishing effort in biomedicine was developed by Biomed Central (BMC, http://www.biomedcentral.com/). Since its inception, BMC has expanded to nearly 200 journals (http://www.biomedcentral.com/info/authors/journaloverview), with over 15,000 scientific articles published. Most BMC papers are indexed in MEDLINE and archived in PMC. Because BMC is a private company, it needs a business model where revenues exceed costs. The main sources of revenue are the article-processing charges that authors must pay after their article is accepted for publication. Reflecting the reality of these costs, the charges have increased from the original $500 to nearly $1,500 for the most expensive journals (http://www.biomedcentral.com/info/about/apcfaq). Individual journals can set their own rates, but must fit within the BMC business model. Most journals waive the charges for scientists who cannot afford them, making up for it by setting the rate for those who pay somewhat higher.

One new innovation at BMC has been institutional memberships, where institutions such as universities pay a fee to join, in turn allowing any member of that institution to publish without paying the usual publishing charge. In the United Kingdom (UK), the government pays an annual fee to BMC that allows any UK researcher to publish in BMC without paying the article-processing charge. Many BMC journals have been publishing long enough to receive impact factors (IFs). Several BMC journals have IFs above 5.0, and most IFs have increased over time for longer-established journals (http://www.biomedcentral.com/info/about/faq? name=impactfactor).

Another journal taking the open-access approach is the Public Library of Science (PLoS, http://www.plos.org/). PLoS has developed a number of journals using the open-access model. Its first was PLoS Biology, which began publication in 2003. Since then, it has launched PLoS Medicine, PLoS Computational Biology, PLoS Genetics, PLoS Pathogens, and PLoS Clinical Trials. One goal of the latter is to reduce publication bias for RCTs by making it easier to publish their results.

Most other journals have not opted for the open-access approach. Lancet has addressed the open-access issue in its pages, noting that the up-front page charges may limit venues of publishing for resource-poor scientists (although BMC and PLoS pledge to waive fees for such scientists) and that open access threatens the survival of nonprofit presses, such as university presses (Horton, 2003). The leadership of JAMA has also taken a negative view, noting that the article-processing charges of BMC and PLoS may not cover the costs of the publishing process, meaning that their business models are not sustainable, especially for journals with low acceptance rates like JAMA at 8% (DeAngelis and Musacchio, 2004). They have also expressed concern that this model may provide incentive for journals to publish more and, as a result, lower their quality. The publisher of BMC, on the other hand, retorted that journals still need to maintain their quality if they want to provide incentive for scientists to publish there (J. Velterop, personal communication).

One journal is actually going in reverse from open publishing. Long hailed as an innovator by making its entire content free on the Web, BMJ began restricting access to nonresearch articles (abridged articles, news stories, letters, etc.) in 2005. The journal said it undertook this action because subscriptions to BMJ had fallen off, resulting in decreased revenue for the production of the journal (Delamothe and Smith, 2003).

One alternative that has emerged to the open-access movement, mainly from nonprofit publishers (typically professional societies), is the *Washington DC Principles for Free Access to Science* (Anonymous, 2004e). These publishers reaffirmed their view that they maintain the copyright on their publications, but advocate a number of principles:

- Selected important articles available free online when published
- Complete contents freely available within months of publication

- Complete contents available for free to scientists in low-income countries
- Content available through online reference linking and major search engines

As such, articles older than 6–12 months are made freely available on most of the Web sites of these journals, which include JAMA, NEJM, and *Annals of Internal Medicine*.

In 2004, the Director of the US National Institutes of Health (NIH) released an analysis of the cost of publishing of NIH research results (Zerhouni, 2004). Based on an estimate that 0.32% of grant funding is devoted to publication costs, he noted that the NIH already provides about $30 million in direct costs for publications through its funded research grants. Zerhouni asserted that adopting a plan to archive all publications in PMC would add only another $2–4 million per year, since it would be built on top of the existing NIH information technology infrastructure. The RFC drew over 6,000 responses. Many were in favor, but both commercial and nonprofit publishers raised concerns about the plan. Among the latter were public documents from the American College of Physicians (Tooker, 2004) and the *New England Journal of Medicine* (Drazen and Curfman, 2004).

A number of public and private funding agencies have begun requiring its funded researchers to submit their papers to public repositories. In 2005, the NIH released a new policy on archiving scientific publications, adopting a voluntary approach whereby NIH-funded researchers were strongly encouraged either themselves or via their publishers to deposit reports of their research into PMC as soon as possible, and within 12 months after final publication (Anonymous, 2005a). Adherence so far has been modest, with only 5% of researchers having voluntarily submitted their papers. One concern was that the manuscript that authors submit may not represent the final version they submitted to the journal, as it may undergo subsequent editing by the journal editors. However, the NIH has now changed its policy effective in April 2008, whereby all manuscripts must be submitted to PMC within 12 months of publication, with instructions on a new NIH Public Access Web site (http://publicaccess.nih.gov/). This brings NIH in line with other public (the UK Medical Research Council) and private funding agencies (Wellcome Trust, http://www.wellcome.ac.uk/ and Howard Hughes Medical Institute, http://www.hhmi.org/) (Kaiser, 2008).

Now that the open-access movement has been around for several years, overviews and research about it have begun to emerge. A number of overviews have laid out the basic issues (Clarke, 2004; Anonymous, 2005d; Funk, 2005; Albert, 2006). Although some articles in the DL literature express great enthusiasm for it as a convergence with the movements to open-source software and open science (Willinsky, 2005), others maintain that a subset of researchers and librarians who are strong advocates are no match for the power of both the commercial and nonprofit publishers (Law, 2006). The latter notes that even though researchers and librarians who advocate open-access publishing have ambivalence about Google for serious research, the search engine may be an unwitting ally in efforts to open accessibility to electronic literature. Esposito (2004) has asserted that existing journals are unlikely to change their models and that new "upstart" media will lead the development of open-access publications.

Schroter and colleagues have published three studies surveying the knowledge and attitudes of authors toward open-access publishing. One study assessed authors who submitted papers to BMJ (Schroter, Tite et al., 2005). Most expressed support for the idea of open-access publishing, but few reported they had submitted to such journals. There was a strong sentiment that the quality of the journal influenced their submission decisions rather than the publishing model. Another study asked authors' opinions of a hypothetical decision by BMJ to restrict access to subscribers for all its online content, including research articles (Schroter, 2006). Only 14% of those surveyed said they would be much less likely to submit in the future if such restricted access were implemented, although two-third said it would diminish their view of the journal. A final study assessed author attitudes from BMJ and two other journals (Schroter and Tite, 2006). Before the survey was administered, less than half were familiar with the terms "open access" and "author pays." Only 10% had submitted to such journals. Open-access journals were viewed with skepticism: 27% thought they had lower impact factors and 46% believed that anyone who paid could get published (i.e., not having peer review). Slightly over half said that open access had low or no priority in their decisions on where to submit, and two-third said they would prefer to submit to a subscription-based journal.

Another study has surveyed senior authors and found that while knowledge about open-access publishing is still scant, with 18% knowing "a lot" or "quite a lot" and 81% having some awareness of it (Rowlands and Nicholas, 2005). About 29% claimed to have published in open-access journals, though the researchers warned that many people interpreted open access to mean free availability at their own institution, which could of course be the result on the institution having a subscription. These researchers also believed that article downloads were a better measure of the usefulness of research than citation counts. They also greatly appreciated electronic tools for tracking down references, rating physical libraries quite low as a place to find them.

A staunch supporter of open access is the European Commission, which has published a report (Dewatripont, Ginsburgh et al., 2006) and policy statement (Anonymous, 2007p), advocating wider access to published scientific literature, especially that funded by governments. This has led to advocacy for support of open-access publishing in the US (http://www.taxpayeraccess.org/).

6.5   Preservation

There are a number of issues related to the preservation of DL materials. One concerns the size of such materials. Although hard disk space is, in modern times, considered "cheap," the computer size of objects becomes important in determinations of how to store massive collections as well as transmit them across networks. Lesk (2005) has compared the longevity of digital materials. He has noted that the longevity for magnetic materials is the least, with the expected lifetime of magnetic tape being 5–10 years. Optical storage has somewhat better longevity, with an expected lifetime of 30–100 years depending on the specific type. Ironically, paper has a life expectancy well beyond all these digital media. Rothenberg (1999) has referred to the Rosetta Stone, which provided help in interpreting ancient Egyptian hieroglyphics and has survived over 20 centuries. He goes on to re-emphasize Lesk's description of the reduced lifetime of digital media in comparison to traditional media, and to note another problem familiar to most long-time users of computers, namely, data can become obsolete not only owing to the medium, but also as a result of data format. Both authors note that storage devices as well as computer applications, such as word processors, have seen their formats change significantly over the last couple of decades. Indeed, it may be harder in the future to decipher a document stored in the WordStar word processing format than an ancient stone or paper document.

One initiative aiming to preserve content is the Lots of Copies Keep Stuff Safe (LOCKSS, http://www.lockss.org) project (Rosenthal, Robertson et al., 2005). As the name implies, numerous digital copies of important documents can be maintained. But the project further concerns itself with the ability to detect and repair damaged copies as well as to prevent subversion of the data. This is done via hashing schemes that assess the integrity of the data in the multiples caches of content and "fix" altered copies.

Of course, some content such as that on the Web is highly dynamic and undergoes constant change. Kahle (1997) estimated that the lifetime of an average Web page was 44 days. He found that the "half-life" of the survival of Web pages may actually be a little longer, at roughly 2 years. This interest in the changing nature of Web pages led Kahle to undertake a project to archive the Internet (http://www.archive.org/) on a periodic basis. A popular feature of this Web site is the Internet Wayback Machine, which allows entry of a URL and its display at different points in time.

Nonetheless, there is an imperative to preserve documents of many types, whatever their medium (Tibbo, 2001). For society in general, there is certainly impetus to preserve historical documents in an unaltered form. And in all of science, certainly health and medicine, there is need to preserve the archive of scientific discoveries, particularly those presenting original experiments and their data. McCray and Gallagher (2001) have written an overview that describes the various principles of DL development, with an emphasis on persistent and accessible content. As noted in Chap. 2, a number of initiatives have been undertaken to insure preservation of scientific information. These include the National Digital Information Infrastructure Preservation Program (NDIIPP) of the US Library of Congress (Friedlander, 2002) and the Digital Preservation Coalition in the United Kingdom (Beagrie, 2002). A Web site has been developed to describe government work in digital preservation generally (http://www.digitalpreservation.gov/).

Rusbridge (2006) has reviewed some of the challenges in digital preservation. A data dictionary for preservation metadata has recently been released (Anonymous, 2005b). Kenney et al. (2006) recently surveyed the archiving approaches of 12 e-journals, which of course have to pay more attention to digital preservation since they do not produce paper copies.

The NLM has also addressed the issue of permanence levels for its archives (Byrnes, 2005). It has developed a Permanence Working Group that focuses on three characteristics of Web documents: identifier validity, resource availability, and content invariance. They have developed a rating system based on these and distilled them into the following four permanence levels:

- *Permanent: unchanging content.* Resource will be kept available permanently. Its identifier will always provide access to the resource. Its content will not change. Example: minutes of meetings.
- *Permanent: stable content.* Resource will be kept available permanently. Its identifier will always provide access to the resource. Its content is subject only to minor corrections or additions. Example: fact sheets.
- *Permanent: dynamic content.* Resource will be kept available permanently. Its identifier will always provide access to the resource. Its content could be revised or replaced. Example: NLM home page.
- *Permanence not guaranteed.* No commitment to keep this resource available. It could become unavailable at any time. Its content and identifier could be changed. Example: frequently asked questions.

6.6 Librarians, Informationists, and Other Professionals

One concern about digital libraries is access to the professionals who have always aided users of physical libraries. For example, reference librarians are still key to assisting researchers, especially when exhaustive searching is required, such as in systematic reviews. One challenge to the role of library professionals is an economic one: as the amount of online content increases in availability to users, and it is used directly with increasing frequency, the amount of time that can be devoted to any user and/or resource shrinks. However, the value of professional assistance to users cannot be denied.

One proposal that caused a stir when it was promoted in an *Annals of Internal Medicine* editorial is the notion of a new information professional for the clinical setting, the *informationist* (Davidoff and Florance, 2000). The medical library community responded to this call by touting the virtue of clinical librarianship and affirming the value of library science training (Schacher, 2001). This term was actually introduced by Garfield (1979a) in the context of having information professionals who understood the laws of information science and was advocated in the early 1990s by Quint (1992). A recent special issue of *Journal of the Medical Library Association* responded to how librarians might take up the challenge in this new era (Shearer, Seymour et al., 2001), with additional elucidation on how education in library and information science (Detlefsen, 2002) and medical informatics (Hersh, 2002) might be structured.

Although the informationist concept continues to generate a fair amount of discussion (and publications), the concept has yet to see widespread adoption.

The original publications cited in the book led to a conference held at the NLM to continue discussion on whether and how such a professional should be developed and function in the clinical setting. The conference resulted in a series of recommendations (Plutchak, 2002; Shipman, Cunningham et al., 2002). Although there has been little research assessing the efficacy of the informationist approach (e.g., in terms of improved clinical care or reduced information-seeking time by clinicians), several new models have emerged. The most mature of these models in the clinical informationist, with the informationist helping to optimize the use not only evidence-based information but also informatics tools at the point of care (Giuse, Koonce et al., 2005). Another approach has been to adapt the model to the biomedical research environment, leading to the clinical bioinformationist model, focusing on molecular biology, genetic analysis, biotechnology, research literature, and databases (Lyon, Giuse et al., 2004). Florance et al. (2002) have described the challenges of integrating information specialists into various biomedical settings. Rosenbloom et al. (2005) have found that informationists have skill levels comparable to physicians trained in research methodology and better than general physicians for selecting pertinent articles for clinical questions.

Recall from Chap. 2 that clinicians have frequent information needs, of the order of two questions for every three patients seen, yet they pursue answers to only one-third of them (Gorman, 1995). This research also showed that the most common source clinicians turned to for answers was another human, most often a colleague or consultant in their referral chain. It was shown in Chap. 7 that relative to overall information needs, computer-based knowledge resources have been used modestly (i.e., the average user seeks answers to clinical questions with online resources only a few times per month). One likely reason for this is the time it takes to obtain an answer: upward of 30 min when one is using MEDLINE and journal literature (Hersh, Crabtree et al., 2000). It is possible that the move toward synoptic information resources, particularly those that adhere to principles of evidence-based medicine, may increase the usage of online knowledge resources (Haynes, 2001).

Another approach to providing knowledge-based information to clinicians might involve the development of technologies that recognize the value of person-to-person consultation and facilitate it. This approach is much less developed than the myriad of online information resources, especially when used in the clinician-to-clinician mode. There are a great many online patient-to-clinician consultation services. Probably the largest of these is NetWellness, which has over 17,000 answered questions in its database (Guard, Fredericka et al., 2000).

Some early clinician-to-clinician consultation services were developed in Iowa (Bergus, Sinift et al., 1998) and the Netherlands (Moorman, Branger et al., 2001). The former used e-mail for physician communications, while the latter used an option within the EMR. A different approach has been taken by others who offer online consultations for a fee, e.g., Partners Medical System (http://econsults. partners.org/) and The Cleveland Clinic (http://www.eclevelandclinic.org/). A review of the Partners consultations found that while only a small number resulted in changed diagnoses (4%), a substantial number (90%) resulted in changes in treatment (Kedar, Ternullo et al., 2003).

Another form of linking to human knowledge is, of course, the reference librarian, described earlier in the book. With the growing amount of online information, the marketplace for others (i.e., nonlibrarians) to fulfill this role has grown. Janes et al. (2001) assessed 20 commercial and noncommercial "expert services" sites that answered information needs for a fee. Three types of questions were developed:

1. Factual questions with verifiable answers
2. Source questions looking for specific information sources
3. Out-of-scope questions explicitly outside the scope of a given service

The response rate for all questions by different services was highly variable, with an overall average of 70%. The rate of correctness for questions with verifiable answers was likewise highly variable, but averaged 69% overall. The subjects with the highest rate of verifiable correctness were Shakespeare (100%) and education (90%). Health questions only had a 50% correct rate.

Another question-answering service that gained a high profile but ultimately was retired was Google Answers (http://answers.google.com/). This service used an "eBay-like" approach, where a user entered some information about the question and a price of how much money he or she was willing to pay (Kenney, McGovern et al., 2003). Google maintained a group of "researchers" who were "experts at finding information." Entering a higher price resulted in more detailed research or a quicker answer, according to the site instructions. The site also allowed other users to search over questions that have been entered. Users of the service were discouraged from entering personal information about themselves, requesting private information about others, seeking assistance in conducting illegal activities, seeking help on school examinations or homework, or trying to sell or advertise products. A preliminary analysis by Kenney et al. (2006) compared the Google Answers service with reference librarians from Cornell University with 24 questions, with the blinded assessment of answers finding a trend toward better answers with the university librarians. These authors also note a concern expressed by professional librarians about the eBay-like approach of the information seeking, in particular with the nonestablishment of a relationship between the patron and the librarian.

6.7 Future Directions

This chapter brings to an end our exploration of the state of the art for IR and DLs. Although access to knowledge-based information is common and even ubiquitous across the globe, the chapters in this section have demonstrated that there are still challenges to improve these systems. In the remainder of the book, we will explore major threads of research in IR, from evaluating the use of systems to developing new approaches for systems and their users.

Part III
Research Directions

Chapter 7
Evaluation

A recurring theme throughout the book thus far is that the information retrieval (IR) world has changed substantially since the first two editions, particularly with the ubiquity of the World Wide Web. From this, one would have expected a substantial increase in the amount and quality of evaluation research. However, this is not the case. While a modest number of new evaluation studies have appeared since the last edition, growth of evaluation research has not paralleled the explosion of new content and systems. This may well be due to the overall success and ubiquity of IR systems in the Web era, i.e., such systems are so ingrained in the lives of users that few believe that the need to evaluate them still exists. This is of course not the case, for much can be learned from looking at how these resources are used and from identifying areas calling for improvement.

In this chapter, we will mainly focus on the evaluation of operational IR systems. (Research system evaluation will be discussed in the context of the research presented in Chap. 8.) We will then focus on two additional issues: research on relevance and on different measures. Our discussion will conclude with a summary of lessons learned and directions for future research.

For the evaluation of operational systems, our discussion will be organized around six questions developed for a systematic review of physician searching and introduced in Chap. 1 (Hersh and Hickam, 1998):

1. Was the system used?
2. For what was the system used?
3. Were the users satisfied?
4. How well did they use the system?
5. What factors were associated with successful or unsuccessful use of the system?
6. Did the system have an impact?

7.1 Usage Frequency

One of the best measurements of the value of IR systems is whether the applications are actually used by their intended audience. One can hypothesize about the pros and cons of different IR systems, but the discussion is moot if the system does not

W. Hersh, *Information Retrieval: A Health and Biomedical Perspective,*
doi: 10.1007/978-0-387-78703-9, © Springer Science + Business Media, LLC 2009

sustain the interest of users in the real world. This is certainly an important issue for developers of commercial systems, since unused systems are unlikely to last long in the marketplace. Clearly, IR systems are used by many people. As noted in Chap. 1, nearly all physicians use the Internet (Anonymous, 2005e), with those who have busier practices likely to use it more (Taylor and Leitman, 2001). In addition, a large majority of others who use the Internet have searched for personal health information (Fox, 2006; Anonymous, 2007m). Furthermore, the National Library of Medicine (NLM) reports about 70,000–80,000 searches per month from around the world on PubMed (http://www.ncbi.nlm.nih.gov/About/tools/restable_stat_pubmed.html).

A number of usage studies were done in the 1980s and 1990s when IR systems were first becoming available in medical setting. Somewhat ironically, such studies were easier to do at that time, since most IR systems required logging in and there were fewer places where they could be accessed. Now, of course, IR systems are available almost everywhere, from desktop computers to wireless laptops and personal digital assistants (PDAs). As such, measuring how often an IR system is used, let alone for a health or biomedical information need, can be challenging at the present.

There were lessons to be learned from the early studies, which were summarized in a systematic review by Hersh and Hickam (1998). A review of about a dozen studies, in a variety of settings and with a variety of users, found usage to be only of the order of 0.3–6.0 times per user per month. This was noted to be in stark contrast with the known two-questions-per-three-patients information needs of clinicians (Gorman, 1995). In addition, a novelty effect was noted, in that usage was lower with a longer duration of observation. Another usage-related finding was a propensity for use of bibliographic resources, in particular MEDLINE, as opposed to full-text resources (such as CD-ROM textbooks).

Data from newer studies do not contradict these older findings. Studies assessing IR system use continue to find usage less than once a day even for newer types of content and devices, including PDA databases (Lapinsky, Wax et al., 2004), evidence-based resources (Westbrook, Gosling et al., 2004; Magrabi, Coiera et al., 2005), an online clinical database (Maviglia, Martin et al., 2002), and infobuttons (Rosenbloom, Geissbuhler et al., 2005; Maviglia, Yoon et al., 2006). One study of a system that provided ratings of quality and relevance by other clinicians was found to be used about twice per day (Haynes, Holland et al., 2006). Studies of PDA use generally in healthcare show have shown that a majority of physicians use these devices quite heavily for clinical care tasks (Garritty and ElEmam, 2006), but their frequency of use of them for IR tasks is comparable to other systems. Even continued studies of physician pursuit of information needs continue to find paper textbooks and other humans to be used more commonly (Arroll, Pandit et al., 2002; Ely, Osheroff et al., 2005). Likewise, at least when measured, bibliographic databases still account for a majority of IR system usage (Nankivell, Wallis et al., 2001). Thus, while IR system in clinical settings is still modest, they are used, and it is unlikely anyone would advocate their not being made available.

There are few studies of nonphysician usage of IR systems for health and biomedical searches. One study looked at reported usage of NLM databases by specific user groups (Wood, Wallingford et al., 1997). The results varied from more than ten times a month (librarian/information services professionals) to one to three times a month (healthcare providers, researchers, educators, students, legal professionals, and media personnel) to less than once a month (patients and healthcare consumers). Although consumers are now well-known users of health-related IR systems, there are no studies of their usage. The closest to such studies comes from analysis of Web searching logs. Spink et al. (2002) have analyzed large numbers of queries posed to the Excite search engine. As these queries solely consist of what the user entered, the information needs behind them are unknown. Furthermore, nothing is known about the individuals who posed them, such as who they are, where they reside, or how many queries they posed. Their analysis found that in 1997, the proportion of "health or sciences" queries was 9.5% of all queries, while by 2001 that proportion dropped to 7.5%. Similarly, Eysenbach and Kohler (2004) have found that about 4.5% of all searches to a Web metasearch engine were on health-related topics.

Another analysis focused on a query log of PubMed rather than a population of individual users (Herskovic, Tanaka et al., 2007). A single day's log from around October 2005 was made available to these researchers. They were able to determine "individuals" by Internet protocol (IP) address. They eliminated from their analysis all users with over 50 queries during the time period, figuring that these were "bot" queries. For the remainder of the data, they determined that there were about 2.7 million queries posed by 624,514 users. The mean number of queries per user was 4.21, while the median number of queries was 2. The three most commonly used words were the PubMed tags [author], [au], and [pmid]. These were followed in frequency by the words cancer, cell, review, and 2005.

A more focused analysis was carried out on 2,272 randomly selected queries. These queries were classified as *informational* (74.4%) vs. *navigational* (22.1%), with the latter appearing to be seeking specific articles. The number of articles in the results set of these queries varied widely (1–4.8 million), with an average of 14,050 and median of 68. Only 11.2% of queries used Boolean operators, with nearly all of them AND. However, another 10.6% of articles had Boolean words (and, or, not) in lowercase and were possibly attempting to use them, although as recalled from Chap. 5, PubMed requires such operators to be in uppercase.

7.2 Types of Usage

In addition to knowing the frequency of system usage, it is also valuable to know what types of information need users address. Many of the studies described in Sect. 7.1 also investigated this issue. Since information resources, users, and settings were heterogeneous, direct comparison is difficult. But taken as a whole, the studies in the Hersh and Hickam (1998) found a relatively consistent picture that questions of therapy are most frequent, followed by overview (or review) and diagnosis.

More recent studies verify these results. Arroll et al. (2002) found that the most common types of questions asked were about treatment (39%), diagnosis (33%), administration (19%), monitoring (4%), prevention (2%), and general review (2%). Another study of faculty physicians found similar result, with questions of therapy (50%), prognosis (14%), epidemiology (13%), and prevention/screening (11%) most common (Schwartz, Northrup et al., 2003). The study of consumers by Fox (2006) found that consumers searching the Web for health information most often were looking for information about a specific disease or medical problem (63%), a certain medical procedure or treatment (47%), or diet or nutrition information (44%).

7.3   User Satisfaction

Another method of evaluating the impact of an IR system is to measure user satisfaction. Of course, researchers are never certain that a user's satisfaction with a system is associated with its successful use. This may be especially problematic when systems are made available with great fanfare, without charge, and in academic settings where peer pressure might motivate their use. Nonetheless, for computer applications in general, Nielsen and Levy (1994) performed a meta-analysis of studies in the human–computer interface literature that showed a general correlation between user satisfaction and successful use of systems. Hersh and Hickam (1998) found a relatively consistent picture for user satisfaction. Although diverse satisfaction-related questions were asked in the included studies, it was found in general that 50–90% of users were satisfied with the system provided them. When users were not satisfied with systems, the general reasons were the time required to use them, concerns over the completeness of information, and difficulties in navigating the software.

One specific form of satisfaction in clinical settings is the belief whether systems made an impact in clinical care. Similar to satisfaction generally, most studies that have measured this aspect have found that most clinicians self-report improvements in delivery of healthcare. One study of usage by family medicine physicians found the belief that care was improved for current patients 56% of the time and would be improved for future patients 70% of the time (Schwartz, Northrup et al., 2003). In another study of an online evidence system in Australia, users reported that nearly half of clinician users reported success in finding answers most or all of the time, while 74% believed the system improved patient care. One study of infobuttons found a self-report that the system answered users' queries 84% of the time and changed patient care decisions 15% of the time (Maviglia, Yoon et al., 2006).

What is the user satisfaction with PDAs for IR tasks? One of the studies in the previous section conducted a focus group to identify shortcomings of PDAs and noted such problems as small text fonts for reading, inadequate search engines, text entry errors, and battery discharge (Lapinsky, Wax et al., 2004). Another study, however, reported positive impact for a PDA-based drug reference in saving time and improving decision making (Rothschild, Lee et al., 2002). It is likely that PDAs are useful for quick and simple access to information, but less valuable for more complex information needs.

7.4 Searching Quality

While usage frequency and user satisfaction are important components in any system evaluation, it is also important to understand how effectively users search with IR systems. As was discussed in Chap. 1, the most commonly used measures used to assess the effectiveness of searchers and databases have been the relevance-based measures of recall and precision. Despite some controversy about the value of these measures in capturing the quality of the interaction with the IR system, considerable knowledge about IR systems has been gained by their use, although newer approaches to evaluation have provided additional perspective.

This section of the chapter is divided into two parts: evaluations that focus on performance of the system and those that focus on the user. As with many classifications in this book, the line between the two is occasionally fuzzy. Within each category, the studies are divided into those that focus predominantly on bibliographic databases, full-text databases, and Web resources. While the discussion focuses on health-related studies, a few important nonhealth evaluation studies are described as well. In addition, since studies of searching have been done for several decades, the discussion will focus on those that assess general techniques and content matter as opposed to specific databases or systems.

7.4.1 System-Oriented Performance Evaluations

System-oriented studies are those that focus on some aspect of the system. That is, even though the searches may have been originated by real users, the research question was oriented toward some aspect of system performance. Many system-oriented retrieval studies were undertaken in the late 1950s and 1960s, but two stand out as setting the historical groundwork for such evaluations. The first of these was actually a series of experiments, commonly called the Cranfield studies, conducted by Cleverdon and associates at the Cranfield College of Aeronautics in England (Cleverdon and Keen, 1966). While these studies have been criticized for some of the methods and assumptions used (Swanson, 1977), they provided a focus for retrieval performance research and the limitations of such studies. The second study, performed by Lancaster (1968), was the first IR evaluation to provide insight into the success and failure of IR systems. Commissioned by the NLM, this study assessed MEDLINE as it was available at the time: with searches composed by librarians on forms that were mailed to the NLM, which ran the actual searches and returned the results by mail. Preceding the advent of interactive searching, this access to MEDLINE was markedly different than from what is available today.

Lancaster's study assessed a total of 299 searches from 21 different academic, research, and commercial sites in 1966–1967. In his protocol, users first completed a searching form and mailed it to the NLM, where librarians undertook a second, manual search on the topic, using *Index Medicus*. The results of both searches were combined and returned to the searcher by mail. The user then judged the combined set of results for relevance. The results showed that the recall and precision for the computer-based searches were 57.7 and 54.4%, respectively, indicating that the manual searches identified many articles that the computer searches did not (and vice versa). For "value" articles (i.e., only those denoted "highly relevant"), recall and precision for the computer-based searches were 65.2 and 25.7%. Lancaster also performed a failure analysis, which is described shortly.

System-oriented evaluations of bibliographic databases have focused on issues such as comparability across different databases, comparability of different approaches with the same database, and optimal strategies for finding articles of specific types. Several studies have assessed how well different databases cover specific topics. McCain et al. (1987) compared different databases for accessing the same topic in medical behavioral sciences. Of the five databases studied, three were bibliographic (MEDLINE, Excerpta Medica, and Psycinfo) and two provided topic citations (Science Citation Index and Social Science Citation Index). The results for the different databases varied widely for recall (18–37%) and precision (50–70%), but clearly each database offered novel relevant and many nonrelevant documents. A more recent study compared five databases (MEDLINE, BIOSIS, EMBASE, NIOSH-TIC, and TOXLINE) for topics related to occupational and environmental toxicology (Gehanno, Paris et al., 1998). The analysis measured recall in a single database followed by combinations of two, three, four, and five databases. Table 7.1 lists the range of recall when searching was done in single and multiple databases and demonstrates that recall improves as the number of databases combined increased.

Some more recent studies have also attempted to compare the value of different databases. Koonce et al. (2004) compared several evidence-based resources for their ability to answer two types of clinical questions: 40 complex questions generated during clinical rounds and 40 general care management questions. Instead of comparing resources against each other, they used all of them to identify the best answer. Their results found that 20% of the complex clinical questions and

Table 7.1 Recall in searching one to five databases for topics related to occupational and environmental toxicology (adapted from Gehanno, Paris et al., 1998)

Number of databases	Range of recall (%)
1	15–59
2	52–84
3	74–93
4	84–99
5	100

47.5% of the general care management questions were completely answered, while 40 and 22.5% of each, respectively, were partially answered. The remainder were unanswered.

Another comparison of "point of care" evidence-based knowledge tools was carried out by Trumble et al. (2007), who looked at the major market segment leaders in this area, assessing them by the quality of their evidence as well as other factors deemed important by an expert panel, such as breadth of information, depth of information, searchability, links to PubMed, and availability of PDA versions. Each product was then ranked by the quality of evidence, the factors deemed most important, and an overall score. The clear leader in all categories was the ACP PIER (http://pier.acponline.org/), followed by *Clinical Evidence* (http://clinicale-vidence.bmj.com/) and *DynaMed* (http://www.ebscohost.com/dynamed/)

Alper et al. (2001) assessed a variety of free and commercial systems for answering the clinical questions of primary care family physicians. Twenty questions were selected for searching from a database of over 1,200 that had been captured observing clinical practice. The selected questions covered a broad array of not only topics but also question types. The study found that four combinations of two databases could answer more than 80% of questions. Two combinations of three databases could answer 90% of questions, while some combinations of four databases answered 95% of questions. This study demonstrated what we have known for decades, which is that no single secondary literature resource answers all questions, and a variety must be available to comprehensively meet information needs.

Other research has focused on comparing different systems accessing the same database. Haynes et al. (1985) undertook a study comparing the performance and time required of 14 different access routes to MEDLINE available in 1986 for six clinical topics. They found that most systems yielded the same quantity of articles both directly and generally relevant, though there were substantial differences in cost, online time required, and ease of use. This study was repeated nearly a decade later, and again, substantial differences were found between systems (Haynes, Walker et al., 1994). The mean number of relevant (1.1–8.4 per search) and nonrelevant (4.9–64.9 per search) citations retrieved varied widely, even though essentially the same search was being run in each system.

Some studies in which the same database was searched have looked at specific features and their impact on retrieval performance. One focus has been the value of MeSH terms in searching MEDLINE. Hersh et al. (1994) compared MEDLINE retrieval using indexing of text (i.e., title and abstract) words only with the indexing of MeSH terms added to text words. Using natural language queries, precision at fixed levels of recall in a MEDLINE test collection was found to improve by about 10% with the MeSH terms also indexed. Srinivasan (1996a) has obtained comparable results. Another study compared the use of MeSH terms in two different commercial products, Dialog and Ovid (Hallett, 1998). Dialog was found to retrieve more references with the same query because of its "double posting," whereby MeSH terms were searched on as whole phrases as well as the individual words within them. This study and the one already cited (Haynes, McKibbon et al., 1985) showed that different results could be obtained for use of the same search terms against the same database.

A third line of system-oriented research with bibliographic databases has focused on the ability to retrieve articles of a specific type. This approach to searching is usually done in the context of evidence-based medicine (EBM), where the searcher is seeking to identify the "best evidence" for a given question. As noted in Chap. 2, what constitutes the best evidence varies according to the question being asked. In the case of articles about interventions, the most common type of question asked of retrieval systems (see Sect. 7.2), the best evidence comes from a randomized controlled trial (RCT). These studies are best accessed by the use of the Publication Type `Randomized Controlled Trial`.

The ability to identify RCTs is particularly important in the production of systematic reviews, especially those that employ meta-analysis. However, the use of the RCT publication type is not perfect. A number of studies have assessed the ability to find RCTs in numerous topic areas. Dickersin et al. (1994), in a systematic review of studies of this question, found that no combinations of search strategies could retrieve all the RCTs identified by exhaustive hand searching. Studies also showed that precision fell drastically as levels of recall increased. More recent studies in the areas of emergency medicine (Langham, Thompson et al., 1999), depression (Watson and Richardson, 1999), rheumatological disorders (Suarez-Almazor, Belseck et al., 2000), medical imaging (Berry, Kelly et al., 2000), and clinical nutrition (Avenell, Handoll et al., 2001) have shown that this problem persists.

Some research has applied more advanced computational approaches, in particular machine learning, to improve the detection of articles likely to contain high-quality evidence. Aphinyanaphongs et al. (2005, 2006) have demonstrated superior retrieval performance over the standard approaches in the NLM Clinical Queries. Cohen et al. (2006) have shown that these techniques can classify articles as likely to have data for systematic reviews, thereby reducing workload for the labor-intensive task of their production.

Other research has assessed identification of methodologically sound studies from databases without the benefit of MEDLINE indexing. Johnson et al. (1995) found that while the MEDLINE publication types were valuable in identifying such studies, search strategies could be devised that enhanced their recall by using the full text of the document or its cited reference fields. Hersh and Price (1998), wishing to identify strategies to retrieve RCTs from unindexed abstracts of conference proceedings, compared a variety of different strategies and found that near-complete recall could be obtained at a price of very poor precision (10–15%). Both this study and a follow-up analysis of the analysis of Wilczynski et al. (1995) found that studies that were not RCTs were sometimes indexed as such and that some that were RCTs were not assigned the appropriate publication type. The latter study also found that studies of other types had similar problems (e.g., studies of diagnostic tests not meeting criteria for being methodologically sound having the word `sensitivity` or `specicity` in their title or abstract).

The second category of system-oriented evaluation focuses on full-text databases, and often their comparison with searching on comparable bibliographic content. The earliest comprehensive study of full-text databases was performed by Tenopir

(1985), who assessed full-text searching of the *Harvard Business Review*. The searches consisted of 40 queries presented to two business school libraries. Tenopir formulated each search and searched on four different levels of text: full text of the documents; abstract words only; controlled vocabulary terms (the documents also had human indexing); and a union of title, abstract, and controlled terms.

Relevance of the retrieved documents was judged by three experts from the business school. The results (see Table 7.2) showed that recall was much higher for full-text searching, but at the cost of markedly diminished precision. Searching less than the full text yielded better precision but less recall. Among the nonfull-text types of searching, controlled vocabulary terms performed somewhat better than use of abstract words, but a combination of these, along with title words, achieved better recall without sacrificing precision. These results demonstrate that indexing more text of a document increases both quality and noise words. They also demonstrate that the use of abstract words and controlled indexing terms can be complementary.

Another well-known study of full-text retrieval was carried out by Blair and Maron (1985). These investigators used the IBM STAIRS system, a full-text, word-based, Boolean system, to evaluate a legal database of 40,000 documents. Fifty-one searches were posed by two attorneys and carried out by paralegal assistants. Searching was repeated until a satisfactory document collection was obtained for a query. After this, additional searching was done by logical (changing ANDs to ORs) and semantic (adding synonyms) expansion. The attorneys who originated the searches made relevance judgments using a four-point scale: vital, satisfactory, marginally relevant, or not relevant. The results (see Table 7.2) showed that recall

Table 7.2 Results of full-text vs. abstract searching in some early studies

Database and condition	Percentage of recall	Percentage of precision
Harvard Business Review (Tenopir, 1985)		
Full text	73.9	18.0
Abstract only	19.3	35.6
Controlled terms	28.0	34.0
Union of all	44.9	37.0
Legal document database (Blair and Maron, 1985)		
All articles	20.0	79.0
Vital and satisfactory articles	25.3	56.6
Vital articles only	48.2	18.3
Medical databases (McKinin, Sievert et al., 1991)		
MEDLINE – indexing terms	42	55
MEDLINE – text words	41	62
MEDIS – full text	78	37
CCML – full text	76	37

was low, far below the 75% level that the attorneys felt was required for optimal searching results.

Full-text searching has also been assessed in the medical domain. McKinin et al. compared searching in two full-text medical databases and MEDLINE (McKinin, Sievert et al., 1991). They took 89 search requests from a university medical library and performed each one on all three systems. Only documents present in all three were used for recall and precision calculations. The articles were judged for relevance by the original requester on a four-point scale: relevant, probably relevant, probably not relevant, not relevant. Their results paralleled those obtained by Tenopir (see Table 7.2), with full-text searching by word-based Boolean methods leading to higher recall at the expense of lower precision in comparison to abstract (i.e., MEDLINE) searching.

The number of studies assessing performance of Web searching systems is surprisingly small. Many of them have focused on the clinical quality of information retrieved rather than measures of retrieval performance. Those that have looked at performance have tended to focus on the quantity of pages retrieved rather than their relevance. The most comprehensive general (i.e., nonmedical) analysis of Web sites focuses on the number of Web pages returned for a group of single-word searches (Search Engine Showdown, http://www.searchengineshow-down.com/). A medical search engine "road test" also took this approach to comparing different clinically oriented Web catalogs (Anonymous, 1997).

Some studies have assessed the ability to search Web resources. Hersh et al. (1998) had a medical librarian enter 50 queries previously known to have answers in the MEDLINE database (Gorman, Ash et al., 1994). The queries were entered into the metasearch engine Metacrawler, with the goal of finding pages oriented toward the healthcare professional (as opposed to the consumer). The results showed that only 26 (52%) of the queries had one or more applicable pages. The proportion of pages having content directly addressing the clinical question (precision) was only 10.7%.

Another study of the ability of Web resources to answer clinical questions looked at how many questions could be answered by specific sites, be they general search engines or medically specific catalogs (Graber, Bergus et al., 1999). Ten questions were posed to nearly 20 sites. One site was able to answer six questions (MDConsult, http://www.mdconsult.com/), while three were able to answer five (HotBot, http://www.hotbot.com/; Excite, http://www.excite.com/; HardinMD, http://www.arcade.uiowa.edu/hardin/md/). Most of the medicine-specific Web catalogs performed poorly.

One problem with studies of Web resources is the rapid change of the Web itself. Nonetheless, these studies do highlight the challenge of finding clinical information on the Web, especially for healthcare professionals. While the Web crawler search engines contain a great deal of nonprofessional and/or low-quality information, the Web catalogs have a hard time keeping track of all the potentially good sites. Furthermore, a great deal of valuable information is hidden in the "invisible Web," virtually inaccessible to the novice user who does not know where to look or lacks a subscription.

7.4.2 User-Oriented Performance Evaluations

Studies assessing the ability of users with IR systems have looked at a variety of measures to define performance; user's self-reports of success were described earlier as user satisfaction studies (Sect. 7.3). A great many have focused on the retrieval of relevant documents, usually as measured by recall and precision, although these measures have been criticized for being less pertinent to user success (see Chap. 3). Other studies have attempted to measure how well users are able to complete a prescribed task, such as answering a clinical question.

In summarizing the first two decades of research on user-oriented evaluation, Fenichel (1980) noted several consistent findings across studies that are probably still pertinent today:

1. There was a correlation between search success, measured in terms of recall, and "search effort," which included number of commands used and time taken.
2. There was considerable variation across users, even with the same system and database. Even experienced users made mistakes that affected searching performance.
3. New users could learn to perform good searches after minimal training.
4. The major problems were related more to the search strategy than to the mechanics of using the system. Users made few errors related to use of the command language.

The main approach to user-oriented evaluation has been through the use of relevance-based measures. One of the original studies measuring searching performance in clinical settings was performed by Haynes et al. (1990). This study also compared the capabilities of librarian and clinician searchers. In this study, 78 searches were randomly chosen for replication by both a clinician experienced in searching and a medical librarian. During this study, each original ("novice") user had been required to enter a brief statement of information need before entering the search program. This statement was given to the experienced clinician and librarian for searching on MEDLINE. All the retrievals for each search were given to a subject domain expert, blinded with respect to which searcher retrieved which reference. Recall and precision were calculated for each query and averaged. The results (Table 7.3) showed that the experienced clinicians and librarians achieved comparable recall, although the librarians had statistically significantly better

Table 7.3 Results from an early study comparing Grateful Med users (adapted from Haynes, McKibbon et al., 1990)

Users	Results (%)	
	Recall	Precision
Novice clinicians	27	38
Experienced clinicians	48	49
Medical librarians	49	58

precision. The novice clinician searchers had lower recall and precision than either of the other groups. This study also assessed user satisfaction of the novice searchers, who despite their recall and precision results said that they were satisfied with their search outcomes. The investigators did not assess whether the novices obtained enough relevant articles to answer their questions, or whether they would have found additional value with the ones that were missed.

A follow-up study yielded some additional insights about the searchers (McKibbon, Haynes et al., 1990), which were described in the last chapter. As was noted, different searchers tended to use different strategies on a given topic. The different approaches replicated a finding known from other searching studies in the past, namely, the lack of overlap across searchers of overall retrieved citations as well as relevant ones. Figure 7.1 shows overlap diagrams, pointing out that the majority of both retrieved documents and relevant documents were retrieved by one searcher only. Thus, even though the novice searchers had lower recall, they did obtain a great many relevant citations not retrieved by the two expert searchers. Furthermore, fewer than 4% of all the relevant citations were retrieved by all three searchers. Despite the widely divergent search strategies and retrieval sets, overall recall and precision were quite similar among the three classes of users.

A later study by the same group assessed different methods of training novice searchers to make them as effective as experts (Haynes, Johnston et al., 1992). It consisted of a randomized trial comparing the basic 2-h training session with the training session plus the addition of a clinical preceptor experienced in searching. There was no difference in searching ability between the two groups, as measured by average number of relevant references retrieved, but both groups improved their performance to the level of experienced searchers by their fourth online search.

Another large-scale attempt to assess recall and precision in clinician searchers was carried out by Hersh and Hickam (1994). These authors attempted not only to assess the capability of expert vs. novice searchers but also provided the latter with access to MEDLINE via Knowledge Finder (KF). This partial-match search system,

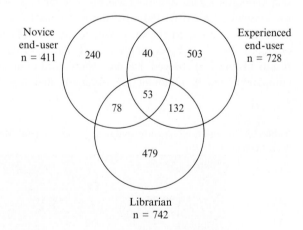

Fig. 7.1 Overlap of relevant articles retrieved by three MEDLINE searchers (adapted from McKibbon et al., 1990)

which represents one of the first commercial implementations of that approach, utilizes non-Boolean "natural language" searches, with relevance ranking of the output. The output sets are usually much larger than those obtained with Boolean systems, with KF setting its default maximum output at 100 references. Hersh and Hickam also compared the performance of the experienced searchers using the full MEDLINE feature set and just text words from the title, abstract, and MeSH heading fields.

As with the studies of Haynes et al., statements of information need were collected online and given for replication to experienced searchers, who were able to use either the NLM's command-line-based ELHILL system or Grateful Med. Most opted for the former. Logs of all searching interactions were also kept. The KF system used in this study was a CD-ROM version containing MEDLINE references from 270 core primary care journals covering a period of 5 years. As with Haynes et al., relevance was assessed by clinicians blinded to the searcher.

One problem with the results of this study (and in fact any study comparing Boolean and natural-language searching) was the large retrieval set obtained by using KF. While advocates of this approach argue that a large output of relevance-ranked documents allows the searcher to choose their own recall and precision (i.e., there are usually more relevant documents near the top of the list, so the further one looks down the retrieval list, the more likely it is that recall will increase and precision will decrease), direct comparison of recall and precision with sets generated from Boolean retrieval is difficult. As seen in Table 7.4, the clinicians who were novices were able to retrieve spectacularly higher recall than any of the expert searchers, although they paid a price in precision (and most likely would not look at all 100 references on the retrieval list anyway). To give a comparison of the novice searchers with retrieval at a level more comparable to that of the experienced searchers, a second set of recall and precision values was calculated with KF's default retrieval lowered to 15, the average size of Boolean retrieval sets. The levels of recall and precision were still comparable among all groups of expert searchers,

Table 7.4 Comparison of Knowledge Finder and ELHILL users (adapted from Hersh and Hickam, 1994)

Group	Retrieved	Results definitely relevant only (%)		Results definitely/ possibly relevant (%)	
		Recall	Precision	Recall	Precision
Novice physicians, using KF	88.8	68.2	14.7	72.5	30.8
Novice physicians, KF top 15	14.6	31.2	24.8	25.5	43.8
Librarians, full MEDLINE	18.0	37.1	36.1	30.8	59.4
Librarians, text words only	17.0	31.5	31.9	27.0	50.3
Experienced physicians, full MEDLINE	10.9	26.6	34.9	19.8	55.2
Experienced physicians, text words only	14.8	30.6	31.4	24.1	48.4

Table 7.5 Overlap among relevant references retrieval by up to five users (adapted from Hersh and Hickam, 1994)

Number of searchers	Relevant references retrieved
1	957 (53.2%)
2	474 (26.4%)
3	190 (10.6%)
4	99 (5.5%)
5	42 (2.3%)

with no statistically significant differences. Thus, the approach used by KF clearly showed the potential to be of value to searchers, certainly novices.

Overlap among retrieval of relevant articles was also assessed, with results similar to those of Haynes et al. As shown in Table 7.5, over half of all relevant references were retrieved by only one of the five searchers, while another quarter were retrieved by two searchers. Well under 10% of relevant references were retrieved by four or five searchers.

This study also compared the searching performance of experienced clinician and librarian searchers. It showed that the difference between both these groups and inexperienced clinician searchers was small and not statistically significant. Related to this finding, there appeared to be no benefit associated with the use of advanced MEDLINE searching features, since both experienced clinicians and librarians achieved comparable recall and precision using text-word searching only. In fact, experienced physicians showed a trend toward better recall when they used text words. There was a statistically significant difference for librarians using MED-LINE features over clinicians using MEDLINE features, indicating that these features are of most benefit to librarians.

One problem with these studies was the unrealistic situation in which the librarian searcher was assessed. As most librarians will note, their work involves more than just the search itself. An equally important aspect is the interview with the user, during which the information needs are explicitly gleaned. Indeed, the study by Saracevic and Kantor (1988b), discussed shortly, notes that performing this interview or having access to it doubles the intermediary searcher's recall. However, most of these studies (and their searches) take place in clinical settings, where detailed interviews by librarians are impractical. Thus, it is valid to compare the end user and the librarian in these settings, if only to use the latter as a point of reference for searching quality.

A number of other studies have focused on recall and precision obtained by clinicians using different IR systems or approaches. Hersh and Hickam (1995a) evaluated medical students searching an online version of *Scientific American Medicine* with a Boolean or natural language interface (as well as an experimental system whose results are discussed in Chap. 8). Twenty-one students searched on 10 queries, which were randomly allocated for each from the 106 queries of the same researchers' study described earlier (Hersh and Hickam, 1994). The users obtained a slightly higher recall (75.3 vs. 70.6%, not statistically significant) and slightly lower precision (14.8 vs. 18.9%, not statistically significant) for the natural language interface. This study also analyzed the relationship between the number of relevant documents and recall, finding that a larger number of relevant documents led, on average, to users obtaining a lower level of recall.

Paris and Tibbo (1998) also compared Boolean and natural language searching with medical documents. Searches were conducted against a database of 1,239 MEDLINE documents indexed by the term `Cystic Fibrosis`. The original queries were formulated by scientists and physicians knowledgeable in the field. From earlier research, the queries had been reformulated in an "optimal" Boolean format to yield the best retrieval. To create natural language queries, the Boolean operators and field limitations were removed. For analysis, the queries were divided into two types: those that used field limiters in the original Boolean queries and those that did not. The results were comparable for both sets. Recall was essentially 100% for queries of both types, most likely because the small document set afforded a broad query statement. Precision was higher for the Boolean searching (40–46% vs. 37–39%), while E (a variant of the F measure) was lower (0.44–0.49 vs. 0.54–0.55).

A final approach to system-oriented evaluation has been through the use of "task-oriented measures." As mentioned at the end of Chap. 1, a number of investigators have looked for alternatives to relevance-based measures for measuring the quality of IR system performance. One approach has been to give users tasks, such as answering a question. Egan et al. (1989) piloted this approach with a statistics textbook, finding significant performance differences with changes in the user interface. Mynatt et al. (1992) used a similar approach to assess the ability of college students to find answers to questions in an online encyclopedia.

Hersh and colleagues have carried out a number of studies assessing the ability of IR systems to help students and clinicians answer clinical questions. The rationale for these studies is that the usual goal of using an IR system is to find an answer to a question. While the user must obviously find relevant documents to answer that question, the quantity of such documents is less important than whether the question is successfully answered. In fact, recall and precision can be placed among the many factors that may be associated with ability to complete the task successfully.

The first study by this group using the task-oriented approach compared Boolean vs. natural language searching in the textbook *Scientific American Medicine* (Hersh, Elliot et al., 1994). Thirteen medical students were asked to answer ten short-answer questions and rate their confidence in their answers. The students were then randomized to one or the other interface and asked to search on the five questions for which they had rated confidence the lowest. The study showed that both groups had low correct rates before searching (average: 1.7 correct out of 10) but were mostly able to answer the questions with searching (average: 4.0 out of 5). There was no difference in the ability to answer questions with one interface or the other. Most answers were found on the first search to the textbook. For the questions that were incorrectly answered, the document with the correct answer was actually retrieved by the user two-thirds of the time and viewed more than half the time.

Another study compared Boolean and natural language searching of MEDLINE with two commercial products, CD Plus (now Ovid) and KF (Hersh, Pentecost et al., 1996). These systems represented the ends of the spectrum in terms of using Boolean searching on human-indexed thesaurus terms (CDP) vs. natural language searching on words in the title, abstract, and indexing terms (KF). Sixteen medical students were recruited and randomized to one of the two systems and given three yes/no clinical questions to answer. The students were able to use each system successfully, answering 37.5% correct before searching and 85.4% correct after searching. There were no significant differences between the systems in time taken, relevant articles retrieved, or user satisfaction. This study demonstrated that both types of system can be used equally well with minimal training.

Further research by this group expanded the analysis to include nurse practitioner (NP) students and a myriad of other possible factors that could influence searching. Most of the results concerning the latter are presented in Sect. 7.5. However, the searching success rates are worth noting here. Each of these studies used only one IR system, the Ovid system used to search MEDLINE but with links to about 80 full-text journals.

The first study focused solely on NP students and used multiple-choice questions from the *Medical Knowledge Self-Assessment Program* (MKSAP, American College of Physicians, Philadelphia) (Rose, 1998). Each of the 24 subjects answered three out of the eight questions used. Before searching, 25 of the 72 questions (34.7%) were answered correctly, and after searching the total of correct responses increased to 42 out of 72 (58.3%).

The second study assessed both medical and NP students, with 29 subjects answering three questions each out of a group of 30 (Hersh, Crabtree et al., 2000). The questions, which were phrased in a short-answer format, were obtained from three sources: MKSAP, the Cochrane Database of Systematic Reviews, and a set expressed in actual clinical practice (Gorman and Helfand, 1995). The main success-related results showed that medical students scored higher before and after searching, but that both groups improved their scores by the same amount.

In the final study, probably the largest study of medical searchers to date, 66 medical and NP students searched five questions each (Hersh, Crabtree et al., 2002). This study used a multiple-choice format for answering questions that also included a judgment about the evidence for the answer. Subjects were asked to choose from one of three answers:

1. Yes, with adequate evidence
2. Insufficient evidence to answer question
3. No, with adequate evidence

Both groups achieved a presearching correctness on questions about equal to chance (32.3% for medical students and 31.7% for NP students). However, medical students improved their correctness with searching (to 51.6%), whereas NP students hardly did at all (to 34.7%). Table 7.6 shows that NP students changed with searching from incorrect to correct answers as often as they did from correct to incorrect. These results were further assessed to determine whether NP students had

Table 7.6 Crosstabulation of number and percentage of answers correct vs. incorrect before and after searching for all (*A*), medical (*M*), and NP (*N*) students

	Postsearch	
Presearch	Incorrect	Correct
Incorrect		
A	133 (41.0%)	87 (26.9%)
M	81 (36.3%)	70 (31.4%)
N	52 (51.5%)	17 (16.8%)
Correct		
A	41 (12.7%)	63 (19.4%)
M	27 (12.1%)	45 (20.2%)
N	14 (13.9%)	18 (17.8%)
Percentages represent percent correct within each group of students (adapted from Hersh, Crabtree et al., 2002)		

trouble answering questions or judging evidence (unpublished data). To assess this, a two-by-two contingency table was constructed that compared designating the evidence correctly (i.e., selecting yes or no when the answer was yes or no and selecting indeterminate when the answer was indeterminate) and incorrectly (i.e., selecting yes or no when the answer was indeterminate and selecting indeterminate when the answer was yes or no). As seen in Table 7.7, NP students had a higher rate of incorrectly judging the evidence. Thus, since medical and NP students had virtually identical rates of judging the evidence correct when answering the question incorrectly, the major difference with respect to questions answered incorrectly between the groups was incorrect judgment of evidence.

Another group to assess ability to use an IR system successfully has been Wildemuth, Friedman, and associates. These researchers used a question-answering approach to assess INQUIRER, a system containing factual databases on several biomedical topics in a medical school curriculum (Wildemuth, de Bliek et al., 1995). The study yielded the following findings:

- Personal knowledge scores (ability to answer questions before searching) were low.
- Database-assisted scores (ability to answer questions with searching) were substantially higher.
- There was no relationship between personal knowledge scores and database-assisted scores, i.e., a searcher's prior knowledge was not associated with better ability to search.
- Database-assisted scores persisted at a higher level long after the course was over and personal knowledge scores had returned to lower levels.

A further analysis of the final point (in the bacteriology domain) showed that personal knowledge scores were low before the bacteriology course (12%), rose right after the course (48%), and decreased 6 months later (25%). However, the database-assisted scores rose linearly over the three assessments from 44 to 57 to 75% (de Bliek, Friedman et al., 1994). Thus information relevant to a problem can

Table 7.7 Crosstabulation of number and percentage of evidence judgments correct vs. incorrect before and after searching for all (A), medical (M), and NP (N) students

	Answer	
Evidence	Incorrect	Correct
Incorrect		
A	138 (42.6%)	0 (0%)
M	84 (37.7%)	0 (0%)
N	54 (53.5%)	0 (0%)
Correct		
A	36 (11.1%)	150 (46.3%)
M	24 (10.8%)	115 (51.6%)
N	12 (11.9%)	35 (34.7%)

Percentages represent percent correct within each group of students (adapted from Hersh, Crabtree et al., 2002)

be retrieved from a database long after the ability to directly recall it from memory has faded.

A subsequent study from this research showed that when INQUIRER was incorporated into a clinical simulation, there was a trend toward better performance when the system was used and a statistically significant benefit when the record containing the correct answer was displayed (Abraham, Friedman et al., 1999). Another study compared a Boolean and a hypertext browsing interface (Friedman, Wildemuth et al., 1996). While both led to improvements in database-assisted scores, the hypertext interface showed a small but statistically significant benefit.

A variant of the task-oriented approach has also been applied to healthcare consumers searching the Web (Eysenbach and Kohler, 2002). This study of 17 users given health questions to search on found an answer was successfully obtained in 4–5 min. Although participants were aware of quality criteria for health-related Web sites (e.g., source, professional design, scientific language), they did not appear to apply these criteria when actually visiting sites.

Several new task-oriented types of studies have appeared in the literature, making use of the much wider diversity of content that is now routinely available. Sintchenko et al. (2004) used infectious disease and intensive care physicians with eight simulated cases to compare efficiency and effectiveness of three different knowledge resources: antibiotics guidelines, laboratory reports, and laboratory reports augmented with clinical decision support. Efficiency was measured in time taken to reach a decision, while effectiveness was measured based on agreement of recommendations with a panel of experts. Another measure assessed was clinical impact score, which was the product of the usage rate of the given resource and the agreement with the expert panel. Intensive care physicians (80–93%) were more likely than infectious disease physicians (31–56%) to use any source of knowledge support. The results in Table 7.8 show each intervention for both groups combined. These results indicate the best agreement and the most impact with laboratory reports augmented with clinical decision support.

Table 7.8 Results of tasks using a variety of different interventions (adapted from Sintchenko, Coiera et al., 2004)

Intervention	Intervention used (%)	Agreement with experts (%)	Confident or highly confident (%)	Time (mean seconds)	Impact score
None (control)	NA	65	68	113	NA
Guidelines	39	67	75	202	0.26
Laboratory report	58	78	78	123	0.45
Laboratory report plus decision support	60	97	73	245	0.58

Westbrook et al. (2005) used clinical scenarios with 44 physicians and 31 clinical nurse consultants (CNCs) to assess an online evidence retrieval system with methods similar to the studies of Hersh et al. described earlier. Westbrook et al. assessed practicing physicians and consulting nurses using a suite of full-text evidence-based resources in addition to MEDLINE. In their study, Westbrook et al. found that physicians started with a higher presearching rate of correctness on the clinical tasks (37 vs. 18%) but that the retrieval system brought both groups up to the same level (50%). They also found that confidence in answers was likely to be higher for correct vs. incorrect answers, although over half of those who had persistently incorrect answers (before and after searching) were likely to have confidence in their answers. In addition, those who answered the scenario incorrectly initially had the same confidence in their answer after searching whether it was correct or incorrect. Both the Hersh et al. and the Westbrook et al. studies demonstrate that retrieval systems, and the confidence they engender, are far from perfect.

McKibbon and Fridsma (2006) used the same questions as Hersh et al. and obtained somewhat similar results. In this study, practicing clinicians were given the questions and allowed to search all their "usual" resources. The results found that the addition of the search system did not improve their answers, as 39.1% of questions were answered correct before searching and 42.1% were answered correct after searching. Users went from incorrect to correct answers with searching at the same frequency of going from correct to incorrect answers. The researchers found great variation in the ability of different resources to answer questions, with Google/Web and the Cochrane database more likely to lead to correct answers and PubMed, Up to Date, and InfoPOEMS more likely to lead to incorrect answers.

7.5 Factors Associated with Success or Failure

Although determining how well users can perform with IR systems is important, additional analysis focusing on why they succeed or fail is important, not only in figuring out how to best deploy such systems but also for the sake of determining how to improve them. This section focuses on two related groups of analyses. In the first group are studies attempting to determine the factors associated with successful use of systems, while the second group consists of analyses of why users fail to obtain optimal results.

7.5.1   Predictors of Success

One of the earliest and most comprehensive analyses of predictors of success was from outside the healthcare domain, but its results set the stage for further work. Saracevic et al. (Saracevic and Kantor, 1988a,b; Saracevic, Kantor et al., 1988) recruited 40 information seekers, each of whom submitted a question to a search intermediary, underwent a taped interview with a reference librarian to describe his or her problem and intended use of the information, and evaluated the retrieved items for relevance as well as the search in general. Each question was searched by nine intermediaries. Up to 150 retrieved items were returned to the users, who rated them as relevant, partially relevant, or not relevant to their information need.

All results were framed in the context of the odds that retrieved items would be judged relevant by the users. Some of the factors that led to statistically significantly higher odds of documents being judged relevant were a well-defined problem posed by a user who was very certain the answer would be found; searches limited to answers in English and requiring less time to complete; questions that were initially not clear or specific but were complex and had many presupposed concepts; and answers that had high utility for the user, as measured by benefits in time, money, or problem resolution. Another finding of interest in this study was a low overlap in search terms used (27%) and items retrieved (17%) for a given question, a finding similar to that of McKibbon et al. (1990) for healthcare searchers. However, Saracevic and Kantor did determine that the more searchers a document was retrieved by, the more likely that document was to be judged relevant.

Also assessing the factors leading to searching success was the study of Wildemuth et al. (1995) described earlier, which evaluated medical student performance in searching factual databases in bacteriology, toxicology, and pharmacology. The authors found that relevance-based measures (recall and precision), term overlap (students selecting terms overlapping with those known to lead to retrieval of records containing the answer), and efficiency (as measured by time) had a positive correlation with successful answering of questions, while personal domain knowledge (as measured by a test in which the system was not used) did not. The positive correlation of search success with relevance and the lack of correlation with personal domain knowledge were also found by Saracevic and Kantor.

In a study of nurses' searching, Royle et al. (1995) asked subjects whether their searches were successful. While 83% of searches were completed to the point of "answering the question," only 42% were deemed "successful." Factors correlating with success included taking more time but rated as worth the time, accessing a bibliographic (as opposed to full text) database, being done for educational (as opposed to patient care) purposes, and being done on disease-related or psychosocial topics.

The most comprehensive analysis of factors relating to searching success has been carried out by Hersh et al. (2002). They developed a comprehensive model of factors that might influence the success of searching. Successful use of the IR system, defined in the study to be the task of successfully answering the clinical question, was the dependent (outcome) variable. The elements of the model made up the independent (predictor) variables and were grouped in several different categories. The first consisted of identifiers for the user and question searched, as well as the order of the question. The next category covered demographic variables, some of which were generic (e.g., age and sex), while others were specific to the study population (e.g., school enrolled and years worked as a nurse). There were also categories for computer experience, computer attitudes, and searching experience. The searching experience factors included not only general amounts of literature and Web searching, but also specific knowledge of and experience with advanced features of MEDLINE.

The model also included assessment of cognitive factors, since these had been shown to be associated with searching performance not only in the studies of Saracevic et al. cited earlier, but in others as well. Three factors were included because they had been found to be associated with successful use of computer systems in general or retrieval systems specifically. The cognitive traits were assessed by validated instruments from the Educational Testing Service (ETS) Kit of Cognitive Factors (Ekstrom, French et al., 1976). The three factors were:

1. *Spatial visualization.* The ability to visualize spatial relationships among objects has been associated with retrieval system performance by nurses (Staggers and Mills, 1994), ability to locate text in a general retrieval system (Gomez, Egan et al., 1986), and ability to use a direct manipulation (3D) retrieval system user interface (Swan and Allan, 1998). This was measured by the ETS *Paper Folding Test* to assess spatial visualization.
2. *Logical reasoning.* The ability to reason from premise to conclusion has been shown to improve selectivity in assessing relevant and nonrelevant citations in a retrieval system (Allen, 1992). This was measured by the ETS *Nonsense Syllogisms Test* to assess logical reasoning.
3. *Verbal reasoning.* The ability to understand vocabulary has been shown to be associated with the use of a larger number of search expressions and high-frequency search terms in a retrieval system (Allen, 1992). This was measured by the ETS *Advanced Vocabulary Test I* to assess verbal reasoning.

Other categories in the model included intermediate search results (i.e., results of searching performance that ultimately influence the user's ability to successfully answer the question). One of these was search mechanics, such as the time taken, the number of Boolean sets used in the searching process, the number of articles retrieved in the "terminal" set, and the number of MEDLINE references and full-text articles viewed by the user. Another intermediate category was user satisfaction, which was measured with the Questionnaire for User Interface Satisfaction (QUIS) 5.0 instrument that measures user satisfaction with a computer system, providing a score from zero (poor) to nine (excellent) on a variety of user preferences (Chin, Diehl et al., 1988). The overall user satisfaction was determined by averaging the scores of all the preferences.

The next group of factors addressed the relevance of the retrieval set. These measures, including recall and precision, were considered to be intermediate outcome measures relative to the ultimate outcome measure of successfully answering the question. This is in distinction to the many retrieval studies that assess recall and precision as the final outcome measures. The final category of factors contains variables associated with the answer, such as the answer itself, the EBM type, whether the user gave the correct answer before or after searching, and the user's certainty of the answer.

As noted in Sect. 7.4, 66 searchers, 45 medical students and 21 NP students, performed five searches each. There were 324 searches analyzed. Several differences between medical and NP students were seen. Use of computers and use of productivity software were higher for NP students, but searching experience was higher for medical students. Medical students also had higher self-rating of knowledge and experience with advanced MEDLINE features. The NP students tended to be older and all were female (whereas only half the medical students were female). Medical students also had higher scores on the three cognitive tests. In searching, medical students tended to have higher numbers of sets, but lower numbers of references viewed. They also had a higher level of satisfaction with the IR system, as measured by QUIS.

Further analysis determined the factors associated with successful searching, as defined by the outcome variable of correct answer after searching. The final model showed that knowing the correct answer before searching, score on the *Paper Folding Test*, past usage of advanced MEDLINE features, and EBM question type were statistically significantly different. For the EBM question type, questions of prognosis had the highest likelihood of being answered correctly, followed by questions of therapy, diagnosis, and harm. The analysis also found that the *Paper Folding Test* and searcher type (medical vs. NP student) demonstrated multicollinearity, i.e., they were very highly correlated, and once one was in the model, the other did not provide any additional statistical significance. Next, a similar analysis was done to find the best model using the 220 searches when the subject did not have the right answer before the MEDLINE search. The final best model was very similar to the model for all questions, with presearching correctness obviously excluded. Again, the *Paper Folding Test* and searcher type demonstrated high multicollinearity.

One surprising finding was that there was virtually no difference in recall and precision between medical and NP students. Likewise, there was no difference in recall and precision between questions that were answered correctly and incorrectly. Other variables having no association with successful searching included time taken to complete the question and certainty that the searcher had in their answer.

A number of conclusions were drawn from this study. First, users spent an average of more than 30 min conducting literature searches and were successful in correctly answering questions less than half the time. Whereas medical students were able to use the IR system to improve question answering, NP students were led astray by the system as often as they were helped by it. The study also found that experience in searching MEDLINE and spatial visualization ability were associated with successful in answering questions. A final finding was that the often-studied measures of recall and precision were virtually identical between medical and NP students and had no association with correct answering of questions. Possible reasons for the limited success of question answering include everything from inadequate training to an inappropriate database (i.e., a large bibliographic database instead of more concise, synthesized references) to problems with the retrieval system to difficulties in judging evidence.

Magrabi et al. (2007) looked at the factors that make IR systems likely to be used by clinicians. In a survey of 227 Australian general practitioners with access to the QuickClinical system described earlier, they found that few factors were associated with usage, including age, level of clinical training, experience, and hours worked. They did find, however, that female clinicians were slightly more likely to search than male physicians. Not surprisingly, those who believed the system improved care were more likely to use it.

7.5.2 Analysis of Failure

The attempt to determine why users do not obtain optimal results with IR systems is called *failure analysis*. A number of such analyses have been carried out over the years. In his original MEDLINE study, Lancaster (1968) performed a detailed failure analysis, which he divided into recall (failure to retrieve a relevant article) and precision (retrieval of nonrelevant article) failures. For both types of failure, Lancaster cataloged problems related to indexing (i.e., problems with the indexing language or assignment of its terms) and retrieval (i.e., problems with search strategy). The particular problems, along with their frequencies, are shown in Table 7.9.

Miller et al. (1988) evaluated end-user searching with Compact Cambridge MEDLINE (now defunct). Search statements were analyzed for identification of errors and "missed opportunities," where better strategies could have resulted in more documents retrieved. Searching errors included the following:

1. Designating a term as a MeSH term when it was not
2. Entering subject terms in the author or unique identifier fields
3. Misspelling a word
4. Using a stop word or truncation symbol in a phrase search
5. Inappropriate back-referencing of an earlier set
6. Entering an author name in incorrect form

Table 7.9 Recall and precision failures in MEDLINE (adapted from Lancaster, 1968)

Recall failures
Indexing language – lack of appropriate terms (10.2%)
Indexing – indexing not sufficiently exhaustive (20.3%), indexer omitted important concept (9.8%), indexing insufficiently specific (5.8%)
Retrieval – searcher did not cover all reasonable approaches to searching (21.5%), search too exhaustive (8.4%), search too specific (2.5%), selective printout (1.6%)

Precision failures
Indexing language – lack of appropriate specific terms (17.6%), false coordinations (11.3%), incorrect term relationships (6.8%)
Indexing – too exhaustive (11.5%)
Retrieval – search not specific (15.2%), search not exhaustive (11.7%), inappropriate terms or combinations (4.3%)
Inadequate user–system interaction (15.3%)

Missed opportunities included the following:

1. Nonuse of truncation
2. Failure to use appropriate MeSH heading
3. Incomplete specification of all fields (e.g., searching for a text word in the title or abstract field only)

Similar findings have been found in other systems and settings. Sewell and Teitelbaum (1986) assessed use of the NLM command-line interface by pathologists and pharmacists at an academic medical center library. They found that most users employed search terms combined with the AND operator. While text words were generally used correctly, MeSH terms were used incorrectly 23% of the time. The most frequent reasons for missed opportunities were failure to use explosions and subheadings appropriately. Wildemuth and Moore (1995) assessed medical student searches of MEDLINE for missed opportunities. Table 7.10 shows the most common of these. By a large margin, the move that would have improved the search most often was use of a MeSH term, followed by better use of Boolean operators and addition of subheadings.

A number of failure analyses focused on the NLM's Grateful Med, which was one of the first systems designed for end users. A large study at the NLM focused on searches retrieving no articles ("no postings") (Kingsland, Harbourt et al., 1993). This was found to occur with 37% of Grateful Med searches performed in April 1987 and 27% of searches from September 1992. The 1987 searches were analyzed in more detail, with the finding that 51% of searches used excessive ANDs, in that no documents contained the intersection of all search terms ANDed together by the searcher. Other reasons for empty sets include inappropriate entering of author names (15%), term misspellings (13%), punctuation or truncation errors (11%), and failed title searches (6%). The investigators did not assess how many "no postings" were due to an absence of material on the topic. Other errors made included the following:

Table 7.10 "Missed opportunities" in 58 MEDLINE searches by medical students (adapted from Wildemuth and Moore, 1995)

Missed opportunity	Frequency
Should have used MeSH term	90
Made an illogical Boolean combination	34
Should have used subheading	31
Should have used a different proximity operator	26
Should have exploded MeSH term	24
Should have limited term to major descriptor	14
Should have added synonyms with OR	12
Should have used term truncation	11
Should have limited term to a specific field	10
Should have used broader term	7
Should have used narrower term	6
Should not have used MeSH term (none available)	3
Should have used full database	2
Should have limited search to specific age groups	2
Other	2

1. Inappropriate use of specialty headings (e.g., using the term `Pediatrics`, which is intended to represent the medical specialty, to search for children's diseases)
2. Incorrect use of subheadings (e.g., using `Management` instead of `Therapy` when searching for articles about treatment of a disease)
3. Not using related terms, either in the form of text words (e.g., adding a term like `cerebr:` or `encephal:` to the MeSH heading `Brain`) or MeSH crossreferences (e.g., adding terms like `Bites and Stings` or `Dust` to `Allergens`)

Walker et al. (1991) assessed 172 "unproductive" Grateful Med searches at McMaster University in 1987–1988, dividing problems into the categories of search formulation (48%), the Grateful Med software itself (41%), and system failure (11%). While half the search formulation problems were due to an absence of material on the topic, the most common errors were found to be use of low postings terms, use of general terms instead of subheadings, and excessive use of AND. Problems specific to Grateful Med included inappropriate use of the title line (i.e., unwittingly typing a term on the title line, thus limiting retrieval to all articles with that term in the title) and the software's automatic combining of words on the subject line(s) with OR, so that the phrase `inammatory bowel disease` was searched as `inammatory` OR `bowel` OR `disease`.

Mitchell et al. (1992) assessed searcher failures of Grateful Med by medical students in biochemistry and pathology courses. An analysis of searches with no postings showed that the most common error was failure to use MeSH terms that could have resulted in retrieval of relevant articles. The most common reasons for excessive postings were searching on only one concept and the OR of words on the subject line described in the preceding paragraph.

Not all failure analyses have looked at bibliographic databases. In their study of full-text retrieval performance described earlier, McKinin et al. (1991) also assessed the reasons for full-text retrieval failures. About two-thirds of the problems were due to search strategy, in that the concepts from the search were not explicitly present in the document or an excessively restrictive search operator was used. The remaining third were due to natural language problems, such as use in the documents of word variants, more general terms, synonyms, or acronyms.

In their assessment of clinicians attempting to use a computer workstation to answer clinical questions, Osheroff and Bankowitz (1993) analyzed the problems users had in dealing with questions they were unable to answer. The most common problem expressed (57% of the time) was poor interaction with the database, either because it was incomplete or because the user entered a poor search. Other problems included noncurrent database (14%), navigational difficulties with the software (15%), and no new information obtained (7%). Even users who obtained partial or full answers to their questions had occasional concerns that their answer was incomplete (63 and 10%, respectively) or complained that the workstation was difficult to navigate (32 and 10%, respectively).

Sievert et al. (2001) looked at how lexical variants of terms affected search results for epistaxis as well as three eye conditions: pink eye, conjunctivitis, and color blindness. They found that bloody nose did not map into epistaxis in MeSH, leading to very poor search results in MEDLINE when using the former. They also noted in consumer-oriented Web resources (which do not use MeSH) that slight variations on the wording of the search (e.g., bloody nose, nose bleed, and nosebleed) led to substantial differences in both number of retrieval and number of relevant pages. They express particular concern for consumers, who are less knowledgeable about medical language than clinicians. Gault et al. (2002) analyzed the MeSH mapping for several different common MEDLINE systems and found substantial variation in how effectively they mapped from user input to MeSH.

Little research has been done of users outside academic medical centers. One exception is a study by McCray and Tse (2003), which assessed search failures (i.e., queries yielding no retrievals) in the NLM's consumer-oriented resources, MEDLINE-plus and ClinicalTrials.gov. About 77% of the MEDLINE-plus queries and 88% of the ClinicalTrials.gov queries were "in scope." Over two-thirds of these in-scope queries were error-free but just retrieved no matches. The most common errors were the same with both databases: misspelled words (16% in MEDLINE-plus and 27% in ClinicalTrials.gov), use of nonalphanumeric characters (14 and 21%, respectively), and inappropriate search operators (14 and 15%, respectively). Another interesting finding of these queries was the minimal use of "consumer" terms, e.g., nose bleed and tube tied, which were used less than 0.4%.

7.6   Assessment of Impact

It was first noted in Chap. 1 that the true measure of an IR system's success should be how much impact it has on the searcher's information problem, be it improving clinical care or the ability to perform research. As we have seen, there have been far more studies of the details of the user–system interaction than of how well that interaction assists in solving a problem, making a correct decision, and so forth. This state of affairs is understandable, given that studies of impact are not only costly and time consuming, but also are potentially contaminated by confounding variables unrelated to the system. Many variables play a role in the outcome of a medical diagnosis and intervention, and even if the use of IR systems is controlled (i.e., physicians are randomized to one system or another), there may be other differences in patients and/or healthcare providers that explain differences in outcome independent of IR system use.

The main approach to assessing impact has been the use of questionnaires asking providers questions such as whether the system led to a change in a decision, action, or outcome. The limitations of this approach, of course, are related to selective recall of those who reply to such surveys and/or potential differences among those who do and do not reply. Three studies have involved administering questionnaires to clinician users of hospital library services.

King (1987) chose random samples of physicians, nurses (registered nurses and NPs only), and other healthcare professionals from eight Chicago-area hospitals to query them on the value of library services in their hospital. The sample sizes were chosen based on the relative numbers of each provider (i.e., 49% physicians, 40% nurses, and 11% other providers). Although the survey response rate was low (57%), it was found that while physicians used the library more often than nurses or other providers, all groups reported that information obtained was of clinical value, led to better-informed decisions, and contributed to higher-quality care more than 90% of the time. Nearly three-quarters of each type of provider reported that the information would definitely or probably persuade the person to handle the case that prompted the library visit in a manner differently from that initially contemplated.

Marshall (1992) performed a similar study in 1992, assessing the impact of the hospital library on physician decision making in the Rochester, New York area. Physicians were recruited to use the library in their hospital and to complete a questionnaire describing its impact. Although Marshall's response rate of 51% was low like King's, those who did respond indicated a generally positive role for the library. More than 80% indicated that they had handled some aspect of a case differently, most frequently in choice of tests, choice of medications, and advice given to the patient from the approach they had considered before consulting the library. Among the aspects of patient care the library information allowed the physicians to avoid were additional tests and procedures, surgery, hospital admission, and even patient mortality.

Mathis et al. (1994) administered a similar survey to library patrons in Michigan and likewise found that 85% of searches were valuable to patient care, with 56% changing the way the case was handled. Among the frequent benefits were change in advice given to patients, avoidance of unnecessary tests and procedures, and modification of drug prescriptions.

Other studies have also attempted to assess whether use of libraries or IR systems led to changes in patient care decisions. Veenstra (1992), for example, found that a clinical medical librarian added to teaching services at Hartford

Hospital was able to find information that affected patient care 40–59% of the time. In their study of Grateful Med introduced in clinical settings, Haynes et al. (1990) found that 47% of system uses led to finding information which changed the course of patient care.

Another approach to assessing impact is the "critical incident technique," in which users are prompted to recall a recent search that was effective or not. Lindberg et al. (1993) analyzed 86% of searches deemed effective by a sample of 552 end-user physicians, scientists, and others. The most common impact of the information obtained was to develop an appropriate treatment plan (45%), followed by recognizing or diagnosing a medical problem or condition (22%), implementing a treatment plan (14%), and maintaining an effective patient–physician relationship (10%).

A more recent application of this technique was used by Westbrook et al. (2005), who performed semistructured interviews with 29 clinicians that generated 85 episodes where the system provided tangible benefit. One-quarter of these led to better provision of clinical care. They also identified a process of "journey mapping" that showed the "journey" clinicians could take from their first initial experiences with systems to their use as key knowledge tools. In another study, these same researchers also surveyed 55,000 users of their system, finding that 41% reported direct experience of a benefit (Westbrook, Gosling et al., 2004).

As noted earlier, the problem with survey data is that such information depends on the memory and self-reporting of those surveyed. In addition, owing to incomplete response rates, the results may not represent a snapshot of the entire population. For this reason, Klein et al. (1994) attempted to determine whether MEDLINE searching had an impact on economic indicators, in this case hospital charges and length of stay (LOS). The investigators used a case-control approach for 192 hospital admissions where MEDLINE searching was known to have been done for patient care reasons. When matched for diagnosis-related group (DRG) and LOS, those that had "early" literature searches (done during the first three-quarters of the standard LOS) had statistically significant lower costs than those done "late." A more recent study with a similar methodology verified that a computerized literature search and librarian support led to reduced hospital charges, LOS, and readmission rate (Banks, Shi et al., 2007). While the case-control nature of these studies means that other confounding variables could explain their results, they do make a compelling case for the value of adding more information to the clinical care process.

In keeping with the philosophy of EBM, could IR systems be evaluated by the appropriate means to assess interventions (i.e., the RCT)? One major impediment to an RCT is that usage of IR systems is heterogeneous. That is, they are used for a variety of information needs. Furthermore, their impact on a given patient's care is usually only indirect or at best one of numerous variables that affect patient outcomes. Other studies in medical informatics have demonstrated that well-designed studies have been used successfully to assess the application of information technology in the healthcare setting for many years (e.g., Tierney, Miller et al., 1993; Bates, Leape et al., 1998; Evans, Pestotnik et al., 1998). But these studies have focused on specific clinical interventions guided by explicit rules in decision support systems. One possibility is to use "surrogate" outcomes, which assess not whether patients actually improve but, rather, whether physicians perform appropriate actions, such as ordering of tests or treatments. This approach has been used to assess the benefit of electronic medical records as documented by a systematic review (Jerant and Hill, 2000). Of course, it has been noted that surrogate outcomes do not always predict actual outcomes, so such findings must be used cautiously (D'Agostino, 2000).

Pluye and colleagues have performed research looking at the impact of IR and other informatics applications on physicians. They began by developing a taxonomy of system impact based on an organizational case study and grouped six types of impact into broader categories of whether the impact was positive or negative (Pluye and Grad, 2004):

- High-positive impact

  o Practice improvement
  o Learning
  o Recall

- Moderate-positive impact

  o Reassurance
  o No impact

- Negative impact

  o Frustration

Next, they performed a systematic review that gathered studies assessing the impact of IR systems on physicians and classified them as to whether they had the above impacts (Pluye, Grad et al., 2005). A number of 26 studies that met their inclusion criteria showed impact in each of the positive categories, with an estimated one-thirds of searches having a positive impact. Many searches, however, showed no impact and a few showed negative impact. Further work compared the impact of IR systems vs. decision support systems, noting that the former were more likely to cause learning and recall, while the latter were associated with practice improvement (Grad, Pluye et al., 2005).

7.7 Research on Relevance

To this point, relevance has merely been defined as a document meeting an information need that prompted a query. This fixed view of relevance makes recall and precision very straightforward to calculate. But as it turns out, relevance is not quite so objective. For example, relevance as judged by physicians has a moderately high degree of variation, as shown in experiments measuring the overlap between judges in assigning relevance of MEDLINE references to queries generated in a clinical setting (Hersh, Buckley et al., 1994). This level of disagreement has been verified in similar assessments (Haynes, McKibbon et al., 1990; Hersh and Hickam, 1993, 1995a; Hersh, Hickam et al., 1994). In each of these studies, the kappa statistic was used to measure inter-rater reliability. This statistic, described in Sect. 7.7.6, is commonly used to assess agreement in diagnostic evaluations, such as X-ray or pathology specimen reading (Kramer and Feinstein, 1981).

Interest in relevance has waxed and waned over the years. There was a great deal of theoretical thinking and research into relevance in the 1960s, culminating in Saracevic's seminal review paper (Saracevic, 1975). That paper summarized all the classifications and research data at that time. Two basic problems, Saracevic noted, were the lack of agreement on the definition of relevance (he identified seven different views of it) and the paucity of experimental data supporting either those definitions or how relevance was being applied in evaluation studies.

There was a rekindling of interest in relevance in the 1990s, most likely owing to the increasing prevalence of IR systems, with a resultant increase in claims and counterclaims about their performance. Schamber et al. (1990) attempted to resurrect debate over the theoretical notions of relevance. Their approach pared Saracevic's categories of relevance down to two: a system-oriented topical view and a user-oriented situational view. These two views are not at odds with Saracevic's classification, since the situational category encompasses several of Saracevic's views that were conceptually similar. The categories of Schamber et al. will be used for the following discussion.

7.7.1   Topical Relevance

The original view of relevance is that of topical relevance, which Saracevic called the system's view of relevance. In this view, a document is relevant because part or all of its topical coverage overlaps with the topic of the user's information need. There is a central but questionable assumption that underlies this view of relevance, noticed by Meadow (1985), which is that the relevance relationship between query and document is fixed. But just because a document is "about" an information need does not mean that it is relevant. A clinician with a patient care problem incorporating the treatment of hypertension with a certain drug most likely will not want to retrieve an article dealing with the use of that drug to treat hypertension in rats. Likewise, a research pharmacologist studying the molecular mechanisms of blood pressure reductions with that drug probably will not want articles about clinical trials with the drug. Furthermore, a medical student or a patient, who knows far less than the clinician or researcher, may not want to retrieve this article at all because its language is too technical.

The topical view of relevance persists, however, for several reasons. First, it is associated with a perception of objectivity, hence reproducibility. Another reason is that quantitative methods to assess IR systems with situational relevance are difficult to perform and interpret. But perhaps the main reason for the survival of topical relevance is that this view has led to relatively easy measures for quantifying performance in IR systems. The notion of a fixed relevance between query and document greatly simplifies the task of IR evaluation, since if the relevance of a document with respect to a document is fixed, then evaluation can be simulated (without human users) quite easily once relevance judgments have been made.

This approach to evaluation has been the modus operandi of a large segment of the IR research world, particularly among those who advocate automated approaches to IR. This approach makes the task of evaluation quite easy in that system users are unnecessary. All that is needed is a test collection consisting of queries, documents, and relevance judgments. When a new system is implemented, or an existing one is modified, evaluation is a simple matter of running the existing queries into the new system and measuring recall and precision. There is reason, however, to question the external validity of the results obtained with this sort of evaluation, which will be explored in greater detail later in this chapter.

7.7.2 Situational Relevance

The second category of relevance attempts to incorporate the user's situation into the judgment. Saracevic called this view the destination's view by, while others have termed variations of it "situational" (Schamber, Eisenberg et al., 1990), "logical" (Cooper, 1973), or "psychological" (Harter, 1992) relevance. The major underlying assumption in this view is that the user's situation and needs cannot be separated from the relevance judgment. Rees (1966) said, "There is no such thing as *the* relevance of a document to an information requirement, but rather the relevance judgment of an individual in a specific judging situation ... at a certain point in time." Cooper (1973) defined the difference between (topical) relevance and utility, arguing that the latter could be measured to assess what value information actually provided to the user.

The case for situational relevance was stated more recently by Schamber et al. (1990), who noted the prevalence of the topical view of relevance but highlighted its problems, especially its use in the making of assertions about the nature and performance of IR systems. These researchers argued that the situational approach, based on the dynamics of human–system interactions, could be used to make systematic and reliable measurements.

Situational relevance can be challenged from two perspectives. The first is in fact very pertinent to IR in the healthcare domain, which is that the user may be distinctly *unqualified* to judge relevance. It was noted in Chap. 2, for example, that many physicians lack the skills to critically appraise the medical literature (Anonymous, 1992). Thus, a user may deem an article relevant to a given issue, yet be unable to recognize that it is flawed or that the results described do not justify the conclusions published.

The second challenge is whether the variance of the situational picture has an impact on retrieval performance measurements. Lesk and Salton (1968) carried out a study in which users originated a query and judged their retrieved documents for relevance. Relevance judgments were also made by another subject expert. Additional sets of relevance judgments were created by taking the intersection and union of both judges' relevance assessments. Recall and precision were then measured based on the original retrieval results, showing that the different judgment sets had little effect on overall results. In other words, algorithms that performed well under one set of relevance judgments performed well under all of them, with the poorly performing algorithms faring poorly under all sets as well. Voorhees (1998) has noted this constancy with data from the Text REtrieval Conference (TREC), as well.

7.7.3   Research About Relevance Judgments

Despite all the disagreement about the nature of relevance, few studies have actually attempted to investigate the factors that influence relevance judgment. Most data on relevance judgments come from two large studies done in the 1960s (Cuadra and Katter, 1967; Rees and Schultz, 1967). Cuadra and Katter (1967) developed a five-category classification scheme of the factors that could affect relevance judgments, which Saracevic later used in his review paper to summarize the results of research from these studies and others (Saracevic, 1975).

The first category was type of document, such as its subject matter and the quantity of it available to the relevance judge. It was found that subject content was the most important factor influencing relevance judgments, indicating that topical relevance does have importance. It was also discovered that specific subject content in a document led to higher agreement among judges. Regarding the amount of document representation available to the relevance judge, it was clear that the title alone led to poor agreement, there were there were conflicting results with respect to whether abstract text or increasing amount of full text was better.

The second category was the query or information needs statement. In general, the more judges knew about a user's information need, the more agreement they had. However, the less they knew about the query, the more likely they were to classify documents as relevant. It was also found that statements in documents that resembled the query statement increased the likelihood of a positive relevance judgment.

The third category was the relevance judge. Increased subject knowledge of the judge and his or her familiarity with subject terminology correlated with consistency of agreement but varied inversely with number of documents judged relevant. Professional or occupational involvement with users' information problem also led to higher rates of agreement, regardless of specific subject knowledge. Differences in intended use of documents (i.e., use for background, updating, etc.) also produced differences in relevance judgments. Level of agreement of the relevance judgment was found to be greater for nonrelevant than for relevant documents.

The fourth category was judgment conditions, such as different definitions of relevance or varied pressures on the judges. Changing the definition of relevance did not appear to lead to different relevance judgments. However, greater time or stringency pressures did have an effect, causing more positive relevance judgments.

In the last category, judgment mode, it was found that judges tend to prefer (i.e., to feel more "comfortable" or "at ease" with) more categories in a rating scale. It was also noted that the end points of scales (i.e., very relevant or very nonrelevant) tended to be used most heavily, although ratings were not normally distributed but rather skewed in one direction. Another finding was that relative scores for a group of document judgments were more consistent than absolute scores. That is, users tended to rank documents for relevance in the same order, even if they chose different categories or scores of relevance.

Research in relevance judgments did not pick up again until the mid-1980s, when Eisenberg (1988) began to investigate methods for estimating relevance. Concerned that fixed, named categories of relevance were problematic, he adapted the technique of *magnitude estimation*, where subjects made their judgments on analog scales without named points. In particular, he used a 100-mm line, with the categories of relevant and nonrelevant as the end points. This approach was found to lessen the problem of relevance judges spreading out their judgments across the fixed, labeled categories of a traditional relevance scale.

This technique has also been used to assess how the order of presentation of documents influences relevance judgments. Eisenberg and Barry (1988) gave subjects a set of 15 documents and an information needs statement. Based on earlier work, the relative relevance of each document was known. The documents were presented in either random, high-to-low, or low-to-high order. A "hedging phenomenon" was observed, wherein judges tended to overestimate the relevance of initial documents in the set ordered "low to high" and to underestimate relevance for the initial documents in the other set.

Subsequent studies of relevance judgments have used more traditional judgment methods. Parker and Johnson (1990), using 47 queries into a database of computer science journal references, found that no difference in relevance judgments occurred with retrieval sets less than or equal to 15 documents (which was the size of Eisenberg's set). But for larger sets, relevant articles ranked beyond the fifteenth document were slightly less likely to be judged relevant than if they had occurred in the first 15.

Florance and Marchionini (1995) provided additional insight into relevance by assessing how three physicians processed the information in a group of retrieved articles on six clinical topics. The order of the presentation not only had a dramatic effect on relevance, but also showed that the information in the articles was complementary and interrelated. The authors identified two strategies these physicians used to process the information. In the *additive* strategy, information from each successive paper reinforced what was present in preceding ones. In the *recursive* strategy, on the other hand, new information led to reinterpretation of previously seen information and reconsideration of the data in the light of new evidence. This work demonstrated that simple topical relevance oversimplifies the value of retrieved documents to users.

Barry (1994) assessed the factors that lead a searcher to pursue a document after its retrieval by an IR system. Looking at users in academic libraries who were asked to evaluate the output of their search during a protocol analysis, Barry found seven general criteria for pursuing a document and measured their frequency:

1. Information content of document (e.g., depth/scope of document, objective accuracy/validity, recency: 35.1%)
2. User's background/experience (e.g., content novelty to user, background experience, user's ability to understand: 21.6%)
3. User's belief and preferences (e.g., subjective accuracy/validity, user's emotional response: 15.8%)
4. Other information sources within the environment (e.g., consensus within field, external verification by other sources, availability via other sources: 14.6%)
5. Sources of the document (e.g., source quality, source reputation/visibility: 7.2%)
6. The document as a physical entity (e.g., obtainability, cost: 2.7%)
7. The user's situation (e.g., time constraints, relationship with author: 2.9%)

This study indicates that the topical content does play an important role in determining relevance to the user, but there are many situational factors, such as novelty to the user and subjective assessment of accuracy and/or validity.

Wang (1994) found similar results in research attempting to model the decision-making process applied to pursuing documents after retrieval. Her model linked document information elements (i.e., title, author, abstract, journal, date of publication, language, media) with criteria (i.e., topicality, novelty, quality, availability, authority) that would lead a user to decide whether to seek a retrieved article. Like Barry, Wang found that while topicality was the reason most likely to lead to pursuit; other factors had significant influence, such as the recency of the article, its availability, and the reputation or authority of the author(s).

Another line of research of relevance judgments looks at the consistency of judges in assigning them. Many studies measuring recall and precision have looked at this phenomenon, obtaining results comparable to those shown in Table 7.11 from the study of Hersh and Hickam (1994). We will discuss these results further in the context of measuring consistency via the kappa statistic in Sect. 7.7.6.

Table 7.11 Overlap of judges on assigning relevance to documents retrieved by clinical questions using MEDLINE (adapted from Hersh, Buckley et al., 1994)

Judge 1	Judge 2		
	Definitely relevant	Probably relevant	Not relevant
Definitely relevant	127	112	96
Probably relevant		97	224
Not relevant			779
Judgments were rated on a three-point scale: definitely relevant, possibly relevant, and not relevant			

7.7.4 Limitations of Relevance-Based Measures

If relevance judgments are situational and inherently variable across judges, then what does this say about the use of recall and precision? One of the harshest critics of these measures has been Swanson (1988a), who has argued that, "An information need cannot be fully expressed as a search request that is independent of innumerable presuppositions of context–context that itself is impossible to describe fully, for it includes among other things the requester's own background of knowledge." Harter (1992) likewise has argued that fixed relevance judgments cannot capture the dynamic nature of the user's interaction with an IR system.

Even if relevance were a relative concept that existed between certain bounds so that measures based on it, such as recall or precision, could be made, there are still a number of limitations associated with the use of these measures to assess user–system interaction. Hersh (1994) has noted that the magnitude of a significant difference (such as between systems) is not known. The beginning of this chapter discussed the notion of statistical significance, which when present ensures that the difference between two values is not merely due to chance. But just because statistical significance exists does not mean that a difference is meaningful. Using a medical example, consider a new drug being used to treat diabetes, and suppose it lowers blood sugar by an average of 5 mg dL^{-1}. Readers with a medical background will note that this value is insignificant in terms of treatment of diabetes or its long-term outcome. Yet one could design a study with a very large sample size that could show statistical significance for the results obtained with this clinically meaningless difference. Yet, clinical significance between different levels of recall and precision has never really been defined for IR. In other words, it is unknown whether the difference between, say, 50 and 60% recall has any significance to a real user whatsoever.

Related to this issue is the assumption that more relevant and fewer nonrelevant articles are better. For example, in some instances complete precision is not totally desired. Belkin and Vickery (1985) have noted that users often discover new knowledge by "serendipity." A famous newspaper columnist, the late Sydney Harris, used to periodically devote columns to "things I learned while looking up something else." Sometimes there is value in learning something new that is peripheral to what one is seeking at the moment. Similarly, at times complete recall is not desired and may even be a distraction, for example, the busy clinician who seeks a quick answer to a question.

A final problem with recall and precision is that they are often applied in a context different from that of the original experiments, or more problematically, in no context at all. The latter case may be akin to testing a medical therapy without a disease. While simulation can be used to achieve meaningful results in IR evaluation, it must go beyond simple batching of queries into a retrieval system. There must be some interaction with the user, even if that user is acting within a simulated setting.

Relevance-based retrieval evaluation has clearly had many benefits, allowing assessment, at least superficially, the value of different approaches to indexing and retrieval. It is clearly useful in the early stages of system development when trying to assess from which indexing and retrieval approaches to choose. Hersh (1994) has stated that conventional recall–precision studies with topical relevance should be done in the early evaluation of a system. The problem comes when investigators attempt to draw conclusions about indexing and retrieval approaches based solely on recall and precision results.

7.7.5   *Automating Relevance Judgments*

Another limitation of relevance judgments is the time and cost it takes to obtain them. A number of researchers have explored whether they, or surrogates for them, can be collected in an automated manner. Soboroff et al. (2001) proposed the measurement of recall and precision without human relevance judgments. Noting past work by Voorhees (1998) demonstrated that differences in judgments did not affect the relative performance of systems, they selected random documents from the retrieval pool of multiple searches on each topic. Their results were most effective when they did not eliminate duplicates from selection (in essence giving more frequently retrieved documents a more likely chance to be selected as relevant). They found that their results were most effective in separating high-performing and low-performing systems from those in the middle, but that they were less successful at identifying the truly best (or worst) systems from among the top (or bottom)-performing systems. Aslam et al. (2006) developed methods for sampling very small numbers of documents (4% of usual pool size) that led to estimates of relevance for the remaining retrieved documents comparable to if they were judged by relevance judges.

Another concern about recall and precision is the completeness of relevance judgments. When using relative recall, we cannot be certain that enough relevant documents have been identified to give a close approximation to absolute recall. Buckley and Voorhees (2004) introduced a new measure, binary preference (bpref), which is based on the number of times judged nonrelevant documents are retrieved before known relevant ones (that, of course, have been judged). Experiments showed that the measure was highly correlated with existing measures, such as MAP, when judgments were complete and more robust to incomplete judgments. Stated simplistically, bpref essentially is a measure that uses only the retrieved documents that have been judged for relevance.

Joachims (2002a, b) introduced a new approach to evaluation for the Web based on *click-through data*. It was based on the premise that the links a user clicks on in the results listing from a Web search engine are a measure of relevance. A search engine or system is therefore "better" if more links are clicked from the output of one over the other. He proposed two types of experiments:

1. *Regular click-through data.* The user's query is sent to two search engines, with the complete rankings from one system or the other randomly presented to the user.
2. *Unbiased click-through data.* The user's query is sent to two search engines, but in this approach the results are mixed (although order within each set is maintained) together.

In both types of experiments, one system was deemed superior to the other when more Web pages from its output are clicked through by users.

In follow-up work, Joachims et al. (2005) looked at the eye movements and click-through behavior of real users, comparing them with the relevance judgments of other real users. They found that the user click-through was relatively highly associated with relevance, but was subject to two modest biases:

1. *Trust bias.* Users are influenced by the ranking order of the search engine, i.e., how much they trust its output.
2. *Quality bias.* Users are influenced by the overall quality of the search engine, i.e., better actual ranking actually influences users clicking.

They conclude that while clicks cannot be thought of as absolute relevance judgments, they are a highly effective relative approximation.

7.7.6 Measures of Agreement

Much IR evaluation involves human judgments. Such judgments may consist of determining whether documents are relevant or indexing terms are appropriately assigned by a person or computer. There are a variety of measures for assessing how well humans agree on these judgments. Probably the best-known and most widely used among these is the *kappa statistic* (Cohen, 1960). There are other measures of agreement and reliability for judgments, which have been described in the textbook by Friedman and Wyatt (2006).

The kappa statistic measures the difference between observed concordance (OC) and expected concordance (EC). Although the kappa statistic can be calculated for more than dichotomous variables, the example here will use a variable that can only have two values (such as relevant or nonrelevant). Table 7.12

Table 7.12 Table to calculate kappa statistic for two observers judging whether an event is X or Y

Observer 1	Observer 2		
	X	Y	Total
X	a	b	$a + b$
Y	c	d	$c + d$
Total	$a + c$	$b + d$	$a + b + c + d$

defines the variables for the following formulas:

$$OC = \frac{a+d}{a+b+c+d} \tag{7.1}$$

$$EC = \frac{\frac{(a+c)(a+b)}{a+b+c+d} + \frac{(b+d)(c+d)}{a+b+c+d}}{a+b+c+d} \tag{7.2}$$

$$Kappa = \frac{OC - EC}{1 - EC} \tag{7.3}$$

In general, the following kappa values indicate the stated amount of agreement (Cohen, 1960):

- Poor < 0.4
- Fair 0.4–0.6
- Good 0.6–0.8
- Excellent > 0.8

Table 7.13 presents sample data to calculate kappa for relevance judgments. The OC is 95/100 = 0.95. The EC is $[(77 \times 78/100) + (23 \times 22/100)]/100 = 0.65$. The kappa is therefore $(0.95–0.65)/(1–0.65) = 0.86$. The kappa value for the relevance judgments presented in Table 7.11 was 0.41 (Hersh, Buckley et al., 1994), with comparable results obtained in other studies (Haynes, McKibbon et al., 1990; Hersh and Hickam, 1992, 1993, 1995a).

Hripcsak and Rothschild (2005) investigated the relationship of kappa to the F measure. They showed that when the number of negative cases is large, and the probability of chance agreement on positive cases is very small, then the two measures will approach each other mathematically. This is therefore useful in situations (more common in assessment of natural language understanding systems) where the true number of negative cases is unknown but large. In addition, there are actually variants of the kappa measure whose assumptions lead to different results in some cases (DiEugenio and Glass, 2004).

Table 7.13 Sample data to calculate kappa

Observer 1	Observer 2		
	Relevant	Nonrelevant	Total
Relevant	75	3	78
Nonrelevant	2	20	22
Total	77	23	100

7.8   What Has Been Learned About IR Systems?

Although the beginning of this chapter lamented that the amount of evaluation research has not kept pace with the growth of IR systems and their use, the sum of research does give many insights into how systems are used, how often they are successful, and where they can be improved. The chapter ends with a review of the research findings in the context of the six questions around which the other sections were organized.

While it is clear that IR systems are being used in clinical settings, their impact is modest, and they are used to meet only a small fraction of clinicians' information needs. This does not mean that the systems are not valuable when they are used, but it does challenge the proponents of computer usage in medicine to implement systems that have more clinically pertinent information and are easier to use. Another consistent finding is that in most settings, bibliographic databases are still used more frequently than full-text resources, but this may change as more textbooks, journals, practice guidelines, and so on become more accessible online. User satisfaction with systems tends to be high, although there are some concerns that usage drops over time and/or when it becomes inconvenient.

System-oriented studies of searching quality have shown that databases vary in coverage by topic. They also show that searching the same database with a different system gives divergent results, an outcome perhaps exacerbated by the new features modern systems have added to make searching simpler for end users. In addition, achieving maximum recall, as needed for identifying RCTs for a meta-analysis, continues to be very difficult. It is likely that full-text searching leads to better recall, but at a significant price of lower precision. The capabilities of Web search engines are still largely unknown, but users must grapple with large amounts of information of varying quality aimed at a diversity of audiences.

User-oriented studies have shown that searchers are generally able to learn to search, but they make significant numbers of errors and have missed many opportunities. Studies of recall and precision show that most searches do not come anywhere close to retrieving all the relevant articles on a given topic. Of course, most searchers do not need to obtain all the relevant articles to answer a clinical question (unless they are doing a systematic review). These studies also find considerable lack of overlap in the relevant articles retrieved when different users search on the same topic. This is important, especially since the quality of the evidence in studies can vary widely, as described in Chap. 2. These studies also show that the type of indexing or retrieval interface may not have a large impact on user performance.

Task-oriented studies show that users improve their ability to answer clinical questions with IR systems, but performance is far from perfect. However quality of searching by users is assessed, systems take a long time to use. Large bibliographic databases such as MEDLINE may be inappropriate for most questions generated in the clinical setting, and the move to "synthesized," evidence-based resources may help in this regard.

Searching ability is influenced by a variety of factors. Although further research is needed to make more definitive statements, the abilities of healthcare personnel vary, with one or more specific cognitive traits (e.g., spatial visualization) possibly explaining the difference. Factors that may not play a significant role at all in search success are recall and precision. Although a searcher obviously needs to retrieve some reasonable amount of relevant documents and not be inundated by nonrelevant ones, the small differences across IR systems and users may not be significant. It is also clear that searchers make frequent mistakes and have missed opportunities that might have led to better results.

Finally, although healthcare IR systems are widely distributed and commercially successful, their true impact on healthcare providers and patient care is unknown. Demonstrating their benefit in the complex healthcare environment is difficult at best, with RCTs showing benefits in patient outcomes unlikely to be performed. On the other hand, as noted in the keynote address at the 1991 Symposium on Computer Applications in Medical Care by David Eddy, no one has ever assessed the impact of elevators on patient care, though they are obviously important. Analogously, no one can deny that medical IR systems are important and valuable, so further research should focus on how they can be used most effectively by clinicians, patients, and researchers.

Chapter 8
System and User Research

In Chap. 7, we saw that while information retrieval (IR) systems are widely used and perform important tasks for their intended audience, their ability to find relevant information and meet the needs of users is far from perfect. Even if one accepts the limitations of recall and precision as evaluation measures, it is clear that new approaches to indexing and retrieval are needed to better steer users to the documents they need. In this chapter, we will explore various research approaches to IR, focusing on two broad categories of research. The first focus will be on the IR system, looking at research that has focused on algorithms and approaches that improve retrieval of content. The second focus will be on the user and how systems can improve his or her retrieval or related task. We will then end with a review of user evaluation of research systems.

8.1 System-Oriented Research

In this section, we will explore research that has attempted to improve IR systems. While the user can never be completely separated from the system, the focus will be on systems and their techniques and algorithms. Within systems, we will focus on three broad aspects, which are those that focus mainly on words in text and statistical operations on them, those that aim for a deeper understanding of the text in order to improve indexing or retrieval, and some specific applications that take advantage of both approaches.

8.1.1 Lexical–Statistical Systems

Lexical–statistical approaches to IR are sometimes called automated retrieval, because they tend to be mainly computer algorithms with very minimal human involvement in indexing or retrieval, or partial-match retrieval, because they tend to

W. Hersh, *Information Retrieval: A Health and Biomedical Perspective.*
doi: 10.1007/978-0-387-78703-9, © Springer Science + Business Media, LLC 2009

rely on incomplete matching between query and document terms. These approaches are described as *lexical* because the unit of indexing tends to be the individual word in the document and *statistical* because they involve operations like weighting of terms and documents. A basic approach for this type of indexing and retrieval was introduced in Chaps. 4 and 5, respectively, because some of these methods are now used in state-of-the-art systems. These methods have actually been used in research systems for almost half a century; this long lag time in acceptance is due partly to their being better suited for end-user searching, which has become prevalent mainly since the advent of the World Wide Web.

Lexical–statistical systems offer many appealing features, especially to novice end users who are less skilled in the use of controlled vocabularies, Boolean operators, and other advanced features of traditional retrieval systems. Lexical–statistical systems do not, for example, require the user to learn a controlled vocabulary, which may express terms in ways not commonly used by clinicians. These systems also do not require the use of Boolean operators, which have shown to be difficult for novices. With some additional features, such as relevance feedback, which also requires little effort on the part of the user, these systems have the potential to be quite valuable in busy clinical settings, where rapid access to information is required.

8.1.1.1   Term Weighting

The basic term-weighting and partial-match approach to indexing approach now widely used and described in Chaps. 4 and 5 was simple and effective. However, it was also limited in that certain advanced features, such as combining terms into phrases or utilizing already retrieved relevant documents to find more, are difficult to conceptualize. For this reason, more advanced approaches were developed. One early approach was the *vector-space model* developed by Salton and McGill (1983). It should be noted that the use of the word *vector* in the term "vector-space model" does not imply that one have a detailed grasp of vector mathematics to understand its principles.

In the vector-space model, documents are represented as N-dimensional vectors, where N is the number of indexing terms in the database. Vectors can be binary or weighted, with term weighting represented by the length of the vector in a given dimension. Queries are also represented as vectors, so that the retrieval process consists of measuring the similarity between a query vector and all the document vectors in the database. The simplest method of doing this is to take the dot or inner product of the query and each document vector. When used with term frequency (TF) and inverse document frequency (IDF) weighting, this reduces to the approach outlined in Sect. 5.2.2. We also saw in Chap. 5 that this basic approach could be extended to include document length normalization to control for the length of documents in relevance ranking and relevance feedback to allow retrieval of more documents similar to ones already retrieved that were relevant.

Although TF*IDF has been a good general weighting scheme, there have been some test collections where other schemes have been found to work better. In the pre-TREC era of smaller test collections, the best document term-weighting measure was found to be TF*IDF (Salton and Buckley, 1988). The TREC era has seen the development of some measures that give better results with its test collections (Zobel and Moffat, 1998). In the early TREC collections, a variant of TF*IDF was found to work better that replaced TF with a logarithmic version (Buckley, Allan et al., 1993):

$$\text{TF}(\text{term}, \text{document}) = \ln(\text{frequency of term in document}) + 1 \qquad (8.1)$$

With the OHSUMED test collection under SMART, however, the best weighting method was found to include another variant of TF, the *augmented normalized term frequency* (Hersh, Buckley et al., 1994):

$$\text{TF}(\text{term}, \text{document}) = 0.5 + 0.5$$
$$\times \frac{\text{frequency of term in document}}{\text{maximum frequency of term in document}} \qquad (8.2)$$

Analysis with this test collection also found that document normalization was not helpful, since most of the MEDLINE references were similar in length and a large number of very short references (those without abstracts) were mostly nonrelevant.

The TREC experiments have led to the discovery of two other term-weighting approaches that have yielded improved results. The first of these was based on a statistical model known as Poisson distributions and has been more commonly called *Okapi weighting* (Robertson and Walker, 1994). This weighting scheme is an improved document normalization approach, yielding up to 50% improvement in mean average precision (MAP) in various TREC collections (Robertson, Walker et al., 1994). One version of Okapi's TF is

$$\text{Okapi TF} = \frac{(\text{frequency of term in document})(k_1 + 1)}{k_1(1 - b) + k_1 b \frac{\text{length of document}}{\text{average document length}} + \text{frequency of term in document}}$$
$$(8.3)$$

The variables k_1 and b are parameters set to values based on characteristics of the collection. Typical values for k_1 are between 1 and 2 and for b are between 0.6 and 0.75. A further simplification of this weighting often used is (Robertson, Walker et al., 1994)

$$\text{Okapi TF} = \frac{\text{frequency of term in document}}{0.5 + 1.5 \frac{\text{length of document}}{\text{average document length}} + \text{frequency of term in document}}$$
$$(8.4)$$

Okapi weighting has its theoretical foundations in probabilistic IR, to be described shortly. As such, its TF*IDF weighting uses a "probabilistic" variant of IDF

$$\text{Okapi IDF} = \log \frac{\text{total number of documents} - \text{number of documents with term} + 0.5}{\text{number of documents with term} + 0.5}$$

(8.5)

The probabilistic model has also led to the newest theoretical approach to term weighting, known as *language modeling*, which will be described later in this section.

The second improved term-weighting approach to come from TREC was *pivoted normalization* (PN) (Singhal, Buckley et al., 1996). Its major effect was to improve document normalization. After empirical analysis of the TREC collections showed that cosine normalization tended to result in shorter documents being over-retrieved and longer documents being under-retrieved, the PN approach learned from existing documents in a given collection what adjustment was optimal for document normalization.

Other techniques for term weighting have achieved varying amounts of success. One approach aimed to capture semantic equivalence of words in a document collection. Called *latent semantic indexing* (LSI), it uses a mathematically complex technique called *singular-value decomposition* (SVD) (Deerwester, Dumais et al., 1990). In LSI, an initial two-dimensional matrix of terms and documents is created, with the terms in one dimension and the documents in the other. The SVD process creates three intermediate matrices, the two most important being the mapping of the terms into an intermediate value, which can be thought to represent an intermediate measure of a term's semantics, and the mapping of this semantic value into the document. The number of intermediate values can be kept small, which allows the mapping of a large number of terms into a modest number of semantic classes or dimensions (i.e., several hundred). The result is that terms with similar semantic distributions (i.e., distributions that co-occur in similar document contexts) are mapped into the same dimension. Thus, even if a term does not co-occur with another, but occurs in similar types of documents it will be likely to have similar semantics. While the optimal number of dimensions is not known, it has been shown for several of the small standard test collections that a few hundred is sufficient (Deerwester, Dumais et al., 1990). Some early evaluation studies showed small performance enhancements for LSI with small document collections (Deerwester, Dumais et al., 1990; Hull, 1994), but these benefits were not realized with larger collections such as TREC (Dumais, 1994). A better use for this technique may be with the automated discovery of synonymy (Landauer and Dumais, 1997).

Another approach to term weighting has been to employ probability theory. This approach is not necessarily at odds with the vector-space model, and in fact its weighting approaches can be incorporated into the vector-space model. The theory underlying probabilistic IR is a model to give more weight to terms likely to occur in relevant documents and unlikely to occur in nonrelevant documents. It is based on Bayes' theorem, a common probability measure that indicates likelihood of an event based on a prior situation and new data. Probabilistic IR is predominantly a relevance feedback technique, since some relevance information about the terms in documents is required. However, it did not show improvement over vector modification techniques in six older test collections (Salton and Buckley, 1990). In the TREC experiments, as noted earlier, some variants on the probabilistic approach were shown to perform better than vector-space relevance feedback with the addition of query expansion (Broglio, Callan et al., 1994; Cooper, Chen et al., 1994; Kwok, Grunfeld et al., 1994; Robertson, Walker et al., 1994; Walczuch, Fuhr et al., 1994).

One modification to probabilistic IR was the *inference model* of Turtle and Croft (1991), where documents were ranked based on how likely they are to infer belief they are relevant to the user's query. This method was also not necessarily incompatible with the vector-space model and in some ways just provided a different perspective on the IR problem. One advantage of the inference model was the ability to combine many types of "evidence" that a document should be viewed by the user, such as queries with natural language and Boolean operators, as well as other attributes, such as citation of other documents. Combining some linguistic techniques, described later in this chapter, with slight modifications of TF*IDF weighting, passage retrieval, and query expansion, this approach performed consistently well in the TREC experiments (Broglio, Callan et al., 1994).

A more recent application of probabilistic IR has been the use of *language modeling* (Hiemstra and Kraaij, 2005). This approach was adapted from other computer tasks, such as speech recognition and machine translation, where probabilistic principles are used to convert acoustic signals into words and words from one language to another, respectively. A key aspect of the language modeling approach is "smoothing" of the probabilities away from a purely deterministic approach of a term being present or absent in a document in a binary fashion. Theoretically, the language modeling approach measures the probability of a query term given a relevant document.

Language modeling was introduced to the IR community by Ponte and Croft (1998), who showed modest performance gains with TREC collections. A variety of enhancements were subsequently found to improve retrieval performance further (Berger and Lafferty, 1999). Zhai and Lafferty (2004) investigated smoothing models and derived a number of new conclusions about this approach to IR. Subsequent work processing text into topic signatures based on mapping to Unified Medical Language System (UMLS) Metathesaurus terms and using those instead of words found 10–20% performance gains with ad hoc retrieval data from the TREC Genomics Track (Zhou, Hu et al., 2007).

Language models also allow the measurement of query "clarity," which is defined as a measure of the deviation between in the query and document language models from the general collection model (Cronen-Townsend, Zhou et al., 2002). Cronen-Townsend et al. found that query clarity was a good predictor of retrieval results from topics in the TREC ad hoc test collections, although application of this technique to real user queries from the TREC Interactive Track failed to uphold this association (Turpin and Hersh, 2004).

8.1.1.2 Stemming

As noted in Chap. 4, most implementations of automated indexing and retrieval use stemming, whereby plurals and common suffixes are removed from words, based on the presumption that the meaning of a word is contained in its stem. Another advantage to stemming is a practical one: the size of inverted files can be decreased, since fewer words have to be stored. This also leads to more efficient query processing. Stemming has disadvantages as well. First, it is purely algorithmic, whereas language can be idiosyncratic. Thus, most implementations do not handle grammatical irregularities. Second, in some instances, the information in the stem may in fact confer meaning. Some aggressive stemmers remove suffixes like -itis, which are not medically insignificant. Later in this chapter, some linguistic alternatives to stemming are described.

A variety of approaches to stemming have been advocated, but the most common approach in IR has been *affix removal* stemming, whereby algorithms specify removal of prefixes or (usually) suffixes. The two most commonly used affix removal algorithms are those by Lovins and Porter. The Lovins stemmer is an iterative longest-match stemmer that removes the longest sequence of characters according to a set of rules (Lovins, 1968). The Porter algorithm, on the other hand, has a series of rules that are performed if various conditions of the word length and suffix are met (Porter, 1980). Another stemmer that has been used in some systems is the S stemmer, whose rules are presented in Table 4.10.

How well do stemming algorithms perform? The data are confounded by a variety of different experimental parameters, such as type of stemmer, test collection, and performance measure used, but it is clear that the benefit of stemming is modest at best and can sometimes be detrimental (Harman, 1991). Two groups have compared stemming with no stemming in TREC ad hoc tasks, finding minimal improvement in performance with its use (Buckley, Salton et al., 1992; Fuller, Kaszkiel et al., 1997). Another analysis has compared different types of stemmers, not only the Lovins, Porter, and S stemmers but also some linguistically based stemmers described in the next chapter, finding minor improvements of a few percentage point increase in MAP overall (Hull, 1996). The latter analysis did find, however, that language idiosyncrasies cause a small number of queries to be affected in a large way, sometimes beneficially but other times detrimentally.

8.1.1.3 Phrases

Combining words into meaningful phrases can enhance precision. This is especially true when broad, high-frequency terms are combined. For example, high and blood and pressure are relatively common words and are likely to appear in many types of medical documents. But when these terms occur adjacently, they take on a very distinct meaning. Recognizing simple common phrases, however, is difficult to do algorithmically, especially without a dictionary or other linguistic resources. Furthermore, many phrases can be expressed in a variety of forms. For example, a document on `high blood pressure` might read, `When blood pressure is found to be high`. ... In addition, a single-word synonym might be substituted, such as `elevated` for `high`.

Of course, recognizing multiword phrases in free text useful to IR has proven difficult. One approach identified important phrases based on statistical co-occurrences of terms, with the goal of finding words that commonly occurred in close proximity to each other (Salton and McGill, 1983; Fagan, 1989). The "synonyms" generated were not true synonyms in the linguistic sense and the phrases generated were not always grammatically or semantically sound. These methods did, however, perform as well as approaches identifying linguistic phrases described later in Sect. 8.1.2.3.

In the TREC experiments, a simpler method of phrase construction was used. Buckley et al. (1993, 1994a) designated phrases as any adjacent nonstop words that occur in 25 or more documents in the training set. This approach conferred modest performance benefit and did better than most of the linguistic approaches discussed below. Harman (2005b) has asserted that further work in phrase construction was not necessary because the same benefits, both linguistically and performance-wise, were achieved with the query expansion techniques described in Sect. 8.1.1.5.

8.1.1.4 Passage Retrieval

Another approach to capturing the importance of term proximity introduced in the 1990s was *passage retrieval*, where documents were broken into smaller passages, which were used to weight the document for retrieval by the query (Salton and Buckley, 1991). The goal of this method was to find sections of documents that matched the query highly under the presumption that these local concentrations of query terms indicated a high likelihood of the document relevance. Salton and Buckley claimed that this process reduced linguistic ambiguity, since the smaller passage was more likely to ensure that words occurring together in the query were also occurring in the same context in the document. To give a medical example, the words `congestive`, `heart`, and `failure` are more likely to represent the concept `congestive heart failure` if they all occur in the same passage rather than scattered in separate parts of the document.

The main problem to this approach was identifying appropriate passages and avoiding having highly relevant areas of documents span across passages. Callan (1994) identified three types of passage in documents that could be used to subdivide documents based on content:

- Discourse passages – based on the structure of documents, such as sections and paragraphs
- Semantic passages – based on changing conceptual content of the text
- Window passages – based on number of words

Interest in passage retrieval has grown with the availability of full-text documents, which provide more text for identifying their topical content. Most implementations start initially with a global match between query and document in the usual manner. This is followed by matching of the query against smaller portions of the document, be they sections, semantic areas, or window contents. Different weighting schemes may be used for the various subdocuments; for example, cosine normalization is typically not helpful at the sentence level, since there is less variation in length.

Salton and Buckley used discourse passages in their original experiments, which were found to work well with the highly structured text of an encyclopedia (Salton and Buckley, 1991), but less ably with the TREC data (Buckley, Allan et al., 1993). Hearst and Plaunt (1993) utilized a vector-based approach to identifying semantic passages based on abrupt changes in document vectors between text sections, a technique that showed modest performance gains. Two groups at TREC found that overlapping text window passages of 200 words provided the best MAP performance gain of around 10–15% (Broglio, Callan et al., 1994; Buckley, Salton et al., 1994b). Passages started 100 words apart and each overlaps the next to avoid the breaking up of potentially relevant passages. Other groups using slightly different approaches also found benefit (Knaus, Mittendorf et al., 1994; Kwok, Grunfeld et al., 1994; Robertson, Walker et al., 1994).

Further work in passage retrieval was used in the TREC 2003 and 2004 High Accuracy Retrieval from Documents (HARD) Tracks (Allan, 2003, 2004). In addition, it was used in the TREC 2006 and 2007 Genomics Tracks described in the next chapter.

8.1.1.5 Relevance Feedback and Query Expansion

Section 5.2.2 introduced the notion of relevance feedback, which aims to discover more relevant documents in the retrieval process by adding terms from documents known to be relevant to a modified query that is rerun against the document collection. Also described was a related approach called query expansion, where the relevance feedback technique is used without relevance information. Instead, a certain number of top-ranking documents are assumed to be relevant and the relevance feedback approach is applied.

Assessing the benefit of relevance feedback can be difficult. Most batch-type studies use the *residual collection method*, in which the documents used for relevance feedback are ignored in the analysis and a new recall–precision table is generated (Salton and Buckley, 1990). For each query, an initial search is performed with some method, such as cosine-normalized TF*IDF. Some top-ranking relevant and nonrelevant documents, typically 15 or 30, are chosen for modification of query vector. At this point, a new recall–precision table could be generated with the new query vector. If, however, the improvements merely reflect reordering of the documents with the existing relevant ones ranked higher, the identification of new relevant documents may not result. In the residual collection method, only the residual documents from those not used in relevance feedback are used in the new recall–precision table.

Another approach to evaluation of relevance feedback techniques came from the early routing task in TREC (which has since been replaced by the Filtering Track). Since this task provided "training" data (i.e., documents known to be relevant to the queries), relevance feedback techniques could be applied to the queries run against the unknown "test" data to follow. The most effective approaches were found to use designation of a "query zone" of a certain number (in this case, 5,000) of documents that are related (e.g., in the same domain), but not all relevant to query and expansion of query terms weighted by Rocchio formula, adding terms and phrases that enhance performance but below the point at which they provide diminishing returns, estimated to be around 300–500 or 5–10% of terms (Buckley, Mitra et al., 2000).

Query expansion techniques have been shown to be among the most consistent methods to improve performance in TREC. They may be viewed as complementary to passage retrieval. While passage retrieval is a precision-enhancing technique that aims to give higher rank to documents in which the query terms are concentrated, presumably promoting their context, query expansion is a recall-enhancing process aiming to broaden the query to include additional terms in top-ranking documents. Based on the increased likelihood of top-ranking documents being relevant, terms present in these documents but not entered in the query should lead to the discovery of additional relevant documents.

In TREC-3, Buckley et al. (1994b) used the Rocchio formula with parameters 8, 8, and 0 (which perform less reweighting for expansion terms than in the relevance feedback experiments cited earlier) along with the addition of the top 500 terms and 10 phrases to achieve a 20% performance gain. Others in TREC have also shown benefit with this approach (Evans and Lefferts, 1993; Broglio, Callan et al., 1994; Buckley, Salton et al., 1994b; Knaus, Mittendorf et al., 1994; Kwok, Grunfeld et al., 1994; Robertson, Walker et al., 1994). Additional work by Mitra et al. (1998) has shown that use of manually created Boolean queries, passage-based proximity constraints (i.e., Boolean constraints must occur within 50–100 words), and term co-occurrences (i.e., documents are given more weight when query terms co-occur) improves MAP performance still further. The value of query expansion (and other lexical–statistical approaches) has been verified by Buckley (2005), who has constructed a table comparing different features of TREC systems with each year's ad hoc retrieval collection.

8.1.1.6 Implementations of Lexical–Statistical Systems

Basic TF*IDF weighting and partial-match retrieval are now part of many commercial search engine products. Although the exact details are proprietary, many Web search engines use various aspects of lexical–statistical approaches. In addition to commercial systems, a number of free research systems are available, many of which are listed in Table 1.4.

One of the first and certainly among the most widely used research systems was SMART, the original test bed for lexical–statistical techniques developed by Salton in the 1960s. First implemented in FORTRAN on a mainframe computer, it underwent several reimplementations on various platforms and the current version is written in C for Unix. A major limitation of SMART is that the system is designed more for batch-style IR experiments than for interactive retrieval. Thus, the basic software has only a command-line interface, although various groups have implemented user interfaces on top of it. The current implementation was designed in a very modular fashion, and thus not only can various existing features (e.g., weighting algorithms, stop lists, stemming, relevance feedback, etc.) be modified, but also new ones can be added.

Some of the other research systems in Table 1.4 provide access to features not available in SMART. For example, MG provides the array of weighting functions assessed by Zobel and Moffat (1998). The Lemur Toolkit (http://www.lemurproject.org/) provides basic indexing and retrieval functionality as well as that of the growing area of language modeling (Lafferty and Zhai, 2001). The search engine-specific portion of Lemur has been extracted out and developed into a system called Indri (http://www.lemurproject.org/indri/).

Another system gaining increasing use not only in IR research but also in operational systems is Lucene, which is part of the open-source Web server Apache (Gospodnetic and Hatcher, 2005). An additional open-source search engine is Zettair. The name comes from zettabyte and IR, with the former representing the quantity of 2 to the 70th power bytes, which is equal to 1,024 exabytes or approximately 10^{21} bytes. Zettair indexes HTML or TREC collections. It was developed for the TREC Terabyte Track, so it is very fast and efficient.

The IR systems of the NLM have generally not used lexical–statistical approaches, with the exception of the "Related Articles" feature of PubMed. However, as noted in Chap. 6, the askMEDLINE interface (http://askmedline.nlm.nih.gov/) is an exception (Fontelo, Liu et al., 2005). Designed mainly for handheld devices, the system allows natural language queries to be entered. The system performs a variety of interactions with the underlying PubMed engine.

8.1.2   Linguistic Systems

In this section, we turn our attention to another major area of research, which is the application of linguistic methods. These methods are based on techniques called *natural language processing* (NLP), which derive from the field of *computational linguistics*. The section begins with an overview of language and computational linguistics, and then turns attention to NLP methods used in IR and their results.

8.1.2.1   Rationale for Linguistic Systems in IR

Although considerable success in indexing and retrieval can be obtained with the use of matching word stems in queries and documents, individual words do not contain all the information encoded in language. One cannot, for example, arbitrarily change the order of words in a sentence and fully understand the original meaning of that sentence (i.e., He has high blood pressure has a clear meaning, whereas Blood has pressure he high does not).

The problem of single words begins with words themselves. Many words have one or more synonyms, which are different words representing the same thing. Some common examples in healthcare include the synonyms high and elevated as well as cancer and carcinoma. Another frequent type of synonym, especially prevalent in healthcare, is the acronym, such as AIDS. Sometimes, acronyms are embedded in multiword terms (AIDS-related complex) or other acronyms (ARC, which stands for AIDS-related complex).

Conversely, many words also exhibit polysemy, which describes a word that has more than one meaning. Consider the word lead, which can represent a chemical, a component of an electrocardiogram, or a verb indicating movement. In discussing polysemy, words are noted to have different senses or meanings. Common words often have many senses. In the *Brown Corpus*, the 20 most commonly used nouns in English have an average of 7.3 senses, while the 20 most common verbs have 12.4 senses (Kucera and Francis, 1967).

There are also problems beyond the synonymy and polysemy of single words. Words combine together to form phrases, which take on meaning beyond the sum of individual words themselves. For example, the words high, blood, and pressure combine in a phrase to take on a highly specific meaning. Furthermore, phrases exhibit synonymy and polysemy as well. For example, another way of describing the disease high blood pressure is hypertension. But the phrase high blood pressure also exhibits polysemy, inasmuch as it can indicate the disease (which is diagnosed by three consecutive elevated blood pressure readings) or a single measurement of elevated blood pressure.

These problems continue up to the most complex levels of language. Thus, certain large phrases have identical words with completely different meaning, such as expert systems used to improve medical diagnosis and medical diagnosis used to improve expert systems, as well as those that have the same meaning but share no common words, such as postprandial abdominal discomfort and epigastric pain after eating.

These problems highlight that the biggest obstacle to computer-based understanding of text is the ambiguity of human language. As such, the major challenge of computational linguistics has been to devise algorithms that disambiguate language as well as possible to allow useful computer applications. Thus, the grand goal of complete understanding of computer-based and unrestricted conversation with computers has been downscaled to applications like IR and related ones described in the next chapter. We will see that those applications, such as text mining and question answering, require specific aspects of NLP to work effectively.

What are the biggest challenges in IR that motivate use of linguistic methods? Mothe and Tanguy (2005) evaluated TREC test collections and noted that the linguistic features of query statements associated with the most difficulty (i.e., lowest MAP) were syntactic link span (i.e., concepts with the longest span of words) and polysemy of query words.

8.1.2.2 Overview of Linguistics

The field concerned with the use and representation of language is *linguistics*. The subfield concerned with computer programs to understand and generate natural language is computational linguistics. It is a practically oriented field, aiming to develop applications in areas such as speech understanding, question-answering systems, database querying, and, of course, IR systems. As will be seen, the goal of complete and unambiguous understanding of language has proved quite difficult to attain, and the success of linguistic methods in IR has been modest. A number of texts provide overviews of linguistics and its computational aspects (Allen, 1995; Kao and Poteet, 2006).

There are three recognized branches of linguistics, which share very little in common except for an interest in the use and understanding of language:

1. *Theoretical linguistics* deals with producing structural descriptions of language. It attempts to characterize organizing principles that underlie all human languages.
2. *Psycholinguistics* deals with how people produce and comprehend natural language. It attempts to characterize language in the ways that it explains human behavior.
3. *Computational linguistics* looks at utilizing language to build intelligent computer systems, such as the types of applications listed in Table 8.1.

Each branch of linguistics deals with language in a different way, but all recognize the different levels of language, starting with the sounds humans make to the complex meaning that is conveyed, as listed in Table 8.2. Most use of linguistic methods in IR focuses on the middle levels of morphology, syntax, and semantics. Phonology is of concern mostly in speech recognition systems, while problems of pragmatics and world knowledge lack solutions that would allow their use in IR.

The next step is to give an overview of the components of English that are addressed in IR systems, beginning with the most basic units and building upward. The lexical–statistical approach to IR considers words or word stems to be the most basic units of written language, but of course they are not. A number of words are composed of more basic units, which are called *morphemes*. Many words are composed of roots and affixes, which can be prefixes and suffixes, and roots. An example of a word with a root, a prefix, and a suffix is the word `pretesting`, with the root `test-`, the prefix `pre-`, and suffix `-ing`.

Table 8.1 Applications of computational linguistics

Abstracting: automated summarization of texts
Data extraction: codifying the information in texts
Information retrieval: retrieval of texts
Machine translation: conversion of texts in one language to another language
Question answering: answering factual queries
User interface: performing computer tasks based on natural language input
Writing assistance: analysis of texts for spelling, grammar, and style

Table 8.2 Levels of language

1. Phonology: analysis of sound units that make up words, most useful in speech understanding systems
2. Morphology: analysis of parts of words, useful in verb tenses, noun singular/plural. Also helpful in breaking down complex words (i.e., `appendic-itis`) and equating noun and verb forms (i.e., verb to `treat` vs. noun `treatment`)
3. Syntax: analysis of relationship of words in a sentence to each other. How words are grouped into phrases, what words modify each other
4. Semantics: meaning of words, phrases, and sentences. What real-world objects each represent
5. Pragmatics: how context affects interpretation of sentences
6. World knowledge: general knowledge of world that must be present to understand discourse

Some words are composed of *bound morphemes*, which are units that cannot occur alone. For example, in the word `arthroscopy`, which refers to the medical procedure of viewing the inside of a joint with a fiber-optic scope, both the prefix `arth-` and the suffix `-oscopy` must be attached to another morpheme. Many bound morphemes have many roots that they can attach to, such as `-itis`, which can combine with virtually any body part to indicate inflammation of that part. The morphemes of a word come together to form *lexemes*, which are the basic word units. Words of different types vary in their value as indexing terms in IR systems. Particles, prepositions, and determiners are less valuable to IR than nouns, verbs, and adjectives, which is why many words from the former group are likely to be on stop word lists.

Words come together to form phrases. As will be seen, phrases reduce the ambiguity of documents and lead to better retrieval in some instances. The phrase that is generally most useful in document retrieval is the noun phrase (NP). NPs vary in complexity from simple one-word nouns to those containing several nouns and adjectives. NPs can be pronouns as well as names or proper nouns (e.g., `Bill Hersh`, `Oregon Health & Science University`). In a multiword NP, the main noun is called the *head*, and the other words are called *modifiers*. The two other important types of phrase are the verb phrase (VP) and prepositional phrase (PP). VPs contain a head verb and optional auxiliary verbs. Head and auxiliary verbs combine in different ways to form tenses (simple past, past perfect). Some verbs take additional words called particles that modify the verb. These overlap with prepositions, but they must immediately follow the verb or object NP. PPs consist of a preposition and NP. They qualify others parts of sentences, and can be attached to a verb (`I gave the stethoscope to Dr. Jones`) or noun (`I gave the stethoscope from Dr. Jones`).

Phrases combine to form sentences, which ask, state, or describe things about the world. The simplest sentences consist of a single NP (the subject) and a VP. The next simplest sentences contain NP–VP–NP, or subject, verb, and object. But sentences can also be very complex, such as a sentence embedded within another (`The patient who was just diagnosed with heart disease felt very depressed`).

As just defined, NLP consists of the computer programs that process language. While NLP techniques make use of many levels of linguistics, often in concert with one another, there are three distinct phases. *Parsing* is the processing of sentences into syntactic categories with the aid of morphological knowledge. *Semantic interpretation* is the attachment of meaning to syntactic interpretation of sentences. *Contextual interpretation* is the understanding of sentences in context.

In parsing, a sentence is analyzed to determine its syntactic structure. This structure is specified by a *grammar*, a set of allowable rules that define how the parts can come together to form larger structures. Each of the words must contain a syntactic category or part-of-speech (POS) that defines the structures in which it can participate. The parsing process requires a lexicon of words (and, if desired, bound morphemes). In recent years, there has been an effort to standardize the labeling of parts of speech. One of the most well-known efforts is the Penn Treebank (http://www.cis.upenn.edu/~treebank/). This project has also generated a large collection of POS-tagged data, with over three million words of text from a variety of sources (Marcus, Santorini et al., 1994). An important large lexicon for healthcare is the SPECIALIST lexicon, developed as part of the UMLS (McCray, Srinivasan et al., 1994).

In the 1990s, the focus of NLP research began to evolve as it was realized that the earlier methods did not lead to general language understanding nor even scale up to allow real-world solutions to language-related computational problems. Recognizing that it was difficult to build and maintain lexicons, grammars, and other linguistic knowledge resources, researchers shifted their focus from "deterministic" NLP to that which was "empirical" or "corpus-based." In the latter approach, which achieved better results, algorithms were developed to extract linguistic knowledge (e.g., POS tagging, grammars, etc.) from natural language corpora rather than requiring system developers to manually encode it. Most approaches have used machine-learning techniques that add probability information to syntactic and semantic processes, aiming to generate the parse most likely to be correct rather than trying to deterministically identify it (Brill and Mooney, 1997). The approaches were found to be successful in computer-based speech recognition in the 1980s (Bahl, Jelineck et al., 1983) and have diffused to other applications of NLP. The probabilistic approach has been highly successful when applied to syntactic parsing (Charniak, 1997).

One area of semantic interpretation highly relevant to IR is word-sense disambiguation (WSD), i.e., determining the sense to which a polysem belongs. A health example is the word cold, which can refer to a temperature or an illness. There are a number of resources that identify the different senses of words, including dictionaries as well as the lexical database WordNet (Fellbaum, 1998). The UMLS Metathesaurus also designates sense for different medical concepts.

It has been suggested that selective use of NLP in IR may be feasible (Strzalkowski, Lin et al., 1999). For example, recognition of nouns and how they come together in NPs may give a better clue to the underlying concepts discussed in a document. Likewise, having some semantic information may allow recognition of synonym equivalence and disambiguation of polysemous terms. In the following section, we explore three approaches – parsing and syntactic analysis, word-sense disambiguation, and semantic analysis – that have been undertaken to exploit linguistic properties of IR databases.

8.1.2.3 Parsing and Syntactic Analysis

Of the NLP steps, the best understood is parsing. It is therefore not surprising that a number of researchers have attempted to enhance IR systems with parsing and other types of syntactic analysis. The motivation for this approach is based on the assumption that by understanding the components of a sentence (i.e., the phrases), one can better understand the underlying conceptual content and presumably better match it to query statements. Early approaches to parsing suffered from two major deficits. First, parsing was viewed as a deterministic process yielding a "correct" parse. There was no attempt to handle the ambiguity arising from multiple or incomplete parses. The second problem was related to computer hardware; until the 1990s, most machines did not have the power to parse databases of the size typically found in IR. Part of this hardware limitation was confounded by the first problem, the deterministic approach to parsing, which in general was computationally intense.

Fagan (1987) pursued a line of research that compared the generation of phrases from word frequencies (statistical phrases, described in Sect. 8.1.1.3) and from parsing (syntactic phrases, with a focus on NPs). He modified the SMART system by adding a parser that derived NPs from the text, which were used along with words to index documents. The same procedure was used for queries. This approach was shown to improve slightly on single-word indexing alone (1.2–8.7%), but performed less well than statistically generated phrases (2.2–22.7%). Salton et al. (1990) subsequently investigated the parser used in Fagan's experiments to determine its effectiveness. They concluded that the benefit for syntactic over statistical phrases was small, and since statistical methods were far more efficient with resources, both in terms of computer algorithm complexity and the human effort required to build parsers and lexicons, deemed them preferable to syntactic methods.

Other IR systems have been based on parsers that do not aim for complete parsing but instead focus on the NP, the area in which the content is likely to represent that present in queries. As such, these systems have focused on the recognition of NPs and their use in indexing and retrieval. The CLARIT system, for example, was designed to recognize NPs, identifying their boundaries rather than completely parsing the entire sentence (Evans, Lefferts et al., 1992). The CLARIT parser applied lexical tagging and an inflectional morphology analyzer to reduce terms to root form. The grammar then identified phrases, with particular emphasis on identifying NPs. The parser could identify just *simplex* NPs, which consisted of the NP head and its modifiers, or both simplex and *complex* NPs, the latter of which contained posthead PPs, relative clauses, and VPs.

CLARIT had several additional features to enhance retrieval after parsing has been completed (Evans and Zhai, 1994). Most simply, it could combine the phrases plus individual words into a vector-space approach, matching them against phrases and words in the user's query for retrieval. Another feature was thesaurus discovery, which could be based on the top-ranking documents (query expansion) or ones denoted by the user to be relevant (relevance feedback). CLARIT also had a comprehensive user interface that allowed the user to generate thesaurus discovery terms, add or delete them from the query, and vary their weighting in the query (Hersh, Campbell et al., 1996).

Another approach to partial parsing was used by Strzalkowski et al. (1999). Similar to CLARIT, their system aimed to recognize simple and complex NPs in concert with other lexical–statistical IR techniques, such as term weighting and query expansion. The architecture of their system separated each technique into "streams" so that each could be relatively weighted to optimize system performance and isolated for analysis in experimentation. None of these techniques, however, performed better than lexical–statistical approaches.

8.1.2.4   Word-Sense Disambiguation

As noted so far, many words, especially commonly used ones, have multiple senses (e.g., AIDS and hearing aids, EKG lead and lead poisoning). Inappropriate retrieval may occur when a query uses one sense and a document uses another. This problem is frequent (Krovetz and Croft, 1992), and efforts to eradicate it may not be successful (Sanderson, 1994). A research question is whether these approaches are amenable to WSD.

One approach to WSD has been to use resources that categorize words into their senses. One such resource is WordNet, a semantic network type of system containing English words, their synonyms, and the senses in which they occur (Fellbaum, 1998). Each set of synonyms in WordNet is called a *synset*. Words can belong to more than one synset; for example, the word cold can be a disease, a temperature, and an emotional state. Synsets are categorized into a semantic hierarchy, with the top-level terms called *unique beginners* (Fellbaum, 1998). Voorhees (1993) analyzed WordNet from the standpoint of improving IR system performance. She noted that while the average number of senses per word is 1.26, some words, which include some used in language with high frequency, have a large number of senses, as many as 27. Likewise, while the average synset contains 1.74 words, the largest one contains 38 words.

Two researchers have used WordNet in attempts to develop algorithms that disambiguate the sense of query words to enhance the retrieval documents where words in the query are used in the same sense as they are in the documents. Voorhees (1993) developed an approach that attempted to identify the *hood* of a synset, which was essentially the largest span of the noun hierarchy and its narrower terms that contained a single synset. The synset identifier became a component of query and document vectors in SMART, with cosine matching providing a ranked retrieval output. Unfortunately, Voorhees found that this approach degraded retrieval performance overall, although selected queries demonstrated benefit.

Further analysis indicated that most queries in these older, smaller test collections were too short to allow disambiguation of their words. Additional experimentation with the longer queries in the TREC collection found that this automated approach did not confer benefit either, although some of the less-developed queries were able to obtain benefit by manual expansion with synsets selected by the user for inclusion (Voorhees, 1994). Richardson and Smeaton (1995) used a somewhat similar approach to WSD with WordNet and obtained comparable results. While their work demonstrated that they could perform WSD reasonably well, this advantage did not translate into improved retrieval performance.

Another approach to WSD did not use any lexical resources but instead employed a thesaurus that was created via automatic means using SVD to determine "synonym" terms (Schutze and Pedersen, 1995). Instead, based on the observation that words occurring close to other words help define its sense, a context vector is created based on clustering techniques that allow words to be disambiguated. Experimental results on a *Wall Street Journal* subset of TREC data found the sense-based approach to improve MAP by 7.4% alone over the word-based baseline and by 14.4% when used in conjunction with regular word-based vectors.

A related challenge to disambiguation of search words in IR systems is author names. In MEDLINE, for example, even though full author names are now entered into each record, there are still authors who share the same name. Furthermore, users searching for author names often just enter just the last name with first or first and middle initials. As such, means for disambiguating author names are essential (Torvik, Weeber et al., 2005).

8.1.2.5 Semantic Analysis

While WSD methods were designed to handle polysemous words, other approaches have been implemented to address the problems of synonymy, which is problematic in all domains, and is certainly a challenge for IR systems in health and biomedicine. The domain specificity of synonyms is sometimes helped by the presence of manually constructed thesauri. Medicine, in particular, has a number of thesauri that contain important terms and their synonyms. Their limitation, however, is that they are often constructed for purposes other than document retrieval. For example, the International Classification of Diseases (ICD) is used mainly for coding medical diagnoses for billing purposes. Many of its terms are not those that physicians are likely to use in documents or queries. Even the Medical Subject Headings (MeSH) vocabulary, which is used for manual indexing and retrieval of medical literature, has a number of expressions of terms that would not normally be used by clinicians.

Aronson (1996) has noted that text strings can map into controlled vocabulary terms in a variety of ways:

- Simple match – text string matches vocabulary term exactly
- Complex match – string maps into more than term (e.g., `intensive care medicine` mapping into `Intensive Care` and `Medicine`)

- Partial match – text string maps into part of a term, which can occur in several ways:

  o Normal – string maps into part of phrase (e.g., `liquid crystal thermography` mapping into `Thermography`)
  o Gapped – string maps with gap either in string or term (e.g., `ambulatory monitoring` mapping into `Ambulatory Cardiac Monitoring`)
  o Overmatch – beginning or end of term includes additional words not in string (e.g., `application` mapping into `Heat/Cold Application` or `Medical Informatics Application`)

- No match – no part of text maps into any term

A number of researchers have developed approaches for mapping concepts from free text into controlled vocabularies for a variety of applications, including IR. One of the earliest efforts to do this in IR was the SAPHIRE system (Hersh, 1991), which utilized the UMLS Metathesaurus. The Metathesaurus provided synonym linkages across medical vocabularies (e.g., the MeSH term `Hypertension` was linked to the ICD-9 term `Elevated Blood Pressure`). Since many terms within these vocabularies contained synonyms, the grand sum of all synonymous terms was large, which enabled SAPHIRE to recognize a wide variety of string forms that mapped into concepts.

The original version of SAPHIRE employed a *concept-matching algorithm* in both indexing and retrieval (Hersh, 1991). The algorithm took as its input any string of text, such as a document sentence or a user query, and returned a list of all concepts found, mapped to their *canonical* or preferred form. This was done by detecting the presence of *word-level synonyms* between words in concepts (e.g., `high` and `elevated`) as well as *concept-level synonyms* between concepts (e.g., `hypertension` and `high blood pressure`). The concept-matching process was purely semantic, with no syntactic methods (e.g., parsing) used. In SAPHIRE's indexing process, the text to be indexed for each document was passed to the concept-matching algorithm. The indexing terms for each document were the concepts matched, which were weighted with IDF and TF redefined for concepts. For retrieval, the user entered a natural language query, and the text was passed to the concept-matching algorithm. Each document with concepts in the list then received a score based on the sum of the weights of terms common to the query and document, with the resulting list of matching documents then sorted based on the score. SAPHIRE was comprehensively evaluated with databases of several different types and in both batch and interactive modes (Hersh and Hickam, 1992, 1993, 1995a; Hersh, Hickam et al., 1992, 1994). In all, SAPHIRE showed performance nearly comparable to, but not better than, word-based methods. While its use of synonyms was shown to be beneficial in some queries, the inability to map free text into vocabulary terms hindered it in others.

Another well-known approach to mapping text into Metathesaurus terms is the MetaMap system (Aronson, 1996, 2001, 2006). MetaMap's general approach is to process input text to generate a wide variety of possible word variants, which are

Table 8.3 Variant generation in MetaMap (adapted from Aronson, 2006)

Variant	Distance score
Spelling variant	0
Inflection	1
Acronym/abbreviation or synonym	2
Derivational variant	3

then used to generate candidate strings for potential matching. It begins by using a POS tagger to assign syntactic tags from the SPECIALIST lexicon to words, which are then grouped into NPs. Next, all possible variants of words within the phrases are generated based on knowledge resources associated with the SPECIALIST lexicon, including lists of acronyms, abbreviation, and synonyms as well as rules for derivational morphology. Table 8.3 lists the types of variants that are generated. Each variant receives a *distance score*, which indicates the extent of variation from the original word and is also shown in Table 8.3.

These scores are used to evaluate candidate terms that are selected for matching. The evaluation scoring process is based on four factors:

1. Centrality – the word that is the NP head gets a score of 1; all other words get a score of 0.
2. Variation – how much the variants in the Metathesaurus string differ from the original text string words, based on the formula

$$\text{Variation} = \frac{4}{\text{Distance} + 4} \tag{8.6}$$

3. Coverage – the amount of words that the Metathesaurus string and the text string have in common, consisting of two components:

   (a) Meta span, the number of words in text string present in Metathesaurus term
   (b) Phrase span, the number of words in Metathesaurus term present in text string

   A *coverage value* is calculated by giving the meta span twice as much as weight as the phrase span. (This value is replaced by a simpler *involvement value* when word order is not utilized.)

4. Cohesiveness – based on the largest number of connected words in the Metathesaurus and text strings, consisting of two components:

   (a) Meta cohesiveness, the sum of squares of the connected components divided by the square of the length of the string
   (b) Phrase cohesiveness, the sum of squares of the connected components divided by the square of the length of the phrase

   A *cohesiveness value* is calculated by giving the meta span twice as much as weight as the phrase span.

Each Metathesaurus term's score is normalized to between 0 and 1,000, and the term candidates are mapped to the disjoint parts of the NP. The program has a variety of parameters, such as how extensively the variant process will be performed, which can be set to tune the algorithm for appropriateness to the function to which it is being applied.

Another use of controlled vocabularies in linguistic systems has been to associate words in the text with controlled vocabulary terms that have been assigned to documents with those words. This approach was originally used with a large physics database that had manually assigned index terms (Fuhr and Knorz, 1984). A number of healthcare applications have used this approach. The MeSH term selection function of the Ovid (http://www.ovid.com/) retrieval system maps the user's input to the MeSH terms that occur most frequently when those words are used in the title and abstract of the MEDLINE record. Another approach in the healthcare domain was implemented by Yang and Chute, who used a technique of linear-least-squares fit to measure the association between words that occur in MEDLINE abstracts and the assigned MeSH terms (Yang and Chute, 1994). This technique required a training set of documents that were used to derive the associations. Using a partitioned MEDLINE test collection, Yang and Chute found enhancement over baseline SMART performance, but only comparable performance to SMART using relevance feedback.

An additional possible use of semantic information is to expand queries with semantically appropriate terms, such as synonyms and other related terms. Evans and Lefferts (1993) introduced expansion via automatically constructed thesauri in TREC, showing modest gains over the TF*IDF baseline but not exceeding other nonlinguistic approaches, such as improved term weighting or query expansion. Voorhees (1994) attempted to use WordNet along its hierarchical and synonym links to expand queries, but as with her WSD experiments, no benefit was seen.

Another approach that achieved modest success in the healthcare domain used MEDLINE test collections to define measures of association between the words in the title and abstract of the MEDLINE record and its assigned MeSH terms (Srinivasan, 1996a,b). In this approach, each MEDLINE record is represented by two vectors, one for words and one for MeSH terms. Initial word-based queries against MEDLINE are expanded to include MeSH terms, which are then used for retrieval by means of the MeSH vectors. Experimental results showed modest performance gains (e.g., 8–9% in average precision), but even better results were obtained by query expansion using the MeSH terms from top-ranking relevant documents. Researchers at NLM have also explored semantically assisted query expansion, with their approach processing queries using MetaMap to identify Metathesaurus terms, which are in turn used to expand queries by means of the INQUERY system (Aronson and Rindflesch, 1997). The NLM researchers achieved comparable results to those of Srinivasan, as seen in Table 8.4.

Table 8.4 Results of MAP using MeSH terms and thesaurus-based query expansion in MED-LINE documents by Srinivasan (1996a,b) and Aronson and Rindflesch (1997)

Method	Srinivasan	Aronson and Rindflesch
Text-only, no MeSH terms	0.52	0.52
MeSH terms	0.56	0.57
MeSH terms with thesaurus-based query expansion	0.57	0.60
Adding document feedback to thesaurus-based query expansion	0.60	(not done)

8.1.3 Applications

Now that we have covered the basic system-oriented research approaches to IR, we can explore some applications of them. In this section, we begin by exploring two important general IR applications, cross-language retrieval and Web searching. This is followed by a discussion more specific to biomedicine, namely, research in biomedical text retrieval and medical image retrieval.

8.1.3.1 Cross-Language Retrieval

English is the *lingua franca* of online information, certainly of scientific and biomedical information. Most international scientific conferences and publications use English as their required language. (Indeed, a German colleague has suggested that if English is not a scientist's first language, it is always his or her second.) However, there is continued growth not only in languages other than English on the Web but also interest in allowing searching across languages, especially in places like Europe where a cacophony of different languages are spoken over a relatively small geographic area.

Cross-language information retrieval (CLIR) is done when queries and documents are in different languages. Despite the preponderance of English in science and on the Web, CLIR capability is desirable in certain instances. Government or business analysts may, for example, desire intelligence from political or business documents in non-English-speaking countries. In healthcare, researchers performing meta-analyses may seek to retrieve randomized controlled trials written in languages other than English. (This task is made somewhat easier by the availability in most major bibliographic databases of translations into English of non-English titles and abstracts.) Cross-lingual capabilities can also be helpful in an educational sense, enabling non-English-speaking individuals to learn English medical terminology.

Evaluation of research in CLIR began at TREC, but then developed into its own independent TREC-like activity for European languages. This spawned the Cross-Language Evaluation Forum (CLEF, http://www.clef-campaign.org/), leaving non-European languages to TREC. Another forum focusing on Asian-language CLIR has been the National Institute for Informatics (NII) Test Collection for IR Systems (NTCIR, http://research.nii.ac.jp/~ntcadm/index-en.html) Project.

As with most IR system-oriented research, CLIR is typically assessed via test collections (Braschler and Schauble, 2000). Experiments can be monolingual (i.e., queries are expressed in one language against a document collection in another) or multilingual (i.e., queries are expressed against documents in more than one language). In the case of multilingual collections, documents may be parallel (i.e., document-for-document translations exist across languages), or comparable (i.e., the documents contain similar conceptual content but are not exact translations). In general, experiments in parallel corpora have found that performance, measured by MAP, is typically 50–75% of what would be obtained when queries and documents are in the same language (Harman, 2005a).

Oard (1997) has classified and reviewed the major approaches to CLIR. He notes that CLIR can be broadly classified into two types of retrieval, controlled vocabulary and free text. The former consists of documents that have been manually indexed into a controlled vocabulary, which itself has been translated into different languages. Although a number of commercial bibliographic databases have thesauri that have been translated into multiple languages, research into their use for CLIR has been minimal (Soergel, 1997). Of note, the MeSH vocabulary from healthcare has been translated into over 20 languages (Nelson, Schopen et al., 2000). Some of the terms from these MeSH translations (only from Roman alphabet or transliterated languages) have begun to appear as "synonyms" in the UMLS Metathesaurus. For example, the Spanish term `corazon` appears as a synonym for the English term `heart`.

Free-text CLIR is further divided by Oard into corpus-based and knowledge-based techniques. Corpus-based techniques take advantage of parallel or comparable corpora, attempting to learn appropriate translations. One approach uses LSI to "shrink" the conceptual space across multilingual collections (Landauer and Littman, 1990). Other work has focused on techniques to align documents across languages at varying levels of similarity (Braschler and Schauble, 2000):

- Same story
- Related story
- Shared aspect
- Common terminology
- Unrelated

Once these alignments have been determined, algorithms can match queries to similar documents or portions of them automatically.

Knowledge-based free-text CLIR techniques typically employ machine-readable resources, such as dictionaries. The earliest work with this approach came from Salton (1970), who used a word-word dictionary to translate words from one language to another. This approach was also used by Hull and Greffenstette (1996) for French queries of the (English) TREC collection. Another approach has been to use EuroWordNet, a version of WordNet extended to several European languages

(Gilarranz, Gonzalo et al., 1997). One limitation of simple word-to-word mapping entails the polysemy of words, since word sense may differ across languages as well as within a language. Some approaches to overcome this problem have included the use of POS tagging and document alignment (Davis and Ogden, 1997) as well as query expansion (Ballesteros and Croft, 1997).

Research for CLIR continues to move forward, led by the tracks in CLEF and NCTIR, many of which parallel those in TREC. A recent special issue of *Information Processing & Management* featured an overview of the state of the art for CLIR (Kishida, 2005) as well as a roadmap for moving forward with additional research (Gey, Kando et al., 2005). The latter, as with many IR applications, made a plea for realistic collections and search tasks in research. The may be aided, at least in CLEF, by the development of JRC-Acquis, a new parallel corpus in all 20 official languages recognized by the European Union (Steinberger, Pouliquen et al., 2006).

The amount of CLIR-related work going on in the healthcare domain has been small, perhaps because of the predominance of English in scientific publications and meetings. Most work has focused on the development of multilingual resources to assist retrieval. Hersh and Donohoe (1998) found that when non-English terms appeared as synonyms in the UMLS Metathesaurus, the SAPHIRE approach could be used to map words in other languages to Metathesaurus concepts. Some analyses have looked at the limitations of non-English languages in the UMLS Metathesaurus, most of which derive from the two-dozen translations of MeSH. Analyses of German (Hersh and Donohoe, 1998) and French (Bodenreider and McCray, 1998) have found problems with small numbers of plural terms and synonyms as well as nonuse of the 8-bit character sets that results in removal of diacriticals (e.g., umlauts) or ligatures (e.g., connected characters). German has additional problems words that come together in phrases to form single words (e.g., `Oesophagus-varizenblutung` or `esophageal bleeding`) that are generally not present in the Metathesaurus, whereas French has problems with removal of diacriticals making words ambiguous, such as the word `côte` (`rib`) and `côté` (`side`) being translated to `cote` (`quotation`).

Other works have looked at Asian languages, with a focus on translating languages such as Chinese and Japanese into English to provide an entry point into English content. Hersh and Zhang (1999) developed a Chinese-based interface to the UMLS Metathesaurus. Asian languages like Chinese differ greatly from Roman languages in that they contain many more than the basic 26 or so alphabet characters. In addition, they generally do not use spaces to indicate word boundaries. (In the case of Chinese, each character is essentially a whole word.) Hiruki et al. (2001) adapted the basic Chinese system to Japanese, a language whose writing is even more complex than Chinese. Their Japanese–English MeSH translator (J-MeSH tool) used a Web browser interface and enables users to accurately find equivalent English medical terms for Japanese medical terms. It accomplished this by first mapping a Japanese term to candidate terms from a Japanese translation of MeSH, then retrieving the English equivalent of the desired candidate term by way of the Metathesaurus concept unique identifier (CUI). Figure 8.1 shows the terms retrieved from entry of the Japanese word for `hypertension`. When one of

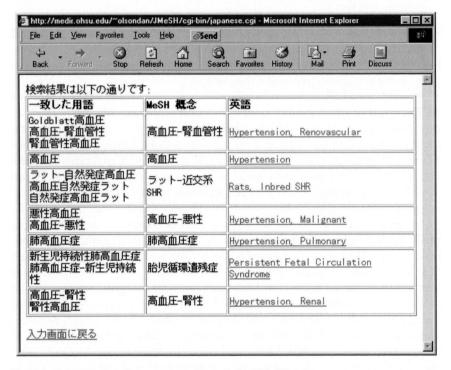

Fig. 8.1 Japanese query for hypertension to the J-MeSH tool

the hyperlinked English terms is selected, another page is shown with the Japanese search term, the English equivalent, the English definition, and parent and child terms in the MeSH hierarchy. This page also provides links that submit the term as a query to CliniWeb, PubMed, or Google. The user can also browse up and down the MeSH hierarchy by clicking on the hyperlinks of the parent and child terms, or return to the candidate terms table page to select a different candidate term. Figure 8.2 shows the page that appears if the user has selected the term Pulmonary Hypertension.

In an approach to CLIR that made use of the UMLS Metathesaurus, Eichmann et al. (1998) attempted to determine how well Spanish and French queries could retrieve English documents. They used the OHSUMED test collection, with its queries translated manually into Spanish and French. They then set out to assess algorithms that used the Metathesaurus to automatically translate those queries back to English and retrieve MEDLINE references from the collection. Their basic approach was to use the SMART system to create a transfer dictionary. This was done by creating "documents" consisting of the Spanish or French word along with all CUIs in which it appeared. This allowed a query to "retrieve" English concepts, with the output ranked by a TF*IDF weighting scheme. The results of their experiments showed that the best approach for Spanish and French was to combine all the refinements just listed except the partial matches, with achievement of 75

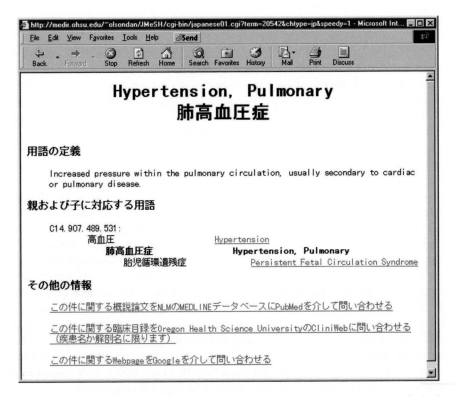

Fig. 8.2 Display of Japanese information for the term `pulmonary hypertension` in the J-MeSH tool

and 64% of the English baseline average precision for Spanish and French, respectively.

A failure analysis provided some further insight. First the researchers noted that there were more Spanish terms than French terms, which could potentially explain the better Spanish results. However, reducing the coverage of the Spanish terms to those also present in French did not change the average precision results. Like Bodenreider and McCray (1998), Eichmann et al. concluded that French coverage in the Metathesaurus was problematic. Another interesting finding was that more French queries performed better than Spanish queries over the English baseline, although many also performed worse.

A more comprehensive approach to CLIR was undertaken with the OHSUMED test collection by Markó et al. (2005), who translated the documents as well as the queries. They utilized their Morphothesaurus system, which translates all language into a common language-independent form of subwords. This then allows querying in any language whose queries can be translated into this form. Their approach looked at translation into German and, with the additional feature of a word adjacency measure that gave higher weight to multiword concepts appearing adjacent to each other, were able to achieve 93% of baseline English performance.

8.1.3.2   Web Searching

With the growth of the Web, it is not surprising that some research has focused specifically on Web searching. However, one unfortunate consequence of the commercialization of Web searching has been the development of proprietary algorithms that cannot be replicated and dissected in evaluations by researchers. A great deal of Web searching research has therefore focused on how users interact with commercial search engines, some of which will be described later in the chapter. In this section, we will focus on the TREC Web Track as well as other system-oriented Web research.

The TREC Web Track emerged with the retiring of the general ad hoc retrieval task after TREC-8 (Hawking and Craswell, 2005). At the same time, the Web Track emerged with a 10-gigabyte, 1.69 million document collection called WT10g for TREC-9, which in essence served as the ad hoc track (Hawking, 2000). Topics were derived from a log of searches posed to the Excite search engine (http://www.excite.com/), with additional narrative added by TREC assessors to make the search topic more explicit. Some of the original queries had misspellings, which were kept in the data to simulate the misspellings made by real users. One general goal of the Web Track has been to determine whether the link information in Web data can lead to more effective retrieval than page content alone. To facilitate the latter, a link connectivity matrix was calculated and distributed with the data. For all the participants in the TREC-9 Web Track, the benefits of link data were found to vary from slight improvements to outright detriment (Hawking, 2000). Performance was found to be resilient for queries with errors, with little effect on MAP.

The TREC 2001 Web Track used the same WT10g collection with two types of query: the standard ad hoc retrieval task and a "home-page-finding" task (Hawking and Craswell, 2001). Topics from the latter were comparable to a "known-item" search task, with 145 home pages defined by assessors from the National Institute of Standards and Technology (NIST). In this task, use of anchor text and link structure was shown to be beneficial. Another task, introduced in TREC 2002, was a "topic-distillation" task, where the goal was to find "entry" pages to Web sites devoted to specified broad topics.

In addition to news tasks, there have been developments of newer, larger, and more realistic Web search test collections. These include:

- .GOV (http://ir.dcs.gla.ac.uk/test_collections/govinfo.html) – based on a crawl of Web sites from the .gov (US government) domain, consisting of about 1.25 million pages. About a million of the pages were in HTML, with the remainder PDF, Word, and other types of documents. Pages were truncated to 100 kilobytes. The size of the collection was about 18 gigabytes.
- .GOV2 (http://ir.dcs.gla.ac.uk/test_collections/gov2-summary.htm) – based on another crawl of .gov Web sites, aiming to be one terabyte in size for the TREC Terabyte Track (http://www-nlpir.nist.gov/projects/terabyte/) that succeeded the Web Track. This collection contained about 25 million documents, with pages

truncated to 256 kilobytes. The pages were either in HTML or the text derived from PDF, Word, and other document types. The size of the collection was 426 gigabytes.

- Blogs (http://ir.dcs.gla.ac.uk/test_collections/blog06info.html) – based on a crawl of Weblog ("blog") feeds for the newer TREC Blog Track. The collection contains about three quarters of a million feeds and is 38 gigabytes in size.

A variety of other research has continued to assess Web search. Craswell et al. (2001) performed additional research on the effectiveness of link-based methods for page-finding tasks. Additional benefit was found from a machine-learning method. Another common Web searching task is finding pages that contain search interfaces to the invisible Web. Most of these pages use HTML forms (an HTML construct allowing entry of data and buttons to submit the form to a server for processing), but there are both false-negatives (a query interface that is not an HTML form) and false-positives (an HTML form that is not a query interface). Scholer et al. (2004) pursued a related approach for page finding, using past queries that retrieved a page as document "surrogates" for that page. Experimental results have found a 7% improvement in retrieval performance. Cope et al. (2003) have also investigated approaches for finding search interfaces, with the best technique using a decision tree to assess the features of pages to predict those representing search interfaces. This approach achieved an accuracy of 85%.

One concern about Web searching is that users enter very few search terms, often no more than one or two words, and do not take advantage of advanced features offered by most search engines, such as Boolean or proximity operators (Jansen, Spink et al., 1998; Spink, Jansen et al., 2002). One analysis of 600 searches using such operators found, however, that when the operators were removed, the search results were largely the same, indicating need for them was probably not necessary (Eastman and Jansen, 2003).

Another approach to improving retrieval has been to take advantage of click-through data, i.e., assuming a page is relevant if a user clicks on the link to it from a page displaying Web search engine results. Joachims (2002a) developed a system that used machine learning to associate words in queries with pages that users were likely to click on to view. Subsequent research has found that while click-throughs are not completely accurate indicators of relevance of a page, they are relatively reliable for that purpose (Joachims, Granka et al., 2007).

Other Web research has looked at its mathematical properties. Two researchers have noted that the distribution of in-links and out-links on the Web follows a power law, i.e., the probability of a page having k links is

$$P(k) = k^{-\gamma}, \tag{8.7}$$

where γ has been found experimentally to vary between 2 and 3 (Albert, Jeong et al., 1999; Broder, Kumar et al., 2000). Albert et al. (1999) also measured the "diameter" (average number of links from one randomly selected page to another) of the Notre Dame University Web site and found it to be 18.6. Broder et al. (2000) found that the larger Web was not completely interconnected and instead consisted of four roughly equal components: a strongly connected core (SCC), IN links to the SCC, OUT links from the SCC, and tendrils not connected to any of the first three. Their analysis also showed that the links from the SCC to the OUT pages tended to be higher in quantity and more diverse than those coming to the SCC from the IN pages. They also found the directed diameters of the SCC to be 28 pages.

Additional research continues to examine the structure of the Web. Pennock et al. (2002) tested the power-law distribution of Web links, which they call the "rich get richer" nature of links on the Web, i.e., a small number of pages have a disproportionate share of links to and from them. They found that while a randomly selected portion of Web pages did indeed follow the power law, certain subsets of Web pages did not. In particular, home pages of companies, universities, newspapers, and scientists tended to follow more of a log-normal distribution. Soboroff (2002) addressed the question of whether the Web collections used in the TREC Web track, WT10g and .GOV, were similar to the Web in general and could thus have their experimental results viewed as generalizable. He indeed found that both collections obeyed the power law, with the slope of 2–3 seen in random collections of Web pages. Other similarities were noted as well.

Fetterly et al. (2003) provided a new analysis of the evolution of Web pages, monitoring 150 million pages on a weekly basis for 11 weeks. Change of pages in the Web is certainly a challenge for IR, since search engines usually lag behind in identifying changes in existing Web pages. This may also be important to users who cite a page for some specific content feature and may not be aware that the page has changed. Their analysis found variable rates of change, but in general, most changes to pages were small. One surprising finding was that large pages changed more frequently and extensively than smaller pages. They also found that pages in the .com and .net top-level domain were more likely to change than those in the .edu and gov domains, and that past changes to a page were a good predictor of future change.

Finally, another concern about Web content is whether the output of search engines presents a skewed or biased view of a topic. Gerhart (2004) has looked at five controversial topics and found the output from Web search engines does not present a diversity of views. Her analysis found that simple queries tended to present the positive views of a controversy, which she attributed to the nature of search engines, current linking practices by authors of Web pages, and the simple queries used by Web searchers. A related concern is that some Web sites, through their robots.txt file (that indicates whether a crawler is given permission to crawl a site or not), give more permissions to more popular search engines (Sun, Zhuang et al., 2007). Recent research has shown, however, that search engines do lead users to a variety of search sites, and not just those with the highest number of in-links (Fortunato, Flammini et al., 2006a,b). On a related note, search engine users tend to be influenced by the "brand" of the search engine, rating results higher from some search engines over others even when the output was identical (Jansen, Zhang et al., 2007).

8.1.3.3   Biomedical Text Retrieval

A variety of research has explored methods to improve IR systems in the biomedical domain. As noted above, early work focused on improving hypertext capabilities (Frisse, 1988), taking advantage of knowledge resources, such as the UMLS Metathesaurus (Evans, Hersh et al., 1991; Hersh and Hickam, 1995b), and improving access to high-quality evidence (Haynes, Wilczynski et al., 1994). A number of early test collections included MED (Salton, 1972), a collection from the NLM (Schuyler, McCray et al., 1989), and OHSUMED (http://ir.ohsu.edu/ohsumed/) (Hersh, Buckley et al., 1994), which was the largest of its kind at the time and is still used for research at present. The latter consists of about 350,000 MEDLINE with 106 topics judged for relevance.

One line of work has looked at methods for reordering search output to identify "important" articles in bibliographic databases such as MEDLINE. Bernstam et al. (2006) assessed a variety of citation-based algorithms that attempted to rank documents deemed important by inclusion in a bibliography about surgical oncology. They compared eight different algorithms: simple PubMed queries, PubMed clinical queries, vector cosine, citation count, journal impact factor, PageRank, and a machine-learning approach based on polynomial support vector machines. The citation-based algorithms were found to be more effective than noncitation-based algorithms at identifying important articles. The most effective strategies were simple citation count and PageRank, which on average identified over six important articles in the first 100 results compared to <1 for the best noncitation-based algorithm. Similar differences were observed between citation-based and noncitation-based algorithms at 10, 20, 50, 200, 500, and 1,000 results. They also assessed citation lag, i.e., how it takes a period of time before citations to appear to an important article. This was found to affect performance of PageRank more than simple citation count. In spite of citation lag, however, the citation-based algorithms were still more effective than noncitation-based algorithms. They concluded that algorithms that were successful on the Web could be applied to biomedical information retrieval, helping to identify important articles within large sets of relevant results. Further work by Aphinyanaphongs et al. (2006) found even better performance with the addition of machine-learning techniques.

Also focused on improving MEDLINE retrieval was the ad hoc retrieval task of the TREC 2004 (Hersh, Bhupatiraju et al., 2006b) and TREC 2005 (Hersh, Cohen et al., 2005) Genomics Tracks. This task modeled the situation of a user with an information need using an IR system to access the biomedical scientific literature. The document collection was based on a 10-year subset of MEDLINE. The rationale for using MEDLINE was that despite being in an era of readily available full-text journals (usually requiring a subscription), many users still entered the biomedical literature through searching MEDLINE. As such, there were still strong motivations to improve the effectiveness of searching MEDLINE.

The MEDLINE subset consisted of 10 years of completed citations from the database inclusive from 1994 to 2003. Records were extracted using the Date Completed (DCOM) field for all references in the range of 19,940,101–20,031,231. This provided a total of 4,591,008 records, which was about one-third of the full MEDLINE database. The data included all the PubMed fields identified in the MEDLINE Baseline record. The subset was provided in the "MEDLINE" format, consisting of ASCII text with fields indicated and delimited by 2–4 character abbreviations. The size of the file uncompressed was about 9.5 gigabytes. In this subset, there were 1,209,243 (26.3%) records without abstracts.

Topics for the ad hoc retrieval task were based on information needs collected from real biologists. In the 2004 track, simple information needs were collected and formatted into 50 topics with the following fields:

- ID – identifier
- Title – abbreviated statement of information need
- Information need – full statement information need
- Context – background information to place information need in context

In the 2005 track, instead of soliciting free-form biomedical questions, a set of five generic topic templates (GTTs) derived from an analysis of the topics from the 2004 track and other known biologist information needs were developed (see Table 8.5). These GTTs consisted of semantic types, such as genes or diseases, placed in the context of commonly queried biomedical questions. After development of the GTTs, biologists were interviewed to obtain specific information needs that conformed to each GTT. The topics did not have to fit precisely into the GTTs, but had to come close, i.e., have all the required semantic types. Ten information needs for each GTT were selected for inclusion in the 2005 track to obtain 50 topics.

Relevance judgments for both years were performed carrying out the usual pooling method of TREC, where the top-ranking results of all official runs

Table 8.5 Generic topic types and example sample topics for the TREC 2005 Genomics Track, with the semantic types in each GTT are italicized (adapted from Hersh, Cohen et al., 2005)

Generic topic type	Example sample topic
Find articles describing standard *methods or protocols* for doing some sort of experiment or procedure	*Method or protocol*: GST fusion protein expression in Sf9 insect cells
Find articles describing the role of a *gene* involved in a given *disease*	*Gene*: DRD4 *Disease*: Alcoholism
Find articles describing the role of a *gene* in a specific *biological process*	*Gene*: Insulin receptor gene *Biological process*: Signaling tumorigenesis
Find articles describing interactions (e.g., promote, suppress, inhibit, etc.) between two or more *genes* in the *function of an organ* or in a *disease*	*Genes*: HMG and HMGB1 *Disease*: Hepatitis
Find articles describing one or more *mutations* of a given *gene* and its biological impact	*Gene with mutation*: Ret *Biological impact*: Thyroid function

submitted by track participants were pooled. The relevance judges in general were individuals who had backgrounds in either biology or medicine. The relevance assessors judged each document for the specific topic as definitely relevant (DR), possibly relevant (PR), or not relevant (NR). For the official results, which required binary relevance judgments, documents that were rated DR or PR were considered relevant. In the 2005 track, articles had to describe a specific gene, disease, impact, mutation, etc. and not just the concept in general. In addition, relevance judges were given more explicit instructions relative to the GTTs:

- Relevant article must describe how to conduct, adjust, or improve a standard, a, new method, or a protocol for doing some sort of experiment or procedure.
- Relevant article must describe some specific role of the gene in the stated disease or biological process.
- Relevant article must describe a specific interaction (e.g., promote, suppress, inhibit, etc.) between two or more genes in the stated function of the organ or the disease.
- Relevant article must describe a mutation of the stated gene and the particular biological impact(s) that the mutation has been found to have.

For both the 2004 and 2005 tracks, the primary measure of performance was MAP. Research groups were also required to classify their runs into one of three categories:

- Automatic – no manual intervention in building queries
- Manual – manual construction of queries but no further human interaction
- Interactive – completely interactive construction of queries and further interaction with system output

In the 2004 track, the best results were obtained by a combination of Okapi weighting (BM25 for term frequency but with standard inverse document frequency), Porter stemming, expansion of symbols by LocusLink and MeSH records, query expansion, and use of all three fields of the topic (title, need, and context) (Fujita, 2004). These achieved a MAP of 0.4075. When the language modeling technique of Dirichlet prior smoothing was added, an even higher MAP of 0.4264 was obtained. Another group achieved high-ranking results with a combination of approaches that included Okapi weighting, query expansion, and various forms of domain-specific query expansion (including expansion of lexical variants as well as acronym, gene, and protein name synonyms) (Buttcher, Clarke et al., 2004). Approaches that attempted to map to controlled vocabulary terms did not fare as well (Aronson, Demmer et al., 2004; Nakov, Schwartz et al., 2004; Seki, Costello et al., 2004). As always in TREC, many groups tried a variety of approaches, beneficial or otherwise, but usually without comparing common baseline or running exhaustive experiments, making it difficult to discern exactly what techniques provided benefit.

Somewhat similar results were obtained in the 2005 track. As with 2004, the basic Okapi with good parameters gives good baseline performance for a number of groups. Manual synonym expansion of queries gave the highest MAP of 0.302 (Huang, Zhong et al., 2005), although automated query expansion did not fare as well (Ando, Dredze et al., 2005; Aronson, Demner-Fushman et al., 2005). Relevance feedback was found to be beneficial, but worked best without term expansion (Zheng, Brady et al., 2005).

Follow-up research with the TREC Genomics Track ad hoc retrieval test collection has yielded a variety of findings. One study assessed word tokenization, stemming, and stop word removal, finding that varying strategies for the first resulted in substantial performance impact while changes in the latter two had minimal impact. Tokenization in genomics text can be challenging due to the use of a wide variety of symbols, including numbers, hyphens, super- and subscripts, and characters in non-English languages (e.g., Greek) (Jiang and Zhai, 2007). Another study, described in Sect. 8.1.1.1, found value for language modeling approaches to term weighting. Other studies have assessed improving the related articles feature of PubMed (Lin and Wilbur, 2007) and categorizing articles containing data for inclusion in comparative effectiveness reviews of drug efficacy (Cohen, Hersh et al., 2006).

8.1.3.4 Medical Image Retrieval

As noted in earlier chapters of this book, although most IR systems and research focus on text, we live in a multimedia world. Indeed, with the proliferation of digital cameras and other easy means for digitizing a wide variety of multimedia, it is only natural that IR turns attention to retrieval of this type of content. As noted in Sect. 4.6.1, images can be indexed by two approaches, textual or semantic (annotating their associated text) or visual or content-based (extracting image features). Another problem in image retrieval research has been the lack of robust test collections and realistic query tasks that allow comparison of system performance (Horsch, Prinz et al., 2004; Müller, Michoux et al., 2004). This was one of the motivations of ImageCLEF (http://www.imageclef.org/), which aims to build test collections for image retrieval research. ImageCLEF arose as a track within CLEF and its collections have mostly had textual annotations in multiple languages. Some participants in ImageCLEF expressed an interest in retrieval of biomedical images, which led to the medical image retrieval task (Hersh, Müller et al., 2006). ImageCLEF has also featured a variety of nonmedical image-related retrieval and classification tasks (Müller, Geissbuhler et al., 2004), which have spawned research efforts with their test collections (e.g., Deselaers, Keysers et al., 2008). Other multimedia challenge evaluations have been organized for video (Smeaton, Over et al., 2006) and music (Orio, 2006) retrieval. (In the latter, music is retrieved by humming a tune and having retrieval based on matching the notes and their duration.)

The conceptual structure of the content of the ImageCLEFmed test collection is shown in Fig. 8.3. The entire *library* consists of multiple collections. Each *collection* is organized into cases that represent a group of related images and annotations. Each *case* consists of a group of images and an optional annotation. Each *image* is part of a case and has optional associated annotations, which consist of metadata, and/or a textual annotation. All the images and annotations are stored in separate

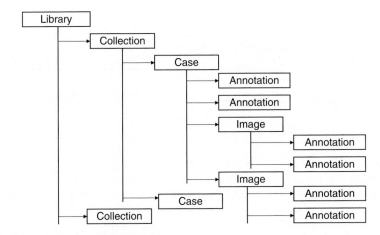

Fig. 8.3 Structure of the ImageCLEFmed test collection

Table 8.6 ImageCLEF medical image retrieval task (ImageCLEFmed), image collections, image and annotation types, and their origins

Collection name	Image type(s)	Annotation type(s)	Original URL
Casimage	Radiology and pathology	Clinical case descriptions	http://www.casimage.com/
Mallinckrodt Institute of Radiology (MIR)	Nuclear medicine	Clinical case descriptions	http://gamma.wustl.edu/home.html
Pathology Education Instructional Resource (PEIR)	Pathology and radiology	Metadata records from HEAL database	http://peir.path.uab.edu/
PathoPIC	Pathology	Image description: long in German, short in English	http://alf3.urz.unibas.ch/pathopic/e/intro.htm
MyPACS	Radiology	Clinical case descriptions	http://www.mypacs.net/
Clinical Outcomes Research Initiative (CORI) Endoscopic Images	Endoscopy	Clinical case descriptions	http://www.cori.org/

files. An XML file contains the connections between the collections, cases, images, and annotations.

The image library for ImageCLEFmed 2005 and 2006 consisted of the first four collections listed in Tables 8.6 and 8.7 (Casimage, MIR, PEIR, and PathoPIC). In 2007, the latter two collections listed in those tables were added (myPACS and CORI). Table 8.6 describes the image collections, their image and annotation types, and their origins, while Table 8.7 lists the numbers of images and annotations

Table 8.7 ImageCLEF medical image retrieval task (ImageCLEFmed), numbers of images and annotations (Including amounts in each language) as well as the archived file size

Collection name	Cases	Images	Annotations	Annotations by language	File size (tar archive)
Casimage	2,076	8,725	2,076	French – 1,899 English – 177	1.28 GB
MIR	407	1,177	407	English – 407	63.2 MB
PEIR	32,319	32,319	32,319	English – 32,319	2.50 GB
PathoPIC	7,805	7,805	15,610	German – 7,805 English – 7,805	879 MB
myPACS	3,577	15,140	3,577	English – 3,577	390 MB
Endoscopic	1,496	1,496	1,496	English – 1,496	34 MB
Total	47,680	66,662	55,485	French – 1,899 English – 45,781 German – 7,805	5.15 GB

Images

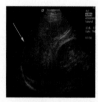 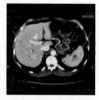 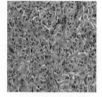

Case annotation

ID: 4272

Description: A large hypoechoic mass is seen in the spleen. CDFI reveals it to be hypovascular and distorts the intrasplenic blood vessels. This lesion is consistent with a metastatic lesion. Urinary obstruction is present on the right with pelvo-caliceal and uretreal dilatation secondary to a soft tissue lesion at the junction of the ureter and baldder. This is another secondary lesion of the malignant melanoma. Surprisingly, these lesions are not hypervascular on doppler nor on CT. Metastasis are also visible in the liver.

Diagnosis: Metastasis of spleen and ureter, malignant melanoma

Clinical Presentation: Workup in a patient with malignant melanoma. Intravenous pyelography showed no excretion of contrast on the right.

Fig. 8.4 Example case from the ImageCLEF test collection

(including amounts in each language) as well as the archived file size. Figure 8.4 shows an example case from the Casimage collection, demonstrating how multiple different images and image types can be part of a case. However, the largest collection, PEIR, is not organized into cases per se (or, using our framework, has one image per case).

Each cycle of ImageCLEFmed for 2005–2007 had 25–30 topics, with each topic classified as amenable to visual, textual, or mixed retrieval methods. Topic creation has mostly been based on identifying general medical queries and applying them in the context of user roles, e.g., clinician, educator, research, etc. (Hersh, Jensen et al., 2005; Müller, Despont-Grosa et al., 2006). All ImageCLEFmed topics contain an information statement in English, French, and German as well as an index image for use by visual retrieval systems. Relevance judgments were performed by physicians who were also students in biomedical informatics. The pools for relevance judging were created by selecting the top-ranking images from submitted runs in their respective years. Judges rated images as definitely relevant (DR), partially relevant (PR), or not relevant (NR). The 3 years of the image collections, topics, and relevance judgments have been folded into a single collection (Hersh, Müller et al., 2007).

A variety of findings have come from the experiments of ImageCLEFmed (Hersh, Müller et al., 2006; Müller, Deselaers et al., 2006, 2007). The first was that mixing visual and textual approaches performed better than those using either approach alone. However, textual approaches were more robust, i.e., they were more resilient to difficult visually oriented topics than visual systems were to difficult textually oriented topics. Visual methods tend to work best when the topic specifies an image modality or highly specific finding, e.g., a certain type of X-ray and/or a type of finding that always appears similar. On the other hand, textual methods tend to work best when a higher-level concept is sought, e.g., images of many modalities for a given disease or clinical finding.

Another conclusion of ImageCLEFmed was that MAP may not be the best measure for the image retrieval task. MAP measures the full range of retrieval results for a topic from low-to-high recall. In the image retrieval task, however, users may be more precision-oriented than recall-oriented. In other words, users may only want a small-to-moderate number of relevant images, and not every last relevant one. This is in distinction to, say, someone carrying out a systematic review who needs to retrieve every last relevant document in a text retrieval system. For some runs, certain techniques achieved very high precision at 10 or 30 images but much lower MAP than other runs with comparable precision at these levels (Jensen and Hersh, 2005; Hersh, Kalpathy-Cramer et al., 2006). Runs with high precision at the top 10 or 30 images may be desirable from the user's standpoint, even though the overall recall (as measured by MAP) is lower. Clearly, further research is necessary to identify which measures are most important to the image retrieval tasks of real users.

The best-performing systems of ImageCLEFmed have applied various types of processing to the images and their annotations. The best results in 2005 and 2006 came from Lacoste et al. (2007), who used several approaches. First, they applied "semantic indexing," which aimed to identify key concepts in certain UMLS semantic type categories in both the image annotations and topic text. They also applied "visual modality filtering" that removed images unlikely to be of the modality specific in the topic. These were combined with a variety of fusion techniques. The best results in 2007 came from Kalpathy-Cramer and Hersh (2007b), who found that detecting the modality of an image, based on an algorithm they had developed (Kalpathy-Cramer and Hersh, 2007a) and applied to visually amenable topics, gave the best performance.

A variety of other research in medical image retrieval has been performed, most of which aims to find conventional and novel ways to connect users to the images they seek. Some of these works have focused on clinical images. A visual retrieval system for spinal diseases is the Spine Pathology and Retrieval System (SPIRS, http://archive.nlm.nih.gov/spirs/) (Hsu, Long et al., 2007). SPIRS allows the user to sketch the contour of interest in an index image and find others that are similar. Textual searching of annotations is allowed as well. A different use case for medical image retrieval is *case finding*, where a clinician might have a new image of a patient not yet diagnosed that he or she wishes to compare to similar images where the diagnosis is known. Although the true benefits of systems for this use case are unknown, one study of physicians making a diagnosis with and without a visual retrieval system performed 29–62% better in making a diagnosis when using such a system (Aisen, Broderick et al., 2003).

Other works have focused on images in the biomedical literature. Yu and Lee (2006) have assessed a variety of approaches to finding images based on their association with sentences in the abstracts that match the query terms entered by users. This approach is based on work classifying the modality of images appearing in bioscience literature (Rafkind, Lee et al., 2006). Kahn (2008) has assessed ability to detect age, gender, and image modality in captions of images from the Goldminer database (Kahn and Thao, 2007) of radiological images.

8.2   User-Oriented Research

The research covered in Sect. 8.1 focused on approaches aimed at improving IR systems. However, an equally important aspect of IR research is how to improve systems for users. We organize this section similar in part to the layout of Part II of the book, covering how to improve content, indexing, and retrieval for the user.

8.2.1   Content

One way to improve systems for users is to facilitate better access to content. A key attribute of innovation in content delivery has been the ability to integrate across resources, although barriers between proprietary collections of content are still an impediment. This section focuses on attempts to improve content delivery beyond what is available commercially, looking at methods innovated in the past but still not implemented in state-of-the-art systems or those still under research. We will focus on two research areas that could serve as foci for integration of clinical information: linkage of knowledge-based content to the electronic health record (EHR) and linkage of users to human knowledge.

8.2.1.1 Linkage to the Electronic Health Record

Most IR applications are stand-alone applications, i.e., the user explicitly launches an application or goes to a Web page. A number of researchers have hypothesized that the use of IR systems can be made more efficient in the clinical setting by embedding them in the EHR. Not only would this allow their quicker launching (i.e., the user would not have to "switch" applications), but also the context of the patient could provide a starting point for a query. Cimino (1996) reviewed the literature on this topic and noted that embedding had been a desirable feature since the advent on the EHR. More recently, however, the ability to link systems and their resources via the Internet, particularly using Web browsers, has made such applications easier to develop and disseminate (Albert, 2007). Cimino noted that the process of linking patient information systems to IR resources consisted of three steps:

1. Identifying the user's question
2. Identifying the appropriate information resource
3. Composing the retrieval strategy

Humphreys (2000) notes that newer technologies enhance the prospects for linking the EMR to knowledge-based information systems. In particular, the Internet and the Web reduce the complexity of integrating disparate legacy systems, provide standards that facilitate development of applications, and allow users of all types to access resources from a variety of locations from the home to the clinical setting. She notes that three levels of integration are required to achieve this vision:

1. Technical connections – the gamut of pure technology-related issues that allow integration, such as hardware, software, telecommunications, access integration, and so on
2. Organizational connections – the means by which organizations license clinical applications and the information they access
3. Conceptual connections – the standardization of the structure of the information and the terminology to describe it

Most IR systems provide a simple mechanism for identifying the user's question: they provide a query box to enter it. Since, however, the EMR contains content about the patient, such as diagnoses, treatments, test results, and demographic data, it is conceivable this information could be leveraged to create a context-specific query. Some early approaches looked at extracting information from dictated reports (Powsner and Miller, 1989; Miller, Gieszczykiewicz et al., 1992), but were limited by the nonspecificity of much of the data in those reports. Cimino et al. (1993) developed *generic queries* that were based on analyses of real queries posed to medical librarians. They subsequently developed *infobuttons* that allowed the user to retrieve specific information. For example, an infobutton next to an ICD-9 code translated the code into a MeSH term using the UMLS Metathesaurus and sent a query to MEDLINE (Cimino, Johnson et al., 1992). Likewise, an infobutton next to a laboratory result generated a MEDLINE search with the appropriate term based on whether the result was abnormal or not (Cimino, Socratorus et al., 1995). The approach has also been extended to radiology results and full-text resources (Zeng and Cimino, 1997). It has even been adapted to allow patients to view some of their own results in a prototype patient-based record system (Baorto and Cimino, 2000).

One challenge for linking clinical information to knowledge-based resources is determining what information to offer the user. This is especially so for clinical narratives which contain a wealth of words and concepts. Mendonça et al. (2001a) assessed narrative reports to determine how to promote the most important concepts on which a user is likely to search. They found that TF*IDF weighting of concepts extracted by a NLP system was effective in promoting those of most interest to real human users. These authors have also developed the means to formulate data extracted from other parts of the clinical record into the types of well-formed questions required in evidence-based medicine (EBM) (Mendonça, Cimino et al., 2001b).

Selecting the appropriate information resource and devising a query to it are also challenging. One system that attempted to provide access to a variety of information resources was SmartQuery (Price, Hersh et al., 2002). This application provided an interface on top of a commercial EHR product, NetAccess, which was a Web-based front end to a mainframe-based results reporting system from Siemens Medical Systems (SMS, http://www.smed.com/). SmartQuery provided context-sensitive links from patient-specific data viewable in NetAccess to online medical knowledge resources that were either freely available or licensed to the local institution. SmartQuery added buttons and checkboxes to the patient data displays in NetAccess. Checkboxes were shown next to each lab test identifier and above displays of dictated reports. To use SmartQuery, the user checked the boxes next to items relevant to his or her question and then clicked an Add button that caused a MeSH term corresponding to the data underlying the displayed information to be added to the list of MeSH terms created from the ICD-9 codes. The user was also able to enter additional terms via a text box. The top of the page contained a series of checkboxes for the different information sources available. With all these options, the user then sent a query by checking the terms of interest and the information sources he or she wanted.

Several studies have now evaluated the approach of linking to medical knowledge from the context of the EHR. Each system uses different approaches and evaluation techniques, but a clear pattern emerges, which is that system usage frequency is comparable with the amount of usage of IR systems generally presented in Chap. 7. Research to date shows these systems have small impact from a frequency standpoint but are valued by users.

One study at Vanderbilt University Medical Center (Rosenbloom, Giuse et al., 2005) provided access to contextual information during patient order entry and laboratory results reviewing. The user was presented with a list of knowledge resources to which he or she could link. A randomized controlled trial was performed to compare access to the linked information vs. the information being available by noncontextual links. The contextually linked information was utilized more frequently, although it was only accessed about twice a month (once every 16 days).

Another study assessed a medication infobutton application, KnowledgeLink, that was implemented and evaluated by Maviglia et al. (2006) within the Partners Healthcare System EHR system. This infobutton worked by providing a "lookup" button where drug names appear in the EHR application, which provided a link to a Web-based information resource with the drug name as the query. The information resources opened in a new browser window so that the user could easily return to the place they left off in the EHR by closing the window. The authors performed a study of KnowledgeLink, assessing its use and impact when linked to two different information resources, Micromedex and SkolarMD. Users were randomized by practice location to have KnowledgeLink link to one or the other reference.

Similar to the previous study, KnowledgeLink was used about twice per month by clinicians, representing 1.2% of all patient encounters. The median session time for usage was short (21 s), but users felt their questions were answered 84% of the time and they altered patient care decisions 15% of the time. Although user satisfaction was quite positive, suggestions for improvements included allowing refinement of the query and the ability to select other target resources. The group assigned to Micromedex as the knowledge resource was more likely to use KnowledgeLink than the one assigned to SkolarMD. Primary care physicians and nurse practitioners used the system more frequently than specialists.

A third evaluation study was performed by Cimino and Zhu (2006), assessing the infobutton system available at Columbia University Medical Center. Not only was usage assessed, but user satisfaction as well. Specific usage rates were not presented due to the changing nature of the system over the study period, but at its peak, usage was about once per month. The most common scenario for use of the system was during laboratory results look up. Users were generally satisfied with the system and believed the information was contextually appropriate nearly all the time.

Additional work by Cimino and colleagues beyond included the development of an "infobutton manager" which keeps track of the various information resources, generic questions that can be asked of them, and contexts in which those questions and resources might be used. The specific context of the patient is derived from the EHR, e.g., demographic information, diagnoses, test results, and so forth. The system then creates specific infobuttons that provide linkage to available resources with queries to find knowledge-based information appropriate to that context. Another outcome of this research has been the actual development of the "infobutton manager" (Cimino and Li, 2003). This tool matches a group of context parameters to information needs and then matches those needs to actual resources. The context parameters include:

- User type – nurse, physician, patient
- Patient age – newborn, infant, child, adolescent, young adult, middle aged, and elderly
- Patient gender – male, female

- Concept of interest – datum (e.g., medication, test result, organism) that generated the user's request, mapped to concepts in the Medical Entities Dictionary (MED)
- Institution – used to determine which resources are available/preferred at a given institution

A form to enter the above data is available (although cannot be used outside the institution) at http://www.dmi.columbia.edu/homepages/ciminoj/howtoUse-Infomanage.html. This system has also been implemented on wireless devices (Lei, Chen et al., 2003).

An additional challenge with infobuttons is that, at this time, most of them work by hard-coding communications between the EHR and information resource. To address this problem, the HL7 standards organization has begun work on a standard API between (a) EHR systems and infobutton managers and (b) infobutton managers and information resources. The idea is that by developing a standard interface between these entities, EHR and information resource vendors will not have to provide customized solutions every time this functionality is implemented. The standard is currently evolving in draft format and a version from 2005 is available publicly (DelFiol, Rocha et al., 2005). There is a growing amount of content available from publishers to be linked into EHRs, including from Elsevier (http://www.clinicaldecisionsupport.com/demo.html), Thomson (http://www.micromedex.com/products/hcs/), and Touchworks (http://www.touchworksemr.com/_htm/Mod_PL.asp).

8.2.1.2   Linkage to Human Knowledge

Recall from Chap. 2 that clinicians have frequent information needs, of the order of two questions for every three patients seen, yet they pursue answers to only one-third of them (Gorman, 1995). This research also showed that the most common source clinicians turned to for answers was another human, most often a colleague or consultant in their referral chain. It was shown in Chap. 7 that relative to overall information needs, computer-based knowledge resources have been used modestly (i.e., the average user seeks answers to clinical questions with online resources only a few times per month). One likely reason for this is the time it takes to obtain an answer: upward of 30 min when one is using MEDLINE and journal literature (Hersh, Crabtree et al., 2000). It is possible that the move toward synoptic information resources, particularly those that adhere to principles of EBM, may increase the usage of online knowledge resources (Haynes, 2001).

Another approach to providing knowledge-based information might involve the development of technologies that recognize the value of person-to-person consultation and facilitate it. This approach is much less developed than the myriad of online information resources, especially when used in the clinician-to-clinician mode. There are a great many online patient-to-clinician consultation services. Probably the largest of these is NetWellness, which has over 17,000 answered questions in its database (Guard, Fredericka et al., 2000). A growing number of commercial Web sites, such as WebMD, offer similar services (http://www.webmd. com/community/experts/). Another system in Sweden has found wide use over a 4-year period (Umefjord, Sandström et al., 2008).

Some early clinician-to-clinician consultation services were developed in Iowa (Bergus, Sinift et al., 1998) and the Netherlands (Moorman, Branger et al., 2001). The former used e-mail for physician communications, while the latter used an option within the EMR. Another approach to online clinical consultation has been the second-opinion service offered by Partners Healthcare, a health system composed of hospitals affiliated with Harvard Medical School (Massachusetts General, Brigham and Women's, and several community hospitals). For a fee, a patient and his or her physician can obtain an Internet-based consultation. A review of the first 79 consultations found that while only a small number resulted in changed diagnoses (4%), a substantial number (90%) resulted in changes in treatment (Kedar, Ternullo et al., 2003).

8.2.2 Indexing

Another focus of research to augment IR systems has been on the indexing process. While Salton and McGill (1983) argued that attempts at human indexing were hopelessly flawed owing to the inconsistency of human indexers, others have noted that human indexers do add value by providing a focus on the most important conceptual aspects in documents (Swanson, 1988a). Inasmuch as many individuals adhere to the latter view, a great deal of research has focused on tools to aid in indexing. While Chap. 9 described some systems that used approaches to recognize concepts as a step in the retrieval process (e.g., SAPHIRE – Hersh, 1991 and MetaMap – Aronson, 2001), the systems described in this section were designed to enhance the NLM's indexing process. This section also describes the Information Sources Map (ISM), a now-defunct component of the UMLS project that attempted to index whole databases, as well as the Semantic Web project.

Initial efforts to augment the indexing process focused on the content of documents as well as the databases in which they resided. As noted in Chap. 5, despite the detailed NLM protocols for human indexing of MEDLINE, indexers have substantial inconsistency (Funk and Reid, 1983; Marcetich, Rappaport et al., 2004). Likewise, indexers do not follow the protocols reliably (Crain, 1987). Humphrey (1992) asserted that human indexers had trouble going from text phrases to identifiable indexing terms and, once terms were found, coordinating them into a group of meaningful descriptors. To address these problems and to assist the human indexer, she initiated the Medindex system, a knowledge-based indexing assistant designed to facilitate correct and consistent indexing for MeSH terms at the NLM (Humphrey, 1988). The system laid the groundwork for future work described next.

In the last decade, the NLM undertook a new approach called the Indexing Initiative (http://ii.nlm.nih.gov/) (Aronson, Bodenreider et al., 2000). The motivation for this initiative came from the realization that not only was human indexing

Fig. 8.5 Overview of components
of NLM Medical Text Indexer
(MTI) (courtesy of National
Library of Medicine)

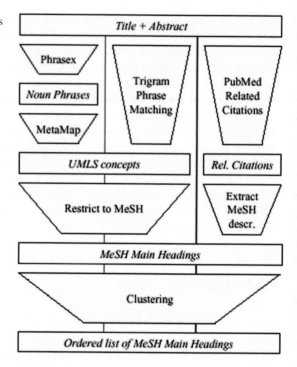

expensive, but also individuals trained to do it well are increasingly difficult to find
and retain. The entire effort is an experimentally driven effort to determine the best
approach to indexing, especially as tools from the UMLS project and other efforts
mature and increasing amounts of full text are available.

At the core of the Indexing Initiative is a system called the Medical Text Indexer
(MTI, http://0-ii.nlm.nih.gov.catalog.llu.edu/mti.shtml) (Aronson, Mork et al., 2004)
(Fig. 8.5). The input to the MTI consists, for now, of titles and abstracts, though full
text will be considered when it is more consistently available. The output is an
ordered list of MeSH main headings. The components of the process are isolated
and parameterized so that the relative behavior of each can be analyzed. There are
three main pathways for generating MeSH terms, which utilize MetaMap, trigram
phrase matching, and PubMed-related citations, respectively. The MetaMap and
trigram phrase-matching pathways generate UMLS Metathesaurus concepts and
then restrict the output to MeSH, whereas the PubMed-related citations pathway
outputs MeSH terms directly. The MeSH terms are then subject to three levels of
filtering:

1. Base – obtaining terms MetaMap and the PubMed-Related Articles function,
   with certain boosting and substitution of some headings
2. Medium – use of additional rules to provide more specificity of headings
3. Strict – restricting output to only terms that are recommended by both MetaMap
   and the PubMed-Related Articles function

One evaluation of MTI with ten indexers found that the system generally provided partial but not complete coverage of all the MeSH terms the indexers might want to employ for a given article (McCray and Aronson, 2002). The system was therefore viewed as a tool to aid indexing in a semiautomated fashion, though it was also being evaluated for deployment where manual indexing is not intended to be employed at all, such as with meeting abstracts in certain fields (e.g., HIV/AIDS, health services research, and space life sciences). A second evaluation of MTI was done when the system was in full operational use and available to all indexers (Aronson, Mork et al., 2004). By this time, the system operated at a rate of about 530 MEDLINE records per hour (3,700 per week, able to keep pace with the 500,000+ records generated annually). Indexers averaged consulting the system about 379 times per day. Aronson et al. estimated MTI was used for about 20% of all articles indexed for MEDLINE. They also noted it was used in an automated fashion to index AIDS/HIV, health services research, and space life sciences abstracts in the NLM gateway.

A subsequent study focused more specifically on which portions of full-text articles were most beneficial for providing terms to indexers (Gay, Kayaalp et al., 2005). A test collection of 500 articles, segmented by section, was used. While title and abstract sections provided a strong baseline performance, incremental benefit was found for using terms from table and figure captions as well as sections labeled as results, results and discussion, conclusions, and no header. A follow-on study explored the user interface to the system and recommended improvements to it (Ruiz and Aronson, 2007).

Another issue addressed by NLM researchers was the ability to index entire databases. A problem always faced by users of IR systems is that a well-phrased search may be executed against the wrong database. Since most other medical databases are not as well known as MEDLINE, searchers may try to use MEDLINE for a topic that is best searched in a different database. The UMLS ISM was designed to address this problem (Masys, 1992). The two major goals of the ISM were to describe electronically available information sources in machine-readable format, so that computer programs can determine which sources are appropriate to a given query, and to provide information on how to connect to those sources automatically. The ISM was essentially a database about databases, indexed by terms in the Metathesaurus.

The ISM component of the UMLS was ultimately abandoned. One of the reasons for this was the sheer increase in volume of information sources. The ISM was undertaken in the pre-Web era, when the number of databases one could access was modest. Keeping track of the additional databases and Web sites that proliferated with the growth of the Web, however, was difficult, if not impossible. Furthermore, the ability of search mechanisms to link to or index multiple sites made the need for an ISM-like system less compelling. In addition, effective systems for using it were never able to be constructed (Miller, Frawley et al., 1995; Mendonça and Cimino, 1999).

8.2.3   Retrieval

Although a large number of research approaches to improving retrieval have been devised, very few of them have been implemented in large-scale systems and, as a result, most systems are accessed via the state-of-the-art means described in Chap. 5. Most IR systems provide little assistance to the user beyond simple online help. Veteran IR researcher Susan Dumais of Microsoft has said, "If in 10 years we are still using a rectangular box and a list of results, I should be fired" (Markoff, 2007). Yet it is not clear what research approaches to IR system interfaces will evolve into widely used systems.

A great deal of user interface design and evaluation comes from the field of *human–computer interaction* (HCI). One of the leading overviews of the field and its proper practice is the textbook by Shneiderman and Plaisant (2005), now in its fourth edition. These authors note that all computer usability (not just IR systems) must take human diversity into account, from physical abilities and physical work-places to cognitive and perceptual abilities. They have formulated a set of eight "golden rules" that should govern the design of human–computer interfaces:

1. Strive for consistency – in terminology, prompts, menus, help screens, color, layout, capitalization, and fonts
2. Cater to universal usability – add features for novices, such as explanations, and for frequent users, such as abbreviations, special keys, hidden commands, and macro facilities
3. Offer informative feedback
4. Design dialogs to yield closure – organize sequences of actions into groups with a beginning, middle, and end
5. Prevent errors – design for error prevention and offer simple error handling when they do occur
6. Permit easy reversal of actions
7. Support internal locus of control – users should sense they are in control of the interface
8. Reduce short-term memory load

Although a variety of techniques have been used to assess HCI, one particular approach commonly used is *usability testing* (Rubin, 1994). A common approach used in such research has been called "think-aloud protocol analysis" (Ericsson and Simon, 1993).

Another well-known writer in the HCI field has compiled a now-annual list of the "top 10 mistakes" made in the creation of Web pages (http://www.useit.com/alertbox/). His list of "all-time" top mistakes includes:

1. Bad search engines, i.e., those that do not provide baseline state-of-the-art functionality
2. PDF files for online reading
3. Not changing the color of visited links
4. Nonscannable text, i.e., a "wall" of text not written for online reading

5. Font size that cannot be changed
6. Page titles with low search engine visibility, i.e., without informative titles
7. Anything that looks like an advertisement
8. Violating design conventions, particularly consistency
9. Opening new browser windows
10. Not answering users' questions, e.g., an e-commerce site not showing a price

A review paper recently summarized known best practices for search user interfaces (Resnick and Vaughan, 2006). The authors identify five domains of best practices and make recommendations within each:

1. Structure of the corpus

    (a) When available, faceted metadata should be attached to records
    (b) If possible, content clustering should be used to identify relationships

2. Matching content

    (a) Employ spell checking, ideally with a domain-specific dictionary
    (b) Consider query expansion algorithms

3. User context and task requirements

    (a) Support searching and browsing
    (b) User should remain in control of how much context displayed
    (c) Customize interface to reflect domain and/or user expertise
    (d) Past queries can be used to frame current needs

4. Interface between search system and user

    (a) Provide large enough query entry box
    (b) Show search terms in context
    (c) Organize large sets of results into clusters
    (d) Provide suggestions for finding results when none retrieved

5. Hardware and bandwidth challenges for mobile devices

    (a) When possible, design alternative versions of content specifically for mobile devices
    (b) When content cannot fit on screen, scrolling is preferable to page switching
    (c) When scrolling is required, use vertical rather than horizontal]

This section describes a number of innovative approaches to enhancing retrieval, some of which are likely to find their way into large-scale systems in the future. Hearst (1999) has grouped user interface enhancements into four categories, which are adopted in this section:

1. Starting the search process
2. Query specification
3. Viewing results in context
4. Aids for relevance feedback

8.2.3.1 Starting Points

Hearst (1999) notes that traditionally, a starting point has been provided by listing available resources. However, this approach is often inadequate, especially for users who are unaware of the structure of the resource(s) or the topics they cover. An alternative approach is to provide an overview of the contents. A variety of approaches have been devised, and the simplest one – the ability to browse through a classification hierarchy – is used quite commonly on the Web (e.g., by Yahoo!, http://www.yahoo.com/). Some systems have provided the ability to browse not only hierarchically, but also by traversing other thesaurus links (Korn and Shneiderman, 1996). Another approach has been to cluster documents topically. One of the best-known approaches of this technique was the Scatter/Gather (Cutting, Pedersen et al., 1992), which grouped documents into topically oriented clusters (based on word similarities). The user was able to focus on specific clusters to further narrow them down, aiming to create an ideal document set. While the original Scatter/Gather approach was text based, a variety of graphical displays have been derived to demonstrate the clustering of topics. One interface employed in the healthcare domain used Kohonen maps, which cluster the concepts in a two-dimensional view (Chen, Houston et al., 1998).

An additional approach to assisting with starting points is to help the user select the appropriate source when a retrieval system searches over multiple databases. This is known to be a challenging research problem (Bartell, Cottrell et al., 1994), but a number of medical metasearch engines have been developed. One example was seen in the ISM portion of the UMLS project described earlier. Other approaches have attempted to help the user focus on certain resources, such as those with a high likelihood of being evidence based. The TRIP database (http://www.tripdatabase.com/) provides word searching over 55 resources in its database, including many of high-profile full-text journals, along with other prominent evidence-based resources, such as the *Cochrane Database of Systematic Reviews* and the *National Guidelines Clearinghouse*. SUMSearch (http://sumsearch.uthscsa.edu/) provides similar coverage of evidence-based resources but provides more detailed searching options. Its interface allows focusing of results to question type (e.g., treatment), resource type, and other limits. Its searching algorithm attempts to adjust for too many or too few results retrieved. For excessive results, searching in large databases (e.g., PubMed) is restricted, while for inadequate results, searching in other databases is added. An evaluation of SUMSearch showed that it did not increase frequency or satisfaction of searching among medical students (Badgett, Paukert et al., 2001). However, a recent study showed it to be more effective in identifying clinical practice guidelines than Google Scholar (Haase, Follmann et al., 2007).

An additional approach to starting points is to provide a variety of options for the user. Oncosifter is a front end to cancer information, allowing entry into the content by a key word interface, a directory interface, and a hierarchical interface (Mane and Thakur, 2003). The latter two provide a browsing interface into controlled terminology. The system also features a personalization interface that allows user profiles to be constructed from various cancer-related terms.

8.2.3.2 Query Formulation

A number of early systems attempted to assist the user with constructing queries. CONIT was one of the first systems that aimed to act as an intelligent intermediary for novice searchers (Marcus, 1983). It performed such tasks as assisting with the syntax of various search systems and mapping from a user's natural language question text to Boolean statements of controlled vocabulary terms or text words. Mapping was done by stemming each natural language term in the query and taking the OR of each term that a stem mapped into, followed by an AND of all the different terms in the query. CONIT-assisted searches were found to achieve performance comparable to that of searches assisted by human intermediaries.

CANSEARCH was one of the first such systems in medicine. It was designed to assist novice physician searchers in retrieving documents related to cancer therapy (Pollitt, 1987). The user did no typing and used only a touch screen to navigate menus related to cancer sites and therapies. (Recall that MEDLINE has a particularly obtuse method of representing cancers, making the newer system all the more valuable.) Once the proper menu items were chosen, a MEDLINE search statement was formed based on rules in the program. The CANSEARCH main menu had the user select the specific cancer, while submenus allowed the designation of more detail, such as the treatment. For instance, if the user chose the site as `breast cancer` and the therapy as `cisplatinum`, then the resulting search statement passed to MEDLINE would be `Breast Neoplasms/Drug Therapy AND Cisplatinum/Therapeutic Use AND Human`.

One of the most comprehensive efforts to provide expert search assistance in the medical domain came from the COACH project at the NLM (Kingsland, Harbourt et al., 1993). COACH was added as an expert assistant to the now-defunct Internet Grateful Med. The rules used by COACH were based on an analysis of failed searches done by end users on the NLM system, as described in Chap. 7. Recall that the biggest problem found was searches with null retrieval (no documents returned). The most common reason for null retrieval was excessive ANDs, such that no documents had all the terms intersected together. Other mistakes commonly made included inappropriate use of specialty headings, improper use of subheadings, and failure to use related terms.

COACH was activated from within Internet Grateful Med after a poor search was obtained. It offered two main modes of operation: assisted increase or assisted focus. The former was invoked when the search yielded no or only a few references. In that instance, COACH may have recommended reducing the number of search terms (or at least those connected by AND), using proper specialty headings where appropriate, or adding related terms or synonyms. The assisted focus mode was called on when an excessive number of references were retrieved. It may have recommended adding a subheading to or designating as a central concept one or more of the search terms.

Another system of historical interest that aimed to implement hypermedia capabilities with the clinician in mind was Frisse's Dynamic Medical Handbook project (Frisse, 1988). This system transformed a well-known reference, the *Washington University Manual of Medical Therapeutics* (Little Brown, Boston), used widely to assist in therapeutic decisions in internal medicine, into a dynamic resource. This reference had a rigid hierarchical structure that lent itself well to a hypermedia design. A combination of lexical–statistical IR and hypertext-based methods led the user to an appropriate starting point for browsing, at which point he or she explored linked nodes to find information.

Frisse also noted several user interface features that were necessary to address the ways in which medical handbooks were typically used. These included the following:

1. Highlighting – to emphasize important concepts and passages
2. Annotating – to add explanatory information
3. Page turners – to rapidly move back and forth between sections
4. Path tracers – to mark the path that led to a section, to preserve content discovered along the way
5. Bookmarks – to allow the user to return later to a specific place
6. Clipboard – to keep information "photocopy," with the source and context specified to allow the user to return to it
7. Agenda keeper – to keep a list of future readings and tasks

The Dynamic Medical Handbook used an approach to retrieval that began with a conventional lexical–statistical approach but modified document weighting to account for terms in linked nodes (Frisse, 1988). Typical of a lexical–statistical IR system, the indexing units were single words and the documents retrieved by a query were those that had one or more words from the query. The uniqueness of Frisse's approach was the use of two weighting components to rank nodes. The *intrinsic* component of the weight consisted of the usual TF*IDF weighting for the words common to each node and the query. The *extrinsic* component, however, was the weights of all immediately linked nodes divided by the number of such nodes. Thus, the formula for the weight of a node was

$$\text{WEIGHT}_i = \sum_j \text{WEIGHT}_{ij} + \frac{1}{y} \sum_d \text{WEIGHT}_d, \qquad (8.8)$$

where WEIGHT_i was the total weight of node i, j was the number of search terms, WEIGHT_{ij} was the weight of all the search terms j in node i, y was the number of immediately linked nodes, d was the index number of immediately linked nodes, and WEIGHT_d was the weight of each linked node.

Muramatsu and Pratt (2001) lament that commercial Web search engines provide little feedback to the user on how queries are transformed. They developed "transparent queries" to give users better feedback on how systems modify queries. The four modifications included:

1. Explicitly defining the meaning of the Boolean operators AND and OR, e.g., "Query matches documents that have ALL of the following words. . ."
2. Showing removed stop words with a red strikeout line and statement that such words have been removed from the query because they are common.

3. Demonstrating stemming by expanding stems with all suffixes (the inverse of stemming) and stating such words were added to the query.
4. Explaining that adjacent words representing phrases were commonly searched in the order they were entered in the query.

A user study found that users understood better the query transformations that had been made of their searches, although they still had significant misunderstandings of what these transformations really did.

McKiernan (2003) has described a variety of novel interfaces to electronic journals. One such interface features a concept browsing interface that allows the user to select, view definitions, and traverse semantic linkages to other concepts (Wiesman, vandenHerik et al., 2004). These concepts are ultimately linked to documents that the user can view.

8.2.3.3   Providing Context

A number of approaches have attempted to provide the user with some sort of context about the document. Hearst (1999) noted that the simplest approach has been through the use of document surrogates that show brief portions of the text. Many Web search engines, for example, show representative sentences from the pages that contain the query terms and words surrounding them. Another state-of-the-art approach has been to highlight query terms in the document. Hearst (1996) has developed the TileBars representation for providing context: the user enters each query topic on a single line and the retrieval interface shows a tile bar next to each document, with the intensity of each tile representing the presence of the topic with each passage of the document. The presence of all topics within a passage indicates a portion of the document that likely will be important to view because all the terms occurred in it.

Another approach to providing context by showing terms is the TopicMap system, available from HighWire Press (http://highwire.stanford.edu/). TopicMaps provide a hierarchy (different from MeSH but incorporating many of its terms) that allow browsing of topics to choose a particular one for searching. The TopicMap interface, shown in Fig. 8.6, displays nearby topics with the one of focus at the center of the display. When other topics are clicked, they move to the center of the display. When the center topic is clicked, a page opens that displays articles indexed on that topic. The search can be limited to a core set of journals, all HighWire journals, or all HighWire journals plus MEDLINE. The TopicMap project is actually led by Topicmaps.Org, an independent consortium interested in developing the applicability of TopicMaps (http://www.topicmaps.org/). This group has developed an XML grammar for interchanging Web-based TopicMaps, called XML TopicMaps (XTM) (Park and Hunting, 2003).

An additional graphical approach to visualization of conceptual relationships is Treemaps, developed by Shneiderman and colleagues at the Human–Computer Interaction Laboratory (HCIL, http://www.cs.umd.edu/hcil/treemap-history/) of

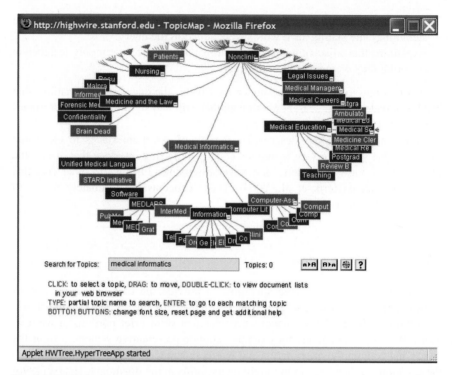

Fig. 8.6 TopicMap view for accessing medical journals (courtesy of HighWire Press)

the University of Maryland. Treemaps allow visualization for hierarchical structures and show attributes of leaf nodes by size and color coding. They enable users to compare sizes of nodes and of subtrees, and are touted to be especially helpful in spotting unusual patterns.

Another approach to showing context has been by the organization of search results via some classification, such as a table of contents or term hierarchy. The SuperBook hypertext statistical textbook organized search results via its table of contents, which would provide users a context for the portion of the book retrieved (Egan, Remde et al., 1989). Alternatively, in the healthcare domain, the DynaCat system used UMLS knowledge and MeSH terms to organize search results (Pratt, Hearst et al., 1999). The goal of DynaCat was to present search results with documents clustered into topical groups, such as the treatments for a disease or the tests used to diagnose it. DynaCat attempted to map the user's queries into one of nine query types, such as treatments, tests, risk factors, etc. Each query type organized search results around MeSH terms in the MEDLINE record for the retrieved documents that contained one of a small number of UMLS semantic types. An evaluation with breast cancer patients and their family members showed that DynaCat allowed them to find more answers to questions in a fixed amount of time and resulted in higher user satisfaction than two other systems, one providing clustering by a table of contents view and the other showing a best-match ranking of the query (Pratt and Fagan, 2000). Further work attempted to generalize the approach beyond the `breast cancer` domain (Pratt and Wasserman, 2001).

An additional approach to showing context has been to display aspects within the document. In biomedicine, for example, Hearst et al. (2007a) have developed the Biotext Search Engine, which allows searching and browsing of images and their captions in scientific articles. A pilot study with biology college and graduate students found positive general acceptance (Hearst, Divoli et al., 2007b). A related approach to showing context within documents is the GoPubMed system, which highlights Gene Ontology (GO) terms within articles (Doms and Schroeder, 2005).

Another means of providing context is to demonstrate the relationship of documents to other documents. One approach that has been shown to be effective is not graphical, and in fact relies on *reference tracing*, in which additional documents are retrieved for the user based on bibliographic citations in ones already obtained and found to be relevant. Chapter 2 demonstrated how citations in papers form networks, showing progression in an area of science. Since authors cite papers relevant to their work, it may be that these cited papers are relevant to someone's searching. Citation retrieval can be thought of as a form of relevance feedback, since it requires at least one relevant paper for the process. Citation retrieval can be *backward* (i.e., papers cited by the relevant one are added to the retrieval list) or *forward* (i.e., papers that cite the relevant one are added to the list). Figure 8.7 depicts this process graphically.

Reference tracing is not a new idea. It was recognized in the 1960s that the bibliographic references in scientific papers could be useful indicators of the significance (Westbrook, 1960) and content (Kessler, 1963) of those papers. In fact, networks of documents and citations were advocated as having many uses in characterizing scientific communications and progress (Price, 1965). The most

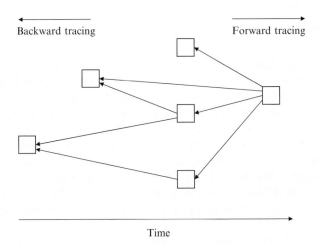

Fig. 8.7 Graphical depiction of reference tracing

practical searching tool to arise out of this early work was the *Science Citation Index* (SCI), which was described in Chap. 4 (Garfield, 1964, 1979b).

The use of citations to enhance IR systems has also been advocated since the 1960s, with some studies looking at health-related applications. Pao and Worthen (1989) evaluated MeSH term searching and citation searching for a cystic fibrosis database. They noted that although MeSH term searching produced a higher number of relevant references per search, there were about 14% of relevant references that could be retrieved only by citation tracing. Pao (1993) looked at 85 searches from a health sciences library and expanded them by the SCI, finding that citation links added at least one relevant item to 85% of the searches. Overall, the citations linked to an average of 24% more relevant materials. Over half the searches had only a handful of additional citations (<10), and of these almost half were relevant. Pao also noted that citation linking can be effective in adding extra relevant citations without excessive loss of precision. As noted in Sect. 8.1.3.3, Bernstam et al. (2006) and Aphinyanaphongs et al. (2006) have assessed citations for reranking the output of search results.

8.2.3.4 Assisting Relevance Feedback and Query Expansion

Operational systems in the healthcare domain employing relevance feedback or query expansion have been few. Probably the most prominent approach has been the ability to find related documents, such as the "Similar Pages" feature of Google or the "Related Articles" feature of PubMed. Another approach has been to use thesaurus relationships to automatically expand query terms. While some research has shown modest benefits with this approach (Srinivasan, 1996c; Aronson and Rindflesch, 1997), other investigations have not (Hersh, Price et al., 2000).

8.2.4 Devices

As noted already, there is growing interest in accessing knowledge-based information from different kinds of devices, in particular handheld personal digital assistants (PDAs). Although these devices are widely used in various aspects of healthcare, it is not clear how valuable they are for IR tasks. A major concern with portable devices has been screen size. A variety of studies have demonstrated that users read 15–25% more slowly from screens that are one-third to two-third the size of regular screens (Duchnicky and Kolers, 1983; Resiel and Shneiderman, 1987), although others have shown no differences (Shneiderman, 1987; Dillon, Richardson et al., 1990). One of the no-difference studies found that users had to navigate more and were more likely to want a different screen size (Dillon, Richardson et al., 1990).

A more recent study compared a Web browser on a larger (1,024 × 768 pixels, approximately 30 lines of content) and a smaller (640 × 480 pixels, approximately

Table 8.8 User success with larger and smaller screen sizes (adapted from Jones, Marsden et al., 1999)

General task	Specific task	Percentage correct	
		With small screen	With large screen
Focused search	Find share price for given company	40	10
	Evaluate performance of company over time	30	0
General search	Find continent with the most public holidays in May 1998	50	20
	Select any intriguing public holiday	80	70

15 lines) display (Jones, Marsden et al., 1999). Users were given four tasks to complete, with two requiring focused searches and two needing more general searches. As shown in Table 8.8, searchers were much more successful with the larger screen. These users were also twice as likely to indicate that the smaller screen impeded task performance. Further analysis showed that users of the smaller screen required many more navigational moves within pages than users of the larger screen. Users of the larger screen, however, were more likely to follow links across pages, whereas users of the smaller screen more often returned to the search interface to query the database again. The authors concluded that Web pages likely to be viewed on smaller devices should place navigational features and key information near the top of the page and reduce the amount of information on pages. Searching is taking place on even smaller devices yet, and one recent study found that users were willing to search on a mobile phone but that the best interface varied by the specific task (Roto, 2006).

Many surveys show widespread usage of PDAs by clinicians (Garritty and El Emam, 2006). One survey of internal medicine physicians showed varying usage for drug information (80%), references for normal lab values (32%), medical textbooks (21%), and billing or coding (21%) (Anonymous, 2002a). While the widespread adoption of handheld devices would imply that they are used successfully, no studies have assessed how well users search knowledge-based resources with them. Perhaps more importantly, no research has attempted to elucidate which types of search and information resources in healthcare are best suited for this platform and which are ill suited. Given that the most popular applications appear to be drug references, disease outlines, and other list-type applications, it may be that these simpler types of application are best suited for these devices.

8.3   User Evaluation of Research Systems

The efficacy of many of the system-oriented approaches described in this chapter has been assessed by a general approach to evaluation that is detailed in this section. Except for some recent studies with real users to be described at the end of the chapter, virtually all evaluation of lexical–statistical systems has been based on "batch-mode" studies using test collections, which were introduced in Chap. 1. These collections typically contain a set of documents, a set of queries, and a binary determination of which documents are relevant to which query. The usual mode of comparing system performance, introduced in Chap. 1, is to generate an aggregate statistic of recall and precision, with the most commonly used metric being MAP.

Some of the test collections have been created with queries captured in the process of real interaction with a system, but others have been built by experimenters for the purpose of doing batch-style evaluation. Likewise, while some relevance judgments have been performed by domain experts, others have not. Nonetheless, these collections have achieved high usage in the research community, and evaluations of IR system performance are typically not considered meaningful to be without their use. However, there are a number of problems with batch-mode studies and the test collections on which they are based:

1. *Lack of real users.* Simulating the behavior of users with batch-style studies does not guarantee that real users will perform identically in front of a computer.
2. *Lack of meaningful measures.* Recall–precision tables do not capture how meaningful the information being retrieved is to the user. Furthermore, research reports often do not provide analyses of statistical significance.
3. *Unrealistic databases.* Until TREC, most test collections were very small, of the order of a few thousand documents. There were concerns not only that such databases might have properties different from those of the large databases used in commercial systems, but also that retrieval algorithms themselves might not be scalable to large databases.
4. *Unrealistic queries.* Most queries in test collections are short statements, which in isolation do not represent the original user's (or anyone else's) information need. Also, recall from Chap. 7 that Saracevic and Kantor (1988b) found a twofold difference in recall when an intermediary searcher had access to a taped transcript of the user's interaction with a librarian, showing that different results can occur when a searcher has access to multiple statements of the same information need.
5. *Unrealistic relevance judgments.* As we saw in Chap. 7, topical relevance judgments can be inconsistent.

8.3.1 Failure Analysis of Research Systems

In 2003, a workshop entitled reliable information access (RIA) was held to address variability in retrieval results (Buckley and Harman, 2004). Two "tracks" addressed different facets and approaches to the problem. A "bottom-up" track carried out a large failure analysis, with six IR systems contributing one run each of 45 topics, with a detailed manual analysis of the results. A "top-down" track performed a number of runs using different variations of query expansion.

The bottom-up analysis found that systems obtained comparable performance (e.g., MAP) scores but performed differently across topics, retrieving different documents and emphasizing different aspects of the topics. However, it was concluded that all systems failed for similar reasons, usually missing some aspect of a topic that would lead to retrieval of more relevant documents. Another conclusion was that if systems could recognize the problem causing the failure, then substantially better retrieval could be obtained. In other words, emphasis on future system development should focus on what current techniques can be applied to which situations, and not on developing new retrieval techniques.

The top-down analysis found that query expansion (also known as blind feedback, i.e., adding terms from highly ranked documents into a query to expand the number of terms and augment retrieval) was highly sensitive to variations in approaches, e.g., the selection of the initial document set for expansion, the number of terms used, and the terms chosen greatly influenced performance.

Another workshop held in 2005 focused on predicting query difficulty (Carmel, Yom-Tov et al., 2005). The TREC Robust Track has also focused on performance on topics that have historically been difficult, assessing methods to recognize such queries and employ methods to improve results (Voorhees, 2006).

8.3.2 Early Studies

One of the first studies to evaluate a lexical–statistical system with real users was performed with CIRT, a front end to an online library catalog at City University in London that featured Boolean and natural language word-based searching, with the latter using term weighting, relevance ranking, and probabilistic relevance feedback (Robertson and Thompson, 1990). In the evaluation study, end users were assisted in using the system by librarian intermediaries, randomized to either Boolean or weighted searching. Users were given offline prints and asked to provide relevance judgments for up to 50 documents. Both user and intermediary filled out questionnaires to document subjective aspects of the system. The results showed essential equivalence between the systems in terms of recall, precision, user effort, cost, and subjective user interactions.

As noted in Chap. 7, Hersh and colleagues compared Boolean and natural language searching with bibliographic and full-text databases using both relevance-based and task-oriented measures (Hersh, Elliot et al., 1994; Hersh and Hickam, 1994, 1995a). These studies showed minimal differences in searching performance between the two approaches.

Turtle achieved different results upon comparing Boolean and natural language searching in two legal databases (Turtle, 1994). Forty-four natural language information need statements were given to expert searchers, who were asked to use the Westlaw Inference Network (WIN) system searching to create Boolean queries. They were allowed to iterate with the system to find an optimal strategy, performing an average of 6.7 searches against the system. Both the natural language statements and the Boolean queries were then run against the databases. Relevance judgments from earlier experiments were used to calculate recall and precision.

In contrast to foregoing studies, Turtle's results showed a marked benefit for natural language over Boolean searching, although no statistical analysis was performed. Nonetheless, recall and precision at 20 documents was about 24–35% higher for the two databases. A clear methodological limitation in this study was its direct comparison of the Boolean and natural language output, since WIN's Boolean output was given in reverse chronological order instead of being ranked. It was unknown whether these results were due to the lack of ordering of the Boolean sets. But since the studies described earlier found no difference in the two types of searching in operational tasks, the ordering of Boolean sets may have had more impact on recall and precision results than the user's ability to successfully interact with the system.

Some investigators have attempted to assess which lexical–statistical system users will actually employ when given a choice. Dumais and Schmitt (1991) assessed an interactive LSI system that allowed two interactive search methods: a *LookUp* function that allowed the user to enter a new query and a *LikeThese* function that provided a new query based on LSI-based relevance feedback. Fifty-seven college students searched ten questions each in a newspaper database. Students were more likely to use LikeThese searches, with or without LookUp searches. The LikeThese searches obtained a higher number of relevant documents in the top-10-ranked items. A look at usage of relevance feedback has also been performed in the interactive portion of the TREC experiments. Users of both the Okapi (Robertson, Walker et al., 1994) and INQUERY (Koenemann, Quatrain et al., 1994) systems were found to use relevance feedback about once per search. Clearly, more studies need to be done in operational settings to determine the benefit and role of all the lexical–statistical techniques that have shown to be beneficial in nonreal-world searching environments.

8.3.3   TREC Interactive Track

As noted in Sect. 8.1, the TREC experiments have for the most part used batch-style searching evaluation with no human involvement in the query process. While some manual modifications of queries have been allowed in various TREC tracks, the emphasis has always been on building automated systems. Nonetheless, most groups in the ad hoc task that employed manual modification of queries found it to enhance results. When users modified INQUERY's automated search statements (produced from processing of the query text), a 15.5% improvement in MAP was seen (Callan, Croft et al., 1995). Likewise, Cooper et al. (1994) had human intermediaries transform queries into word lists by searching on a non-TREC newspaper database, which resulted in a 10% MAP improvement in searches on the TREC database. Similarly, Beaulieu et al. (1996) found that for the Okapi system, automated runs performed better than manual ones. The human difficulties in these experiments were attributed to the difficulty users had in building training queries.

An overview of user-evaluation activities at TREC, including the Interactive Track, has been provided by Dumais and Belkin (2005). The TREC Interactive Track shifted into full gear in TREC-5, when it adopted an *instance recall* task (Hersh, 2001). Recognizing that the number of relevant documents retrieved was not a good indicator of a user's performance with an IR system, the track moved toward a task-oriented approach. The approach chosen was to measure how well users could define instances (called "aspects" in TRECs 5–6 but "instances" subsequently) of a topic. For example, How many stars have been discovered by the Hubble Telescope? or How many countries import Cuban sugar? The database for searching was the 1991–1994 *Financial Times* database, consisting of 210,158 news articles. In the searching experiments, users were asked to save the documents that contained instances and record the specific instances identified. As with the development of document relevance judgments, assessors at NIST devised a set of "correct" instances and the documents they occurred in based on the results submitted from participating sites. This allowed instance recall to be measured:

$$\text{Instance recall} = \frac{\text{number of relevant instances in saved documents}}{\text{number of relevant instances for topic}} \quad (8.9)$$

One of the challenges for the Interactive Track was to define the degree of standardization of experiments across sites. Certainly, one of the values of TREC in general was the standardization of tasks, queries, and test collections. Counter to this, however, were not only the varying research interests of different participating groups, but also the diversity of users, settings, and available systems. As such, attempts to have a common control system to be matched with the different groups' experimental systems were not successful.

There were, however, a number of standardized procedures undertaken. In particular, common data were collected about each user and each of the searches. The data elements were collected from common questionnaires used by all sites or extracted from search logs. Searchers were also given an explicit amount of time for searching: 20 min in TREC-6 and TREC-8 and 15 min in TREC-7. Sites were also asked to provide a narrative of one user's search on one topic each year.

With TREC-9, a new task was adopted: question answering (Hersh and Over, 2000). The TREC-9 Interactive Track continued many of the other standard approaches adopted for TREC-6 through TREC-8, although one change was an expansion of the collection used to include more documents from several additional news sources. The correct answers to the questions were determined by NIST assessors, with searcher results judged as either completely correct, partially correct, or incorrect. Most sites required the answer to be completely correct in their data analysis.

Most participating research groups have assessed specific research questions in their experiments over the years in the Interactive Track. Hersh and colleagues, for example, compared Boolean and natural language searching interfaces in TREC-7 and compared weighted schemes shown to be more effective in batch studies with real users in TREC-8 and TREC-9. This group also attempted to determine the factors associated with successful searching, similar to the experiments they performed using MEDLINE described in Sect. 7.4.2 (Rose, Crabtree et al., 1998; Hersh, Crabtree et al., 2000, 2002).

The studies comparing Boolean and natural language also built on work initiated earlier in the medical domain that showed little difference between the two types of interfaces (Hersh, Elliot et al., 1994; Hersh and Hickam, 1994, 1995a). The TREC-7 study of Hersh et al. (2001) compared these two approaches with the instance recall task. A group of highly experienced information professionals (mostly librarians) was recruited to take part. The Web-based interfaces used are shown in Figs. 8.8 and 8.9. Both interfaces used the MG system (see Table 1.3) as the underlying retrieval system.

Users performed virtually identical on both systems, similar to most earlier studies comparing these two types of interface. However, there were other differences between the systems. Topics using the natural language interface resulted in more documents being shown to the user (viewed). However, fewer documents

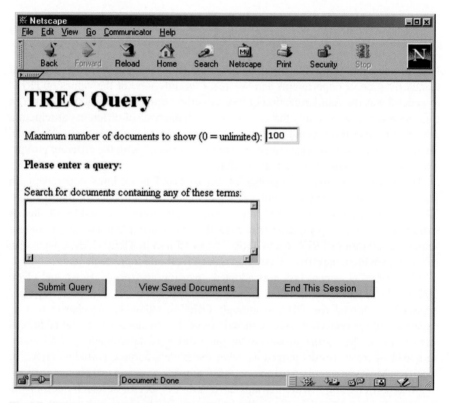

Fig. 8.8 The natural language interface for TREC Interactive Track experiments of Hersh, Turpin et al. (2001)

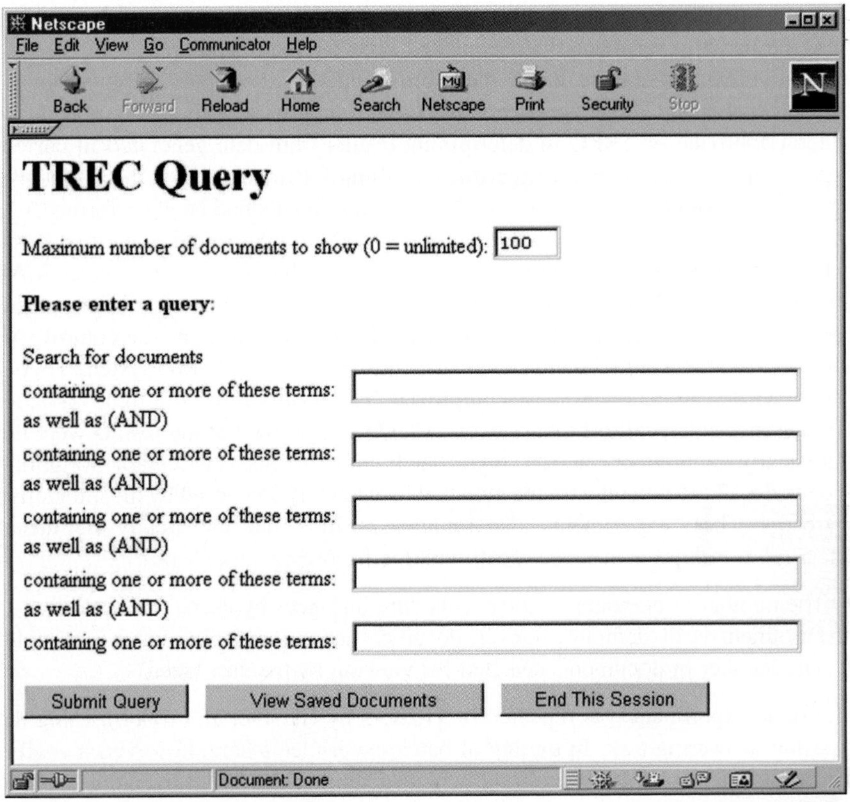

Fig. 8.9 The Boolean interface for TREC Interactive Track experiments of Hersh, Turpin et al. (2001)

were actually selected for viewing (seen) when that interface was used, probably because users had to spend more time scrolling through the document titles shown. This group of highly experienced searchers also clearly preferred the Boolean interface, no doubt in part owing to their familiarity with it.

In TREC-8 and TREC-9, Hersh and colleagues addressed the question of whether results from batch searching experiments are comparable to those obtained by real users. That is, are the results found when batch-style experiments and measures like MAP are used congruent with those obtained by real users with retrieval tasks using the same systems? To test this question, three-part experiments were performed. First, previous TREC Interactive Track data were used to determine the "best-performing" system under batch experiments. This was done by creating a test collection that designated documents with instances as relevant and running traditional batch experiments to generate MAP results. These experiments found that Okapi weighting (TREC-8) and Okapi plus PN weighting (TREC-9) performed much better than "baseline" TF*IDF weighting. Next, the interactive user experiments were carried out, with the best-performing system serving as the "experimental" intervention and the TF*IDF system as the "control." In the final step, the batch experiments were repeated with the data generated from the new interactive experiments, to verify the results held with the topics employed in the user experiments. (The experiments had to be done this way to accommodate the general approach of TREC in determining results from data generated in current experiments. Thus, the batch experiments calling for the data from the interactive experiments could not take place until those experiments had been performed.)

In the TREC-8 instance recall task, Hersh et al. (2000a) found in the first batch experiment that Okapi weighting performed best, achieving an 81% better MAP than TF*IDF weighting. So for the user experiments that followed, Okapi weighting served as the experimental system and TF*IDF weighting as the control. All subjects used the natural language interface (see Fig. 8.8) to the MG system. Highly experienced searchers were again employed. The results showed a trend to better average instance recall for Okapi over TF*IDF weighting, but the results were not statistically significant. In the final batch experiments, the Okapi weighting achieved a 17.6% benefit with the data that had actually been used by the interactive searchers. These experiments also found a positive and statistically significant linear relationship for instance recall with the following variables:

- The number of documents saved as having instances by users
- Document recall (defining a relevant document has one having one instance or more)
- The number of documents selected for viewing by the user (seen)

The same experiment was repeated in TREC-9 by Hersh et al. (2000b), using the question-answering task. In the initial batch experiments here, however, a combination of Okapi plus PN weighting achieved the highest MAP over the TF*IDF baseline, 58%. The user experiments thus employed Okapi plus PN weighting as the experimental system. The same user types as well as the same natural language interface to the MG system were used. In the user experiments, the proportion of questions answered correctly was virtually identical between systems, 43.0% for TF*IDF weighting and 41.0% for Okapi plus PN weighting. In both the TREC-8 and TREC-9 experiments, use of the same user interface precluded measuring user satisfaction differences between systems. The results of the final batch experiments were comparable to those of the TREC-8 experiment: the Okapi plus PN weighting achieved a 31.5% MAP improvement over the TF*IDF weighting.

A follow-up experiment attempted to determine why the "improved" (Okapi weighting in TREC-8 and Okapi plus PN weighting in TREC-9) systems failed to lead to better performance over the TF*IDF system in the hands of real users (Turpin and Hersh, 2001). Analysis of the search output found that the users retrieved more relevant documents as well as more instances in the top 10 documents with the improved systems. However, the overall number of relevant documents retrieved was comparable for both systems, although the improved system retrieved fewer nonrelevant documents. Further analysis showed that the average length of documents retrieved by the improved systems was over twice as long. This was to be expected, given that the document length normalization in Okapi and PN weighting give additional weight to longer documents. The most likely explanation from these experiments was that the TF*IDF system provided users access to shorter documents, albeit fewer relevant ones, enabling users to achieve comparable performance with the outcomes measures: instance recall and correctness of answering questions.

Further work has explored the discordant results between batch and user searching. Allan et al. (2005) found that as "system accuracy" (as measures by clusters containing increasing amounts of relevant content) increased, subject time and number of answers found to a question increased. However, another study by Turpin and Scholer (2006) found that time required to find the first relevant document and the proportion of queries with no relevant answer had no association with MAP of the underlying system. The only measure that was associated with finding the first relevant document was whether the first document in the system output was relevant (i.e., precision at one document). These results have significant meaning for the myriad of batch experiments performed in TREC and other IR evaluations. Namely, the MAP of systems without human users in the loop is a very limited and possibly misleading measure of performance. Of course, the TREC Interactive Track and subsequent experiments were limited to certain tasks, topics, users, and databases. However, further research must determine how well the results of batch experiments correlate with the performance of real users.

Other groups used the TREC Interactive Track to assess different research questions. Belkin et al. (2000) attempted to determine the utility to users of relevance feedback. Their initial experiments (TREC-5) looked at the value of basic relevance feedback, i.e., the ability to designate documents as relevant and to add some of their terms to the query to generate a new list of document outputs. Their observational study found that users preferred interactive to automatic relevance feedback, i.e., they wanted to use relevance feedback as a device to add new terms to their queries rather than have it blindly suggest more documents. The next experiments (TREC-6) added features to the system, including the ability to specify the use of documents for feedback in a positive or negative way. In addition, the user was given control over terms added to the query, i.e., relevance feedback was used as a *term suggestion* device. Users were randomized to have access to only the positive feedback functions or to both the positive and negative feedback functions. There was a trend toward improved instance recall with the latter system as well as the number of documents saved, but the results were not statistically significant, possibly owing to the small sample size. A follow-up experiment with similar interfaces (TREC-7) showed similar results.

Other researchers investigated relevance feedback as well. Robertson et al. (1998) found that it slightly enhanced instance recall in the Okapi system, though a simple TF*IDF approach outperformed both. Yang et al. (2000) assessed different approaches to relevance feedback. The main focus of their experiments was to compare the use of the whole document for relevance feedback vs. selection by the user of specific passages in documents. They hypothesized that the user would do better with the latter, more focused approach. Their results showed no significant difference, but a definite trend in favor of the whole-document approach.

Additional research in the TREC Interactive Track looked at the presentation of search results. Wu et al. (2000) used the instance recall tasks to assess the value of users' clustering of documents (TREC-7) or classifications of terms (TREC-8). The value of clustering was assessed by comparing a system that grouped the document list by clusters with one that just provided a straight ranked list. The list approach yielded better instance recall than the cluster approach, but the difference was not statistically significant. Feedback showed that users liked the cluster approach but had difficulty understanding exactly how it worked. Analysis of the value of term classification also showed no differences between the two approaches.

In the TREC-9 question-answering interactive task, Wu et al. (2001) identified a user interface difference that affected results. They compared two systems that differed in how they displayed their document output (or "surrogates"). One system displayed "answer-indicative sentences" that showed three sentences containing the highest number of words from the query. The other displayed the title and first 20 words of the document. Users had a higher rate of answering questions correctly with the former system (65 vs. 47%). A follow-up experiment with a different locally developed test collection showed comparable results.

Other researchers investigated presentation of search results as well. In the TREC-7 instance recall task, Allan (1997) found that separate "aspect windows" allowing a user to maintain different queries and result sets did not improve performance over a baseline TF*IDF system, but a 3D interface highlighting documents belonging to the different instances produced an improvement that was statistically significant. Belkin et al. (2000) compared displays that showed single documents vs. six documents tiled at a time, with no differences in the results.

8.4 Summary

This chapter has summarized the major research carried out on IR systems and users. As IR becomes more mainstream, the findings from research like this make their way into state-of-the-art systems like those described in Part II of the book. Evaluative results, mostly coming from the TREC initiative, show consistent benefit for a variety of approaches, such as certain types of term weighting, passage retrieval, and query expansion. However, the sections describing the results of Web and interactive searching results should temper those conclusions, since it is not clear that the approaches studied provide much benefit for real users. In a summary of the value of TREC, Sparck-Jones (2006) advocated that in its earlier days, TREC focused on generalizing and not particularizing its results. However, given the mainstreaming of IR, she advocates that TREC and related research now focus on particularizing, with an emphasis on real users and the tasks that motivate their use of IR systems.

Chapter 9
Related Topics

In this chapter, we will expand our discussion to topics beyond information retrieval (IR) but that still require the processing of text. We will see that these techniques have different purposes than the retrieval of documents but still require good basic IR techniques to succeed. The context of these topics can be gleaned from Fig. 1.6, where we move down the funnel from trying to find probably relevant information to finding definitely relevant information and turning it into actionable knowledge. The four topics we will explore include information extraction and text mining, question-answering, text categorization, and document summarization.

9.1 Information Extraction and Text Mining

As we have seen in the first eight chapters of this book, the general goal of IR systems is the retrieval of documents from textual databases, which will then be read and applied to the task for which they were retrieved, such as a search for more information on a disease by a clinician or a patient or an attempt by a researcher to identify earlier studies. Sometimes, however, there is a desire to do more with textual data, such as to extract facts or obtain actionable knowledge from the content.

The name usually given to the process of identifying facts and knowledge from large collections of text is *information extraction* (IE) (McCallum, 2005). In an overview article, Cowie and Lehnert (1996) noted that IE can make use of IR techniques to narrow down the amount of information for the IE process, but the IE is fundamentally different in that it aims to provide the user with facts and knowledge rather than with documents. Another name that has been given to the IE process is *text mining* (Weiss, Indurkhya et al., 2005; Fan, Wallace et al., 2006; Feldman and Sanger, 2007). There have also been overviews of text mining in the biomedical domain as well as in books (Ananiadou and McNaught, 2006; Kao and Poteet, 2006) and articles (Cohen and Hersh, 2005; Hoffmann, Krallinger et al., 2005; Krallinger and Valencia, 2005; Hunter and Cohen, 2006; Jensen, Saric et al.,

W. Hersh, *Information Retrieval: A Health and Biomedical Perspective*,
doi: 10.1007/978-0-387-78703-9, © Springer Science + Business Media, LLC 2009

2006; Roberts, 2006). IE or text mining can also be viewed as one aspect of data mining, which is sometimes called *knowledge discovery from databases* (KDD). The genomics community has called text mining of the published literature "mining the bibliome" to demonstrate its similarity to data mining of the genome (Alfred, 2001). Whatever one chooses to call it, IE and text mining draw on techniques from many areas. They make use not only of IR techniques, but also of natural language processing (NLP), machine learning, and other aspects of artificial intelligence.

In the biomedical domain, there have been two distinct threads of research in IE and text mining. One has focused on processing the electronic health record (EHR), in particular from its clinical narratives, with the goal of extracting attributes about the patient and/or his or her care. Often, the goal is the "secondary use" of clinical data for tasks such as clinical decision support, quality assurance, clinical research, and public health surveillance (Safran, Bloomrosen et al., 2007). The other major thread has been the processing of medical literature to improve efficiency or augment discovery in biomedical research. This work is particularly motivated by modern "high-throughput" biotechnologies that generate massive amounts of data about the sequence and functions of genes, proteins, and other biological entities (Mobasheri, Airley et al., 2004; Troyanskaya, 2005). Even though both these threads make use of common basic techniques, their data and goals for use are sufficiently different to warrant separate discussion.

9.1.1   Patient-Specific Information

We noted in Chap. 2 that IR focuses mostly on knowledge-based information. Patient-specific information is quite different from knowledge-based information because it is generated and used for different purposes. Patient-specific information is produced as a result of an encounter between a patient and the healthcare system. Its main purpose is to document the clinical encounter. However, with the increasing computerization of medical records, as well as the incentives to control costs and ensure quality, there is increasing desire to tap the information in the clinical record for other purposes, such as the secondary uses described above (Safran, Bloomrosen et al., 2007).

One reason to attempt to extract such information is that the data historically used for secondary purposes, the coded information in charts, are usually generated for billing purposes and do not capture the richness or complexities of the actual patient and the course of his or her disease (Jollis, Ancukiewicz et al., 1993). Research has also shown a discordance between the data in coded and free-text portions of the medical record (Stein, Nadkarni et al., 2000). If clinical narrative data are to be used in this fashion, however, they must be encoded to allow application in decision support rules and/or database analysis. Thus, if the information in clinical narratives is going to be used for these purposes, IE techniques must be employed to extract such encoding.

9.1.1.1 Challenges in Processing the Clinical Narrative

For general IR tasks, the goal of processing a text is to select descriptors that represent the subject matter. Whether the traditional approaches of human indexing and word indexing that were discussed in Chap. 4 or the newer innovations such as term-weighting and linguistic techniques that were introduced in Chap. 8, the goal of these indexing processes is to identify the topical content of the document so that it will be retrievable by someone searching for documents on that topic.

As noted earlier, however, the goal of processing the clinical narrative is usually different. While document retrieval is occasionally the aim of searching patient reports, the goal is more likely to be retrieval of specific factual information, such as whether a patient had a particular symptom, physical finding, or test result. The requirement for accuracy is much higher, however, because this information is used in the care of individual patients (e.g., alerting the clinician to the presence of some potentially dangerous combination of attributes) or groups of patients (e.g., assessing the outcomes of a population treated with a drug having potentially serious side effects). While the consequences of an inappropriate indexing term in an IR system are modest (e.g., leading to a false hit in retrieval), the consequences of erroneous fact extraction from a clinical narrative can be an inappropriate recommendation in the care of a patient or an incorrect assessment of the efficacy of a treatment in a population. Another problem is that while documents in journals and textbooks are typically edited, spell-checked, and otherwise polished for easy reading, clinical narratives are usually written or dictated quickly in a telegraphic, elliptical style with misspellings and grammatical incompleteness. As a result of these problems, Hripcsak et al. (1995) have noted that such information is usually "locked" in the clinical narrative.

Problems in processing the clinical narrative occur in all three phases of NLP described in Chap. 8: parsing, semantics, and contextual interpretation. The major challenge for parsing the clinical narrative arises from the incomplete sentences that predominate in clinical texts. For example, Marsh and Sager (1982) assessed a set of hospital discharge summaries and found that about half of the sentences were syntactically incomplete. Table 9.1 lists the major categories of incomplete sentence types they found, in decreasing order of frequency.

Another problem related to parsing is that words may not be in the lexicon. There are a variety of reasons for this, from spelling errors to names of people, devices, or

Table 9.1 Categories of syntactic incompleteness in medical records (adapted from Marsh and Sager, 1982)

Category	Example
Deleted verb and object (or subject and verb), leaving a noun phrase	Stiff neck and fever
Deleted tense and verb "be"	Brain scan negative
Deleted subject, tense, and verb "be"	Positive for heart disease and diabetes
Deleted subject	Was seen by local doctor

Table 9.2 Amount and proportion of words in categories (adapted from Hersh, Campbell et al., 1997)

Category	Amount	Averages	
		Documents	Frequency
Initials and embedded metacharacters	1,344 (1.1%)	157.7	158.1
In one of six medical vocabularies	42,721 (34.2%)	827.5	1,658.5
In names list or Unix spell checker	32,100 (25.7%)	75.6	140.6
Algorithmically recognizable	12,592 (10.1%)	15.0	18.2
Recognizable in context	7,311 (5.8%)	9.1	12.2
Otherwise unrecognized	28,925 (23.1%)		
Correctly spelled real word	12,912 (10.3%)	23.7	28.1
Probably correctly spelled	9,101 (7.3%)	5.8	6.6
Incorrectly spelled	6,171 (4.9%)	2.2	2.4
Garbage word	70 (0.1%)	1.4	1.4
Unknown	671 (0.5%)	1.6	1.7
Total	124,993 (100%)	311.6	613.9

other entities to novel words that clinicians create when they generate narratives. Hersh et al. (1997) analyzed all the words in a corpus of 560 MB of clinical narratives from a university teaching hospital. The 238,898 documents contained a total of 124,993 unique words, which were classified into categories as shown in Table 9.2. Only about 60% of the words occurred in one of six major medical vocabularies including the Unified Medical Language System (UMLS) Metathesaurus, a large list of names, or the Unix spell checker utility. A small percentage of characters were artifacts of the system (initials and embedded metacharacters), but the remaining (nearly 40%) were content words that a lexicon based on the aforementioned medical words, general words, and names would not contain. An analysis of these words discovered that they could represent the following categories:

- Algorithmically recognized by a grammar (e.g., 3 year (age) or 3 × 5 cm (dimension))
- Recognized in context (Dr. William Hersh or Lloyd Center)
- Medical words not in any vocabulary (e.g., dipsticked or righthandedness)
- Incorrectly spelled or otherwise unknown

Semantically, there are problems with words that are used differently in medical language and general English usage. Macleod et al. (1987) found that some words are used differently in medical narratives, such as the word appreciated, which acts as a synonym for detected or identified (e.g., PMI not appreciated). In addition, they noted that other words were used idiosyncratically, such as eye drops (drops is a noun, not a verb) and mass felt at 3 o' clock (the mass is felt at the position of 3 o' clock, not the time). Some words were also difficult to semantically interpret owing to the syntactic incompleteness. For example,

May halt penicillamine could be interpreted to indicate that that penicil-lamine may be discontinued or that it will be definitely discontinued in May.

Medical narrative language is also full of synonymy, leading Evans to assert that the "surface strings" of clinical findings cannot capture the underlying structure (Evans, 1988). He points to the phrases epigastric pain after eating and postprandial stomach discomfort, which mean the same thing yet have no words in common. A related problem is that clinical narratives typically use many abbreviations, some of which can be ambiguous. For example, the abbreviation PCP can stand for the drug phencyclidine, the disease *Pneumocystis carinii* pneumonia, or an individual, the primary care physician.

Contextually, there are many problems as well. Medical charts are typically full of elliptical sentences (e.g., Complains of chest pain. Increasing frequency, especially with exertion. Usually associated with shortness of breath and nausea/vomiting.) The example series of sentences represents a single clinical entity, which is chest pain due to angina pectoris, but the components of the finding are spread across three sentences.

Another contextual problem, also of concern in IR, is that parts of the document may not be relevant for IE. For example, a section of narrative may be engaging in discussion or speculation. While some types of narrative (e.g., history and physical reports or discharge summaries) are well structured, others (e.g., progress notes) are not. The repercussions of extracting discussion or speculation as "facts" could be detrimental to systems that used the extracted data operationally.

There are also a number of practical problems in processing clinical text, as noted by Friedman (2005). First, the extraction of facts requires a higher degree of accuracy than retrieval of documents, which are not expected to all be relevant. Second, clinical text may not be readily available or, even if it is, there may be concerns about patient confidentiality. Third, text from different sources may not be interoperable, in that it may be encoded using standards such as XML and HL7 in one system, but not another. Fourth, language may contain varying amounts of synonymy and polysemy. Abbreviations are a particular problem in clinical narratives. Fifth, some clinical terms may be rare and thus not encoded in rules or other structures. Finally, clinical narratives are usually processed for a specific clinical function, and the simple detection of facts may not be enough for decision support, clinical research, quality measurement, or other uses.

Fortunately, there are some aspects of clinical narratives that do make processing easier. The first is that they follow a fairly regular grammar, which linguists called a *subgrammar*. Thus, even though the wording is cryptic and the sense of words ambiguous, there is some regularity to the use of language in clinical narratives. Sager asserts that virtually all clinical narrative statements can be represented by one of six information formats, a fact exploited heavily in the Linguistic String Project (Sager, Friedman et al., 1987). Another aspect of the clinical narrative that can help with processing is the predictable discourse, especially in portions like the physical examination, where most physicians follow a consistent pattern in presenting the findings (Archbold and Evans, 1989).

9.1.1.2   Applications of Extraction from the Clinical Narrative

The approaches undertaken to extract content from the clinical narrative have varied in scope and domain. Simple, domain-specific approaches focus on a specific area and can usually handle many of the idiosyncrasies of that area but are difficult to generalize to other domains. Comprehensive approaches, on the other hand, scale better but are much harder to build and maintain. This section covers a number of approaches that have been implemented and are described in the literature. After describing some early approaches, this section focuses on two NLP systems that have achieved operational use in EHR systems.

Since the evaluations have been small in size and have utilized different data sets, there is unfortunately no way to compare the different systems. There are actually a number of challenges to evaluation research for the clinical narrative (Friedman and Hripcsak, 1998). One challenge is determining metrics for such evaluation. A common approach is to adapt recall and precision, where recall becomes the proportion of findings correctly determined from all correct findings and precision becomes the proportion of findings correctly determined from all findings suggested by the system. Recall and precision can be calculated at the level of individual findings across all documents in the collection or at the level of individual documents. However, as with IR, these are limited measures in that they do not give the entire picture of how an IE system might perform for a real-world task. Another challenge to evaluation systems for processing the clinical narrative is that patient record text is much more difficult to share across research sites text owing to concerns about privacy and confidentiality of the personally identifiable health information it contains.

The best-known early effort in clinical text processing was Sager's Linguistic String Project (LSP) (Sager, Friedman et al., 1987). This effort was based on the notion of *sublanguage analysis*, in that technical documents in a single field (such as clinical medical narratives) were found to utilize only a subset of English grammar and vocabulary. If these sublanguages could be recognized and incorporated into algorithms, then accurate extraction could occur without having to process general English. Sager et al. (1987) noted that most statements in the medical record could be reduced to six information formats:

1. General medical management
2. Treatment other than medication
3. Medication
4. Test and result
5. Patient state
6. Patient behavior

These formats contained enough semantic information to allow the extracted information to be loaded into a relational database. Appropriate information formats could be qualified by various modifiers, such as time, levels of uncertainty, and severity.

The key to each information format's operation was the lexicon, which contained words with their English and sublanguage classifications. The classes not only represented syntactic information about the words but also placed semantic restrictions on them that enable the information formats to be interpreted semantically. The LSP lexicon contained 40 healthcare sublanguage classes and 14 English semantic subclasses. An example of the Medication information format is shown in Fig. 9.1. The top-level tree contained slots for the classes INST (institution), PT (patient), MEDINFO (medical information), and VTR (treatment verb). Each slot allowed all terms from each of its classes. The VTR class, for example, allowed verbs about treatment (e.g., treated, injected). These verbs were distinct from the VMD class of medical management verbs (e.g., examined, admitted). The medical information slot was actually a subtree that had four slots for the classes H-RX (medication name), QN (dose), H-RXFREQ (medication frequency), and H-RXMANNER (route of administration).

The most substantial evaluation of the LSP system was performed for asthma discharge summaries (Sager, Lyman et al., 1994). A list of 13 important details of asthma management was developed, with the measures of recall and precision adapted based on a gold standard of human review of the documents. The 59 discharge summaries were divided into a training set and a test set, with the former used to update the dictionary, modify the grammar, and develop the database queries. The recall for the testing set was 82.1%, while the precision was 82.5%. When minor errors (e.g., a misplaced word or part of a finding not retrieved) were eliminated, the recall and precision rose to 98.6 and 92.5%, respectively.

Despite the LSP's heavy reliance on syntactic methods, part of its ability to handle domain-specific language processing came from its knowledge about the semantics of terms in medical usage. It might have been possible to set aside the use of complex syntactic information and just focus on semantic information and relationships. This sort of approach was developed by computational linguists (Hendrix, Sacerdoti et al., 1978; DeJong, 1979; Lebowitz, 1983) and formed the basis of the Medical Language Extraction and Encoding (MedLEE) system to perform clinical finding extraction without extensive parsing (Friedman, Alderson et al., 1994). In MedLEE, the rewrite rules for the syntax are replaced with semantic categories. The first domain of use for MedLEE was radiology reports. A radiology finding consists of the central finding, a body location, and finding modifiers. After

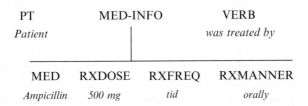

Fig. 9.1 The Medication information format for the statement, Patient was treated by Ampicillin 500 mg tid orally (adapted from Sager, Friedman et al., 1987)

findings are identified in reports, they are stylistically regularized and mapped to controlled terminology using a thesaurus.

The first evaluation of MedLEE assessed its ability to recognize findings from four diseases in 230 randomly selected chest X-ray (CXR) reports (Friedman, Alderson et al., 1994). Physicians who read the actual reports and denoted the findings provided the gold standard. Recall and precision were found to be 70 and 87%, respectively. When additional terminology was added to the queries to enhance their retrieval capability, recall increased to 85%, while precision remained unchanged. A further analysis of the data found that orienting the grammar to identifying the largest well-formed segment of the sentence led to better performance than attempting to process the entire sentence (Friedman, Hripcsak et al., 1998). Additional enhancements to the grammar were required to adapt the system for CXR reports in infants.

Hripcsak et al. (1995) assessed MedLEE based on its ability to automatically detect clinical decisions that might be used in decision support applications. Six radiologists and six internists were given radiology reports and asked to state whether six clinical conditions were present or absent. The level of disagreement between the radiologists, the internists, and the radiology text processor was assessed via a "distance" measure, defined as the number of conditions per report in which there was disagreement on the conditions. The average distance across all physicians was 0.24, and the confidence interval for this measurement contained MedLEE's average distance from each physician, which was 0.26. Thus, the system's performance fell within the normal level of variation among physicians. This study also found that the sensitivity for detecting the six conditions was 81% for the physicians and 85% for MedLEE. The specificity was 98% for both. This study also looked at the distance of lay persons as well as a system using simple word matching (i.e., no NLP), finding much greater distance for each.

There was also effort to move MedLEE outside the realm of radiology reports. Friedman (1997) assessed the challenges in adapting the system to hospital discharge summaries. Unlike the incremental changes required for mammography and neuroradiology reports, extension to discharge summaries required 23 new semantic categories, nearly 300 new grammar rules, and about 6,000 new entries to the lexicon. New information representations were required, such as drug dose abbreviations (e.g., 10 mg PO tid) and temporal phrases (e.g., 2 days after admission). Although evaluation has been incomplete, the general impression from early work in this area has been that unrestricted IE is more difficult than focused detection of explicit findings.

Another promising application of MedLEE was in the parsing of progress note text. Barrows et al. (2000) adapted MedLEE to the terse, highly abbreviated text that ophthalmologists enter after an outpatient visit. They found that MedLEE had lower recall but higher precision than a specialized parser that had been developed for glaucoma. For six specific findings, MedLEE achieved a recall of 80–100% and a precision of 100%. More recently, MedLEE has been expanded to automated coding of clinical documents generally (Friedman, Shagina et al., 2004; Chen, Hripcsak et al., 2006) as well as the incorporation of temporal data, something that IE systems have not historically done well (Zhou and Hripcsak, 2007; Zhou, Parsons et al., 2008).

Another long-standing effort in IE has come from Haug and colleagues at the University of Utah (Haug, Koehler et al., 1994). Early efforts for this system also focused on the CXR report domain (Haug, Ranum et al., 1990). Fiszman et al. (2000) carried out an evaluation for this task that was organized similar to the study of Hripcsak et al. above. Physicians, lay persons, their system, and two keyword algorithms were assessed for their ability to detect three pneumonia-related concepts (pneumonia, infiltrate compatible with acute bacterial pneumonia, and aspiration) as well as an inference that acute bacterial pneumonia was present. Similar to Hripcsak et al., the performance of the IE system was within the confidence interval of the physicians. A follow-up study compared different classification algorithms for inferring pneumonia and found them all to perform comparably and within the range of performance of the physicians (Chapman, Fiszman et al., 2001). Recent efforts have focused on adapting the MetaMap system (Aronson, 2001) along with a negation detection algorithm (Chapman, Bridewell et al., 2001) to improve completeness of a problem list (Meystre and Haug, 2006) and identify patients for a trauma registry (Day, Christensen et al., 2007).

Other work in clinical narrative IE has focused on classification of text in reports for syndromic surveillance and automated or semiautomated annotation. With an aim to detect syndromes earlier in their development than would be noted clinically, a real-time system has been in place in Pittsburgh, Salt Lake City, and other locations to process emergency department chief complaints. Unfortunately, the sensitivity of detecting these findings has only been in the range of 30–75%, although the specificity has been above 90–95% (Chapman, Dowling et al., 2005). A similar approach has been taken for automated annotation of findings in pathology reports (Liu, Mitchell et al., 2005) and has also been shown to improve agreement among human annotators of emergency department reports (Chapman, Dowling et al., 2008).

An offshoot of this work brought the surveillance task back to IR, as the system was adapted to monitor entries into a health-related search engine to assess for correlation with other influenza surveillance data (Johnson, Wagner et al., 2004). Although the correlation was relatively strong, the timeliness did not improve over usual surveillance techniques. A related attempt to apply this approach has used Google Adwords to create a sponsored link to click for more information on influenza (Eysenbach, 2006). Analysis showed the correlation to other surveillance data was high and timely compared with traditional surveillance methods.

A variety of other researchers have applied IE techniques for an array of clinical applications. Some approaches have assessed the quality of healthcare or its documentation. For example, Hazlehurst, Frost et al. (2005) and Hazlehurst, Sittig et al. (2005) have assessed how well clinicians adhere to the recommended guidelines for the ask–advise–assess–assist–arrange approach to smoking cessation, finding judgment of the automated system indistinguishable from human assessments. Brown et al. (2006) have similarly assessed nine quality indicators for spine disability examinations in Veteran's Administration (VA). Pakhomov et al. have applied IE for identification of patients with heart failure (Pakhomov, Weston et al., 2007) and the classification of foot examination findings (Pakhomov, Hanson et al., 2008).

A number of European groups have developed systems to process the clinical narrative as well, with an additional focus on cross-language issues. Baud et al. (1998) developed a *morphosemantic* parser that processed text down to the level of morphemes, including bound morphemes, to break them into the finest level of semantic granularity possible. One advantage to this approach was that it allowed translation across languages, although it was harder than word-level parsing because of the idiosyncrasies of language (Baud, Rassinoux et al., 1999). Schulz and Hahn (2000) have also taken an approach focused on the morpheme level, with a more concentrated focus on the German language. Recent efforts have focused on generalizing the approach to multiple languages (Namer and Baud, 2007). One application of the morphosemantic parser has been its application to the parsing of physician orders (Lovis, Chapko et al., 2001). This approach was analyzed in a laboratory evaluation and was found to achieve a 7% reduction in the time required to enter orders compared to a conventional system. Users rated the parser as easier to learn and use than the conventional system.

There have also been a number of small challenge evaluations in this area that provided tasks and standardized test collections for comparison of systems. Two of these projects have come from the Informatics for Integrating Biology and the Bedside (i2b2, http://www.i2b2.org/) project of Partners Health Care, while the third came from the Computational Medical Center of the University of Cincinnati (http://www.computationalmedicine.org/).

In the first i2b2 project, the challenge was to deidentify from eight categories of private health information (PHI) (Uzuner, Luo et al., 2007). These included patients, physicians, locations, hospitals, dates, identifiers, phone numbers, and ages. A training set of 669 annotated records were provided, with another 220 records used for testing. Evaluation was measured at the instance level of PHI, with the deidentification being either correct (C) or one of the following types of errors:

- Substitution (S) – PHI type, content, or extent was incorrect
- Insertion (I) – non-PHI was identified as PHI
- Deletion (D) – PHI was marked as non-PHI

Instance-level recall was defined as the C/C + S + D and instance-level precision was defined as C/C + S + I, with a balanced F measure combining the two. Seven groups participated, with best recall, precision, and F measure being 0.99, 0.98, and 0.98, respectively. ifferent groups employed a variety of approaches, but all made use of a combination of global (e.g., sentence position) and local features (e.g., lexical cues, templates, or special characters), trained with some sort of machine-learning algorithm.

A second challenge of the i2b2 project was to identify smoking status from discharge records (Uzuner, Goldstein et al., 2008). Smoking status could be past smoker, current smoker, smoker, nonsmoker, or unknown, with the largest category being the last one. There were 398 training records and 104 test records. Recall, precision, and F were calculated on the correctness of the status designation, with results presented both as microaveraged (giving equal weight to each individual record) and macroaveraged (giving equal weight to each category). The best F measure results for each measurement were 0.90 and 0.76, respectively, indicating a diversity of results among the different categories. As with the deidentification task, most groups aimed to identify features in text for the categories and apply machine-learning techniques to them.

The Computational Medical Center challenge focused on the automated assignment of ICD-9 codes to a set of de-identified radiology reports, with 978 training reports and 976 test reports (Pestian and Brew, 2007). The main evaluation measure was a macroaveraged (over all assignments) balanced F measure, although a microaveraged (average of assignments for each code) F measure was calculated as well. In addition, a cost-sensitive accuracy measure was developed, which parameterized the cost of overcoding (false positives) and undercoding (false negatives), since these could have different value in different circumstances. For the experiments, overcoding was penalized threefold over undercoding (under the presumption that overcoding may lead to prosecution for fraud). A total of 44 research groups participated, with best scores for macroaverage F, microaverage F, and cost-sensitive accuracy being 0.77, 0.89, and 0.92, respectively. One of the best-performing groups used a combination of approaches that included MetaMap, NegEx, and "stacking" of the output from a variety of machine-learning algorithms (Aronson, Bodenreider et al., 2007).

9.1.1.3 Systems for Processing the Clinical Narrative

Many of the earlier-mentioned applications focused on a research task that was carried out by using multiple systems, usually parameterized for the specific task. Some of these systems, however, have been developed as standalone systems, with a small number in use in operational settings. For example, the MetaMap Transfer System (MMTx, http://mmtx.nlm.nih.gov/) makes available the MetaMap system for mapping biomedical text to UMLS Thesaurus terms (Aronson, 2001). Also available is NegEx (http://www.dbmi.pitt.edu/chapman/NegEx.html), a system for detecting negation of medical terms (Chapman, Bridewell et al., 2001). Another system used in a number of locations is the Mayo Clinic Vocabulary Server, which maps text to controlled medical terminologies (Elkin, Brown et al., 2006).

The largest integration of an IE system into an operational EHR system has been the use of MedLEE at Columbia-Presbyterian Medical Center (Friedman, Hripcsak et al., 1995). A major challenge was achieving interoperability with all the other components of the EHR system, such as the clinical database for storing all data on the patient (Johnson, 1996), the terminology knowledge base for managing encoded concepts (Cimino, Clayton et al., 1994), and the event monitor for detecting events and triggering messages for actions based on those events (Hripcsak, Clayton et al., 1996). This required translating output to the Health Level 7 (HL7) format for data transfer into other components of the EMR. It also required reducing the amount of information coming from MedLEE to facilitate subsequent retrieval. Other requirements for adapting to the real-world environment included more robust error handling, since MedLEE output was stored alongside other real data for real patients, and more efficiency in the parsing process, since the system was required to operate on large quantities of data. The Web site and an operational demo version of MedLEE are available at http://lucid.cpmc.columbia.edu/medlee/. The system of Haug et al. has also seen some use in the operational EHR at the University of Utah.

If these systems are ever to achieve widespread and generalizable use in operational settings, an additional requirement will be the development of a comprehensive clinical vocabulary. Such terminology systems will need to provide more than just simple lists of terms, but rather need to capture the complexity of clinical findings. While lists of terms are usually adequate to represent diagnoses and procedures, term lists fare worse in describing clinical findings. For example, medical students learning history taking quickly memorize the mnemonic PQRST, which represents the attributes of symptoms: provocative-palliative factors, quality, radiation, severity, temporal factors. These attributes are not insignificant for research, as it is known, for example, that the attributes of chest pain (e.g., radiation to the back vs. radiation down the arm) have significant value in diagnosing myocardial infarction.

The vocabulary that comes closest to meeting the foregoing requirements, which also has the broadest coverage of clinical content, is the Systematized Nomenclature of Medicine–Clinical Terms (SNOMED CT) (Anonymous, 2007r). Originally developed by the College of American Pathologists (CAP, http://www.snomed.org/), resulting from a merger of SNOMED Reference Terminology (SNOMED RT) and the National Health Service Clinical Terms projects, development has now moved to an international body, the International Health Terminology Standards Development Organisation (IHTSDO, http://www.ihtsdo.org/). A browser for SNOMED CT and some other clinical terminologies is available through the National Cancer Institute Terminology Browser (http://nciterms.nci.nih.gov/NCIBrowser/Dictionary.do).

Almost unique among the widely used clinical terminologies, SNOMED CT is *compositional* or *multiaxial*. These terms mean that concepts represented in SNOMED CT can be built from structured aggregations of other concepts, defined by relationships (akin to atoms coming together to form molecules). Although the representation of concepts in SNOMED can get complicated, an overriding goal is the practical representation of clinical information. Indeed, one of the challenges of SNOMED CT (or any compositional clinical vocabulary) is to balance the precoordination of concepts, which provides the convenience of designating a commonly used term, with postcoordination, which allows construction of concepts that are not explicitly represented.

Elkin et al. (2003) have explored the tradeoff between the ease of use of precoordinated concepts with the expressivity allowed by postcoordination. A not uncommon problem that can arise is when simpler concepts are postcoordinated into an equivalent precoordinated concept, which can make the two to appear different to a computer system that does not "know" that the left foot is the structure `foot` with laterality `left`. Elkin et al. promote that systems must impose discipline to insure that equivalent composition expressions are represented as such. This requires consistent use of attributes such as topography, morphology, and etiology. Another limitation of SNOMED is that the system itself does not prevent meaningless compositional aggregations, such as `fractured blood caused` by `Staphylococcus aureus`.

The hierarchies in SNOMED CT are listed in Table 9.3. Figure 9.2 shows representation of the term `myocardial infarction`. Each SNOMED CT term has a fully specified name, which is not necessarily the preferred term that may be used by a clinician. However, each fully specified name is unique. All fully specified names, preferred terms, and synonyms have unique DescriptionIDs. More than one concept may have a same (i.e., polysemous) term, e.g., both `Cold sensation quality` and `Common cold` have a term `cold`. SNOMED CT concepts also have relationships, which can be of four types: defining, qualifying, historical, and additional.

SNOMED CT users are also encouraged to create "subsets" of the vocabulary, which allow (Anonymous, 2007s):

- Organizing it into relevant chunks that act as "favorites" for different groups of end users
- Constraining choices, where required, to particular defined categories (e.g., national data sets, cancer registry data sets)
- Encouraging structured clinical data entry

Table 9.3 The hierarchies of SNOMED CT (adapted from Anonymous, 2007r)

Clinical finding
Physical force
Procedure
Event
Observable entity
Environments/geographical locations
Body structure
Social context
Organism
Situation with explicit context
Substance
Staging and scales
Pharmaceutical/biologic product
Linkage concept
Specimen
Qualifier value
Special concept
Record artifact
Physical object

The clinical finding hierarchy includes disorders, which is where names of diseases occur

Fig. 9.2 Representation of the
concept myocardial infarction in
SNOMED CT (adapted from
Anonymous, 2007r)

Concept:
- ConceptID: 22298006
- Fully specified name: myocardial infarction (disorder)

Descriptions:
- Preferred term: myocardial infarction
- Synonym: cardiac infarction
- Synonym: heart attack
- Synonym: infarction of heart

Relationships:
- Defining relationships (is a)
    - Concept: structural disorder of heart
        • Associated morphology: Infarct
        • Finding site: myocardium structure
    - Concept: injury of anatomical site
        • Associated morphology: infarct
        • Finding site: myocardium structure
    - Concept: myocardial disease
        • Associated morphology: infarct
        • Finding site: myocardium structure
- Allowable qualifiers
    - Qualifier: onset
    - Qualifier: severity
    - Qualifier: episodicity
    - Qualifier: course

- Supporting background processes that might trigger decision support (e.g., conditions that contraindicate the use of a drug)
- Achieving a consistent representation of disease where important

Some researchers have evaluated the coverage of SNOMED for clinical problem lists. Wasserman and Wang (2003) evaluated 8,378 coded diagnoses and problems at a large academic medical center, finding 1,266 unique surface forms and the ten most frequent diagnoses accounting for 40.5% of all diagnoses. Over 88% of all diagnoses and problems were found in SNOMED CT and most not present were missing synonyms. Concept coverage was therefore found to be 98.5%. Elkin et al. (2006) performed a similar analysis of nearly 5,000 most common terms used at another large academic medical center. They found that SNOMED was able to capture over 92% of such terms. Expanding synonymy and missing modifiers would have expanded the coverage even greater.

One of the challenges to terminologies is to develop both an interface terminology that provides means for users to enter terms and a reference terminology that provides definitions as well as mappings to internal representations (Rosenbloom, Miller et al., 2006). Evaluation of interface terminologies must include how well they support correct, complete, and efficient encoring or review of terms by humans (Rosenbloom, Miller et al., 2008). Indeed, there are many challenges generally to building (Rubin, Lewis et al., 2006) and evaluating (Arts, Cornet et al., 2005) terminology systems and ontologies.

Even if the structural issues concerning vocabularies are resolved, additional challenges remain. As noted earlier, Hersh et al. (1997) found that many words used in clinical narratives were not present in the major medical vocabularies, although some could be discovered algorithmically. Humphreys et al. (1997) assessed coverage at the concept level, assessing the UMLS Metathesaurus and three additional vocabularies (SNOMED, Read Clinical Terms, and the Logical Observations, Identifiers, Names, and Codes (LOINC) terminology) for over 41,000 terms submitted by 63 individuals from their clinical information systems. About 58% of the terms had exact meaning matches with terms in the collection, 41% had related concepts, and 1% had no match whatsoever. For the 28% of the terms that were narrower in meaning than a concept in the controlled vocabularies, 86% shared lexical items with the broader concept but had additional modifiers. The single vocabulary with the largest coverage was SNOMED.

How can clinical vocabularies be augmented beyond the tedious addition of terms? A number of researchers have suggested ways. Hersh et al. (1996) carried out preliminary work using a parser to identify modifiers occurring with ten noun phrase (NP) heads in a corpus of 842 MB of clinical narrative text. While many of the individual words in the NPs occurred in the major vocabularies, the NPs themselves did not exist as terms but could be formed compositionally from their words. Another challenge in vocabulary maintenance is identifying synonymy. Hole and Srinivasan (2000) used a variety of approaches to detect potential synonyms; the most fruitful approach was to identify lexical-level synonyms not detected by baseline means and compare terms with some but not all words in common. A final challenge is specifying relationships, which has also been assessed with research approaches (Vizenor, Bodenreider et al., 2006).

9.1.1.4 Alternatives to Processing the Clinical Narrative

Given the challenges of clinical narrative processing described in this chapter, we might be tempted to look for approaches that avoid the use of ambiguous natural language in the first place. A number of researchers have attempted to develop *structured data entry* systems featuring forms that allow direct input of coded data. Of course, form-based input is a tradeoff, sacrificing clinician's "freedom of expression" for the unambiguous structure of coded data.

Systems have been implemented over the years for a variety of constrained domains, including the `obstetric ultrasound` (Greenes, 1982), `cardiovascular exam` (Cimino and Barnett, 1987), and for following clinical guidelines (Henry, Douglas et al., 1998). Larger-scale systems have also been implemented in the past, without long-lasting usage (Greenes, Barnett et al., 1970; Fischer, Stratmann et al., 1980) and some companies attempting to market approaches have come and gone (e.g., Oceania Corp.). More recent efforts have attempted to utilize the pointing devices and graphical displays of modern microcomputers as well as more sophisticated coding structures. One of the more comprehensive current efforts is the Open System Development Environment

(OpenSDE, http://www2.eur.nl/fgg/mi/OpenSDE/, http://sourceforge.net/projects/opensde/) (Los, vanGinneken et al., 2005). OpenSDE has been recently applied in the pediatrics (Bleeker, Derksen-Lubsen et al., 2006) and coronary surgery (Venema, vanGinneken et al., 2007) domains.

9.1.1.5   Future Directions for Processing the Clinical Narrative

We have described a wide variety of approaches to extract clinical findings. For narrative processing systems, each one described, from the simplest to complex, was shown to extract appropriate findings at a fairly high rate of accuracy (e.g., 80–95%). However, this leads to a number of larger questions. Will these systems be able to process the remaining 5–20% accurately? If so, how much work will be required to get them to the level of accuracy of a human reader? If not, will systems still be useful for research or quality assurance purposes if they have an inherent level of inaccuracy? Also, will these systems be generalizable to the larger medical environment beyond the research-oriented institutions where they were developed?

For clinical vocabularies and structured data entry systems, there are larger questions as well. For the former, will comprehensive clinical nomenclatures be developed that can scale up to all the types of information desired for capture? For the latter, will clinicians accept structured data entry and provide the comprehensiveness and quality currently entered into the clinical narrative? Despite the problems noted with all the foregoing data extraction and capture systems, these are not questions that can be ignored. As patients, clinicians, health systems, researchers, and others continue to demand more information about the quality of healthcare, impetus will exist to tap the data in clinical findings, whether in narrative or structured data entry form.

9.1.2   Knowledge-Based Information

As noted above, the purpose for IE and text mining of knowledge-based information operates on different information and usually has a different task. With the concomitant growth of scientific literature as well as data-intensive "high-throughput" biotechnologies, the need for tools to manage the burgeoning literature is acute (Mobasheri, Airley et al., 2004). However, the use of IE and text mining of knowledge-based information is not limited to genomics, and some efforts have focused on clinical knowledge (Payne, Mendonça et al., 2007). A number of overviews have been written in books (Ananiadou and McNaught, 2006; Kao and Poteet, 2006) and articles (Cohen and Hersh, 2005; Hoffmann, Krallinger et al., 2005; Krallinger and Valencia, 2005; Hunter and Cohen, 2006; Jensen, Saric et al., 2006; Roberts, 2006). These overviews demonstrate that IE shares some problems with IR, such as ambiguity of text, but also faces some distinct problems, such as focusing on the portion of text or other information as to where the "important" information to extract is. In this section, we will explore four major application areas of research – knowledge acquisition, literature-based discovery (LBD), curation and annotation, and analysis of scientific texts. We will then describe some available systems that have been developed and end with a discussion of test collections and evaluation challenges.

9.1.2.1   Knowledge Acquisition

The goal of knowledge acquisition from knowledge-based information is to identify facts that can be used to identify, summarize, or model the content of literature. The initial step in this process is *named entity recognition* (NER), i.e., the recognition in text of entities such as genes, proteins, cellular components, disease processes, drugs, etc. Of course, just recognizing entities is not enough; they must be "normalized" to controlled vocabulary terms. Furthermore, to truly recognize knowledge, the relationships among different entities (e.g., genes causing disease, proteins interacting with cellular processes, drugs acting on certain locations in the cell) must also be extracted. Once concepts and relationships have been recognized, the knowledge can be used for other applications, such as LBD and curation.

Much initial work in biomedical text mining focused on NER. Some major approaches to concept recognition have included identification of NPs through part-of-speech tagging, exemplified by Tanabe and Wilbur (2002), and training of classifiers, as seen in the GAPSCORE algorithm (Chang, Schutze et al., 2004). Some researchers have applied dictionary-based lookup methods (e.g., Cohen, 2005). Identifying relationships between concepts is more challenging, requiring correct extraction of not only the relationship but also its constituent concepts. As such, most systems have focused on narrow domains (akin to clinical narrative extraction systems described above), such as the Textpresso system (Müller, Kenny et al., 2004).

Other works have focused on taking advantage of Medical Subject Headings (MeSH) terms in the biomedical literature to identify concepts associated with gene expression. Masys et al. (2001) were among the first to provide profiles of MeSH terms for differentially regulated genes in microarray experiments. Djebbari et al. (2005) extended this approach to identify "overrepresented" MeSH terms in gene sets.

One of the major challenges of genomic knowledge acquisition is the ambiguity (i.e., synonymy and polysemy) of gene and other entity names. There has historically been no control over gene names; they tend to be assigned by the researchers who discover them. A leading geneticist has noted this problem and called for better approaches to naming genes (O'Neill, 2003). Genes have characteristics that may present even more challenges than names of other entities:

- Genes often have multiple names, with different names preferred by different research subcommunities.
- In some species, genes are named using common words or named entities, e.g., Sleeping Beauty (Ivics, Hackett et al., 1997).

- Genes have homology across species, in which genes produce the same or a similar protein (e.g., insulin is produced in the mouse, rat, human, etc.), yet the naming of homologs is not consistent.
- Genes produce products (proteins) that may carry the same name of the gene. Some research communities adopt conventions, such as capitalizing or italicizing the name when it represents the gene or the product. This is usually problematic for retrieval systems that tend to case-fold (usually converting all uppercase letters to lowercase) and use only ASCII characters (eliminating italicization).
- Some disorders are caused by specific alleles of a gene, which furthermore may be variably expressed, such that the occurrence of the gene name can indicate little about the process in which it takes part.

Several studies have investigated gene-naming problems. Tuason et al. (2004) systematically assessed ambiguity in gene names across four species: mouse, worm, fly, and yeast. This analysis was extended to 17 more organisms by Chen et al. (2005). Table 9.4 shows the results obtained across 21 organisms (Chen, Liu et al., 2005). It should be noted there was substantial variation across different organisms. For official symbols, there was virtually no ambiguity within species or with English words or the Metathesaurus. The substantial (14.2%) ambiguity across species was believed to be due to homologous genes. The ambiguity with English words and Metathesaurus terms was generally low with one exception, which was between gene names and Metathesaurus terms. Analysis of the latter showed that 80% of the ambiguity was due to gene names being given the same name as the resulting phenotype from expression of the gene, e.g., the gene `limb deformity` results in deformed limbs. Chen et al. also looked at the terms authors preferred to use in the papers they wrote, finding an overwhelming preference for gene synonyms (74.7%) over official symbols (17.7%) and official names (7.6%).

Fundel and Zimmer (2006) focused on the four organisms of Tuason et al. as well as the rat, looking more deeply at the problem and assessing how it might be improved with human curation. All these studies looked at ambiguities within the organism, with general English words, with terms in the UMLS Metathesaurus, and across the organisms. For each gene, they also assessed the ambiguity of official symbols, all symbols, and all symbols and names.

Table 9.4 Percentage of ambiguity of gene names (adapted from Chen, Liu et al., 2005)

Percentage of ambiguity	Official symbols only (%)	All symbols (official and aliases) (%)	All names (including all symbols) (%)
Within species	0.02	5.0	5.6
Across species	14.2	13.4	16.0
English words	0.6	1.1	1.8
UMLS Metathesaurus terms	1.0	3.0	13.1

The organization responsible for the naming of human genes is the Human Genome Organization (HUGO, http://www.hugo-international.org/). The NCBI databases on human genes, e.g., Online Mendelian Inheritance in Man (OMIM, http://www.ncbi.nlm.nih.gov/entrez/query.fcgi?db=OMIM), adhere to the HGNC, although as noted above, authors in the literature do not always do so.

Less work has been done using knowledge extraction for clinical topics. Chen and Friedman (2004) and Lussier et al. (2006) have adapted MedLEE to detect phenotypic information from the biomedical literature. Borlawsky has applied the same system to extract diseases, therapies, and drugs from Cochrane Collaboration reviews (Borlawsky, Friedman et al., 2006). Chen et al. (2008) have combined the use of MedLEE to detect drug–disease interactions in clinical narratives and biomedical literature.

9.1.2.2   Literature-Based Discovery

Another line of research has looked at processing the medical literature to facilitate scientific discovery. This area does not necessarily require NLP, but has been shown to be automated by it. Much of the focus has been on disconnected threads in the literature. For example, there might be studies that identify diseases or syndromes that result in certain manifestations and others that identify treatments that improve such manifestations, yet the treatment has never been assessed for this particular disease or syndrome. Swanson showed this (manually) to be the case in two instances:

1. Articles on Raynaud's Disease found blood viscosity to be abnormally high, while others on the fish oil eicosapentaenoic acid found this substance to reduce blood viscosity, yet the latter had never been considered as a treatment for the former (Swanson, 1986).
2. Articles on migraine found the disease to be implicated by spreading depression in the cortex of the brain, while others found magnesium to be effective in inhibiting such depression (usually in the context of treating a different condition, epilepsy) (Swanson, 1988b).

When first identified, the two literatures in each instance were completely disconnected, and no researcher had thought of the potential for treatment. After identification of these potential linkages, clinical trials found effectiveness for both treatments (Swanson and Smalheiser, 1997). Additional disconnected complementary literatures have also been discovered in a variety of clinical areas (Weeber, Vos et al., 2003; Srinivasan, 2004; Srinivasan and Libbus, 2004). Some more recent work has incorporated genomic information (Hettne, Weeber et al., 2007; Seki and Mostafa, 2007). An overview of the tools available for LBD has been written (Weeber, Kors et al., 2005). In addition, a system called ARROWSMITH has been developed to facilitate further exploration (http://arrowsmith.psych.uic.edu/) (Smalheiser and Swanson, 1998). ARROWSMITH combines terms common to two different literatures (the A-literature and C-literature of Fig. 9.3) with so-called

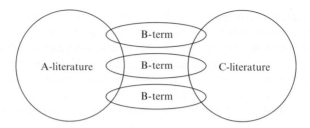

Fig. 9.3 The components of literature-based discovery (adapted from Smalheiser and Swanson, 1998)

B-terms that may offer conceptual explanations for linkage of the literatures. One of the challenges in using ARROWSMITH is the large number of B-terms generated, and further work has focused on methods to prune them automatically to a more manageable size (Torvik and Smalheiser, 2007).

9.1.2.3 Curation and Annotation

As our knowledge in genomics, systems biology, and related areas grows, there is an increased need for annotation of the functions of various biologic entities such as genes and proteins. Manual curation is extremely labor intensive and, given the rapid growth of the volume of scientific research, probably prohibitively expensive. As such, another area where use of IE and text mining could be of value is in curation of scientific databases. As noted below, the use case for the major challenge evaluation in this area is to automate or semiautomate identification of terms and relationships for curation.

A variety of approaches over the last decade have been developed to annotate genes (Raychaudhuri, Chang et al., 2002), proteins (Xie, Wasserman et al., 2002), and gene function (Vinayagam, König et al., 2004; Theodosiou, Angelis et al., 2007). Other work has looked at annotating text of gene function, which could also be considered a form of summarization (see Sect. 9.4). The TREC 2003 Genomics Track featured a task devoted to predicting the text of Gene Reference into Function (GeneRIF) annotations in the LocusLink (now called Entrez Gene, http://www.ncbi.nlm.nih.gov/sites/entrez?db=gene) database (Hersh and Bhupatiraju, 2003). While the TREC 2003 task found little ability to find GeneRIF text beyond selecting the article title, later work showed improvement through use of Gene Ontology (GO) annotations (Lu, Cohen et al., 2006).

Wilbur et al. (2006) have looked at factors related to annotation and their consistency across annotators based on guidelines for annotation. The factors included focus, polarity, certainty, evidence, and trend. They noted a 70–80% agreement across the different factors and concluded that annotation based on their guidelines was reproducible and amenable to automation.

9.1.2.4 Analysis of Scientific Texts

Some research has focused on analyzing scientific texts, which can provide interesting insights as well as aid the kinds of applications just described. As findings and conclusions in scientific literature are not always completely certain, some work has focused on speculation or hedging. Light et al. (2004) investigated detection of speculative sentences in biomedical literature and found that humans could reliably detect it and an automated classifier could mimic their performance reasonably well for three biomedical topics. Medlock and Briscoe (2007) were similarly able to detect and automatically classify hedging in *Drosophila genome* literature.

Related work has focused on where important information for IE is likely to occur in biomedical articles and whether titles and abstracts alone are sufficient for IE. Schuemie et al. (2004) have assessed occurrences of gene symbol–gene name combinations that can resolve gene-symbol ambiguity. The most information-rich section in general is the Results section of papers, yet that only accounts for 30–40% of all information. The authors conclude that all sections are needed and that titles and abstracts alone are insufficient for IE. This has been further verified in an analysis of biological molecular interaction literature (McIntosh and Curran, 2007). Other work has assessed the ability of systems to identify "rhetorical zones" in biomedical articles, which could be used to assist IE (Mullen, Collier et al., 2005).

An additional line of work has assessed the ability of biomedical literature to suggest synonymy and help disambiguate abbreviations and acronyms. A variety of approaches have been used for synonym detection of genes, proteins, and other entities (Yu and Agichtein, 2003; Cohen, Hersh et al., 2005) as well as map abbreviations and acronyms to their full forms (Chang, Schutze et al., 2002; Yu, Kim et al., 2007). Xu et al. (2007) have used profiles based on associated MEDLINE records to disambiguate gene symbols.

9.1.2.5 Biomedical Text-Mining Systems

A variety of biomedical text-mining systems are available, some commercial and others that are open source and more thoroughly explained in the scientific literature. Some commercial applications include IBM WebSphere (http://www-306. ibm.com/software/websphere/), SAS Text Miner (http://www.sas.com/technologies/analytics/datamining/textminer/), and Vivisimo (http://vivisimo.com/).

A compendium of open-source text-mining tools is available (http://arrowsmith. psych.uic.edu/arrowsmith_uic/tools.html). Some of the best-known systems include:

- Medminer (http://discover.nci.nih.gov/textmining/main.jsp) – a system to extract and organize relevant sentences in the literature based on a gene, gene–gene, or gene–drug query (Tanabe, Scherf et al., 1999)
- Chilibot (http://www.chilibot.net/) – creates relationship networks among entities in biomedical literature (Chen and Sharp, 2004)

- Medpost (ftp://ftp.ncbi.nlm.nih.gov/pub/lsmith/MedPost/medpost.tar.gz) – a part-of-speech tagger for biomedical text (Smith, Rindflesch et al., 2004)
- Bitola (http://www.mf.uni-lj.si/bitola/) – interactive system to identify candidate genes for diseases (Hristovski, Peterlin et al., 2005)
- MetaMap (http://mmtx.nlm.nih.gov/) – the National Library of Medicine (NLM) tool for mapping text to UMLS Metathesaurus terms (Aronson, 2006)
- Whatizit (http://www.ebi.ac.uk/webservices/whatizit/info.jsf) – a text-mining pipeline implemented as a series of Web services (Rebholz-Schuhmann, Arregui et al., 2008)

9.1.2.6   Evaluation of Biomedical Text Mining

Most of the earlier approaches have been accompanied by evaluation. However, as lamented by this author, most research has been very system-focused and based upon small and unrealistic data sets (Hersh, 2005). Larger-scale, user-oriented, and task-based evaluation is necessary to determine the best uses for IE and text mining to augment scientific discovery and its annotation. Furthermore, as with IR systems, differences in performance found in system-level evaluations may not translate to improvement in user-oriented evaluations, as shown in the case of protein annotation (Caporaso, Deshpande et al., 2008). A user-questionnaire study found that curation could be speeded up by one-third, but only with near-perfect NLP, although what curators valued most was high precision (Alex, Grover et al., 2008). Another study of users documented a preference for high precision in what is displayed (Divoli, Hearst et al., 2008).

Although a number of test corpora have been developed for biomedical text mining, there have been few challenge evaluations. One notable exception is the Critical Assessment of Information Extraction in Biology (BioCreAtIvE) (Hirschman, Yeh et al., 2005). This challenge evaluation was an outgrowth of an earlier effort aiming to identify articles containing experimental evidence for *Drosophila* gene products (Yeh, Hirschman et al., 2003). The first BioCreAtIvE took place in 2004 and had two general tasks: extraction of gene and protein names (Task 1A) (Yeh, Morgan et al., 2005) and their mapping to standardized gene identifiers (Task 1B) (Hirschman, Colosimo et al., 2005) as well as mapping sentences in full-text articles to Gene Ontology annotations (Task 2) (Blaschke, Leon et al., 2005). A total of 27 research groups from 10 countries participated. Many groups achieved balanced F scores in the range of 0.8–0.9, although the results of functional annotation were much lower. The tagged corpora continue to be available for research use (http://biocreative.sourceforge.net/biocreative_1.html). A second Bio-CreAtIvE challenge evaluation was held in 2007 with similar tasks of gene mention tagging, gene normalization, and extraction of protein-protein interactions from text (http://biocreative.sourceforge.net/biocreative_2.html).

A variety of other corpora have been made available and widely used. Probably the most frequently employed of these is the GENIA corpus (http://www-tsujii.is.s.u-tokyo.ac.jp/GENIA/) (Kim, Ohta et al., 2003). This annotated corpus contains

2,000 MEDLINE abstracts collected using the search terms human, transcription factors, and blood cells. Technical term information such as the names of substances, biological sources, and other terms relevant to biological events are marked up with their semantic class in an XML format. The original version of the corpus provided part-of-speech tagging as well and was recently extended to include biological events, such as regulation and binding (Kim, Ohta et al., 2008). Another corpus for research is the Bio Information Extraction Resource (BioInfer, http://mars.cs.utu.fi/BioInfer/), a collection of 1,110 sentences tagged for gene, protein, and RNA relationships (Pyysalo, Ginter et al., 2007a). Both GENIA and BioInfer have recently been reformatted to adhere to the Stanford dependency scheme (Pyysalo, Ginter et al., 2007b). Another collection of literature available for text mining consists of more than 30,000 articles that have been published by Biomed Central (http://www.biomedcentral.com/info/about/datamining/). It should be noted that most of the above corpora are relatively small, at least compared to IR test collections, such that generalization of results with them may not be justified.

9.2 Text Categorization

The goal of *text categorization* is to assign documents into specific categories, usually based on their subject matter or document type (Lewis, 1995; Sebastiani, 2005). In the former type of category, a news producer or scientific journal may aim to assign documents to specific subject headings. In the latter type of category, documents may be classified as having certain attributes. One common categorization task in biomedicine is the determination of whether a document has experimental data suitable for extraction into a database or results appropriate for evidence-based medicine (EBM). Related to text categorization is *document routing or filtering*, which differs in that the goal is to identify relevant documents from a new stream based on queries modified by those already retrieved and determined to be relevant. The document-routing task can be viewed as a form of relevance feedback, since all documents are returned to the user in a ranked order. With filtering, however, a categorization decision is made, which is whether or not to return a document to the user. The early TREC forums featured a routing task, while a filtering track was introduced in TREC-5 (Lewis, 1996).

Text categorization and document filtering are usually evaluated with some sort of *utility score* that includes a penalty for nonrelevant documents that are retrieved:

$$\text{Utility} = (u_r * \text{relevant documents retrieved}) \\ + (u_{nr} * \text{nonrelevant documents retrieved}), \tag{9.1}$$

where u_r and u_{nr} are relative utilities of the value of retrieving relevant and nonrelevant documents, respectively. In the TREC Filtering Track, the values of u_r and u_{nr} were usually set at 2 and -1 (Robertson and Soboroff, 2001).

The early test collections for routing and filtering came from Reuters news service data (http://www.reuters.com/). As such, the task motivating initial text categorization research was the classification of news stories by topic, people, places, and so forth. An early widely used resource was the Reuters-21578 collection, which was later superseded by a new collection of more recent documents and categories (Lewis, Yang et al., 2004). Other document collections have been used for text categorization research in TREC and other settings, including MEDLINE records from the OHSUMED test collection (Robertson and Hull, 2000).

The TREC Filtering Track simulated two types of filtering, adaptive and batch (Robertson and Hull, 2000). In *adaptive filtering*, the documents are "released" to the system one at a time, and only documents chosen for retrieval can be used to modify the filtering query. In *batch filtering*, all documents and their relevance judgments can be used at once. Similar to other TREC tasks and tracks, participants in the filtering track have used a variety of methods, which yield a wide spectrum of performance (Robertson and Hull, 2000). In general, most approaches have aimed to optimize document weighting and then identify a threshold that maximizes inclusion of relevant document and discards nonrelevant ones. Some have used machine-learning techniques, such as neural networks or logistic regression, although their results have not exceeded simpler term-weighting approaches.

Yang (1999) performed a large-scale comparison of different approaches to text categorization. A baseline method used a simple word-matching approach between category words and documents, with no learning. The most effective methods, each achieving comparable performance, were:

1. k-Nearest neighbor (kNN): the documents most similar (i.e., the nearest neighbors) to the training documents were ranked and top k documents used to rank the best-fitting categories
2. Linear least-squares fit (LLSF): a multivariate regression model was used to map document vectors into categories
3. Neural network: a neural network was used to map document words into categories

Text categorization techniques have also been applied in a variety of biomedical examples. Yang and Chute (1994) found the LLSF method to be far more effective than simple word matching for retrieval of MEDLINE documents and classification of surgical reports into 281 International Classification of Diseases-9-CM (ICD-9-CM) categories. Larkey and Croft (1996) performed similar experiments with a collection of discharge summaries classified into ICD-9-CM codes, finding that a combination of kNN, relevance feedback, and Bayesian classifiers worked more effectively in combination than any single one individually. Ruch (2006) has found that MEDLINE references can be effectively categorized into MeSH and GO categories, with the former being easier due to its broader coverage and terms expressed as they are commonly used within the literature.

Another approach has used the measure of *term strength*, defined as the probability of finding a term in a document that is closely related to, or relevant to, any document in which the term has already occurred (Wilbur and Yang, 1996). Used mainly as a relevance feedback device, this approach has been found to perform comparable to LLSF. Perhaps the most important aspect of this approach is its use in the "related articles" feature of PubMed (see Chap. 5).

A major biomedical text categorization effort was the categorization task of the TREC Genomics Track, run in 2004 and 2005. The mail goal of the task was to "triage" articles for human annotators in the Mouse Genome Informatics (MGI) system (http://www.informatics.jax.org/). Systems were required to classify full-text documents from a 2-year span (2002–2003) of three journals, with the first year's (2002) documents comprising the training data and the second year's (2003) documents making up the test data.

One of the goals of MGI is to provide structured, coded annotation of gene function from the biological literature. Human curators identify genes and assign Gene Ontology and other codes about gene function with another code describing the type of experimental evidence supporting assignment of the code. The huge amount of literature requiring curation creates a challenge for MGI, as their resources are not unlimited. As such, they employ a three-step process to identify the papers most likely to describe gene function:

1. *About mouse.* The first step is to identify articles about mouse genomics biology. The full text of articles from several hundred journals is searched for the words *mouse*, *mice*, or *murine*. Articles passing this step are further analyzed for inclusion in MGI. At present, articles are searched in a Web browser one at a time because full-text searching is not available for all the journals included in MGI.
2. *Triage.* The second step is to determine whether the identified articles should be sent for curation. MGI curates articles not only for GO terms, but also for other aspects of biology, such as gene mapping, gene expression data, phenotype description, and more. The goal of this triage process is to limit the number of articles sent to human curators for more exhaustive analysis. Articles that pass this step go into the MGI system with a tag for GO, mapping, expression, etc. The rest of the articles do not go into MGI.
3. *Annotation.* The third step is the actual curation with GO and other terms. In the case of GO codes, curators identify genes for which there is experimental evidence to warrant assignment of codes, with another code for each indicating the type of experimental evidence. There can more than one gene assigned GO codes in a given paper and there can be more than one GO code assigned to a gene.

The TREC Genomics text categorization tasks focused on triage of articles since this function was believed by MGI to have the most value in automating. In addition, challenge evaluations such as Biocreative (described earlier) were already investigating annotation. The triage task basically considered designating whether or not an article should be designated for sending to a curator for annotation. Performance was assessed by the utility measure in (9.1), with the parameters u_r and u_{nr} tuned for each specific triage subtask. In TREC 2004, the triage task was to assign articles for GO annotation, whereas in 2005, the task was expanded to include triage for inclusion in databases about tumor biology (Krupke, Naf et al., 2005), embryologic gene expression (Hill, Begley et al., 2004), and alleles of mutant phenotypes (Strivens and Eppig, 2004).

The documents for the categorization task consisted of articles from three journals over 2 years published by Highwire Press (http://www.highwire.org/). The journals available and used by the task were *Journal of Biological Chemistry* (JBC), *Journal of Cell Biology* (JCB), and *Proceedings of the National Academy of Science* (PNAS). Each of the papers from these journals was provided in SGML format based on Highwire's Document Type Definition (DTD). Articles from the year 2002 were assigned as training data and articles from 2003 were assigned as test data.

The results from different groups are summarized in Table 9.5 and papers describing the task (Hersh, Cohen et al., 2005; Cohen and Hersh, 2006). These groups used a variety of NLP and machine-learning tasks, with a wide range of results. One notable finding across all groups was the GO triage task was substantially more difficult than the tumor biology, embryologic gene expression, or alleles of mutant phenotypes tasks. Very little could be done to improve triage of articles for GO annotation beyond the presence of the MeSH term `Mice`. Some additional work has used a subset of the TREC Categorization data to assess the detection of figures and their types for use as features (Shatkay, Chen et al., 2006).

Besides the TREC Genomics Track categorization task, there has only been a small amount of other work in text categorization that has focused on biomedical topics. One exception is effort of Cohen et al. (2006), who attempted to determine whether automated classification of document citations could be useful in reducing the time spent by experts reviewing journal articles for inclusion in updating systematic reviews of drug class efficacy for treatment of disease. They developed a voting perceptron-based automated citation classification system that classified articles as containing high-quality, drug class-specific evidence or not. Performance was assessed using crossvalidation experiments. They found that at the level of 95% recall, there was a reduction in the number of articles needing manual review in 11 of 15 drug review topics by as much as 50%. They concluded that automated document citation classification could be a useful tool in maintaining systematic reviews of the efficacy of drug therapy. Further work will refine the classification system and determine the best manner to integrate the system into the production of systematic reviews.

Table 9.5 Best and median utility scores for each subtask of the TREC Genomics text categorization task (adapted from Hersh, Cohen et al., 2005)

Subtask	Best utility	Median utility
A (allele)	0.871	0.7773
E (expression)	0.8711	0.6413
G (GO annotation)	0.587	0.4575
T (tumor)	0.9433	0.761

Another effort has focused on the identification of high-quality articles for use in EBM. Aphinyanaphongs et al. (2005, 2006) have shown that machine-learning approaches can improve on the identification of such articles (as determined by their inclusion in EBM publications such as *ACP Journal Club*) over the techniques used by the MEDLINE Clinical Queries algorithms of Haynes et al. (1994). These authors have also found ways to express these queries using Boolean operators, so they can be used in exact-match retrieval systems (Aphinyanaphongs and Aliferis, 2004). The work of these authors has also been extended to identifying unproven cancer treatments on the Web (Aphinyanaphongs and Aliferis, 2007).

A number of new interesting, if not controversial, techniques have emerged from text categorization research. One of these is plagiarism detection (a topic no doubt of interest to students!). Schleimer et al. (2003) describe a system for "document fingerprinting" that enables copies of documents and subdocuments within them. A growing cat-and-mouse environment has emerged as Web-based services make the purchase of term papers easier than ever, while the tools for detecting them are also more powerful due to their availability to crawl Web sites and compare student papers already entered into its database from the local purchaser and, sometimes, beyond. The controversies behind these tools have been enumerated by Foster (2002).

Another controversial use of text categorization is the prediction of author gender based on writing style (Ball, 2003). A group of researchers developed algorithms to predict author gender for a group of 566 English-language texts with about 80% accuracy (Koppel, Argamon et al., 2002; Argamon, Koppel et al., 2003). The controversy in their work was that it "confirmed" a number of gender stereotypes, e.g., men talk more about objects vs. women talking more about relationships and female writers using more pronouns. Their algorithms are also able to discern fiction vs. nonfiction with about 98% accuracy.

A more recent use of text categorization has spam email detection, i.e., classifying email as spam (Cormack and Lyman, 2007). Some of this work has emanated from the TREC Spam Track, which was started in TREC 2005 (Cormack and Lynam, 2005). Major challenges in evaluation spam detection have included the ever-changing approaches used by senders of spam as well as the difficulty in obtaining test collections due to private nature of individuals' email.

9.3   Question-Answering

One of the most common uses of an IR system is to answer questions, and such users may be more interested in finding answers rather than documents. Interest in this research problem led to formation of the TREC Question-Answering (QA) Track starting in TREC-8 and continuing ever since (Voorhees, 2005). Despite work on computer-generated answering to questions dating back decades (e.g., the LUNAR system to answer questions in a database about lunar rocks from space missions; Woods, 1970), the IR and biomedical informatics communities have only recently shown interest in this area.

9.3.1 TREC Question-Answering Track

A variety of tasks have been specified in the QA Track over the years, but a number of common themes have emerged. The original types of questions in the topics were *closed-class questions*, which assumed a definite answer in something like an NP, i.e., a fact, as opposed to a procedural answer. The questions came for a variety of sources, including track participants, NIST staff and assessors, and search engine question logs. Sample examples of questions include Who was the first American in Space? and Where is the Taj Mahal? Correct answers had to provide not only the document that answered the question, but also a span of text that contained the answer, with NIST assessors judging the submitted strings for correctness. Performance was measured by the mean reciprocal rank (MRR):

$$\text{MRR} = \frac{1}{\text{Rank of answer passage}} \qquad (9.2)$$

In early years of the QA Track, there were two subtasks: answers limited to 50-byte span and answers limited to 250-byte span. The best results for both tasks showed an MRR of around two-third. While most groups doing both tasks scored higher on the 250-byte task (i.e., it was easier), the best overall MRR sometimes came from the 50-byte task. When the answer was found, the document containing it tended to be ranked high. In general, traditional best-match document retrieval approaches worked reasonably well in the 250-byte task, but more linguistic processing was required for the 50-byte task. Examples of linguistic knowledge used for the latter included trying to identify people or organizations for "who" questions and time designations for "when" questions.

Some of the wrong answers to the sample questions above demonstrated the challenge of the task. In looking for answers to where the Taj Mahal was located, many of the newswire stories in the collection referred to the Taj Mahal Casino in Atlantic City, New Jersey, not the tomb in Agra, India. Likewise for the other question, one document referred to former California Governor Jerry Brown as someone "who has been called the first American in space" and some searches returned that answer accordingly.

In 2000, a 5-year plan for QA under the auspices of several U.S. government research agencies was developed (Burger, Cardie et al., 2000). This led in TREC 2001 for a new type of question to be added, list questions. In these questions, systems had to provide multiple instances, i.e., a list of answers. An example of this type of question was What are nine countries that have imported Cuban sugar? The list task run was scored by a measure of accuracy (i.e., the proportion of instances correct), with the range of the top 10 performing groups varying from 15 to 76%.

Another change after the release of the plan, implemented in TREC 2002, was a modification in closed-class questions to become "factoid" questions. These questions required return of a single exact answer, with questions ranked by the system's confidence in its answers. Answers for questions were assigned one of the following judgments: incorrect, not supported (answer correct but document does not support answer), not exact (returned string contains more than just answer or is missing bits of it), and correct. The latter was modified later into categories of locally correct (answer correct but later document contradicts it) and globally correct (answer correct and no later document contradicts it). A third type of question was added in TREC 2003, the definition question. In this type of question, several aspects of the definition were designated as "nuggets," with a subset of nuggets classified as "vital" to adequately provide the definition.

Performance was assessed via modification of recall and precision and their aggregation into an F score. Recall was calculated as the proportion of vital nuggets retrieved, i.e., vital nuggets retrieved/total vital nuggets. Precision was calculated as the number of correct vital nuggets provided, with a penalty for answers exceeding an allowable length, in this case 100 bytes. To encourage groups to pursue all three question types in TREC 2003, a combined score was derived for closed-class, list, and definition questions.

The most consistent performing group over the years in the QA Track has been Language Computer Corp. (LCC, http://www.languagecomputer.com/). A summary of their approach documents many components required for accurate question-answering (Moldovan, Pasca et al., 2003). These include:

- Keyword preprocessing – spelling correction and splitting or binding of words
- Construction of question representation – parsing of question to capture concepts and their dependencies
- Derivation of expected answer type – disambiguating semantic category of expected answers
- Selection of key words for searching
- Expansion of key words for searching based on morphological, lexical, or semantic alternations
- Retrieval of documents and passages – based on a Boolean query derived from previous steps
- Passage postfiltering – precision is enhanced by removing passages that do not satisfy semantic constraints of questions
- Identification of candidate answers – search within passages for answers based on expected types
- Answer ranking – based on relevance score calculated from lexical and proximity features
- Answer formulation – system selects candidate answers with highest relevance scores

Several loops of feedback within the modules have been shown to improve system performance on the TREC test collections. In addition, unlike IR, various applications of NLP in the different modules have provided measurable benefit, especially NER. Error analysis has shown that the most common errors based on TREC collections were in the derivation of the expected answer type, e.g., `area` was interpreted to mean a geographic region and not a geometric quantity, and incomplete keyword expansion, e.g., the word `murder` was not expanded to include synonyms such as `homicide`.

9.3.2 Biomedical Question-Answering

Early work in biomedical QA assessed its feasibility. For example, Zweigenbaum (2003) explored the task and resources for it. He noted that medical QA had some different attributes than general QA. For example, biomedical language is highly specialized, some sources are considered trustworthy and others are not, and the availability of sources is modest, at least relative to the types of content for general QA. Rinaldi et al. (2004) explored the steps necessary to convert a general QA system to answering questions about genomics. They found that the key challenges were selecting the appropriate part of the document for extracting information, handling the technical language of genomics and its synonymy and polysemy, and being able to accurately parse text.

Other research has focused in the clinical domain, with a particular emphasis on answering questions in EBM. These types of questions may be more amenable to QA techniques because they tend to fit a semantic pattern, i.e., the patient–intervention–comparison–outcome (PICO) format introduced in Chap. 2, and they often have an answer. Niu and colleagues, however, have noted a number of challenges. For example, while NER has been shown to be essential for general QA (Moldovan, Pasca et al., 2003), there are several aspects of clinical questions that are not named entities, such as some outcomes of clinical studies (Niu, Hirst et al., 2003). The latter may be nouns (e.g., `death`), verbs (e.g., `improve`), or adjectives (e.g., `adverse`), and sometimes the outcome is even something that did not occur (e.g., `no difference in death rates`). This placed importance on the proper identification of semantic classes in medical texts based on the PICO framework (Niu and Hirst, 2004) and the ability to detect the correct clinical outcome and its polarity (Niu, Zhu et al., 2006).

This foundational work has led to systems being developed and evaluated to perform QA of EBM questions. Demner-Fushman and Lin (2007) developed a system that aimed to answer EBM questions. They implemented a system based on a suite of "knowledge extractors" aiming to process the text of MEDLINE abstracts into the PICO framework, determine the strength of evidence of the article, and determine the EBM task, i.e., treatment, diagnosis, prognosis, or harm. These attributes are then matched up against EBM questions that come from users. An evaluation found the system improved substantially over the PubMed baseline in terms of ranking documents overall as well as putting answers to the questions into the top 5 documents retrieved.

Sneiderman et al. (2007) compared a variety of research and operational systems available at NLM for finding answers to EBM questions, including PubMed, Essie (Ide, Loane et al., 2007), SemRep Summarization (Fiszman, Rindflesch et al., 2004a), and a prototype called CQA-1.0 that used elements of the PICO approach described in the previous paragraph. In addition, the authors explored fusion of results from combinations of these systems. They developed three sets of five questions each, which they called general questions (similar to definition questions in the TREC QA Track), specific questions (requiring yes/no or factoid answers), and intermediate questions (requiring more than an overview but are not focused enough for an exact answer). Based on a variety of measures (e.g., mean average precision, precision at N documents, and others), the fusion approaches performed best. However, Essie performed best individually for general questions, while CQA-1.0 performed best individually for intermediate and specific questions. The authors concluded that both the structuring based on the PICO format and the robust concept detection are required for robust clinical QA.

The MedQA system (http://monkey.ims.uwm.edu:8080/MedQA/) has been designed to answer definition questions (Yu, Lee et al., 2007). These are the approximately half of questions from the Ely et al. taxonomy that begin with the word "What." MedQA performs a number of steps to provide its answers:

- Question classification – assuring the question is of a format it can answer and parsing the NP for searching
- Document retrieval – from MEDLINE and several high-quality Web sources
- Answer extraction – identifying the sentences that provide answers
- Summarizing – removal of redundant sentences containing answers
- Answer formulation – generating a coherent summary
- Presentation – providing the summary to the user

MedQA was evaluated using 12 questions extracted from an archive of clinical questions at the NLM (http://clinques.nlm.nih.gov/). Four physicians participated, posing questions to MedQA or three other search systems: PubMed, Google, and OneLook (http://www.onelook.com/), a commercial dictionary site. The results showed that the highest quality (subjectively assessed) answer and ease of use came from Google, although MedQA had the lowest time spent to find an answer and number of actions required to obtain it.

9.3.3 TREC Genomics Track Entity-Based Question-Answering Task

Another initiative that exploring question-answering in the biomedical domain has been the TREC Genomics Track. In 2006 and 2007, the track implemented a task that covered *entity-based question-answering* (Hersh, Cohen et al., 2006, 2007). The rationale for this was that what many information seekers, especially users of the biomedical literature, really desire is something in the middle between IR and IE, i.e., a system that attempts to provide short, specific answers to questions and puts them in context by providing supporting information and linking to original sources. As such, the track developed a new task that focused on retrieval of short passages (from phrase to sentence to paragraph in length) that specifically addressed an information need, along with linkage to the location in the original source document. Figure 9.4 shows the relationship among passages, the entities they contained, and the documents in which they occurred.

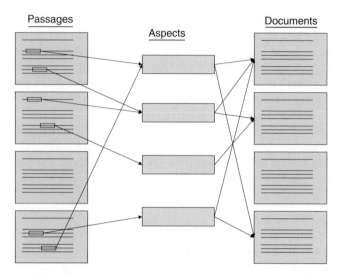

Fig. 9.4 Relationship among passages, the entities they contained, and the documents in which they occurred in the TREC Genomics entity-based question-answering task

Topics were expressed as questions and systems were measured on how well they retrieved relevant information at the passage, aspect, and document levels. Systems were required to return passages linked to source documents, while relevance judges not only rated the passages, but also grouped them by aspect. For this task, aspect was defined similar to its definition in the TREC Interactive Track aspectual recall task (Hersh, 2001), representing answers that covered a similar portion of a full answer to the topic question. The track also drew upon experience in passage retrieval from the previous TREC High Accuracy Retrieval from Documents (HARD) Track (Allan, 2003, 2004).

The documents for this task came from a new full-text biomedical corpus, as track members had also advocated a move from bibliographic (MEDLINE) to full-text documents (journal articles). Permission was obtained from a number of publishers who used Highwire Press (http://www.highwire.org/) for electronic distribution of their journals. Those publishers agreed to allow use of their full text in HTML format, which preserved formatting, structure, table and figure legends, etc. The document collection was derived from 49 journals and contained 162,259 documents, which was about 12.3 GB in size when uncompressed. In addition to the full-text data, the NLM provided MEDLINE records for the full-text documents in the collection.

Some additional files were made available:

- A text file, metadata.txt listed the original URL of the article, the file name in this collection, and its size in kilobytes. The name of each document file was its PMID plus the extension.html, which facilitated accessing the associated MEDLINE record.

- Another file, legalspans.txt, contained all "legal spans" for all documents in the collection. Legal spans were defined as any contiguous text > 0 characters in length not including any HTML paragraph tags, defined as any tag that started with <P or </P (case insensitive). There were a total of 12,641,127 legal spans in the collection. These were used to define allowed passages in the pooling and evaluation process, and to limit the size of the passages that needed reviewing by the expert judges.

Retrieved passages could contain any span of text that did not include any part of an HTML paragraph tag (i.e., one starting with <P or </P). Because there was some confusion about the different types of passages, the following terms were defined:

- *Nominated passage.* This was the passage that systems nominated in their runs and were scored in the passage retrieval evaluation. To be legal, these passages had to be a subset of a maximum-length legal span.
- *Maximum-length legal span.* These were all the passages obtained by delimited the text of each document by the HTML paragraph tags. As noted below, nominated passages could not cross an HTML paragraph boundary. So these spans represented the longest possible passage that could be designated as relevant. These spans were also used to build pools for the relevance judges. The judges did not need to designate the entire span as relevant and could select just a part of the span as the relevant passage.
- *Relevant passage.* These were the spans that the judges designated as definitely or possibly relevant.

These span definitions can be illustrated with the following example:

```
0000000000011111111112222222222333333333344444444445
01234567890123456789012345678901234567890123456789 0
Aaa. <p> Bbbbb <b>cc</b> ddd. <p><p><p> Eee ff ggg.
```

The last line of the example is sample text from an HTML file hypothetically named 12345.html (i.e., having PMID 12345). The numbers above the text represent the tens (top line) and ones (middle) digits for the file position in bytes. The maximum-length legal spans in this example are from bytes 0–4, 8–29, and 39–50. Let us consider the span 8–29 further. This is a maximum-length legal span because there is an HTML paragraph tag on either side of it. If a system nominated a passage that exceeded these boundaries, it will be disqualified for further analysis or judgment. But anything within the maximum-length legal span, e.g., 8–19, 18–19, or 18–28, could be nominated or relevant passages.

9.3.3.1   TREC 2006 Genomics Track

The first running of the task took place in 2006, with the topics expressed as questions (Hersh, Cohen et al., 2006). They were derived from the set of biologically relevant questions based on the Generic Topic Types (GTTs, described in Sect. 8.1.3.3) developed for the 2005 track (Hersh, Cohen et al., 2005). The questions (and GTTs) all had the general format of containing one or more biological objects and processes and some explicit relationship between them. The biological objects might be genes, proteins, gene mutations, etc. The biological process could be physiological processes or diseases. The relationships could be anything, but were typically verbs such as *causes*, *contributes to*, *affects*, *associated with*, or *regulates*. The GTTs, questions patterns for them, and examples are shown in Table 9.6.

The relevance assessments were done by the usual TREC method of pooling the top-ranking passages from different groups that submitted official runs. For each topic, a pool of passages was created that consisted of maximum-length spans from those passages there were retrieved. The relevance judges were experts (usually having a PhD) who were provided with guidelines and a training session to improve the judging process. To assess relevance, judges were instructed to break down the question into required elements (e.g., the biological entities and processes that make up the GTT) and isolate the minimum contiguous substring that answered the question. In general, a passage was definitely relevant if it contained all required elements of the question and it answered the question. A passage was possibly relevant if it contained the majority of required elements, missing elements were within the realm of possibility (i.e., more general terms are mentioned that probably include the missing elements), and it possibly answered the question.

After determining the "best" answer passages, judges were instructed to group them into related concepts and then assign one or more MeSH terms (possibly with subheadings) to capture similarities and differences among retrieved passage aspects. They were told to use the most specific MeSH term, with the option of adding subheadings, similar to the NLM literature indexing process. If one term was insufficient to denote all aspects of the gold standard passage, judges assigned additional MeSH terms. All passages judged as definitely or possibly relevant were required to have a gold standard passage and at least one MeSH term. For all the topics, the mean number of relevant passages was 35 (range 3–593), with a mean

Table 9.6 Generic topic types used in the TREC 2006 Genomics Track

GTT	Question pattern	Example
Find articles describing the role of a gene involved in a given disease.	What is the role of gene in disease?	What is the role of DRD4 in alcoholism?
Find articles describing the role of a gene in a specific biological process.	What effect does gene have on biological process?	What effect does the insulin receptor gene have on tumorigenesis?
Find articles describing interactions (e.g., promote, suppress, inhibit, etc.) between two or more genes in the function of an organ or in a disease.	How do genes interact in organ function?	How do HMG and HMGB1 interact in hepatitis?
Find articles describing one or more mutations of a given gene and its biological impact.	How does a mutation in gene influence biological process?	How does a mutation in Ret influence thyroid function?

relevant passage length of 400 characters (range 27–6,928). There were an average of 22 distinct relevant aspects per topic (range 7–96).

For this entity-based, question-answering task, there were three levels of retrieval performance measured: passage retrieval, aspect retrieval, and document retrieval. Each of these provided insight into the overall performance for a user trying to answer the given topic questions. Each was measured by some variant of MAP:

- *Passage-level MAP.* This measure used a variation of MAP, computing individual precision scores for passages based on character-level precision, using a variant of a similar approach used for the TREC 2004 HARD Track (Allan, 2004). For each nominated passage, the number of characters that overlapped with those deemed relevant by the judges in the gold standard was determined. For each relevant retrieved passage, precision was computed as the fraction of characters overlapping with the gold standard passages divided by the total number of characters included in all nominated passages from this system for the topic up until that point. Similar to regular MAP, remaining relevant passages that were not retrieved (no overlap with any nominated passages) were added into the calculation as well, with precision set to 0 for these relevant nonretrieved gold standard passages. Then, the mean of these average precisions over all topics was calculated to compute the MAP for passages.
- *Aspect-level MAP.* Aspect retrieval was measured using the average precision for the aspects of a topic, averaged across all topics. To compute this, for each submitted run, the ranked passages were transformed to two types of values, either the aspect(s) of the gold standard passage that the submitted passage overlapped with or the value "not relevant." This resulted in a ranked list, for each run and each topic, of lists of aspects per passage; nonrelevant passages had empty lists of aspects. Because of the uncertainty of the value for a user of a repeated aspect (e.g., same aspect occurring again further down the list), they discarded these from the output to be analyzed. For the remaining aspects of a topic, precision for the retrieval of each aspect was computed as the fraction of relevant passages for the retrieved passages up to the current passage under consideration. These fractions at each point of first aspect retrieval were then averaged together to compute the average aspect precision. Taking the mean over all topics produced the final aspect-based MAP.
- *Document-level MAP.* For the purposes of this measure, any PMID that had a passage associated with a topic ID in the set of gold standard passages was considered a relevant document for that topic. All other documents were considered not relevant for that topic. System run outputs were collapsed by PMID document identifier, with the documents appearing in the same order as the first time the corresponding PMID appeared in the nominated passages for that topic. For a given system run, average precision was measured at each point of correct (relevant) recall for a topic. The MAP was the mean of the average precisions across topics.

As shown in Table 9.8, document MAP scores were highest, followed by aspect, and then passage, although these scores were not directly comparable since they measured precision at recall of different things. There was a general, though far from perfect, correlation them. It was clear from the results and techniques of the top-performing groups in passage retrieval that certain approaches were quite effective. In particular, "trimming" passages to shorten them was done in all the runs with the highest passage MAP. Indeed, because noncontent manipulations of passages had substantial effects on passage MAP, an alternative passage MAP (passage2) that calculated MAP as if each character in each passage were a ranked document was developed for additional analysis and use in the TREC 2007 Genomics Track.

A further analysis showed that four factors were associated with the best performance in passage MAP (Rekapalli, Cohen et al., 2007):

- Normalization of keywords in the query into root forms
- Use of the Entrez Gene thesaurus for synonym terms expansion
- Unit of text retrieved using respective IR algorithms at sentence level
- Passage "trimming" to best sentence

9.3.3.2   TREC 2007 Genomics Track

The TREC 2007 Genomics Track continued with the same task and document collection, but some modifications to the topics and relevance judging were made, along with adoption of a new official measure of passage retrieval performance (Hersh, Cohen et al., 2007). There were 36 official topics for the track in 2007, which were in the form of questions asking for lists of specific entities. As in the past, information needs were gathered from working biologists. In addition to asking about information needs, there biologists were asked if their desired answer was a list of a certain type of entity, such as genes, proteins, diseases, mutations, etc., and if so, to designate that entity type. An example topic was:

What [GENES] are genetically linked to alcoholism?

Answers to this question were passages that related one or more entities of type GENE to alcoholism. For example, a valid and relevant answer to this topic would be, The DRD4 VNTR polymorphism moderates craving after alcohol consumption (from PMID 11950104). And the GENE entity supported by this statement would be DRD4. Table 9.7 shows the entities, their definitions, potential sources of terms, and topics with each entity type.

Relevance judging was once again by pooling of top-ranking passages retrieved by participating groups. Judges were required to have significant domain knowledge, typically in the form of a PhD in a life science. They were trained using a 12-page manual and a 1-h videoconference. They were given the following instructions:

1. Review the topic question and identify key concepts.
2. Identify relevant paragraphs and select minimum complete and correct excerpts.
3. Develop controlled vocabulary for entities based on the relevant passages and code entities for each relevant passage based on this vocabulary.

Table 9.7 TREC 2007 Genomics Track entities, their definitions, potential sources of terms, and topics with each entity type

Entity type	Definition	Potential source of terms	Topics with entity type
Antibodies	Immunoglobulin molecules having a specific amino acid sequence by virtue of which they interact only with the antigen (or a very similar shape) that induced their synthesis in cells of the lymphoid series (especially plasma cells).	MeSH	1
Biological substances	Chemical compounds that are produced by a living organism.	MeSH	3
Cell or tissue types	A distinct morphological or functional form of cell, or the name of a collection of interconnected cells that perform a similar function within an organism.	MeSH	2
Diseases	A definite pathologic process with a characteristic set of signs and symptoms. It may affect the whole body or any of its parts, and its etiology, pathology, and prognosis may be known or unknown.	MeSH	1
Drugs	A pharmaceutical preparation intended for human or veterinary use.	MEDLINEplus	2
Genes	Specific sequences of nucleotides along a molecule of DNA (or, in the case of some viruses, RNA) which represent functional units of heredity.	iHoP, Harvester	11
Molecular functions	Elemental activities, such as catalysis or binding, describing the actions of a gene product or bioactive substance at the molecular level.	GO	2
Mutations	Any detectable and heritable change in the genetic material that causes a change in the genotype and which is transmitted to daughter cells and to succeeding generations.	MeSH	1
Pathways	A series of biochemical reactions occurring within a cell to modify a chemical substance or transduce an extracellular signal.	BioCarta, KEGG	2
Proteins	Linear polypeptides that are synthesized on ribosomes and may be further modified, crosslinked, cleaved, or assembled into complex proteins with several subunits.	MeSH	5
Strains	A genetic subtype or variant of a virus or bacterium.	Ad hoc	2

(continued)

Table 9.7 (continued)

Signs or symptoms	A sensation or subjective change in health function experienced by a patient, or an objective indication of some medical fact or quality that is detected by a physician during a physical examination of a patient.	MeSH	1
Toxicities	A measure of the degree and the manner in which something is toxic or poisonous to a living organism.	MeSH	2
Tumor types	An abnormal growth of tissue, originating from a specific tissue of origin or cell type, and having defined characteristic properties, such as a recognized histology.	MeSH	1

There were an average of 124.8 relevant passages containing an average of 72.3 aspects from 69.2 relevant documents per topic. The mean relevant passage length was 968, with an average of 1.63 aspects per relevant passage.

The performance measures were similar to those used in 2006, with the exception of an alternative passage MAP (passage2) that calculated MAP as if each character in each passage were a ranked document. In essence, the output of passages was concatenated, with each character being from a relevant passage or not. Table 9.8 shows the minimum, median, mean, and maximum for the official results from the TREC 2006–2007 Genomics Track task.

The level of performance of the top systems for 2007 was somewhat lower than for 2006. This may have been due to list entity-type questions being more difficult to answer than the GTT questions. This would not be unexpected since list entity questions were more open-ended, involved more different entity types, and were closer to natural language than the GTT question used in 2006. The top systems did consistently well on all measures, and the measures were highly correlated. Unlike the 2006 track, the aspect MAP measure was a meaningful measure of system topic coverage in 2007. While the range of the average number of aspects per relevant passages was low (1–3), the number of aspects per topic was relatively high (could be over 300). Therefore, for a system to do well on the aspect MAP measure, a number of passages with complementary aspect information would have to be retrieved and ranked highly since, for most topics, almost no single passages would cover all the required entities.

9.4 Text Summarization

Another important area related to IR is text summarization, which is the process of distilling the most important information from documents to produce a shorter version for specific users and/or tasks (Mani and Maybury, 1999). There is a long history of research in automated summarization dating back to the 1950s (Luhn,

Table 9.8 Overall results from TREC 2006–2007 Genomics Track task (adapted from Hersh, Cohen et al., 2006, 2007)

	Passage2 MAP	Passage MAP	Aspect MAP	Document MAP
TREC 2006				
Min	0.0007	0.0019	0.0110	0.0198
Median	0.0345	0.0316	0.1581	0.3083
Mean	0.0392	0.0347	0.1643	0.2887
Max	0.1486	0.1012	0.4411	0.5439
TREC 2007				
Min	0.0008	0.0029	0.0197	0.0329
Median	0.0377	0.0565	0.1311	0.1897
Mean	0.0398	0.0560	0.1326	0.1862
Max	0.1148	0.0976	0.2631	0.3286

1958; Edmunson, 1969). Now, however, there are a variety of commercial text summarization systems available, including the AutoSummarize facility in the Microsoft Word application (Microsoft Corp., http://www.microsoft.com/).

Manually generated summaries of documents have been around for centuries. Probably the best-known summary of a document is the abstract that accompanies a scientific paper. In essence, however, all documents are summaries in the sense that even full documents are abstractions of reality, as noted by Mani (2001). However, he does point out that summarization, as the term is commonly used, usually refers to a condensed version of a longer document. Mani also has created a diagram that shows all the parameters that modify the output of an automatic summarization system (see Fig. 9.5).

There are two types of output from text summarization systems: *extracts*, consisting of material copied from one or documents; and *abstracts*, consisting of material not present in the original document(s), such as more general terms or paraphrased content. Summaries may be of single or multiple documents. Mani and Maybury (1999) have noted three important characteristics of automatically generated summaries:

1. Reduction – the compression or condensation rate, measuring the length of the summary, usually in words, divided by the length of the original source
2. Informativeness – how the relevant information is to the user
3. Well-formedness – how well extracts avoid gaps, ambiguous anaphors, and incoherent reductions in lists and tables and the readability of output produced from abstracts

Afantenos et al. (2005) have reviewed automatic summarization in the context of biomedicine. In addition to highlighting important work, they presented a list of factors influencing the output of summarization systems:

- Input factors

  o Single vs. multiple document

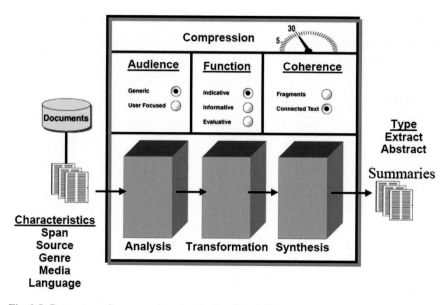

Fig. 9.5 Parameters of automated summarization (Mani, 2001)

- ○ Language
- ○ Text vs. multimedia

- • Purpose factors

  - ○ Informative vs. indicative – former aims to substitute for longer document, whereas latter just describes what the document covers
  - ○ Generic vs. user-oriented former takes into account all information in document, whereas latter is focused toward needs of a user as expressed by a query
  - ○ General purpose vs. domain-specific – former employs generic techniques, whereas latter utilizes resources from a given domain

- • Output factors

  - ○ Abstract vs. extract
  - ○ Quality – how well does summary meet intended purpose?
  - ○ Length – how long is summary?

An ideal summarization would allow these parameters to be set and then create an appropriate summary.

The growing amount of textual information on the Web and in the scientific literature has increased interest in text summarization. A prototypical use case comes from the biological world. Many scientists increasingly use so-called "high-throughput" biotechnologies that generate massive amounts of data. A gene microarray, for example, may measure 10,000 genes or gene polymorphisms

(Mobasheri, Airley et al., 2004). Likewise, genome-wide association studies may find associations between gene variations and phenotypic characteristics in living organisms (Christensen and Murray, 2007). Both these kinds of studies may identify dozens or even hundreds of genes about which information must be obtained. Yet there may be hundreds or even thousands of articles about each gene and/or its variants. Although the state of the art of text summarization is not to this point yet, a system that could properly summarize information from documents about each gene could be extraordinarily useful to scientists performing this kind of biomedical research.

Of the two general summarization tasks, extraction has proved easier than abstraction. Extraction systems have often focused on using machine-learning techniques to learn the best features of informative sentences for summarization. Some of the features used to determine which sentences to extract include the following:

1. Location – in document or specific part (e.g., section, title, introduction, or conclusion)
2. Thematic – presence of statistically important terms in sentence (e.g., those with high TF*IDF)
3. Fixed phrases – those giving cues (e.g., "in summary") or emphasis (e.g., "in particular") to important sentences
4. Weight – added to text units containing terms in title, heading, opening paragraph, or user's interests
5. Cohesion – text units connected based on repetition or presence of synonyms

Abstraction usually requires some sort of NLP. Documents are usually processed to slot important features into a template or to recognize key concepts. From this representation, summaries are generated into some narrative form based on the other factors desired, including length.

There are many other comparable use cases outside biomedicine (Teufel and Moens, 2002). One of the leading available systems for summarization is MEAD (Radev, Jing et al., 2000), which has been used in a variety of applications, including news summarization (Radev, Otterbacher et al., 2005). MEAD is available as part of the CLAIRLIB system (http://www.clairlib.org/).

Evaluation of summarization systems has been challenging. Although we noted in earlier chapters that relevance and the evaluation of IR systems was somewhat subjective, evaluation of what constitutes a "good" summary is probably even more so. Radev et al. (2003) have explored the challenges in evaluation of summarization, noting there are two general approaches:

1. Intrinsic – evaluation independent of purpose summary aims to serve. Factors that can be assessed include the grammatical quality, such as the integrity of sentences and readability, or word or phrase overlap with some gold standard summary created by a human. The latter is very challenging, since human summarizers tend to create very different summaries and the overlap of words or phrases is not a guarantee that there is true conceptual overlap.

2. Extrinsic – evaluation of summary for a specific task, usually by human judges.

Radev et al. (2003) also provide a classification of evaluation measures:

- Coselection measures – measures of selection of extracts judged by humans to represent important sentences. These include recall, precision, kappa, and relative utility. The first three were defined in Chap. 1, while the latter is used by having judges assign a relative score (usually on a 1–10 scale) for sentences and include them in a cluster of similar sentences. These measures cannot be used with abstracts.
- Similarity measures – measures of similarity with manual summaries. These include the cosine measure, introduced in this chapter, and the longest common subsequence, which measures the minimum number of steps needed to transform one string into another.
- Relevance correlation – measures the relative decrease in retrieval performance of summaries when they replace full documents in IR experiments. This approach was motivated by work of Sparck-Jones and Sakai (2001), who found that document summaries achieved good precision when substituted for full documents, although the results were not as good for recall.

Interest in information summarization evaluation has led to the development of the Document Understanding Conference (DUC, http://duc.nist.gov/). Organized by NIST, it is run similar to TREC. DUC has been guided by a roadmap developed by leading researchers in the field (Carbonell, Harman et al., 2000). DUC has also allowed assessment of various evaluation measures for summarization. A summary of results from DUC 2001–2004 noted that baseline approaches such as using the first sentence of a document were difficult to outperform, although it was also found that there was a variety of "performance" of human summarizers, i.e., those having their summaries reviewed the same processes as automated systems, with the latter falling within the range of performance of the former (Nenkova, 2005).

The main task of DUC in recent years has been aimed to model "real-world complex question-answering" as suggested by Amigo et al. (2004). This has been operationalized by providing a topic and set of relevant documents, with systems required to create an approximately 250-word summary that summarizes the topic based on the documents. DUC 2007 added an "update" task that required a shorter 100-word summary under the assumption of the user having read an earlier set of documents. The documents for DUC have been derived from the AQUAINT corpus (Graff, 2002).

A variety of evaluation approaches have been used. One is an assessment of summary quality by the NIST assessors who develop the topics (http://duc.nist.gov/duc2007/quality-questions.txt). They rate several factors on a 1 (very poor) to 5 (very good) scale, including the following:

1. *Grammaticality*. The summary should have no datelines, system-internal formatting, capitalization errors, or obviously ungrammatical sentences that make the text difficult to read.

2. *Nonredundancy*. There should be no unnecessary repetition in the summary, e.g., whole sentences that are repeated, or repeated facts, or the repeated use of a noun or NP when a pronoun is sufficient.
3. *Referential clarity*. It should be easy to identify who or what the pronouns and NPs in the summary are referring to. If a person or other entity is mentioned, their role in the story should be clear.
4. *Focus*. The summary should have a focus; sentences should only contain information that is related to the rest of the summary.
5. *Structure and coherence*. The summary should be well structured and well organized. It should not just be a heap of related information, but should build from sentence to sentence to a coherent body of information about a topic.

Other approaches look at language overlap with important words or phrases from "gold standard" summaries. An initial approach was the ROUGE system, which measures *n*-gram overlap from summaries generated by human experts (Lin and Hovy, 2003; Lin, 2004). More recently, ROUGE has been enhanced to calculate overlap of *basic elements*, which are NP heads or NPs that contain an attribute defined by a relationship (e.g., indicted|1991|time). Another approach has been the *pyramid method*, which has multiple human assessors create *summarization content units* (SCUs), weighted by how many assessors nominate the SCU (Nenkova and Passonneau, 2004). Other assessors then judge the presence or absence of the SCU in the automatically generated summary, calculating a pyramid score based on the summation of weights for SCUs present in the summary. Recent work has focused on developing automated approaches based on overlap between the words in the summary and SCUs (Harnly, Nenkova et al., 2005). Correlation between the measures of subjective assessment of summary quality and these word-overlap approaches has been in the range of 0.7–0.8 (Dang, 2006).

A variety of researchers have looked at automatic summarization in the biomedical domain. One large body of work came from the Personalized Search and Summarization over Multimedia Information (PERSIVAL, http://persival.cs.columbia.edu/) digital library project. Their approach used discharge summaries with mapping of terms in the cardiology domain to UMLS Metathesaurus concepts to retrieve and summarize articles (Elhadad, Kan et al., 2005). A less patient-specific approach has been taken in the Centrifuser system, which attempts to derive features of documents (e.g., topicality, content type, readability, etc.) and can be used to process the output of results from Web search engines (Kan, McKeown et al., 2001). This system processing Google output was compared with the regular output of three Web search engines (Google, Yahoo, and About.com) in a usability test employing 13 subjects searching on three medical topics: diabetes, hypertension, and asthma (Kushniruk, Kan et al., 2002). All four systems performed comparably, with strengths and weaknesses identified of each.

Additional work on summarization has come from researchers at the NLM, looking at both summaries of biomedical literature (Fiszman, Rindflesch et al., 2004a) and consumer health information (Fiszman, Rindflesch et al., 2004b). Both systems use a relatively common approach that proceeds through a number of steps.

The first step is to map document text into semantic propositions, consisting of two concepts and a relationship between them, e.g., `proton-pump inhibitors treat Zollinger-Ellison Syndrome`. The propositions are then transformed into a small set of specified predicates consisting of two semantic types linked by one of six relationships, such as CAUSES, TREATS, and LOCATIO-N_OF. These are then connected into a "conceptual condensate" that links the concepts together in a single graph. This is followed by a pruning operation that eliminates general concepts (i.e., those near the top of the terminology hierarchy). From this point, a narrative summary can be generated. An analysis of the approach applied to four conditions from a medical encyclopedia found that the text could be reduced 98% in size with an 87% precision (rate of correctness) (Fiszman, Rindflesch et al., 2004b). The precision for biomedical literature was lower, at 66% (Fiszman, Rindflesch et al., 2004a).

Other work has focused on the use case described earlier of summarizing information about genes. Ling et al. (2007) developed a system for developing a semistructured summary of a gene from articles in the biomedical literature. They evaluated their system using ROUGE with summaries developed by experts, finding it performed better than generic approaches such as those available in MEAD. Yang et al. (2007, 2008) developed a system that processed a list of genes (such as those upregulated in a microarray experiment) to cluster them and extract the most informative sentences, which were in turn linked to their MED-LINE records (and thus linked to their full text). They found that meaningful clusters could be generated and that users designated the nominated sentences as more informative than the article titles from PubMed.

References

Abbasi, K. (2004). Let's dump impact factors. *British Medical Journal,* 329. http://bmj.bmjjournals.com/cgi/content/full/329/7471/0-h.

Abraham, V., Friedman, C., et al. (1999). Student and faculty performance in clinical simulations with access to a searchable information resource. *Proceedings of the AMIA 1999 Annual Symposium,* Washington, DC. Hanley & Belfus. 648–652.

Adam, D. (2002). The counting house. *Nature,* 415: 726–728.

Afantenos, S., Karkaletsis, V., et al. (2005). Summarization from medical documents: a survey. *Artificial Intelligence in Medicine,* 33: 157–177.

Agger, B. (1990). *The Decline of Discourse: Reading, Writing, and Resistance in Postmodern Capitalism.* London, England. Taylor & Francis.

Agnew, G. and Kniesner, D. (2001). ViDe User's Guide: Dublin Core Application Profile for Digital Video, Video Development Initiative (ViDE). http://www.vide.net/workgroups/video-access/resources/vide_dc_userguide_20010909.pdf.

Agosti, M. (2008). *Information Access through Search Engines and Digital Libraries.* Dordrecht, The Netherlands. Springer.

Aisen, A., Broderick, L., et al. (2003). Automated storage and retrieval of thin-section CT images to assist diagnosis: system description and preliminary assessment. *Radiology,* 228: 265–270.

Aksnes, D. (2003). Characteristics of highly cited papers. *Research Evaluation,* 12: 159–170.

Aksnes, D. (2006). Citation rates and perceptions of scientific contribution. *Journal of the American Society for Information Science and Technology,* 57: 169–187.

Albert, K. (2006). Open access: implications for scholarly publishing and medical libraries. *Journal of the Medical Library Association,* 94: 253–262.

Albert, K. (2007). Integrating knowledge-based resources into the electronic health record: history, current status, and role of librarians. *Medical Reference Services Quarterly,* 26(3): 1–19.

Albert, R., Jeong, H., et al. (1999). Diameter of the World Wide Web. *Nature,* 401: 130–131.

Alderson, P. (2004). Absence of evidence is not evidence of absence. *British Medical Journal,* 328: 476–477.

Alex, B., Grover, C., et al. (2008). Assisted curation: does text mining really help? *Pacific Symposium on Biocomputing,* Big Island, Hawaii. World Scientific. 556–567.

Alfred, J. (2001). Mining the bibliome. *Nature Reviews – Genetics,* 2: 401.

Allan, J. (1997). Building hypertext using information retrieval. *Information Processing and Management,* 33: 145–160.

Allan, J. (2003). HARD Track overview in TREC 2003 – high accuracy retrieval from documents. *The Twelfth Text REtrieval Conference – TREC 2003,* Gaithersburg, MD. Naitonal Institute of Standards and Technology. 24–37. http://trec.nist.gov/pubs/trec12/papers/HARD.OVERVIEW.pdf.

Allan, J. (2004). HARD Track overview in TREC 2004 – high accuracy retrieval from documents. *The Thirteenth Text REtrieval Conference (TREC 2004),* Gaithersburg, MD. National Institute of Standards and Technology. http://trec.nist.gov/pubs/trec13/papers/HARD.OVERVIEW.pdf.

Allan, J., Aslam, J., (2003). Challenges in information retrieval and language modeling. *SIGIR Forum*, 37(1): 31–47. http://www.sigir.org/forum/S2003/ir-challenges2.pdf.

Allan, J., Carterette, B., et al. (2005). When will information retrieval be "good enough?": user effectiveness as a function of retrieval accuracy. *Proceedings of the 28th International ACM SIGIR Conference on Research and Development in Information Retrieval*, Salvador, Brazil. ACM Press. 443–440.

Allen, B. (1992). Cognitive differences in end-user searching of a CD-ROM index. *Proceedings of the 15th Annual International ACM SIGIR Conference on Research and Development in Information Retrieval*, Copenhagen, Denmark. ACM Press. 298–309.

Allen, J. (1995). *Natural Language Understanding*. Redwood City, CA. Benjamin-Cummings.

Almind, T. and Ingwersen, P. (1998). Informetric analyses on the World Wide Web: methodological approaches to 'webometrics'. *Journal of Documentation*, 53: 404–426.

Alper, B., Stevermer, J., et al. (2001). Answering family physicians' clinical questions using electronic medical databases. *Journal of Family Practice*, 50: 960–965.

Altman, D., Chalmers, I., et al. (2001). *Systematic Reviews in Healthcare: Meta-Analysis in Context*. Oxford, England. Blackwell.

Altman, L. (1996). The Ingelfinger rule, embargoes, and journal peer review—Part 1. *Lancet*, 347: 1382–1386.

Altman, M. and King, D. (2007). A proposed standard for the scholarly citation of quantitative data. *D-Lib Magazine*, 13(3/4). http://www.dlib.org/dlib/march07/altman/03altman.html.

Amigo, E., Gonzalo, J., et al. (2004). An empirical study of information synthesis task. *Proceedings of the 41st Annual Meeting of the Association for Computational Linguistics*, Barcelona, Spain. http://acl.ldc.upenn.edu/acl2004/main/pdf/303_pdf_2-col.pdf.

Ananiadou, S. and McNaught, J., eds. (2006). *Text Mining for Biology And Biomedicine*. Boston, MA. Artech House.

Anderson, N., Tarczy-Hornoch, P., (2006). On the persistence of supplementary resources in biomedical publications. *BMC Bioinformatics*, 7: 260. http://www.biomedcentral.com/1471–2105/7/260.

Anderson, P. and Allee, N., eds. (2004). *The MLA Encyclopedic Guide to Searching and Finding Health Information on the Web*. New York, NY. Neal-Schuman.

Ando, R., Dredze, M., et al. (2005). TREC 2005 Genomics Track experiments at IBM Watson. *The Fourteenth Text REtrieval Conference Proceedings (TREC 2005)*, Gaithersburg, MD. National Institute for Standards and Technology. http://trec.nist.gov/pubs/trec14/papers/ibm-tjwatson.geo.pdf.

Andrews, J. (2003). An author co-citation analysis of medical informatics. *Journal of the Medical Library Association*, 91: 47–56. http://www.pubmedcentral.nih.gov/articlerender.fcgi?artid=141187.

Angell, M. and Kassirer, J. (1991). The Ingelfinger rule revisited. *New England Journal of Medicine*, 325: 1371–1373.

Anonymous (1948). Streptomycin treatment of pulmonary tuberculosis. *British Medical Journal*, 30: 769–782.

Anonymous (1989). International Publishers Association (IPA) resolution on use of permanent papers in published works. *International Publishers' Bulletin*, 5: 9–10. http://www.librime.com/ipa_en.htm.

Anonymous (1992). Evidence-based medicine: a new approach to teaching the practice of medicine. Evidence-Based Medicine Working Group. *Journal of the American Medical Association*, 268: 2420–2425.

Anonymous (1997). Search engine road test: top three returns. *Medicine on the Net*, 3(4): 3.

Anonymous (1998). Quality First: Better Health Care for All Americans. Department of Health & Human Services. http://www.hcqualitycommission.gov/final/. Accessed: July 1, 2002.

Anonymous (2000). Organization of National Library of Medicine Bibliographic Databases. National Library of Medicine. http://www.nlm.nih.gov/pubs/techbull/mj00/mj00_buckets.html. Accessed: July 1, 2002.

Anonymous (2001a). AMA Survey Finds Upsurge in Physician Usage and Regard for Internet. American Medical Association. http://www.ama-assn.org/ama/pub/article/1616–4692.html. Accessed: July 1, 2002.

Anonymous (2001b). *Crossing the Quality Chasm: A New Health System for the 21st Century.* Washington, DC. National Academy Press.

Anonymous (2001c). The future of the electronic scientific literature. *Nature*, 413: 1–3.

Anonymous (2001d). Initial sequencing and analysis of the human genome. *Nature*, 409: 860–921.

Anonymous (2001e). Virtual "Treatments" Can Be Real-World Deceptions. Federal Trade Commission. http://www.ftc.gov/bcp/conline/pubs/alerts/mrclalrt.htm. Accessed: July 1, 2002.

Anonymous (2002a). ACP-ASIM Survey Finds Nearly Half of U.S. Members Use Handheld Computers. American College of Physicians. http://www.acponline.org/college/pressroom/handheld_survey.htm. Accessed: July 1, 2002.

Anonymous (2002b). Credibility on the Web. Consumers International. http://www.consumersinternational.org/newsdocs/{FAC5B4E3-2CC7-483A-9C46-92F8A0305602}.doc.

Anonymous (2002c). EBM: unmasking the ulgy truth. *British Medical Journal*, 325: 1496–1498.

Anonymous (2002d). Invisible Web: What it is, Why it exists, How to find it, and its Inherent Ambiguity. University of California Berkeley Library. http://www.lib.berkeley.edu/TeachingLib/Guides/Internet/InvisibleWeb.html.

Anonymous (2002e). Risks and benefits of estrogen plus progestin in healthy postmenopausal women – principal results from the women's health initiative randomized controlled trial. *Journal of the American Medical Association*, 288: 321–333.

Anonymous (2003). The Selection, Appraisal and Retention of Digital Scientific Data – ERPA-NET/CODATA Workshop Final Report. Lisbon, Portugal, Biblioteca Nacional. http://www.erpanet.org/events/2003/lisbon/LisbonReportFinal.pdf.

Anonymous (2004a). Addressing the limitations of structured abstracts. *Annals of Internal Medicine*, 140: 480–481.

Anonymous (2004b). Index medicus to cease as print publication. *NLM Technical Bulletin.* May-June, e2: 338. http://www.nlm.nih.gov/pubs/techbull/mj04/mj04_im.html.

Anonymous (2004c). Is GSK guilty of fraud? *Lancet*, 363: 1919.

Anonymous (2004d). MEDLINE/PubMed Subsets and Filters. Bethesda, MD, National Library of Medicine. http://locatorplus.gov/medlinesubsets.html.

Anonymous (2004e). Washington D.C. Principles For Free Access to Science – A Statement from Not-for-Profit Publishers. Washington, DC, Washington D.C Principles For Free Access to Science. http://www.dcprinciples.org/statement.pdf.

Anonymous (2005a). Authors' Manual: Abridged Policy, Submission Process and FAQ. Bethesda, MD, National Institutes of Health. http://publicaccess.nih.gov/publicaccess_manual.pdf.

Anonymous (2005b). Data Dictionary for Preservation Metadata – Final Report of the PREMIS Working Group. Dublin, OH, Online Computer Library Center. http://www.oclc.org/research/projects/pmwg/premis-final.pdf.

Anonymous (2005c). Fact Sheet – Medical Subject Headings (MeSH). Bethesda, MD, National Library of Medicine. http://www.nlm.nih.gov/pubs/factsheets/mesh.html.

Anonymous (2005d). Open access in medical publishing: trends and countertrends. *Canadian Medical Association Journal*, 172: 149.

Anonymous (2005e). Physician Internet Use Statistics. http://www.max.md/pdf/PhysicianInternetUseStatistics.pdf.

Anonymous (2005f). Policy on Enhancing Public Access to Archived Publications Resulting from NIH-Funded Research. Washington, DC, National Institutes of Health. http://grants.nih.gov/grants/guide/notice-files/NOT-OD-05–022.html.

Anonymous (2005g). Using Dublin Core – Dublin Core Qualifiers, Dublin Core Metadata Initiative. http://dublincore.org/documents/usageguide/qualifiers.shtml.

Anonymous (2006a). Charting a Course for the 21st Century – NLM's Long Range Plan 2006–2016. Bethesda, MD, National Library of Medicine. http://www.nlm.nih.gov/pubs/plan/lrp06/report/default.html.

Anonymous (2006b). Fact Sheet – PubMed: MEDLINE Retrieval on the World Wide Web. Bethesda, MD, National Library of Medicine. http://www.nlm.nih.gov/pubs/factsheets/pubmed.html.

Anonymous (2006c). Fatally Flawed – Refuting the Recent Study on Encyclopedic Accuracy by the Journal Nature. Chicago, IL, Encyclopedia Brittanica. http://corporate.britannica.com/britannica_nature_response.pdf.

Anonymous (2006d). Key MEDLINE Indicators. Bethesda, MD, National Library of Medicine. http://www.nlm.nih.gov/bsd/bsd_key.html.

Anonymous (2006e). Mass Digitization: Implications for Information Policy. Washington, DC, U. S. National Commission on Libraries and Information Science. http://www.nclis.gov/digitization/MassDigitizationSymposium-Report.pdf.

Anonymous (2006f). Overview: nature's peer review trial. *Nature*. http://www.nature.com/nature/peerreview/debate/nature05535.html.

Anonymous (2006g). Publication Characteristics (Publication Types) – Scope Notes. Bethesda, MD, National Library of Medicine. http://www.nlm.nih.gov/mesh/pubtypes2007.html.

Anonymous (2006h). Qualifier Hierarchies. Bethesda, MD, National Library of Medicine. http://www.nlm.nih.gov/mesh/subhierarchy2007.html.

Anonymous (2006i). Uniform Requirements for Manuscripts Submitted to Biomedical Journals: Writing and Editing for Biomedical Publication, International Committee of Medical Journal Editors. http://www.icmje.org/icmje.pdf.

Anonymous (2006j). What's the Difference Between MEDLINE and PubMed? Bethesda, MD, National Library of Medicine. http://www.nlm.nih.gov/pubs/factsheets/dif_med_pub.html.

Anonymous (2007a). 7/07 Health Information Site & 9/07 Pharmacy Site Ratings Methodology. Bethesda, MD, Health Improvement Institute. http://www.healthratings.org/2007/flash/pdfs/methodology3.pdf.

Anonymous (2007b). Agenda for Developing E-Science in Research Libraries – Final Report and Recommendations. Washington, DC, Association for Research Libraries. http://www.arl.org/bm~doc/ARL_EScience_final.pdf.

Anonymous (2007c). Appendices, in Anonymous, ed. *PubMed Help*. Bethesda, MD. National Library of Medicine. http://www.ncbi.nlm.nih.gov/books/bv.fcgi?rid=helppubmed.section.pubmedhelp.Appendices.

Anonymous (2007d). ClinicalTrials.gov Data Element Definitions. Bethesda, MD, National Library of Medicine. http://prsinfo.clinicaltrials.gov/definitions.html.

Anonymous (2007e). The Dublin Core Metadata Element Set. Bethesda, MD, National Information Standards Organization. http://www.niso.org/standards/resources/Z39-85-2007.pdf.

Anonymous (2007f). Fact Sheet – Errata, Retraction, Duplicate Publication, Comment, Update and Patient Summary Policy for MEDLINE. Bethesda, MD, National Library of Medicine. http://www.nlm.nih.gov/pubs/factsheets/errata.html.

Anonymous (2007g). Fact Sheet – MEDLINE. Bethesda, MD, National Library of Medicine. http://www.nlm.nih.gov/pubs/factsheets/medline.html.

Anonymous (2007h). Fact Sheet – MEDLINE Journal Selection. Bethesda, MD, National Library of Medicine. http://www.nlm.nih.gov/pubs/factsheets/jsel.html.

Anonymous (2007i). Frequently Asked Questions About Indexing. Bethesda, MD, National Library of Medicine. http://www.nlm.nih.gov/bsd/indexfaq.html.

Anonymous (2007j). Health Web Site Accreditation Standards, Version 2.0. Washington, DC, URAC. http://www.urac.org/docs/programs/HealthWebSiteAccreditationStandards.pdf.

Anonymous (2007k). Health Website Rating (HWR) Project – HII Health Website Rating Instrument (HWRI). Bethesda, MD, Health Improvement Institute. http://www.healthratings.org/2007/flash/pdfs/instrument3.pdf.

Anonymous (2007l). MEDLINE/PubMed Data Element (Field) Descriptions. Bethesda, MD, National Library of Medicine. http://www.nlm.nih.gov/bsd/mms/medlineelements.html.

Anonymous (2007m). Number of "Cyberchondriacs" – Adults Who Have Ever Gone Online for Health Information – Increases to an Estimated 160 Million Nationwide. Rochester, NY, Harris Interactive. http://www.harrisinteractive.com/harris_poll/index.asp?PID=792.

Anonymous (2007n). OLDMEDLINE Data. Bethesda, MD, National Library of Medicine. http://www.nlm.nih.gov/databases/databases_oldmedline.html.

Anonymous (2007o). Principles of MEDLINE Subject Indexing. Bethesda, MD, National Library of Medicine. http://www.nlm.nih.gov/bsd/disted/mesh/indexprinc.html.

Anonymous (2007p). Scientific Information in the Digital Age: Access, Dissemination and Preservation. Brussels, Belgium, European Commission. http://ec.europa.eu/research/science-society/document_library/pdf_06/communication-022007_en.pdf.

Anonymous (2007q). Searching PubMed, in Anonymous, ed. *PubMed Help*. Bethesda, MD. National Library of Medicine. http://www.ncbi.nlm.nih.gov/books/bv.fcgi?rid=helppubmed. section.pubmedhelp.Searching_PubMed.

Anonymous (2007r). SNOMED Clinical Terms User Guide. Northbrook, IL, College of American Pathologists. http://www.cap.org/apps/docs/snomed/documents/snomed_ct_user_guide.pdf.

Anonymous (2007s). SNOMED CT – The Language of the NHS Care Records Service – A Guide for NHS Staff in England. London, England, National Health Service. http://www.connecting-forhealth.nhs.uk/systemsandservices/data/snomed/snomed-ct-a.pdf.

Anonymous (2007t). *Stopwords*, in Anonymous, ed. *PubMed Help*. Bethesda, MD. National Library of Medicine. http://www.ncbi.nlm.nih.gov/books/bv.fcgi?highlight=stopwords&rid=helppubmed.table.pubmedhelp.T43.

Anonymous (2007u). *Thesaurus of Psychological Index Terms*, 11th Edition. Washington, DC. American Psychological Association.

Anonymous (2007v). The universal protein resource (UniProt). *Nucleic Acids Research*, 35: D193–D197.

Anonymous (2007w). Worldwide Internet Audience has Grown 10 Percent in Last Year, According to comScore Networks. Reston, VA, comScore Networks. http://www.comscore.com/press/release.asp?press=1242.

Anonymous (2008). Information Behaviour of the Researcher of the Future. London, England, Centre for Information Behaviour and the Evaluation of Research. http://www.bl.uk/news/pdf/googlegen.pdf.

Antelman, K. (2004). Do open-access articles have a greater research impact? *College and Research Libraries*, 65: 372–382. http://www.ala.org/ala/acrl/acrlpubs/crljournal/crl2004/crlseptember/antelman.pdf.

Antman, E., Lau, J., et al. (1992). A comparison of results of meta-analyses of randomized controlled trials and recommendations of clinical experts: treatments for myocardial infarction. *Journal of the American Medical Association*, 268: 240–248.

Aphinyanaphongs, Y. and Aliferis, C. (2004). Learning Boolean queries for article quality filtering. *MEDINFO 2004 – Proceedings of the Eleventh World Congress on Medical Informatics*, San Francisco, CA. IOS Press. 263–267. http://discover1.mc.vanderbilt.edu/discover/public/Publications/Boolean_Queries.pdf.

Aphinyanaphongs, Y. and Aliferis, C. (2007). Text categorization models for identifying unproven cancer treatments on the web. *MEDINFO 2007 – Proceedings of the Twelfth World Congress on Health (Medical) Informatics*, Brisbane, Australia. IOS Press. 968–972.

Aphinyanaphongs, Y., Statnikov, A., et al. (2006). A comparison of citation metrics to machine learning filters for the identification of high quality MEDLINE documents. *Journal of the American Medical Informatics Association*, 13: 446–455.

Aphinyanaphongs, Y., Tsamardinos, I., et al. (2005). Text categorization models for high-quality article retrieval in internal medicine. *Journal of the American Medical Informatics Association*, 12: 207–216.

Apps, A. and MacIntyre, R. (2006). Why openURL? *D-Lib Magazine*, 12(5). http://www.dlib.org/dlib/may06/apps/05apps.html.

Archbold, A. and Evans, D. (1989). On the topical structure of medical charts. *Proceedings of the 13th Annual Symposium on Computer Applications in Medical Care*, Washington, DC. IEEE. 543–547.

Argamon, S., Koppel, M., et al. (2003). Gender, genre, and writing style in formal written texts. *Text*, 23: 321–346.

Arms, W. (2001). *Digital Libraries*. Cambridge, MA. MIT Press.

Arms, W., Hillmann, D., et al. (2002). A spectrum of interoperability: the site for science prototype for the NSDL. *D-Lib Magazine*, 8(1). http://www.dlib.org/dlib/january02/arms/01arms.html.

Arnold, S. (2007). Google Version 2.0 – The Calculating Predator. Tetbury, UK. Infonortics. http://www.infonortics.com/publications/google/google-predator.html.

Aronsky, D., Ransom, J., et al. (2005). Accuracy of reference in five biomedical informatics journals. *Journal of the American Medical Informatics Association*, 12: 225–228.

Aronson, A. (1996). MetaMap: Mapping Text to the UMLS Metathesaurus. Bethesda, MD, National Library of Medicine. http://ii.nlm.nih.gov/resources/metamap.pdf. Accessed: July 1, 2002.

Aronson, A. (2001). Effective mapping of biomedical text to the UMLS Metathesaurus: the MetaMap program. *Proceedings of the 2001 AMIA Annual Symposium*, Washington, DC. Hanley & Belfus. 17–21.

Aronson, A. (2006). MetaMap: Mapping Text to the UMLS Metathesaurus. Bethesda, MD, National Library of Medicine. http://ii.nlm.nih.gov/resources/metamap.pdf.

Aronson, A., Bodenreider, O., et al. (2000). The NLM indexing initiative. *Proceedings of the AMIA 2000 Annual Symposium*, Los Angeles, CA. Hanley & Belfus. 17–21.

Aronson, A., Bodenreider, O., et al. (2007). From indexing the biomedical literature to coding clinical text: experience with MTI and machine learning approaches. *Proceedings of the ACL BioNLP'07 Workshop*, Prague, Czech Republic. Association for Computational Linguistics. 105–112. http://www.lhncbc.nlm.nih.gov/lhc/docs/published/2007/pub2007040.pdf.

Aronson, A., Demmer, D., et al. (2004). Knowledge-intensive and statistical approaches to the retrieval and annotation of genomics MEDLINE citations. *The Thirteenth Text REtrieval Conference: TREC 2004*, Gaithersburg, MD. National Institute of Standards and Technology. http://trec.nist.gov/pubs/trec13/papers/nlm-umd-ul.geo.pdf.

Aronson, A., Demner-Fushman, D., et al. (2005). Fusion of knowledge-intensive and statistical approaches for retrieving and annotating textual genomics documents. *The Fourteenth Text REtrieval Conference Proceedings (TREC 2005)*, Gaithersburg, MD. National Institute for Standards and Technology. http://trec.nist.gov/pubs/trec14/papers/nlm-umd.geo.pdf.

Aronson, A., Mork, J., et al. (2004). The NLM indexing initiative's medical text indexer. *MEDINFO 2004 – Proceedings of the Eleventh World Congress on Medical Informatics*, San Francisco, CA. IOS Press. 268–272. http://ii.nlm.nih.gov/resources/aronson-medinfo04. wheader.pdf.

Aronson, A. and Rindflesch, T. (1997). Query expansion using the UMLS metathesaurus. *Proceedings of the 1997 AMIA Annual Fall Symposium*, Nashville, TN. Hanley & Belfus. 485–489.

Arroll, B., Pandit, S., et al. (2002). Use of information sources among New Zealand family physicians with high access to computers. *Journal of Family Practice*, 51: 8. http://www. jfponline.com/content/2002/08/jfp_0802_0706a.asp.

Arts, D., Cornet, R., et al. (2005). Methods for evaluation of medical terminological systems – a literature review and a case study. *Methods of Information in Medicine*, 44: 616–625.

Aslam, J., Pavlu, V., et al. (2006). A statistical method for system evaluation using incomplete judgments. *Proceedings of the 29th Annual International ACM SIGIR Conference on Research and Development in Information Retrieval*, Seattle, WA. ACM Press. 541–548.

Atkins, D. (2007). Creating and synthesizing evidence with decision makers in mind: integrating evidence from clinical trials and other study designs. *Medical Care*, 45: S16–S22.

Avenell, A., Handoll, H., et al. (2001). Lessons for search strategies from a systematic review, in The Cochrane Library, of nutritional supplementation trials in patients after hip fracture. *American Journal of Clinical Nutrition*, 73: 505–510.

Babu, A., Kymes, S., et al. (2003). Eponyms and the diagnosis of aortic regurgitation: what says the evidence? *Annals of Internal Medicine*, 138: 736–742.

Bachmann, L., Coray, R., et al. (2002). Identifying diagnostic studies in MEDLINE: reducing the number needed to read. *Journal of the American Medical Informatics Association*, 9: 653–658. http://www.jamia.org/cgi/content/full/9/6/653.

Bachrach, C. and Charen, T. (1978). Selection of MEDLINE contents, the development of its thesaurus, and the indexing process. *Medical Informatics*, 3: 237–254.

Badgett, R., Paukert, J., et al. (2001). Teaching clinical informatics to third-year medical students: negative results from two controlled trials. *BMC Medical Education*, 1: 3. http://www.biomed-central.com/1472–6920/1/3.

Baeza-Yates, R. and Ribeiro-Neto, B., eds. (1999). *Modern Information Retrieval*. New York. McGraw-Hill.

Bahl, L., Jelineck, F., et al. (1983). A maximum-likelihood approach to continued speech recognition. *IEEE Transactions on Pattern Analysis and Machine Intelligence*, 5: 179–190.

Bailar, J. (1986). Science, statistics, and deception. *Annals of Internal Medicine*, 104: 259–260.

Bailey, C. (2006). Strong copyright + DRM + weak net neutrality = digital dystopia? *Information Technology and Libraries*, 25: 116–127. http://www.digital-scholarship.com/cwb/DigitalDys-topia.pdf.

Baker, T. and Dekker, M. (2003). Identifying metadata elements with URIs. *D-Lib Magazine*, 9(7/8). http://www.dlib.org/dlib/july03/baker/07baker.html.

Balas, E. and Boren, S. (2000). Managing clinical knowledge for health care improvement, 65–70, in vanBemmel, J. and McCray, A., eds. *Yearbook of Medical Informatics 2000 – Patient-Centered Systems*. Stuttgart, Germany. Schattauer.

Balk, E., Bonis, P., et al. (2002). Correlation of quality measures with estimates of treatment effect in meta-analyses of randomized controlled trials. *Journal of the American Medical Association*, 287: 2973–2982.

Ball, P. (2003). Computer program detects author gender. *Nature*. http://www.nature.com/nsu/030714/030714–13.html.

Ballesteros, L. and Croft, W. (1997). Phrasal translation and query expansion techniques for cross-language information retrieval. *Proceedings of the 20th Annual International ACM SIGIR Conference on Research and Development in Information Retrieval*, Philadelphia, PA. ACM Press. 84–91.

Banks, D., Shi, R., et al. (2007). Decreased hospital length of stay associated with presentation of cases at morning report with librarian support. *Journal of the Medical Library Association*, 95: 381–387.

Banks, M. (2005). The excitement of Google Scholar, the worry of Google Print. *Biomedical Digital Libraries*, 2: 2. http://www.bio-diglib.com/content/2/1/2.

Baorto, D. and Cimino, J. (2000). An "infobutton" for enabling patients to interpret on-line Pap smear reports. *Proceedings of the AMIA 2000 Annual Symposium*, Los Angeles, CA. Hanley & Belfus. 47–51.

Bar-Hillel, Y. and Carnap, R. (1953). Semantic information. *British Journal for the Philosophy of Science*, 4: 147–157.

Barabási, A. (2002). *Linked: The New Science of Networks*. Cambridge, MA. MIT Press.

Barabási, A. and Oltvai, Z. (2004). Network biology: understanding the cell's functional organization. *Nature Reviews – Genetics*, 5: 101–113.

Barnes, M. and Gary, R. (2003). *Bioinformatics for Geneticists*. West Sussex, England. Wiley.

Barr, C., Komorowski, H., et al. (1988). Conceptual modeling for the unified medical language system. *Proceedings of the 12th Annual Symposium on Computer Applications in Medical Care*, Washington, DC. IEEE. 148–151.

Barrett, T., Troup, D., et al. (2007). NCBI GEO: mining tens of millions of expression profiles–database and tools update. *Nucleic Acids Research*, 35: D760–D765.

Barroso, L., Dean, J., et al. (2003). Web search for a planet: the Google Cluster Architecture. *IEEE Micro*, 23(2): 22–28. http://labs.google.com/papers/googlecluster-ieee.pdf.

Barrows, R., Busuioc, M., et al. (2000). Limited parsing of notational text visit notes: ad-hoc vs. NLP approaches. *Proceedings of the AMIA 2000 Annual Symposium*, Los Angeles, CA. Hanley & Belfus. 51–55.

Barrows, R. and Traverso, J. (2006). Search considered integral. *ACM Queue*, 4(4). http://acmqueue.com/modules.php?name=Content&pa=showpage&pid=389.

Barry, C. (1994). User-defined relevance criteria: an exploratory study. *Journal of the American Society for Information Science*, 45: 149–159.

Bartell, B., Cottrell, G., et al. (1994). Automatic combination of multiple ranked retrieval systems. *Proceedings of the 17th Annual International ACM SIGIR Conference on Research and Development in Information Retrieval*, Dublin, Ireland. Springer-Verlag. 173–181.

Bates, D., Leape, L., et al. (1998). Effect of computerized physician order entry and a team intervention on prevention of serious medication errors. *Journal of the American Medical Association*, 280: 1311–1316.

Bates, M. (2002). After the dot-bomb: getting web information right this time. *First Monday*, 7: 7. http://firstmonday.org/issues/issue7_7/bates.

Battelle, J. (2005). *The Search – How Google and Its Rivals Rewrote the Rules of Business and Transformed Our Culture*. New York, NY. Penguin Group.

Baud, R., Lovins, C., et al. (1998). Morpho-semantic parsing of medical expressions. *Proceedings of the AMIA 1998 Annual Symposium*, Orlando, FL. Hanley & Belfus. 760–764.

Baud, R., Rassinoux, A., et al. (1999). The power and limits of a rule-based morpho-semantic parser. *Proceedings of the AMIA 1999 Annual Symposium*, Washington, DC. Hanley & Belfus. 22–26.

Beagrie, N. (2002). An update on the Digital Preservation Coalition. *D-Lib Magazine*, 8. http://www.dlib.org/dlib/april02/beagrie/04beagrie.html.

Beall, J. (2006). Metadata and data quality problems in the digital library. *Journal of Digital Information*, 6(3): 355. http://jodi.tamu.edu/Articles/v06/i03/Beall/Beall.pdf.

Beaulieu, M., Robertson, S., et al. (1996). Evaluating interactive systems in TREC. *Journal of the American Society for Information Science*, 47: 85–94.

Becker, E., Buhse, W., et al. (2004). *Digital Rights Management: Technological, Economic, Legal and Political Aspects*. New York, NY. Springer.

Bednarz, A. and Dubie, D. (2006). Desktop search tools seen raising red flags. *Network World*. Apr 17, 2006. http://www.networkworld.com/news/2006/041706-desktop-security.html.

Belew, R. (2000). *Finding Out About – A Cognitive Perspective on Search Engine Technology and the WWW*. Cambridge, UK. Cambridge University Press.

Belis, M. and Guiasu, S. (1968). A quantitative-qualitative measure of information in cybernetic systems. *IEEE Transactions on Information Theory*, 14: 593–594.

Belkin, N. (2000). Helping people find what they don't know. *Communications of the ACM*, 43: 58–61.

Belkin, N., Cool, C., et al. (2000). Iterative exploration, design and evaluation of support for query reformulation in interactive information retrieval. *Information Processing and Management*, 37: 403–434.

Belkin, N. and Croft, W. (1992). Information filtering and information retrieval: two sides of the same coin? *Communications of the ACM*, 35: 29–38.

Belkin, N., Keller, A., et al. (2000). Support for question-answering in interactive information retrieval: Rutger's TREC-9 interactive track experience. *The Ninth Text REtrieval Conference (TREC-9)*, Gaithersburg, MD. National Institute of Standards and Technology. 463–474.

Belkin, N. and Vickery, A. (1985). *Interaction in the Information System: A Review of Research from Document Retrieval to Knowledge-Based System*. London, England. The British Library.

Benson, D., Karsch-Mizrachi, I., et al. (2007). GenBank. *Nucleic Acids Research*, 35: D21–D25.

Benson, H., Dusek, J., et al. (2006). Study of the therapeutic effects of intercessory prayer (STEP) in cardiac bypass patients: a multicenter randomized trial of uncertainty and certainty of receiving intercessory prayer. *American Heart Journal*, 151: 934–942.

Benson, K. and Hartz, A. (2000). A comparison of observational studies and randomized, controlled trials. *New England Journal of Medicine*, 342: 1878–1886.

Berger, A. and Lafferty, J. (1999). Information retrieval as statistical translation. *Proceedings of the 22nd Annual International ACM SIGIR Conference on Research and Development in Information Retrieval*, Berkeley, CA. ACM Press. 222–229.

Bergus, G., Sinift, S., et al. (1998). Use of an e-mail curbside consultation service by family physicians. *Journal of Family Practice*, 47: 357–360.

Berland, G., Elliott, M., et al. (2001). Health information on the Internet: accessibility, quality, and readability in English and Spanish. *Journal of the American Medical Association*, 285: 2612–2621.

Berners-Lee, T., Hall, W., et al. (2006). Creating a science of the web. *Science*, 313: 769–771.

Bernstam, E., Herskovic, J., et al. (2006). Using citation data to improve retrieval from MEDLINE. *Journal of the American Medical Informatics Association*, 13: 96–105.

Bernstam, E., Sagaram, S., et al. (2005). Usability of quality measures for online health information: can commonly used technical quality criteria be reliably assessed? *International Journal of Medical Informatics*, 74: 675–683.

Bernstam, E., Shelton, D., et al. (2005). Instruments to assess the quality of health information on the World Wide Web: what can our patients actually use? *International Journal of Medical Informatics*, 74: 13–20.

Bernstein, L., Barriere, S., et al. (1982). Utilization of antibiotics: analysis of appropriateness of use. *Annals of Emergency Medicine*, 11: 21–24.

Berry, E., Kelly, S., et al. (2000). Identifying studies for systematic reviews. An example from medical imaging. *International Journal of Technology Assessment in Health Care*, 16: 668–672.

Besser, H. (2002). The next stage: moving from isolated digital collections to interoperable digital libraries. *First Monday*, 7: 6. http://www.firstmonday.dk/issues/issue7_6/besser/.

Biermann, J., Golladay, G., et al. (1999). Evaluation of cancer information on the internet. *Cancer*, 86: 381–390.

Birney, E. and Clamp, M. (2004). Biological database design and implementation. *Briefings in Bioinformatics*, 5: 31–38.

Black, N., vanRooyen, S., et al. (1998). What makes a good reviewer and a good review for a general medical journal? *Journal of the American Medical Association*, 280: 231–233.

Blackman, S. (2006). Nature has Wikipedia in its cites. *The Scientist*, 20(2): 18–19. http://www.the-scientist.com/article/display/23079/.

Blair, D. (1980). Searching biases in large interactive document retrieval systems. *Journal of the American Society for Information Science*, 31: 271–277.

Blair, D. (2002). Some thoughts on the reported results of TREC. *Information Processing and Management*, 38: 445–451.

Blair, D. and Maron, M. (1985). An evaluation of retrieval effectiveness for a full-text document-retrieval system. *Communications of the ACM*, 28: 289–299.

Bland, J. and Altman, D. (2000). The odds ratio. *British Medical Journal*, 320: 1468.

Blaschke, C., Leon, E., et al. (2005). Evaluation of BioCreAtIvE assessment of task 2. *BMC Bioinformatics*, 6: S16. http://www.biomedcentral.com/1471–2105/6/S1/S16.

Bleeker, S., Derksen-Lubsen, G., et al. (2006). Structured data entry for narrative data in a broad specialty: patient history and physical examination in pediatrics. *BMC Medical Informatics & Decision Making*, 6: 29. http://www.biomedcentral.com/1472–6947/6/29.

Blum, B. (1984). *Information Systems for Patient Care*. New York. Springer-Verlag.

Blythe, J. and Royle, J. (1993). Assessing nurses' information needs in the work environment. *Bulletin of the Medical Library Association*, 8: 433–435.

Bodenreider, O. (2004). The Unified Medical Language System (UMLS): integrating biomedical terminology. *Nucleic Acids Research*, 32: D267–D270.

Bodenreider, O. and McCray, A. (1998). From French vocabulary to the Unified Medical Language System: a preliminary study. *MEDINFO 98 – Proceedings of the Ninth World Congress on Medical Informatics*, Seoul, South Korea. IOS Press. 670–674.

Bodenreider, O. and Nelson, S. (2004). RxNav: a semantic navigation tool for clinical drugs. *MEDINFO 2004 – Proceedings of the Eleventh World Congress on Medical Informatics*, San Francisco, CA. IOS Press. 1530.

Bogue, M., Grubb, S., (2007). Mouse Phenome Database (MPD). *Nucleic Acids Research*, 35: D643–D649.

Bohannon, R. (1990). Information accessing behaviour of physical therapists. *Physiotherapy Theory and Practice*, 6: 212–225.

Bombardier, C., Laine, L., et al. (2000). Comparison of upper gatrointestinal toxicity of rofecoxib and naproxen in patients with rheumatoid arthritis. *New England Journal of Medicine*, 343: 1520–1528.

Bordage, G. (2001). Reasons reviewers reject and accept manuscripts: the strengths and weaknesses in medical education reports. *Academic Medicine*, 76: 889–896.

Borgman, C. (1999). What are digital libraries? Competing visions. *Information Processing and Management*, 35: 227–244.

Borlawsky, T., Friedman, C., et al. (2006). Generating executable knowledge for evidence-based medicine using natural language and semantic processing. *Proceedings of the AMIA 2006 Annual Symposium*, Washington, DC. American Medical Informatics Association. 56–60.

Bourne, P. (2005). Ten simple rules for getting published. *PLoS Computational Biology*, 1(5): e57.

Bourne, P. and Korngreen, A. (2006). Ten simple rules for reviewers. *PLoS Computational Biology*, 2(9): e110.

Bourque, P., Dupuis, R., et al. (1999). The guide to the Software Engineering Body of Knowledge. *IEEE Software*, 16(6): 35–44.

Bradford, S. (1948). *Documentation*. London, England. Crosby Lockwood.

Braschler, M. and Schauble, P. (2000). Using corpus-based approaches in a system for multilingual information retrieval. *Information Retrieval*, 3: 273–284.

Brennan, T., Rothman, D., et al. (2006). Health industry practices that create conflicts of interest: a policy proposal for academic medical centers. *Journal of the American Medical Association*, 295: 429–433.

Brenner, S. and McKinin, E. (1989). CINAHL and MEDLINE: a comparison of indexing practices. *Bulletin of the Medical Library Association*, 77: 366–371.

Brickley, D. and Guha, R. (2004). RDF Vocabulary Description Language 1.0: RDF Schema. World Wide Web Consortium. http://www.w3.org/TR/rdf-schema/. Accessed: April 26, 2004.

Brill, E. and Mooney, R. (1997). An overview of empirical natural language processing. *AI Magazine*, 18: 13–24.

Brin, S. and Page, L. (1998). The anatomy of a large-scale hypertextual web search engine. *Computer Networks and ISDN Systems*, 30: 107–117. http://infolab.stanford.edu/pub/papers/google.pdf.

Brinkley, J. and Rosse, C. (1997). The Digital Anatomist distributed framework and its applications to knowledge-based medical imaging. *Journal of the American Medical Informatics Association*, 4: 165–183.

Brinkley, J. and Rosse, C. (2002). Imaging informatics and the Human Brain Project: the role of structure, 111–128, in Haux, R. and Kulikowski, C., eds. *Yearbook of Medical Informatics 2002*. Stuttgart, Germany. Schattauer. http://sig.biostr.washington.edu/publications/online/Yearbook_MI_2002.pdf.

Broder, A. (2002). A taxonomy of web search. *SIGIR Forum*, 36(2): 3–10. http://www.acm.org/sigir/forum/F2002/broder.pdf.

Broder, A., Kumar, R., et al. (2000). Graph structure in the web. *Computer Networks*, 33: 309–320. http://www9.org/w9cdrom/160/160.html.

Broglio, J., Callan, J., et al. (1994). Document retrieval and routing using the INQUERY system. *Overview of the Third Text REtrieval Conference (TREC-3)*, Gaithersburg, MD. National Institute of Standards and Technology. 29–38.

Brown, S., Speroff, T., et al. (2006). eQuality: electronic quality assessment from narrative clinical reports. *Mayo Clinic Proceedings*, 81: 1472–1481.

Bruce, T. and Hillmann, D. (2004). The continuum of metadata quality: defining, expressing, exploiting, 238–256, in Hillmann, D. and Westbrooks, E., eds. *Metadata in Practice*. Chicago, IL. American Library Association.

Bryant, S. (2004). The information needs and information seeking behaviour of family doctors. *Health Information and Libraries Journal*, 21: 84–93.

Buckley, C. (2005). *The SMART Project at TREC*, 301–320, in Voorhees, E. and Harman, D., eds. *TREC: Experiment and Evaluation in Information Retrieval*. Cambridge, MA. MIT Press.

Buckley, C., Allan, J., et al. (1993). Automatic routing and ad-hoc retrieval using SMART: TREC-2. *The Second Text REtrieval Conference (TREC-2)*, Gaithersburg, MD. National Institute of Standards and Technology. 45–56.

Buckley, C. and Harman, D. (2004). Reliable Information Access Final Workshop Report. Bedford, MA, MITRE Corp. https://rrc.mitre.org/pubs/ria_final.pdf.

Buckley, C., Mitra, M., et al. (2000). Using clustering and superconcepts within SMART: TREC 6. *Information Processing and Management*, 36: 109–131.

Buckley, C., Salton, G., et al. (1992). Automatic retrieval with locality information using SMART. *The First Text REtrieval Conference (TREC-1)*, Gaithersburg, MD. National Institute of Standards and Technology. 59–72.

Buckley, C., Salton, G., et al. (1994a). The effect of adding relevance information in a relevance feedback environment. *Proceedings of the 17th Annual International ACM SIGIR Conference on Research and Development in Information Retrieval*, Dublin, Ireland. Springer-Verlag. 292–300.

Buckley, C., Salton, G., et al. (1994b). Automatic query expansion using SMART: TREC 3. *Overview of the Third Text REtrieval Conference (TREC-3)*, Gaithersburg, MD. National Institute of Standards and Technology. 69–80.

Buckley, C. and Voorhees, E. (2004). Retrieval evaluation with incomplete information. *Proceedings of the 27th Annual International ACM SIGIR Conference on Research and Development in Information Retrieval*, Sheffield, England. ACM Press. 25–32.

Buckley, C. and Voorhees, E. (2005). *Retrieval System Evaluation*, 53–75, in Voorhees, E. and Harman, D., eds. *TREC: Experiment and Evaluation in Information Retrieval*. Cambridge, MA. MIT Press.

Buetow, K. (2005). Cyberinfrastructure: empowering a "third way" in biomedical research. *Science*, 308: 821–824.

Bunyan, L. and Lutz, E. (1991). Marketing the hospital library to nurses. *Bulletin of the Medical Library Association*, 79: 2131–2133.

Burger, J., Cardie, C., et al. (2000). Issues, Tasks and Program Structures to Roadmap Research in Question & Answering (Q&A). http://www-nlpir.nist.gov/projects/duc/papers/qa.Roadmap-paper_v2.doc. Accessed: July 1, 2002.

Burnham, J. (1990). The evolution of editorial peer review. *Journal of the American Medical Association*, 263: 1323–1329.

Burnham, J. (2006). Scopus database: a review. *Biomedical Digital Libraries*, 3: 1. http://www.bio-diglib.com/content/3/1/1.

Bush, V. (1945). As we may think. *Atlantic Monthly*, 176: 101–108.

Bush, V. (1967). *Science is Not Enough*. New York. Morrow.

Buttcher, S., Clarke, C., et al. (2004). Domain-specific synonym expansion and validation for biomedical information retrieval (MultiText experiments for TREC 2004). *The Thirteenth Text REtrieval Conference: TREC 2004*, Gaithersburg, MD. National Institute of Standards and Technology. http://trec.nist.gov/pubs/trec13/papers/uwaterloo-clarke.geo.pdf.

Butte, A. and Kohane, I. (2006). Creation and implications of a phenome-genome network. *Nature Biotechnology*, 1: 55–62.

Byrnes, M. (2005). Permanence levels and the archives for NLM's permanent web documents. *NLM Technical Bulletin*. Mar–Apr, e4: 343. http://www.nlm.nih.gov/pubs/techbull/ma05/ma05_archive.html.

Cabana, M., Rand, C., et al. (1999). Why don't physicians follow clinical practice guidelines? A framework for improvement. *Journal of the American Medical Association*, 282: 1458–1465.

Calishain, T. and Dornfest, R. (2004). *Google Hacks – Tips & Tools for Smarter Searching*, Second Edition. Sebastapol, CA. O'Reilly.

Callaham, M., Baxt, W., et al. (1998). Reliability of editors' subjective quality ratings of peer reviews of manuscripts. *Journal of the American Medical Association*, 280: 229–231.

Callaham, M., Wears, R., et al. (2002). Journal prestige, publication bias, and other characteristics associated with citation of published studies in peer-reviewed journals. *Journal of the American Medical Association*, 287: 2847–2850.

Callaham, M., Wears, R., et al. (1998). Positive-outcome bias and other limitations in the outcome of research abstracts submitted to a scientific meeting. *Journal of the American Medical Association*, 280: 254–257.

Callan, J. (1994). Passage level evidence in document retrieval. *Proceedings of the 17th Annual International ACM SIGIR Conference on Research and Development in Information Retrieval*, Dublin, Ireland. Springer-Verlag. 302–310.

Callan, J., Allan, J., et al. (2007). Meeting of the MINDS: an information retrieval research agenda. *SIGIR Forum*, 41(1): 25–34.

Callan, J., Croft, W., et al. (1995). TREC and TIPSTER experiments with INQUERY. *Information Processing and Management*, 31: 315–326.

Candela, L., Castelli, D., et al. (2007). Setting the foundations of digital libraries – the DELOS Manifesto. *D-Lib Magazine*, 13(3/4). http://www.dlib.org/dlib/march07/castelli/03castelli.html.

Candler, C., Uijtdehaage, S., et al. (2003). Introducing HEAL: the Health Education Assets Library. *Academic Medicine*, 78: 249–253. http://www.healcentral.org/publications/Academic_Medicine_C_Mar_2003.pdf.

Canese, K. (2004). New PubMed spell checking feature. *NLM Technical Bulletin*. Nov–Dec, e12: 341. http://www.nlm.nih.gov/pubs/techbull/nd04/nd04_spell.html.

Canese, K. (2005). RSS feeds available from PubMed. *NLM Technical Bulletin*. May–June, e2: 344. http://165.112.6.70/pubs/techbull/mj05/mj05_rss.html.

Canese, K. (2006). PubMed limits page updated. *NLM Technical Bulletin*. Mar–Apr, e2: 349. http://165.112.6.70/pubs/techbull/ma06/ma06_limits.html.

Caporaso, J., Deshpande, N., et al. (2008). Intrinsic evaluation of text mining tools may not predict performance on realistic tasks. *Pacific Symposium on Biocomputing*, Big Island, Hawaii. World Scientific. 640–651.

Carbonell, J., Harman, D., et al. (2000). Vision Statement to Guide Research in Question & Answering (Q&A) and Text Summarization. http://www.ai.mit.edu/people/jimmylin/papers/Carbonell00.pdf.

Card, S. (2003). *Information Foraging Theory*. Palo Alto, CA. Palo Alto Research Center. http://hci.ucsd.edu/220/UP-2003–0101-Card-UM-NextGen.pdf.

Carmel, D., Yom-Tov, E., et al. (2005). Predicting query difficulty – methods and applications. *SIGIR Forum*, 39(2): 25–28. http://www.acm.org/sigir/forum/2005D/2005d_sigirforum_carmel.pdf.

Carson, S., Cohen, A., et al. (2007). *Making Clinical Trial Results Databases Useful for Systematic Reviews*. Bethesda, MD. Lister Hill National Center for Biomedical Communications, National Library of Medicine.

Caruso, D. (2000). Digital Commerce; If the AOL-Time Warner deal is about proprietary content, where does that leave a noncommercial directory it will own? *New York Times*. Jan 17, 2000.

Case, D. (2006). *Looking for Information: A Survey of Research on Information Seeking, Needs, and Behavior,* Second Edition. San Diego. Academic Press.

Cha, K. and Wirth, D. (2001). Does prayer influence the success of in vitro fertilization-embryo transfer? Report of a masked, randomized trial. *Journal of Reproductive Medicine*, 46: 781–787. http://www.reproductivemedicine.com/Features/2001/2001Sep.htm.

Chalmers, I. (1990). Under-reporting scientific research is scientific misconduct. *Journal of the American Medical Association*, 263: 1405–1408.

Chan, A., Hrobjartsson, A., et al. (2004). Empirical evidence for selective reporting of outcomes in randomized trials: comparison of protocols to published articles. *Journal of the American Medical Association*, 291: 2457–2465.

Chang, J., Schutze, H., et al. (2002). Creating an online dictionary of abbreviations from MEDLINE. *Journal of the American Medical Informatics Association*, 6: 612–620.

Chang, J., Schutze, H., et al. (2004). GAPSCORE: finding gene and protein names one word at a time. *Bioinformatics*, 20: 216–225.

Chapman, W., Bridewell, W., et al. (2001). A simple algorithm for identifying negated findings and diseases in discharge summaries. *Journal of Biomedical Informatics*, 34: 301–310.

Chapman, W., Dowling, J., et al. (2008). Evaluation of training with an annotation schema for manual annotation of clinical conditions from emergency department reports. *International Journal of Medical Informatics*, 77: 107–113.

Chapman, W., Dowling, J., et al. (2005). Classification of emergency department chief complaints into 7 syndromes: a retrospective analysis of 527,228 patients. *Annals of Emergency Medicine*, 46: 445–455.

Chapman, W., Fiszman, M., et al. (2001). A comparison of classification algorithms to automatically identify chest x-ray reports that support pneumonia. *Journal of Biomedical Informatics*, 34: 4–14.

Charen, T. (1976). *MEDLARS Indexing Manual, Part I: Bibliographic Principles and Descriptive Indexing, 1977*. Springfield, VA. National Technical Information Service.

Charen, T. (1983). *MEDLARS Indexing Manual, Part II*. Springfield, VA. National Technical Information Service.

Charniak, E. (1997). Statistical techniques for natural language parsing. *AI Magazine*, 18: 33–44.

Chatterjee, A. (2003). Vaccine and immunization resources on the World Wide Web. *Clinical Infectious Diseases*, 36: 355–362.

Chen, E., Hripcsak, G., et al. (2006). Disseminating natural language processed clinical narratives. *Proceedings of the AMIA 2006 Annual Symposium*, Washington, DC. American Medical Informatics Association. 126–130.

Chen, E., Hripcsak, G., et al. (2008). Automated acquisition of disease drug knowledge from biomedical and clinical documents: an initial study. *Journal of the American Medical Informatics Association*, 15: 87–98.

Chen, H., Houston, A., et al. (1998). Internet browsing and searching: user evaluations of category map and concept space techniques. *Journal of the American Society for Information Science*, 49: 582–608.

Chen, H. and Sharp, B. et al. (2004). Content-rich biological network constructed by mining PubMed abstracts. *BMC Bioinformatics*, 5: 147. http://www.biomedcentral.com/1471–2105/5/147.

Chen, L., Liu, H., et al. (2004). Extracting phenotypic information from the literature via natural language processing. *MEDINFO 2004 – Proceedings of the Eleventh World Congress on Medical Informatics*, San Francisco, CA. IOS Press. 758–762.

Chen, L., Liu, H., et al. (2005). Gene name ambiguity of eukaryotic nomenclatures. *Bioinformatics*, 21: 248–256.

Chen, Y., Chattopadhyay, A., et al. (2007). The online bioinformatics resources collection at the University of Pittsburgh Health Sciences Library System – a one-stop gateway to online bioinformatics databases and software tools. *Nucleic Acids Research*, 35: D780–D785.

Chin, J., Diehl, V., et al. (1988). Development of an instrument measuring user satisfaction of the human-computer interface. *Proceedings of CHI '88 – Human Factors in Computing Systems*, New York. ACM Press. 213–218.

Chong, S. and Normile, D. (2006). How young Korean researchers helped unearth a scandal. *Science*, 311: 22–25.

Choudhry, N., Fletcher, R., et al. (2005). Systematic review: the relationship between clinical experience and quality of health care. *Annals of Internal Medicine*, 142: 260–273.

Christensen, K. and Murray, J. (2007). What genome-wide association studies can do for medicine. *New England Journal of Medicine*, 356: 1094–1097.

Chueh, H. and Barnett, G. (1997). "Just-in-time" clinical information. *Academic Medicine*, 72: 512–517.

Cimino, J. (1996). Linking patient information systems to bibliographic resources. *Methods of Information in Medicine*, 35: 122–126.

Cimino, J. (1998). Desiderata for controlled medical vocabularies in the twenty-first century. *Methods of Information in Medicine*, 37: 394–403.

Cimino, J. (2006). Use, usability, usefulness, and impact of an infobutton manager. *Proceedings of the AMIA 2006 Annual Symposium*, Washington, DC. American Medical Informatics Association. 151–155.

Cimino, J., Aguirre, A., et al. (1993). Generic queries for meeting clinical information needs. *Bulletin of the Medical Library Association*, 81: 195–206.

Cimino, J. and Barnett, G. (1987). The physician's workstation: recording a physical examination using a controlled vocabulary. *Proceedings of the 11th Annual Symposium on Computer Applications in Medical Care*, Washington, DC. IEEE. 287–291.

Cimino, J., Clayton, P., et al. (1994). Knowledge-based approaches to the maintenance of a large controlled medical terminology. *Journal of the American Medical Informatics Association*, 1: 35–50.

Cimino, J., Johnson, S., et al. (1992). The MEDLINE button. *Proceedings of the 16th Annual Symposium on Computer Applications in Medical Care*, Baltimore, MD. McGraw-Hill. 81–85.

Cimino, J. and Li, J. (2003). Sharing infobuttons to resolve clinicians' information needs. *Proceedings of the AMIA 2003 Annual Symposium*, Washington, DC. Hanley & Belfus. 815.

Cimino, J., Li, J., et al. (2002). Theoretical, empirical and practical approaches to resolving the unmet information needs of clinical information system users. *Proceedings of the 2002 AMIA Annual Symposium*, San Antonio, TX. Hanley & Belfus. 170–174.

Cimino, J., Socratorus, S., et al. (1995). Internet as clinical information system: application development using the World Wide Web. *Journal of the American Medical Informatics Association*, 2: 273–284.

Cimino, J. and Zhu, X. (2006). The practical impact of ontologies on biomedical informatics. *Methods of Information in Medicine*, 45(Supp 1): 124–135.

Clark, T., Martin, S., et al. (2004). Globally distributed object identification for biological knowledgebases. *Briefings in Bioinformatics*, 5: 59–70.

Clarke, M. (2004). Open sesame? Increasing access to medical literature. *Pediatrics*, 114: 265–268.

Clarke, M., Alderson, P., et al. (2002). Discussion sections in reports of controlled trials published in general medical journals. *Journal of the American Medical Association*, 287: 2799–2801.

Cleverdon, C. and Keen, E. (1966). *Factors Determining the Performance of Indexing Systems (Vol. 1: Design, Vol. 2: Results)*. Cranfield, England. Aslib Cranfield Research Project.

Clifford, T., Moher, D., et al. (2001). Absence of associations between funding source, trial outcome, and quality score: a benefit of financial disclosure. *Fourth International Congress on Peer Review in Biomedical Publication*, Barcelona, Spain. American Medical Association. http://www.ama-assn.org/public/peer/peerhome.htm.

Cochrane, A. (1972). *Effectiveness and Efficiency: Random Reflections on Health Services*. London, England. Nuffield Provincial Hospital Trust.

Cockburn, A. (2001). *Writing Effective Use Cases*. Boston. Addison-Wesley.

Cogdill, K. (2003). Information needs and information seeking in primary care: a study of nurse practitioners. *Journal of the Medical Library Association*, 91: 203–214.

Cohen, A. (2005). Unsupervised gene/protein entity normalization using automatically extracted dictionaries. *Linking Biological Literature, Ontologies and Databases: Mining Biological Semantics, Proceedings of the BioLINK2005 Workshop*, Detroit, MI. Association for Computational Linguistics. 17–24. http://acl.ldc.upenn.edu/W/W05/W05–1303.pdf.

Cohen, A. and Hersh, W. (2005). A survey of current work in biomedical text mining. *Briefings in Bioinformatics*, 6: 57–71.

Cohen, A. and Hersh, W. (2006). The TREC 2004 Genomics Track categorization task: classifying full-text biomedical documents. *Journal of Biomedical Discovery and Collaboration*, 1: 4. http://www.j-biomed-discovery.com/content/1/1/4.

Cohen, A., Hersh, W., et al. (2005). Using co-occurrence network structure to extract synonymous gene and protein names from MEDLINE abstracts. *BMC Bioinformatics*, 6: 103. http://www.biomedcentral.com/1471–2105/6/103.

Cohen, A., Hersh, W., et al. (2006). Reducing workload in systematic review preparation using automated citation classification. *Journal of the American Medical Informatics Association*, 13: 206–219.

Cohen, A., Stavri, P., et al. (2004). A categorization and analysis of the criticisms of evidence-based medicine. *International Journal of Medical Informatics*, 73: 35–43.

Cohen, J. (1960). A coefficient of agreement for nominal scales. *Educational and Psychological Measurement*, 20: 37–46.

Cohen, J. (2001). Dose discrepancies between the physicians' desk reference and the medical literature, and their possible role in the high incidence of dose-related adverse drug events. *Archives of Internal Medicine*, 161: 957–964.

Colaianni, L. (1992). Retraction, comment, and errata policies of the U.S. National Library of Medicine. *Lancet*, 340: 536–537.

Coletti, M. and Bleich, H. (2001). Medical subject headings used to search the biomedical literature. *Journal of the American Medical Informatics Association*, 8: 317–323.

Collins, F. and McKusick, V. (2001). Implications of the Human Genome Project for medical science. *Journal of the American Medical Association*, 285: 540–544.

Collins, F., Morgan, M., et al. (2003). The Human Genome Project: lessons from large-scale biology. *Science*, 300: 286–290.

Concato, J., Shah, N., et al. (2000). Randomized, controlled trials, observational studies, and the hierarchy of research designs. *New England Journal of Medicine*, 342: 1887–1892.

Connelly, D., Rich, E., et al. (1990). Knowledge resource preferences of family physicians. *Journal of Family Practice*, 30: 353–359.

Cooper, R., Schriger, D., et al. (2003). The quantity and quality of scientific graphs in pharmaceutical advertisements. *Journal of General Internal Medicine*, 18: 294–297.

Cooper, W. (1973). On selecting a measure of retrieval effectiveness. *Journal of the American Society for Information Science*, 24: 87–100.

Cooper, W., Chen, A., et al. (1994). Experiments in the probabilistic retrieval of documents. *Overview of the Third Text REtrieval Conference (TREC-3)*, Gaithersburg, MD. National Institute of Standards and Technology. 127–134.

Copas, J. and Shi, J. (2000). Meta-analysis, funnel plots and sensitivity analysis. *Biostatistics*, 1: 247–262.

Cope, J., Craswell, N., et al. (2003). Automated discovery of search interfaces on the web. *Proceedings of the Fourteenth Australasian Database Conference on Database Technologies*, Adelaide, Australia. Australian Computer Society. 181–189.

Corcoran-Perry, S. and Graves, J. (1990). Supplemental information-seeking behavior of cardiovascular nurses. *Research in Health and Nursing*, 13: 119–127.

Cormack, G. and Lyman, T. (2007). Online supervised spam filter evaluation. *ACM Transactions on Information Systems*, 25(3): Article 11.

Cormack, G. and Lynam, T. (2005). TREC 2005 spam track overview. *The Fourteenth Text REtrieval Conference (TREC 2005) Proceedings*, Gaithersburg, MD. National Institute for Standards and Technology. http://trec.nist.gov/pubs/trec14/papers/SPAM.OVERVIEW.pdf.

Corrao, S., Colomba, D., et al. (2006). Improving efficacy of PubMed Clinical Queries for retrieving scientifically strong studies on treatment. *Journal of the American Medical Informatics Association*, 13: 485–487.

Courant, P. (2006). Scholarship and academic libraries (and their kin) in the world of Google. *First Monday*, 11(8). http://www.firstmonday.org/issues/issue11_8/courant/index.html.

Couzin, J. (2006). And how the problems eluded peer reviewers and editors. *Science*, 311: 23–24.

Couzin, J. and Unger, K. (2006). Scientific misconduct – cleaning up the paper trail. *Science*, 312: 38–43.

Covell, D., Uman, G., et al. (1985). Information needs in office practice: are they being met? *Annals of Internal Medicine*, 103: 596–599.

Cover, T. and Thomas, J. (2006). *Elements of Information Theory*. Hoboken, NJ. Wiley.

Cowie, J. and Lehnert, W. (1996). Information extraction. *Communications of the ACM*, 39: 80–91.

Coyle, K. (2005). Descriptive metadata for copyright status. *First Monday*, 10(10). http://www.firstmonday.org/issues/issue10_10/coyle/.

Craig, I., Plume, A., et al. (2007). Do open access articles have greater citation impact? A critical review of the literature. *Journal of Informetrics*, 1: 239–248.

Crain, C. (1987). Appendix A — Protocol study of indexers at the National Library of Medicine, in Carbonell, J., Evans, D., Scott, D. and Thomason, R., eds. *Final Report on the Automated Classification Retrieval Project, Grant N01-LM-4-3529*. Bethesda, MD. National Library of Medicine.

Craswell, N., Hawking, D., et al. (2001). Effective site finding using link anchor information. *Proceedings of the 24th Annual International ACM SIGIR Conference on Research and Development in Information Retrieval*, New Orleans, LA. ACM Press. 250–257.

Crichlow, R., Winbush, N., et al. (2004). The accessibility and accuracy of web references in five major medical journals. *Journal of the American Medical Association*, 292: 2723–2724.

Crocco, A., Villasis-Keever, M., et al. (2002). Analysis of cases of harm associated with use of health information on the internet. *Journal of the American Medical Association*, 287: 2869–2871.

Croft, W. (2003). Salton Award Lecture – Information retrieval and computer science: an evolving relationship. *Proceedings of the 26th Annual International ACM SIGIR Conference on Research and Development in Information Retrieval*, Toronto, Canada. ACM Press. 2–3.

Cronen-Townsend, S., Zhou, Y., et al. (2002). Predicting query performance. *Proceedings of the 25th Annual International ACM SIGIR Conference on Research and Development in Information Retrieval*, Tampere, Finland. ACM Press. 299–306.

Cuadra, C. and Katter, R. (1967). *Experimental Studies of Relevance Judgments*. Santa Monica, CA. Systems Development Corp.

Cui, L. (1999). Rating health web sites using the principles of citation analysis: a bibliometric approach. *Journal of Medical Internet Research*, 1(1): e4. http://jmir.org/1999/1/e4.

Cummings, A., Witte, M., et al. (1992). University Libraries and Scholarly Communication: A Study Prepared for the Andrew W. Mellon Foundation. Association of Research Libraries. http://etext.lib.virginia.edu/subjects/mellon/. Accessed: July 1, 2002.

Curfman, G., Morrissey, S., et al. (2005). Expression of concern: Bombardier et al., "Comparison of upper gastrointestinal toxicity of rofecoxib and naproxen in patients with rheumatoid arthritis". *New England Journal of Medicine*, 353: 2318–2319.

Curley, S., Connelly, D., et al. (1990). Physicians use of medical knowledge resources: preliminary theoretical framework and findings. *Medical Decision Making*, 10: 231–241.

Cutting, D., Pedersen, J., et al. (1992). Scatter/Gather: a cluster-based approach to browsing large document collections. *Proceedings of the 15th Annual International ACM SIGIR Conference on Research and Development in Information Retrieval*, Copenhagen, Denmark. ACM Press. 318–329.

D'Agostino, R. (2000). Debate: the slippery slope of surrogate outcomes. *Controlled Clinical Trials in Cardiovascular Medicine*, 1: 76–78.

Dang, H. (2006). Overview of DUC 2006. *Document Understanding Conference (DUC) 2007*, New York, NY. http://www-nlpir.nist.gov/projects/duc/pubs/2006papers/duc2006.pdf.

Darmoni, S. and Thirion, B. (2000). A standard metadata scheme for health resources. *Journal of the American Medical Informatics Association*, 7: 108–109.

Davidoff, F., DeAngelis, C., et al. (2001). Sponsorship, authorship, and accountability. *Annals of Internal Medicine*, 135: 463–466.

Davidoff, F. and Florance, V. (2000). The informationist: a new health profession? *Annals of Internal Medicine*, 132: 996–998.

Davies, K. (2006). Search and deploy. *Bio-IT World*. Oct 16, 2006. http://www.bio-itworld.com/issues/2006/oct/biogen-idec/.

Davis, H. (2006). *Google Advertising Tools*. Sebastopol, CA. O'Reilly.

Davis, M. and Ogden, W. (1997). Free resources and advanced alignment for cross-language text retrieval. *The Sixth Text REtrieval Conference (TREC-6)*, Gaithersburg, MD. National Institute of Standards and Technology. 385–402.

Dawes, M. and Sampson, U. (2003). Knowledge management in clinical practice: a systematic review of information seeking behavior in physicians. *International Journal of Medical Informatics*, 71: 9–15.

Dawes, M., Summerskill, W., et al. (2005). Sicily statement on evidence-based practice. *BMC Medical Education*, 5(1): 1. http://www.biomedcentral.com/1472–6920/5/1.

Dawkins, R. (1976). *The Selfish Gene*. New York. Oxford University Press.

Day, S., Christensen, L., et al. (2007). Identification of trauma patients at a level 1 trauma center utilizing natural language processing. *Journal of Trauma Nursing*, 14: 79–83.

Dean, J. and Ghemawat, S. (2008). MapReduce: simplified data processing on large clusters. *Communications of the ACM*, 51(1): 107–113.

DeAngelis, C., Drazen, J., et al. (2004). Clinical trial registration: a statement from the International Committee of Medical Journal Editors. *Journal of the American Medical Association*, 292: 1363–1364.

DeAngelis, C., Drazen, J., et al. (2005). Is this clinical trial fully registered? A statement from the International Committee of Medical Journal Editors. *Journal of the American Medical Association*, 293: 2927–2929.

DeAngelis, C. and Musacchio, R. (2004). Access to JAMA. *Journal of the American Medical Association*, 291: 370–371.

DeBakey, M. (1991). The National Library of Medicine: evolution of a premier information center. *Journal of the American Medical Association*, 266: 1252–1258.

deBliek, R., Friedman, C., et al. (1994). Information retrieved from a database and the augmentation of personal knowledge. *Journal of the American Medical Informatics Association*, 1: 328–338.

Dee, C. and Blazek, R. (1993). Information needs of the rural physician: a descriptive study. *Bulletin of the Medical Library Association*, 81: 259–264.

Deerwester, S., Dumais, S., et al. (1990). Indexing by latent semantic analysis. *Journal of the American Society for Information Science*, 41: 391–407.

De Jong, G. (1979). Prediction and substantiation: a new approach to natural language processing. *Cognitive Science*, 3: 251–273.

de Lacey, G., Record, C., et al. (1985). How accurate are quotations and references in medical journals? *British Medical Journal*, 291: 884–886.

Delamothe, T., Mullner, M., et al. (1999). Pleasing both authors and readers: a combination of short print articles and longer electronic ones may help us do this. *British Medical Journal*, 318: 888–889.

Delamothe, T. and Smith, R. (2003). Paying for bmj.com. *British Medical Journal*, 327: 241–242.

DelBimbo, A. (1999). *Visual Information Retrieval*. San Francisco, CA. Morgan Kaufmann.

DelFiol, G., Rocha, R., (2005). HL7 Infobutton Standard API Proposal. Ann Arbor, MI. Health Level Seven. http://cslxinfmtcs.csmc.edu/hl7/arden/2005–05-AMS/HL7-Infobutton-API-2–10–05.doc.

Demeter, J., Beauheim, C., et al. (2007). The Stanford microarray database: implementation of new analysis tools and open source release of software. *Nucleic Acids Research*, 35: D766–D770.

Demner-Fushman, D. and Lin, J. (2007). Answering clinical questions with knowledge-based and statistical techniques. *Computational Linguistics*, 33: 63–103.

Derry, S., Loke, Y., et al. (2001). Incomplete evidence: the inadequacy of databases in tracing published adverse drug reactions in clinical trials. *BMC Medical Research Methodology*, 1: 7. http://www.biomedcentral.com/1471–2288/1/7.

DerSimonian, R., Charette, L., et al. (1982). Reporting on methods in clinical trials. *New England Journal of Medicine*, 306: 1332–1337.

Deselaers, T., Keysers, D., et al. (2008). Features for image retrieval: an experimental comparison. *Information Retrieval*, 11(2): 77–107.

Detlefsen, E. (2002). The education of informationists, from the perspective of a library and information sciences educator. *Journal of the Medical Library Association*, 90: 59–67.

Devereaux, P., Bhandari, M., et al. (2005). Need for expertise based randomised controlled trials. *British Medical Journal*, 330: 88.

Dewatripont, M., Ginsburgh, V., et al. (2006). Study on the economic and technical evolution of the scientific publication markets in Europe. Brussels, Belgium, European Commisssion. http://ec.europa.eu/research/science-society/pdf/scientific-publication-study_en.pdf.

Dickersin, K. (1990). The existence of publication bias and risk factors for its occurrence. *Journal of the American Medical Association*, 263: 1385–1389.

Dickersin, K. and Min, Y. (1993). Publication bias: a problem that won't go away. *Annals of the New York Academy of Sciences*, 703: 135–148.

Dickersin, K. and Rennie, D. (2003). Registering clinical trials. *Journal of the American Medical Association*, 290: 516–523.

Dickersin, K., Scherer, R., et al. (1994). Identifying relevant studies for systematic reviews. *British Medical Journal*, 309: 1286–1291.

Diehn, M., Sherlock, G., et al. (2003). SOURCE: a unified genomic resource of functional annotations, ontologies, and gene expression data. *Nucleic Acids Research*, 31: 219–223.

DiEugenio, B. and Glass, M. (2004). The kappa statistic: a second look. *Computational Linguistics*, 30: 95–101.

Dillon, A., Richardson, J., et al. (1990). The effect of display size and text splitting on reading lengthy text from the screen. *Behaviour and Information Technology*, 9: 215–227.

Divoli, A., Hearst, M., et al. (2008). Evidence for showing gene/protein name suggestions in bioscience literature search interfaces. *Pacific Symposium on Biocomputing*, Big Island, Hawaii. World Scientific. 568–579.

Djebbari, A., Karamycheva, S., et al. (2005). MeSHer: identifying biological concepts in microarray assays based on PubMed references and MeSH terms. *Bioinformatics*, 15: 3324–3326.

Dolin, R., Boles, M., et al. (2001). Kaiser Permanente's "metadata-driven" national clinical intranet. *MEDINFO 2001 – Proceedings of the Tenth World Congress on Medical Informatics*, London, England. IOS Press. 319–323.

Doms, A. and Schroeder, M. (2005). GoPubMed: exploring PubMed with the gene ontology. *Nucleic Acids Research*, 33: W783–W786.

Dong, P., Loh, M., et al. (2005). The "impact factor" revisited. *Biomedical Digital Libraries*, 2: 7. http://www.bio-diglib.com/content/2/1/7.

Downey, D., Dumais, S., et al. (2007). Models of searching and browsing: languages, studies, and applications. *International Joint Conference on Artificial Intelligence 2007*, Hyderabad, India. http://www.ijcai.org/papers07/Papers/IJCAI07–440.pdf.

Doyle, J., Alderson, D., et al. (2005). The "robust yet fragile" nature of the internet. *Proceedings of the National Academy of Sciences*, 102: 14497–14502.

Drazen, J. and Curfman, G. (2004). Public access to biomedical research. *New England Journal of Medicine*, 351: 1343.

Duchnicky, R. and Kolers, P. (1983). Readability of text scrolled on visual display terminals as a function of window size. *Human Factors*, 25: 683–692.

Dumais, S. (1994). Latent semantic indexing (LSI): TREC-3 Report. *Overview of the Third Text REtrieval Conference (TREC-3)*, Gaithersburg, MD. National Institute of Standards and Technology. 219–230.

Dumais, S. and Belkin, N. (2005). The TREC interactive tracks: Putting the user into search, 123–152, in Voorhees, E. and Harman, D., eds. *TREC - Experiment and Evaluation in Information Retrieval*. Cambridge, MA. MIT Press.

Dumais, S. and Schmitt, D. (1991). Iterative searching in an online database. *Proceedings of the Human Factors Society 35th Annual Meeting,* San Francisco. 398–403.

Durack, D. (1978). The weight of medical knowledge. *New England Journal of Medicine*, 298: 773–775.

Dushay, N. (2006). NSDL Metadata Primer. Boulder, CO. National Science Digital Library. http://metamanagement.comm.nsdl.org/outline.html.

Eastman, C. and Jansen, B. (2003). Coverage, relevance, and ranking: the impact of query operators on web search engine results. *ACM Transactions on Information Systems*, 21: 383–411.

Edhlund, B. (2005). *Basic Principles of Pubmed*. Morrisville, NC. Lulu Press.

Edhlund, B. (2006). *PubMed and EndNote*. Morrisville, NC. Lulu Press.

Edmunson, H. (1969). New methods in automatic extracting. *Journal of the Association for Computing Machinery*, 16: 264–285.

Egan, D., Remde, J., et al. (1989). Formative design-evaluation of Superbook. *ACM Transactions on Information Systems*, 7: 30–57.

Egger, M., Bartlett, C., et al. (2001). Are randomised controlled trials in the BMJ different? *British Medical Journal*, 323: 1253–1254.

Egger, M., Smith, G., et al. (1997). Bias in meta-analysis detected by a simple, graphical test. *British Medical Journal*, 315: 629–634.

Egger, M., Zellweger-Zahner, T., et al. (1997). Language bias in randomised controlled trials published in English and German. *Lancet*, 350: 326–329.

Eggers, S., Huang, Z., et al. (2005). *Mapping Medical Informatics Research*, 36–62, in Chen, H., Fuller, S., Friedman, C. and Hersh, W., eds. *Medical Informatics: Knowledge Management and Data Mining in Biomedicine*. New York, NY. Springer-Verlag.

Eichmann, D., Ruiz, M., et al. (1998). Cross-language information retrieval with the UMLS metathesaurus. *Proceedings of the 21st Annual International ACM SIGIR Conference on Research and Development in Information Retrieval*, Melbourne, Australia. ACM Press. 72–80.

Eisenberg, M. (1988). Measuring relevance judgments. *Information Processing and Management*, 24: 373–389.

Eisenberg, M. and Barry, C. (1988). Order effects: a study of the possible influence of presentation order on user judgments of document relevance. *Journal of the American Society for Information Science*, 39: 293–300.

Ekstrom, R., French, J., et al. (1976). *Manual for Kit of Factor-Referenced Cognitive Tests*. Princeton, NJ. Educational Testing Service.

Elhadad, N., Kan, M., et al. (2005). Customization in a unified framework for summarizing medical literature. *Artificial Intelligence in Medicine*, 33: 179–198.

Elkin, P., Brown, S., et al. (2003). A formal representation for messages containing compositional expressions. *International Journal of Medical Informatics*, 71: 89–102.

Elkin, P., Brown, S., et al. (2006). Evaluation of the content coverage of SNOMED CT: ability of SNOMED clinical terms to represent clinical problem lists. *Mayo Clinic Proceedings*, 81: 741–748.

Ellerbeck, E., Jencks, S., et al. (1995). Quality of care for medicare patients with acute myocardial infarction: a four-state pilot study from the cooperative cardiovascular project. *Journal of the American Medical Association*, 273: 1509–1514.

Elstein, A., Shulman, L., et al. (1978). *Medical Problem Solving: An Analysis of Clinical Reasoning*. Cambridge, MA. Harvard University Press.

Ely, J., Burch, R., et al. (1992). The information needs of family physicians: case-specific clinical questions. *Journal of Family Practice*, 35: 265–269.

Ely, J., Levy, B., et al. (1999). What clinical information resources are available in family physicians' offices? *Journal of Family Practice*, 48: 135–139.

Ely, J., Osheroff, J., et al. (2005). Answering physicians' clinical questions: obstacles and potential solutions. *Journal of the American Medical Informatics Association*, 12: 217–224.

Ely, J., Osheroff, J., et al. (1999). Analysis of questions asked by family doctors regarding patient care. *British Medical Journal*, 319: 358–361.

Ely, J., Osheroff, J., et al. (2002). Obstacles to answering doctors' questions about patient care with evidence: qualitative study. *British Medical Journal*, 324: 710–713.

Ely, J., Osheroff, J., et al. (2000). A taxonomy of generic clinical questions: classification study. *British Medical Journal*, 321: 429–432.

Ely, J., Osheroff, J., et al. (2007). Patient-care questions that physicians are unable to answer. *Journal of the American Medical Informatics Association*, 14: 407–414.

Epstein, W. (2004). Confirmational response bias and the quality of the editorial processes among American social work journals. *Research on Social Work Practice*, 14: 450–458.

Ericsson, K. and Simon, H. (1993). *Protocol Analysis: Verbal Reports as Data, Revised Edition*. Cambridge, MA. MIT Press.

Esposito, J. (2004). The devil you don't know: the unexpected future of open access publishing. *First Monday*, 9(8). http://www.firstmonday.org/issues/issue9_8/esposito/.

Evans, A., McNutt, R., et al. (1993). The characteristics of peer reviewers who produce good quality reviews. *Journal of General Internal Medicine*, 8: 422–428.

Evans, D. (1988). Pragmatically-structured, lexical-semantic knowledge bases for unified medical language systems. *Proceedings of the 12th Annual Symposium on Computer Applications in Medical Care*, Washington, DC. IEEE. 169–173.

Evans, D., Hersh, W., et al. (1991). Automatic indexing of abstracts via natural language processing using a simple thesaurus. *Medical Decision Making*, 11: S108–S115.

Evans, D. and Lefferts, R. (1993). Design and evaluation of the CLARIT TREC-2 system. *The Second Text REtrieval Conference (TREC-2)*, Gaithersburg, MD. National Institute of Standards and Technology. 137–150.

Evans, D., Lefferts, R., et al. (1992). CLARIT TREC design, experiments, and results. *The First Text REtrieval Conference (TREC-1)*, Gaithersburg, MD. National Institute of Standards and Technology. 251–286.

Evans, D. and Zhai, C. (1994). Noun-phrase analysis in unrestricted text for information retrieval. *Proceedings of the 34th annual meeting on Association for Computational Linguistics*, Santa Cruz, CA. Association for Computational Linguistics. 17–24.

Evans, J., Nadjari, H., et al. (1990). Quotational and reference accuracy in surgical journals: a continuing peer review problem. *Journal of the American Medical Association*, 263: 1353–1354.

Evans, R., Pestotnik, S., et al. (1998). A computer-assisted management program for antibiotics and other antiinfective agents. *New England Journal of Medicine*, 338: 232–238.

Eysenbach, G. (2000a). Consumer health informatics. *British Medical Journal*, 320: 1713–1716.

Eysenbach, G. (2000b). Report of a case of cyberplagiarism – and reflections on detecting and preventing academic misconduct using the Internet. *Journal of Medical Internet Research*, 2: e4.

Eysenbach, G. (2006). Infodemiology: tracking flu-related searches on the web for syndromic surveillance. *Proceedings of the AMIA 2006 Annual Symposium*, Washington, DC. American Medical Informatics Association. 244–248.

Eysenbach, G. and Diepgen, T. (1998). Towards quality management of medical information on the internet: evaluation, labelling, and filtering of information. *British Medical Journal*, 317: 1496–1502.

Eysenbach, G. and Kohler, C. (2002). How do consumers search for and appraise health information on the World Wide Web? Qualitative study using focus groups, usability tests, and in-depth interviews. *British Medical Journal*, 324: 573–577.

Eysenbach, G. and Kohler, C. (2004). Health-related searches on the internet. *Journal of the American Medical Association*, 291: 2946.

Eysenbach, G., Powell, J., et al. (2002). Empirical studies assessing the quality of health information for consumers on the World Wide Web: a systematic review. *Journal of the American Medical Association*, 287: 2691–2700.

Eysenbach, G., Tuische, J., et al. (2001). Evaluation of the usefulness of internet searches to identify unpublished clinical trials for systematic reviews. *Medical Informatics and the Internet in Medicine*, 26: 203–218.

Fagan, J. (1987). Experiments in Automatic Phrase Indexing Document Retrieval: A Comparison of Syntactic and Non-Syntactic Methods. Department of Computer Science. Ph.D. Thesis. Cornell University.

Fagan, J. (1989). The effectiveness of a non-syntactic approach to automatic phrase indexing for document retrieval. *Journal of the American Society for Information Science*, 40: 115–132.

Fail, D. and Pedersen, J. (2005). Sponsored search: a brief history. *Bulletin of the American Society for Information Science and Technology*, 32(2): 12–13. http://www.asis.org/Bulletin/Dec-05/pedersen.html.

Fallis, D. and Fricke, M. (2002). Indicators of accuracy of consumer health information on the internet: a study of indicators relating to information for managing fever in children in the home. *Journal of the American Medical Informatics Association*, 9: 73–79.

Fallows, D. (2005). Search Engine Users. Washington, DC, Pew Internet & American Life Project. http://www.pewinternet.org/pdfs/PIP_Searchengine_users.pdf.

Fallows, D., Rainie, L., et al. (2004). Data Memo on Search Engines. Washington, DC, Pew Internet & American Life Project. http://www.pewinternet.org/pdfs/PIP_Data_Memo_Search-engines.pdf.

Fan, W., Wallace, L., et al. (2006). Tapping the power of text mining. *Communications of the ACM*, 49(9): 76–82.

Feinstein, A. (1995). Meta-analysis: statistical alchemy for the 21st century. *Journal of Clinical Epidemiology*, 48: 71–79.

Feinstein, A. and Horwitz, R. (1997). Problems in the "evidence" of "evidence-based medicine". *American Journal of Medicine*, 103: 529–535.

Feldman, R. and Sanger, J. (2007). *The Text Mining Handbook: Advanced Approaches in Analyzing Unstructured Data*. New York, NY. Cambridge University Press.

Fellbaum, C., ed. (1998). *WordNet: An Electronic Lexical Database*. Cambridge, MA. MIT Press.

Fenichel, C. (1980). The process of searching online bibliogrpahic databases: a review of research. *Library Research*, 2: 107–127.

Fensel, D., Wahlster, W., et al. eds. (2002). *Spinning the Semantic Web: Bringing the World Wide Web to Its Full Potential*. Cambridge, MA. MIT Press.

Ferguson, T. (2002). From patients to end users: quality of online patient networks needs more attention than quality of online health information. *British Medical Journal*, 324: 555–556.

Fetterly, D., Manasse, M., et al. (2003). A large-scale study of the evolution of web pages. *Proceedings of the Twelfth International Conference on the World Wide Web*, Budapest, Hungary. ACM Press. 669–678.

Fidel, R. and Soergel, D. (1983). Factors affecting online bibliographic retrieval: a conceptual framework for research. *Journal of the American Society for Information Science*, 34: 163–180.

Field, M. and Lohr, K., eds. (1990). *Clinical Practice Guidelines: Directions for a New Program*. Washington, DC. National Academy Press.

Fischer, P., Stratmann, W., et al. (1980). User reaction to PROMIS: issues related to acceptability of medical innovations. *Proceedings of the 4th Annual Symposium on Computer Applications in Medical Care*, New York, IEEE. 1722–1730.

Fisher, C. (2006). Public health. Clinical trials results databases: unanswered questions. *Science*, 311: 180–181.

Fiszman, M., Chapman, W., et al. (2000). Automatic detection of acute bacterial pneumonia from chest x-ray reports. *Journal of the American Medical Informatics Association*, 7: 593–604.

Fiszman, M., Rindflesch, T., et al. (2004a). Abstraction summarization for managing the biomedical research literature. *Proceedings of the HLT-NAACL Workshop on Computational Lexical Semantics*, Boston, MA. North American Association for Computational Linguistics. 76–83. http://lhncbc.nlm.nih.gov/lhc/docs/published/2004/pub2004015.pdf.

Fiszman, M., Rindflesch, T., et al. (2004b). Summarization of an online medical encyclopedia. *MEDINFO 2004 – Proceedings of the Eleventh World Congress on Medical Informatics*, San Francisco, CA. IOS Press. 506–510.

Flamm, B. (2002). Review of Cha, KY, Wirth, DP, Lobo, RA. Does prayer influence the success of in vitro fertilization-embryo transfer? *The Scientific Review of Alternative Medicine*, 6: 47–50.

Flamm, B. (2004). The Columbia University 'miracle' study: flawed and fraud. *Skeptical Inquirer*. http://www.csicop.org/si/2004–09/miracle-study.html.

Flanagin, A., Carey, L., et al. (1998). Prevalence of articles with honorary authors and ghost authors in peer-reviewed medical journals. *Journal of the American Medical Association*, 280: 222–224.

Flesch, R. (1948). A new readability yardstick. *Journal of Applied Psychology*, 32: 221–233.

Fletcher, R. (2003). Adverts in medical journals: caveat lector. *Lancet*, 361: 10–11.

Fletcher, R. and Fletcher, S. (1979). Clinical research in general medical journals: a 30-year perspective. *New England Journal of Medicine*, 301: 180–183.

Florance, V. (1992). Medical knowledge for clinical problem solving: a structural analysis of clinical questions. *Bulletin of the Medical Library Association*, 80: 140–149.

Florance, V., Giuse, N., et al. (2002). Information in context: integrating information specialists into practice settings. *Journal of the Medical Library Association*, 90: 49–58.

Florance, V. and Marchionini, G. (1995). Information processing in the context of medical care. *Proceedings of the 18th Annual International ACM SIGIR Conference on Research and Development in Information Retrieval*, Seattle. ACM Press. 158–163.

Foltz, A. and Sullivan, J. (1996). Reading level, learning presentation preference, and desire for information among cancer patients. *Journal of Cancer Education*, 11: 32–38.

Fomous, C., Mitchell, J., et al. (2006). 'Genetics home reference': helping patients understand the role of genetics in health and disease. *Community Genetics*, 9: 274–278.

Fontanarosa, P., Rennie, D., et al. (2004). Postmarketing surveillance – lack of vigilance, lack of trust. *Journal of the American Medical Association*, 292: 2647–2650.

Fontelo, P., Ackerman, M., et al. (2003). The PDA as a portal to knowledge sources in a wireless setting. *Telemedicine Journal and e-Health*, 9: 141–147.

Fontelo, P., Liu, F., et al. (2005). askMEDLINE: a free-text, natural language query tool for MEDLINE/PubMed. *BMC Medical Informatics and Decision Making*, 5: 5. http://www.biomedcentral.com/1472–6947/5/5.

Fontelo, P., Nahin, A., et al. (2005). Accessing MEDLINE/PubMed with handheld devices: developments and new search portals. *Proceedings of the 38th Annual Hawaii International Conference on System Sciences*, Big Island, Hawaii. IEEE Computer Society. 158b. http://csdl. computer.org/comp/proceedings/hicss/2005/2268/06/22680158b.pdf.

Fortunato, S., Boguna, M., et al. (2005). How to Make the Top Ten: Approximating PageRank from In-degree. Bloomington, IN, Indiana University. http://arxiv.org/pdf/cs.IR/0511016.

Fortunato, S., Flammini, A., et al. (2006a). The egalitarian effect of search engines. *WWW 2006*, Edinburgh, UK. International World Wide Web Conference Committee. http://arxiv.org/ PS_cache/cs/pdf/0511/0511005.pdf.

Fortunato, S., Flammini, A., et al. (2006b). Topical interests and the migration of search engine bias. *Proceedings of the National Academy of Sciences*, 103: 12684–12689.

Foster, A. (2002). Plagiarism-detection tool creates legal quandary. *Chronicle of Higher Education*. May 17, 2002. http://chronicle.com/free/v48/i36/36a03701.htm.

Foulonneau, M., Habing, T., et al. (2006). Automated capture of thumbnails and thumbshots for use by metadata aggregation services. *D-Lib Magazine*, 12(1). http://www.dlib.org/dlib/january06/foulonneau/01foulonneau.html.

Fox, C. (1992). Lexical analysis and stop lists, 102–130, in Frakes, W. and Baeza-Yates, R., eds. *Information Retrieval: Data Structures and Algorithms*. Englewood Cliffs, NJ. Prentice-Hall.

Fox, J., McMillan, S., et al. (2007). Conducting research on the web: 2007 update for the bioinformatics links directory. *Nucleic Acids Research*, 35: W3–W5.

Fox, S. (2006). Online Health Search 2006. Washington, DC, Pew Internet & American Life Project. http://www.pewinternet.org/pdfs/PIP_Online_Health_2006.pdf.

Frakes, W. (1992). Stemming algorithms, 131–160, in Frankes, W. and Baeza-Yates, R., eds. *Information Retrieval: Data Structures and Algorithms*. Englewood Cliffs, NJ. Prentice-Hall.

Frakes, W. and Baeza-Yates, R., eds. (1992). *Information Retrieval: Data Structures and Algorithms*. Englewood Cliffs, NJ. Prentice-Hall.

Frankel, M., Elliot, R., et al. (2000). Defining and Certifying Electronic Publication in Science. American Association for the Advancement of Science. http://www.aaas.org/spp/dspp/sfrl/ projects/epub/define.htm. Accessed: July 1, 2002.

Freiman, J., Chalmers, T., et al. (1978). The importance of beta, the type II error and sample size in the design and interpretation of the randomized controlled trial. *New England Journal of Medicine*, 299: 690–694.

Friedlander, A. (2002). The National Digital Information Infrastructure Preservation Program: expectations, realities, choices, and progress to date. *D-Lib Magazine*, 8. http://www.dlib.org/ dlib/april02/friedlander/04friedlander.html.

Friedman, C. (1997). Towards a comprehensive medical language processing system: methods and issues. *Proceedings of the 1997 AMIA Annual Fall Symposium*, Nashville, TN. Hanley & Belfus. 595–599.

Friedman, C. (2005). Semantic text parsing for patient records, 423–448, in Chen, H., Fuller, S., Friedman, C. and Hersh, W., eds. *Medical Informatics: Knowledge Management and Data Mining in Biomedicine*. New York, NY. Springer.

Friedman, C., Alderson, P., et al. (1994). A general natural-language text processor for clinical radiology. *Journal of the American Medical Informatics Association*, 1: 161–174.

Friedman, C. and Hripcsak, G. (1998). Evaluating natural language processors in the clinical domain. *Methods of Information in Medicine*, 37: 334–344.

Friedman, C., Hripcsak, G., et al. (1995). Natural language processing in an operational clinical system. *Natural Language Engineering*, 1: 83–108.

Friedman, C., Hripcsak, G., et al. (1998). An evaluation of natural language processing methodologies. *Proceedings of the AMIA 1998 Annual Symposium*, Orlando, FL. Hanley & Belfus. 855–859.

Friedman, C., Shagina, L., et al. (2004). Automated encoding of clinical documents based on natural language processing. *Journal of the American Medical Informatics Association*, 11: 392–402.

Friedman, C., Wildemuth, B., et al. (1996). A comparison of hypertext and Boolean access to biomedical information. *Proceedings of the 1996 AMIA Annual Fall Symposium*, Washington, DC. Hanley & Belfus. 2–6.

Friedman, C. and Wyatt, J. (2001). Publication bias in medical informatics. *Journal of the American Medical Informatics Association*, 8: 189–191.

Friedman, C. and Wyatt, J. (2006). *Evaluation Methods in Biomedical Informatics*. New York, NY. Springer.

Friedman, P. (1990). Correcting the literature following fraudulent publication. *Journal of the American Medical Association*, 263: 1416–1419.

Friedman, T. (2003). Is Google God? *New York Times*. June 29, 2003. 13. http://www.nytimes.com/2003/06/29/opinion/29FRIE.html.

Frisse, M. (1988). Searching for information in a hypertext medical handbook. *Communications of the ACM*, 31: 880–886.

Fromme, E., Eilers, K., et al. (2004). How accurate is clinician reporting of chemotherapy adverse effects? A comparison with patient-reported symptoms from the Quality-of-Life Questionnaire C30. *Journal of Clinical Oncology*, 22: 3485–3490.

Fry, E. (1977). Fry's readability graph: clarifications, validity, and extension to level 17. *Journal of Reading*, 21: 242–252.

Fuhr, N. and Knorz, G. (1984). Retrieval test evaluation of a rule-based automatic indexing (AIR/PHYS), 391–408, in vanRijsbergen, C., ed. *Research and Development in Information Retrieval*. Cambridge. Cambridge University Press.

Fujita, S. (2004). Revisiting again document length hypotheses – TREC 2004 Genomics Track experiments at Patolis. *The Thirteenth Text REtrieval Conference: TREC 2004*, Gaithersburg, MD. National Institute of Standards and Technology. http://trec.nist.gov/pubs/trec13/papers/patolis.geo.pdf.

Fuller, M., Kaszkiel, M., et al. (1997). MDS TREC-6 report. *The Sixth Text REtrieval Conference (TREC-6)*, Gaithersburg, MD. National Institute of Standards and Technology. 241–257.

Fundel, K. and Zimmer, R. (2006). Gene and protein nomenclature in public databases. *BMC Bioinformatics*, 7: 372. http://www.biomedcentral.com/1471-2105/7/372.

Funk, M. (2005). Open Access – A Primer. Chicago, IL, Medical Library Association. http://www.mlanet.org/pdf/resources/oa_primer_mfunk.pdf.

Funk, M. and Reid, C. (1983). Indexing consistency in MEDLINE. *Bulletin of the Medical Library Association*, 71: 176–183.

Gagliardi, A. and Jadad, A. (2002). Examination of instruments used to rate quality of health information on the Internet: chronicle of a voyage with an unclear destination. *British Medical Journal*, 324: 569–573.

Gantz, J., Reinsel, D., et al. (2007). The Expanding Digital Universe: A Forecast of Worldwide Information Growth Through 2010. Hopkinton, MA, EMC Corp. http://www.emc.com/about/destination/digital_universe/pdf/Expanding_Digital_Universe_IDC_WhitePaper_022507.pdf.

Garcia-Berthou, E. and Alcaraz, C. (2004). Incongruence between test statistics and P values. *BMC Medical Research*, 4: 13. http://www.biomedcentral.com/1471–2288/4/13.

Gardner, M. and Bond, J. (1990). An exploratory study of statistical assessment of papers published in the British medical journal. *Journal of the American Medical Association*, 263: 1355–1357.

Garfield, E. (1964). "Science Citation Index" – a new dimension in indexing. *Science*, 144: 649–654.

Garfield, E. (1979a). Bradford's law and related statistical patterns, 476–483, in Garfield, E., ed. *Essays of an Information Scientist: 1979–1980.*Vol 4. Philadelphia. Institute for Scientific Information.

Garfield, E. (1979b). The citation index as a search tool, 41–61, in Garfield, E., ed. *Citation Indexing – Its Theory and Application in Science, Technology, and Humanities.* New York. Wiley.

Garfield, E. (1994). The impact factor. *Current Contents*, 25: 3–7.

Garfield, E. (2006). The history and meaning of the journal impact factor. *Journal of the American Medical Association*, 295: 90–93.

Garfield, E. and Welljams-Dorof, A. (1990). The impact of fraudulent research on the scientific literature: the Stephen Breuning case. *Journal of the American Medical Association*, 1990: 1424–1426.

Garfunkel, J., Lawson, E., et al. (1990). Effect of acceptance or rejection on the author's evaluation of peer review of medical manuscripts. *Journal of the American Medical Association*, 263: 1376–1378.

Garfunkel, J., Ulshen, M., et al. (1990). Problems identified by secondary review of accepted manuscripts. *Journal of the American Medical Association*, 263: 1369–1371.

Garfunkel, J., Ulshen, M., et al. (1994). Effect of institutional prestige on reviewers' recommendations and editorial decisions. *Journal of the American Medical Association*, 272: 137–138.

Garg, A., Adhikari, N., et al. (2005). Effects of computerized clinical decision support systems on practitioner performance and patient outcomes: a systematic review. *Journal of the American Medical Association*, 293: 1223–1238.

Garritty, C. and El Emam, K. (2006). Who's using PDAs? Estimates of PDA use by health care providers: a systematic review of surveys. *Journal of Medical Internet Research*, 8: e7. http://www.jmir.org/2006/2/e7/.

Garrow, J., Butterfield, M., et al. (1998). The reported training and experience of editors in chief of specialist clinical medical journals. *Journal of the American Medical Association*, 280: 286–287.

Gault, L., Shultz, M., et al. (2002). Variations in Medical Subject Headings (MeSH) mapping: from the natural language of patron terms to the controlled vocabulary of mapped lists. *Journal of the Medical Library Association*, 90: 173–180. http://pubmedcentral.gov/articlerender.fcgi?artid=100762.

Gay, C., Kayaalp, M., et al. (2005). Semi-automatic indexing of full text biomedical articles. *Proceedings of the AMIA 2005 Annual Symposium*, Washington, DC. Hanley & Belfus. http://ii.nlm.nih.gov/resources/amia05.fulltext.w.footer.pdf.

Gazmararian, J., Baker, D., et al. (1999). Health literacy among Medicare enrollees in a managed care organization. *Journal of the American Medical Association*, 281: 545–551.

Gehanno, J., Paris, C., et al. (1998). Assessment of bibliographic databases performance in information retrieval for occupational and environmental toxicology. *Occupational and Environmental Medicine*, 55: 562–566.

Gerhart, S. (2004). Do web search engines suppress controversy? *First Monday*, 9: 1. http://www.firstmonday.dk/issues/issue9_1/gerhart/.

Gey, F., Kando, N., et al. (2005). Cross-language information retrieval: the way ahead. *Information Processing and Management*, 41: 415–432.

Ghemawat, S., Gobioff, H., et al. (2003). The Google file system. *Proceedings of the19th ACM Symposium on Operating Systems Principles*, Lake George, NY. ACM Press. http://labs.google.com/papers/gfs-sosp2003.pdf.

Gilarranz, J., Gonzalo, J., et al. (1997). An approach to conceptual text retrieval using the EuroWordNet multilingual semantic database. *AAAI Spring Symposium on Cross-Language Text and Speech Retrieval*, Palo Alto, CA. AAAI. http://www.ee.umd.edu/medlab/filter/sss/papers/gilarranz2.ps.

Giles, J. (2005). Internet encyclopaedias go head to head. *Nature*, 438: 900–901. http://www.nature.com/nature/journal/v438/n7070/full/438900a.html.

Giuse, N., Huber, J., et al. (1994). Information needs of health care professionals in an AIDS outpatient clinic as determined by chart review. *Journal of the American Medical Informatics Association*, 1: 395–403.

Giuse, N., Koonce, T., et al. (2005). Evolution of a mature clinical informationist model. *Journal of the American Medical Informatics Association*, 12: 249–255.

Giustini, D. (2005). How Google is changing medicine. *British Medical Journal*, 331: 1487–1488.

Giustini, D. (2006). How web 2.0 is changing medicine. *British Medical Journal*, 333: 1283–1284.

Glantz, S. (1980). Biostatistics: how to detect, correct, and prevent errors in the medical literature. *Circulation*, 61: 1–7.

Glass, G. (1976). Primary, secondary, and meta-analysis of research. *Educational Research*, 10: 3–8.

Glasziou, P. and Irwig, L. (1998). Meta-Analysis of diagnostic tests, 2579–2585, in Armitage, P. and Colton, T., eds. *Encyclopaedia of Biostatistics, Vol. 4*. Chichester. Wiley.

Glasziou, P., Irwig, L., et al. (2001). *Systematic Reviews in Health Care: A Practical Guide*. Cambridge, UK. Cambridge University Press.

Godby, C., Young, J., et al. (2004). A repository of metadata crosswalks. *D-Lib Magazine*, 10(12). http://www.dlib.org/dlib/december04/godby/12godby.html.

Godlee, F., Gale, C., et al. (1998). Effect on the quality of peer review of blinding reviewers and asking them to sign their reports. *Journal of the American Medical Association*, 280: 237–240.

Golder, S., McIntosh, H., et al. (2006). Developing efficient search strategies to identify reports of adverse effects in MEDLINE and EMBASE. *Health Information and Libraries Journal*, 23: 3–12.

Goldsmith, L. and Hall, R. (2006). A socratic dialogue on impact factors. *Journal of Investigative Dermatology*, 126: 1923–1924.

Gomez, L., Egan, D., et al. (1986). Learning to use a text editor: some learner characteristics that predict success. *Human-Computer Interaction*, 2: 1–23.

Goncalves, M., Fox, E., et al. (2004). Streams, structures, spaces, scenarios, societies (5S): a formal model for digital libraries. *ACM Transactions on Information Systems*, 22: 270–312.

Gonzales, R., Bartlett, J., et al. (2001). Principles of appropriate antibiotic use for treatment of acute respiratory infections in adults: background, specific aims, and methods. *Annals of Internal Medicine*, 134: 479–486.

Gorman, P. (1993). Does the medical literature contain the evidence to answer the questions of primary care physicians? Preliminary findings of a study. *Proceedings of the 17th Annual Symposium on Computer Applications in Medical Care*, Washington, DC. McGraw-Hill. 571–575.

Gorman, P. (1995). Information needs of physicians. *Journal of the American Society for Information Science*, 46: 729–736.

Gorman, P., Ash, J., et al. (1994). Can primary care physicians' questions be answered using the medical literature? *Bulletin of the Medical Library Association*, 82: 140–146.

Gorman, P. and Helfand, M. (1995). Information seeking in primary care: how physicians choose which clinical questions to pursue and which to leave unanswered. *Medical Decision Making*, 15: 113–119.

Gospodnetic, O. and Hatcher, E. (2005). *Lucene in Action*. Greenwich, CT. Manning Publications.

Gotzsche, P. and Olson, O. (2001). Misleading publications of major mammography screening trials in major medical journals. *Fourth International Congress on Peer Review in Biomedical Publication*, Barcelona, Spain. American Medical Association. http://www.ama-assn.org/public/peer/peerhome.htm.

Graber, M., Bergus, G., et al. (1999). Using the World Wide Web to answer clinical questions: how efficient are different methods of information retrieval? *Journal of Family Practice*, 49: 520–524.

Graber, M., Roller, C., et al. (1999). Readability levels of patient education material on the World Wide Web. *Journal of Family Practice*, 48: 58–61.

Grad, R., Pluye, P., et al. (2005). Assessing the impact of clinical information-retrieval technology in a family practice residency. *Journal of Evaluation in Clinical Practice*, 11: 576–586.

Graff, D. (2002). The AQUAINT Corpus of English News Text. Philadelphia, PA, Linguistic Data Consortium. http://www.ldc.upenn.edu/Catalog/CatalogEntry.jsp?catalogId= LDC2002T31.

Graham, R., Perriss, R., et al. (2005). DICOM demystified: a review of digital file formats and their use in radiological practice. *Clinical Radiology*, 60: 1133–1140.

Gravois, S., Fisher, W., et al. (1995). Information-seeking practices of dental hygienists. *Bulletin of the Medical Library Association*, 83: 446–452.

Gray, J. (2003). What next? A dozen information technology research goals. *Journal of the ACM*, 50: 41–57.

Gray, J. (2004). Evidence based policy making. *British Medical Journal*, 329: 988–989.

Greenberg, J., Pattuelli, M., et al. (2002). Author-generated Dublin core metadata for web resources: a baseline study in an organization. *Journal of Digital Information*, 2: 2. http://jodi. ecs.soton.ac.uk/Articles/v02/i02/Greenberg/.

Greenes, R. (1982). OBUS: a microcomputer system for measurement, calculation, reporting, and retrieval of obstetric ultrasound examinations. *Radiology*, 144: 879–883.

Greenes, R., Barnett, G., et al. (1970). Recording, retrieval, and review of medical data by physician-computer interaction. *New England Journal of Medicine*, 282: 307–315.

Greenes, R., McClure, R., et al. (1992). The findings-diagnosis continuum: implications for image descriptions and clinical databases. *Proceedings of the 16th Annual Symposium on Computer Applications in Medical Care*, Baltimore, MD. McGraw-Hill. 383–387.

Greenwald, R. (2005). And a diagnostic test was performed. *New England Journal of Medicine*, 353: 2089–2090.

Gregoire, G., Derderian, F., (1995). Selecting the language of the publications included in a meta-analysis: is there a Tower of Babel bias? *Journal of Clinical Epidemiology*, 48: 159–163.

Grossman, D. and Frieder, O. (2004). *Information Retrieval Algorithms and Heuristics*, Second Edition. New York, NY. Springer.

Guard, R., Fredericka, T., et al. (2000). Health care, information needs, and outreach: reaching Ohio's rural citizens. *Bulletin of the Medical Library Association*, 88: 374–381.

Guimera, R., Uzzi, B., et al. (2005). Team assembly mechanisms determine collaboration network structure and team performance. *Science*, 308: 697–702.

Gupta, A., Gross, C., et al. (2001). Disclosure of financial conflict of interest in published research: a study of adherence to uniform requirements. *Fourth International Congress on Peer Review in Biomedical Publication*, Barcelona, Spain. American Medical Association. http://www.ama-assn.org/public/peer/peerhome.htm.

Guyatt, G. and Rennie, D. (2001). *Users' Guide to the Medical Literature: Essentials of Evidence-Based Clinical Practice*. Chicago. American Medical Association.

Guyatt, G., Rennie, D., et al. (2001). *Users' Guide to the Medical Literature: A Manual for Evidence-Based Clinical Practice*. Chicago. American Medical Association.

Haase, A., Follmann, M., et al. (2007). Developing search strategies for clinical practice guidelines in SUMSearch and Google Scholar and assessing their retrieval performance. *BMC Medical Research Methodology*, 7(28). http://www.biomedcentral.com/1471–2288/7/28.

Hafner, K. (2006). Researchers Yearn to Use AOL Logs, but They Hesitate. New York Times. August 23, 2006. http://www.nytimes.com/2006/08/23/technology/23search.html.

Hallett, K. (1998). Separate but equal? a system comparison study of MEDLINE's controlled vocabulary MeSH. *Bulletin of the Medical Library Association*, 86: 491–495.

Halpern, S., Karlawish, J., et al. (2002). The continuing unethical conduct of underpowered clinical trials. *Journal of the American Medical Association*, 288: 358–362.

Hammersley, B. (2005). *Developing Feeds with RSS and Atom*. Sebastopol, CA. O'Reilly.

Hammond, T., Hannay, T., et al. (2004). The role of RSS in science publishing: syndication and annotation on the web. *D-Lib Magazine*, 10(12). http://www.dlib.org/dlib/december04/hammond/12hammond.html.

Hammond, T., Hannay, T., et al. (2005). Social bookmarking tools (I) – a general review. *D-Lib Magazine*, 11(4). http://www.dlib.org/dlib/april05/hammond/04hammond.html.

Hansell, S. (2006). Online Trail Can Lead To Court. New York Times. February 4, 2006. C1. http://www.nytimes.com/2006/02/04/technology/04privacy.html.

Hargens, L. (1990). Variation in journal peer review systems: possible causes and consequences. *Journal of the American Medical Association*, 263: 1348–1352.

Harman, D. (1991). How effective is suffixing? *Journal of the American Society for Information Science*, 42: 7–15.

Harman, D. (2005a). Beyond English, 153–182, in Voorhees, E. and Harman, D., eds. *TREC: Experiment and Evaluation in Information Retrieval*. Cambridge, MA. MIT Press.

Harman, D. (2005b). The TREC Ad Hoc Experiments, 79–98, inVoorhees, E. and Harman, D., eds. *TREC: Experiment and Evaluation in Information Retrieval*. Cambridge, MA. MIT Press.

Harnly, A., Nenkova, A., et al. (2005). Automation of summary evaluation by the pyramid method. *Recent Advances in Natural Language Processing 2005*, Borovets, Bulgaria. http://www1.cs.columbia.edu/~becky/DUC2006/pyramidpubs/aabo-ranlp.pdf.

Harter, S. (1992). Psychological relevance and information science. *Journal of the American Society for Information Science*, 43: 602–615.

Hatch, C. and Goodman, S. (1998). Perceived value of providing peer reviewers with abstracts and preprints of related published and unpublished papers. *Journal of the American Medical Association*, 280: 273–274.

Haug, C., Gotzsche, P., et al. (2005). Registries and registration of clinical trials. *New England Journal of Medicine*, 353: 2811–2812.

Haug, P., Koehler, S., et al. (1994). A natural language understanding system combining syntactic and semantic techniques. *Proceedings of the 18th Annual Symposium on Computer Applications in Medical Care*, Washington, DC. Hanley & Belfus. 247–251.

Haug, P., Ranum, D., et al. (1990). Computerized extraction of coded findings from free-text radiologic reports. *Radiology*, 174: 543–548.

Hawking, D. (2000). Overview of the TREC-9 web track. *The Ninth Text REtrieval Conference (TREC-9)*, Gaithersburg, MD. National Institute of Standards and Technology. 87–102.

Hawking, D. and Craswell, N. (2001). Overview of the TREC-2001 web track. *The Tenth Text REtrieval Conference (TREC 2001)*, Gaithersburg, MD. National Institute of Standards and Technology. 61–67.

Hawking, D. and Craswell, N. (2005). The very large collection and web tracks, 199–232, in Voorhees, E. and Harman, D., eds. *TREC: Experiment and Evaluation in Information Retrieval*. Cambridge, MA. MIT Press.

Haynes, R. (2001). Of studies, syntheses, synopses, and systems: the "4S" evolution of services for finding current best evidence. *ACP Journal Club*, 134: A11–A13.

Haynes, R. (2002). What kind of evidence is it that Evidence-Based Medicine advocates want health care providers and consumers to pay attention to? *BMC Health Services Research*, 2: 3. http://www.biomedcentral.com/1472–6963/2/3.

Haynes, R. (2004). What has evidence based medicine done for us? *British Medical Journal*, 329: 987–988.

Haynes, R. (2005). bmjupdates+, a new free service for evidence-based clinical practice. *Evidence-Based Nursing*, 8: 39.

Haynes, R., Cotoi, C., et al. (2006). Second-order peer review of the medical literature for clinical practitioners. *Journal of the American Medical Association*, 295: 1801–1808.

Haynes, R., Holland, J., et al. (2006). McMaster PLUS: a cluster randomized clinical trial of an intervention to accelerate clinical use of evidence-based information from digital libraries. *Journal of the American Medical Informatics Association*, 13: 593–600.

Haynes, R., Johnston, M., et al. (1992). A randomized controlled trial of a program to enhance clinical use of MEDLINE. *Online Journal of Controlled Clinical Trials*, Doc No 56.

Haynes, R. and McKibbon, K. (1987). Grateful Med. *M.D. Computing*, 4: 47–57.

Haynes, R., McKibbon, K., et al. (1985). Computer searching of the medical literature: an evaluation of MEDLINE searching systems. *Annals of Internal Medicine*, 103: 812–816.

Haynes, R., McKibbon, K., et al. (1990). Online access to MEDLINE in clinical settings. *Annals of Internal Medicine*, 112: 78–84.

Haynes, R., Mulrow, C., et al. (1990). More informative abstracts revisited. *Annals of Internal Medicine*, 113: 69–76.

Haynes, R. and Walker-Dilks, C. (2005). Having trouble deciding what's most important to read? Look to the stars. *ACP Journal Club*, 143(1): A10. http://www.acpjc.org/shared/about_stars. htm.

Haynes, R., Walker, C., et al. (1994). Performance of 27 MEDLINE systems tested by searches with clinical questions. *Journal of the American Medical Informatics Association*, 1: 285–295.

Haynes, R., Wilczynski, N., et al. (1994). Developing optimal search strategies for detecting clinically sound studies in MEDLINE. *Journal of the American Medical Informatics Association*, 1: 447–458.

Hazlehurst, B., Frost, H., et al. (2005). MediClass: a system for detecting and classifying encounter-based clinical events in any electronic medical record. *Journal of the American Medical Informatics Association*, 12: 517–529.

Hazlehurst, B., Sittig, D., et al. (2005). Natural language processing in the electronic medical record: assessing clinician adherence to tobacco treatment guidelines. *American Journal of Preventive Medicine*, 29: 434–439.

Hearst, M. (1996). Improving full-text precision on short queries using simple constraints. *Proceedings of the 5th Annual Symposium on Document Analysis and Information Retrieval (SDAIR)*, Las Vegas, NV. University of Nevada, Las Vegas. 217–232.

Hearst, M. (1999). User interfaces and visualization, 257–323, in Baeza-Yates, R. and Ribeiro-Neto, B., eds. *Modern Information Retrieval*. New York. ACM Press.

Hearst, M., Divoli, A., et al. (2007a). Biotext search engine: beyond abstract search. *Bioinformatics*, 23: 2196–2197.

Hearst, M., Divoli, A., et al. (2007b). Exploring the efficacy of caption search for bioscience journal search interfaces. *Proceedings of the ACL BioNLP'07 Workshop*, Prague, Czech Republic. Association for Computational Linguistics. http://biotext.berkeley.edu/papers/bionlp07. pdf.

Hearst, M. and Plaunt, C. (1993). Subtopic structuring for full-length document access. *Proceedings of the 16th Annual International ACM SIGIR Conference on Research and Development in Information Retrieval*, Pittsburgh, PA. ACM Press. 59–68.

Heath, B., McArthur, D., et al. (2005). Metadata lessons from the iLumina digital library. *Communications of the ACM*, 48(7): 68–74.

Helfand, M., Morton, S., et al. (2005). Challenges of summarizing better information for better health: the evidence-based practice center experience. *Annals of Internal Medicine*, 142(12 Part 2).

Hemila, H. (1997). Vitamin C intake and susceptibility to the common cold. *British Journal of Nutrition*, 77: 59–72.

Henderson, G. (2005). Google Scholar: a source for clinicians? *Canadian Medical Association Journal*, 172: 1549–1550.

Hendrix, G., Sacerdoti, E., et al. (1978). Developing a natural language interface to complex data. *ACM Transactions on Database Systems*, 3: 105–147.

Henry, D., Doran, E., et al. (2005). Ties that bind: multiple relationships between clinical researchers and the pharmaceutical industry. *Archives of Internal Medicine*, 165: 2493–2496.

Henry, S., Douglas, K., et al. (1998). A template-based approach to support utilization of clinical practice guidelines within an electronic health record. *Journal of the American Medical Informatics Association*, 5: 237–244.

Henzinger, M., Motwani, R., et al. (2002). Challenges to web search engines. *SIGIR Forum*, 36: 11–22. http://www.acm.org/sigir/forum/F2002/henzinger.pdf.

Hersh, A., ML, M. S., et al. (2004). National use of postmenopausal hormone therapy: annual trends and response to recent evidence. *Journal of the American Medical Association*, 291: 47–53.

Hersh, W. (1991). Evaluation of Meta-1 for a concept-based approach to the automated indexing and retrieval of bibliographic and full-text databases. *Medical Decision Making*, 11: S120–S124.

Hersh, W. (1994). Relevance and retrieval evaluation: perspectives from medicine. *Journal of the American Society for Information Science*, 45: 201–206.

Hersh, W. (1999). "A world of knowledge at your fingertips": the promise, reality, and future directions of on-line information retrieval. *Academic Medicine*, 74: 240–243.

Hersh, W. (2001). Interactivity at the Text Retrieval Conference (TREC). *Information Processing and Management*, 37: 365–366.

Hersh, W. (2002). Medical informatics education: an alternative pathway for training informationists. *Journal of the Medical Library Association*, 90: 76–79.

Hersh, W. (2005). Evaluation of biomedical text mining systems: lessons learned from information retrieval. *Briefings in Bioinformatics*, 6: 344–356.

Hersh, W. and Bhupatiraju, R. (2003). TREC Genomics Track overview. *The Twelfth Text REtrieval Conference (TREC 2003)*, Gaithersburg, MD. NIST. 14–23. http://trec.nist.gov/pubs/trec12/papers/GENOMICS.OVERVIEW3.pdf.

Hersh, W., Bhupatiraju, R., et al. (2006a). Adopting e-learning standards in health care: competency-based learning in the medical informatics domain. *Proceedings of the AMIA 2006 Annual Symposium*, Washington, DC. American Medical Informatics Association. CD-ROM.

Hersh, W., Bhupatiraju, R., et al. (2006b). Enhancing access to the bibliome: the TREC 2004 genomics track. *Journal of Biomedical Discovery and Collaboration*, 1: 3. http://www.j-biomed-discovery.com/content/1/1/3.

Hersh, W., Bhuptiraju, R., et al. (2004). TREC 2004 genomics track overview. *The Thirteenth Text REtrieval Conference (TREC 2004)*, Gaithersburg, MD. National Institute for Standards and Technology. http://trec.nist.gov/pubs/trec13/papers/GEO.OVERVIEW.pdf.

Hersh, W., Brown, K., et al. (1996). Cliniweb: managing clinical information on the World Wide Web. *Journal of the American Medical Informatics Association*, 3: 273–280.

Hersh, W., Buckley, C., et al. (1994). OHSUMED: an interactive retrieval evaluation and new large test collection for research. *Proceedings of the 17th Annual International ACM SIGIR Conference on Research and Development in Information Retrieval*, Dublin, Ireland. Springer-Verlag. 192–201.

Hersh, W., Campbell, E., et al. (1996). Empirical, automated vocabulary discovery using large text corpora and advanced natural language processing tools. *Proceedings of the 1996 AMIA Annual Fall Symposium*, Washington, DC. Hanley & Belfus. 159–163.

Hersh, W., Campbell, E., et al. (1997). Assessing the feasibility of large-scale natural language processing in a corpus of ordinary medical records: a lexical analysis. *Proceedings of the 1997 AMIA Annual Fall Symposium*, Nashville, TN. Hanley & Belfus. 580–584.

Hersh, W., Cohen, A., et al. (2007). TREC 2007 Genomics Track overview. *The Sixteenth Text REtrieval Conference (TREC 2007)*, Gaithersburg, MD. National Institute for Standards and Technology. http://ir.ohsu.edu/genomics/trec-07-genomics.pdf.

Hersh, W., Cohen, A., et al. (2006). TREC 2006 Genomics Track overview. *The Fifteenth Text REtrieval Conference (TREC 2006)*, Gaithersburg, MD. National Institute for Standards and Technology. 52–78. http://trec.nist.gov/pubs/trec15/papers/GEO.OVERVIEW.pdf.

Hersh, W., Cohen, A., et al. (2005). TREC 2005 Genomics Track overview. *The Fourteenth Text REtrieval Conference – TREC 2005*, Gaithersburg, MD. National Institute for Standards and Technology. http://trec.nist.gov/pubs/trec14/papers/GEO.OVERVIEW.pdf.

Hersh, W., Crabtree, M., et al. (2002). Factors associated with success for searching MEDLINE and applying evidence to answer clinical questions. *Journal of the American Medical Informatics Association*, 9: 283–293.

Hersh, W., Crabtree, M., et al. (2000). Factors associated with successful answering of clinical questions using an information retrieval system. *Bulletin of the Medical Library Association*, 88: 323–331.

Hersh, W. and Donohoe, L. (1998). SAPHIRE international: a tool for cross-language information retrieval. *Proceedings of the AMIA 1998 Annual Symposium*, Orlando, FL. Hanley & Belfus. 673–677.

Hersh, W., Elliot, D., et al. (1994). Towards new measures of information retrieval evaluation. *Proceedings of the 18th Annual Symposium on Computer Applications in Medical Care*, Washington, DC. Hanley & Belfus. 895–899.

Hersh, W., Gorman, P., et al. (1998). Applicability and quality of information for answering clinical questions on the web. *Journal of the American Medical Association*, 280: 1307–1308.

Hersh, W. and Hickam, D. (1992). A comparison of retrieval effectiveness for three methods of indexing medical literature. *American Journal of the Medical Sciences*, 303: 292–300.

Hersh, W. and Hickam, D. (1993). A comparison of two methods for indexing and retrieval from a full-text medical database. *Medical Decision Making*, 13: 220–226.

Hersh, W. and Hickam, D. (1994). The use of a multi-application computer workstation in a clinical setting. *Bulletin of the Medical Library Association*, 82: 382–389.

Hersh, W. and Hickam, D. (1995a). An evaluation of interactive Boolean and natural language searching with an on-line medical textbook. *Journal of the American Society for Information Science*, 46: 478–489.

Hersh, W. and Hickam, D. (1995b). Information retrieval in medicine: the SAPHIRE experience. *Journal of the American Society for Information Science*, 46: 743–747.

Hersh, W. and Hickam, D. (1998). How well do physicians use electronic information retrieval systems? A framework for investigation and review of the literature. *Journal of the American Medical Association*, 280: 1347–1352.

Hersh, W., Hickam, D., et al. (1994). A performance and failure analysis of SAPHIRE with a MEDLINE test collection. *Journal of the American Medical Informatics Association*, 1: 51–60.

Hersh, W., Hickam, D., et al. (1992). Word, concepts, or both: optimal indexing units for automated information retrieval. *Proceedings of the 16th Annual Symposium on Computer Applications in Medical Care*, Baltimore, MD. McGraw-Hill. 644–648.

Hersh, W., Jensen, J., et al. (2005). A qualitative task analysis of biomedical image use and retrieval. *MUSCLE/ImageCLEF Workshop on Image and Video Retrieval Evaluation*, Vienna, Austria. http://muscle.prip.tuwien.ac.at/workshop2005_proceedings/hersh.pdf.

Hersh, W., Kalpathy-Cramer, J., et al. (2006). Medical image retrieval and automated annotation: OHSU at ImageCLEF 2006. *Evaluation of Multilingual and Multi-modal Information Retrieval – Seventh Workshop of the Cross-Language Evaluation Forum, CLEF 2006*, Alicante, Spain. Lecture Notes in Computer Science. Springer 660–669. http://www.clef-campaign.org/2006/working_notes/workingnotes2006/hershCLEF2006.pdf.

Hersh, W., Müller, H., et al. (2006). Advancing biomedical image retrieval: development and analysis of a test collection. *Journal of the American Medical Informatics Association*, 13: 488–496.

Hersh, W., Müller, H., et al. (2007). Consolidating the ImageCLEF medical task test collection: 2005–2007. *Proceedings of the Third MUSCLE/ImageCLEF Workshop on Image and Video Retrieval Evaluation*, Budapest, Hungary. 31–39. http://www.billhersh.info/muscle-07-image.pdf.

Hersh, W. and Over, P. (2000). TREC-9 interactive track report. *The Ninth Text REtrieval Conference (TREC-9)*, Gaithersburg, MD. National Institute of Standards and Technology. 41–50.

Hersh, W., Pentecost, J., et al. (1996). A task-oriented approach to information retrieval evaluation. *Journal of the American Society for Information Science*, 47: 50–56.

Hersh, W. and Price, S. (1998). Identifying randomized controlled trials in conference proceedings abstracts. *Proceedings of the Sixth Annual Cochrane Colloquium*, Baltimore, MD. 52.

Hersh, W., Price, S., et al. (2000). Assessing thesaurus-based query expansion using the UMLS metathesaurus. *Proceedings of the AMIA 2000 Annual Symposium*, Los Angeles, CA. Hanley & Belfus. 344–348.

Hersh, W. and Rindfleisch, T. (2000). Electronic publishing of scholarly communication in the biomedical sciences. *Journal of the American Medical Informatics Association*, 7: 324–325.

Hersh, W., Turpin, A., et al. (2000a). Do batch and user evaluations give the same results? *Proceedings of the 23rd Annual International ACM SIGIR Conference on Research and Development in Information Retrieval*, Athens, Greece. ACM Press. 17–24.

Hersh, W., Turpin, A., et al. (2000b). Further analysis of whether batch and user evaluations give the same results with a question-answering task. *The Ninth Text REtrieval Conference (TREC-9)*, Gaithersburg, MD. National Institute of Standards and Technology. 407–416.

Hersh, W., Turpin, A., et al. (2001). Challenging conventional assumptions of automated information retrieval with real users: Boolean searching and batch retrieval evaluations. *Information Processing and Management*, 37: 383–402.

Hersh, W. and Zhang, L. (1999). Teaching English medical terminology using the UMLS metathesaurus and World Wide Web. *Proceedings of the AMIA 1999 Annual Symposium*, Washington, DC. Hanley & Belfus. 1078.

Herskovic, J., Tanaka, L., et al. (2007). A day in the life of PubMed: analysis of a typical day's query log. *Journal of the American Medical Informatics Association*, 14: 212–220.

Hesse, B., Nelson, D., et al. (2005). Trust and sources of health information: the impact of the internet and its implications for health care providers: findings from the first Health Information National Trends Survey. *Archives of Internal Medicine*, 165: 2618–2624.

Hettne, K., Weeber, M., et al. (2007). Automatic mining of the literature to generate new hypotheses for the possible link between periodontitis and atherosclerosis: lipopolysaccharide as a case study. *Journal of Clinical Peridontology*, 34: 1016–1024.

Hibble, A., Kanka, D., et al. (1998). Guidelines in general practice: the new Tower of Babel? *British Medical Journal*, 317: 862–863.

Hiemstra, D. and Kraaij, W. (2005). A language-modeling approach to TREC, in Voorhees, E. and Harman, D., eds. *TREC: Experiment and Evaluation in Information Retrieval*. Cambridge, MA. MIT Press.

Higgins, J., Green, S., et al. (2006). *Cochrane Handbook for Systematic Reviews of Interventions*. Oxford, England, Cochrane Collaboration. http://www.cochrane.org/resources/handbook/Handbook4.2.6Sep2006.pdf.

Hildreth, C. (1989). *The Online Catalogue: Developments and Directions*. London, England. The Library Association.

Hill, D., Begley, D., et al. (2004). The mouse Gene Expression Database (GXD): updates and enhancements. *Nucleic Acids Research*, 32: D568–D571.

Hillmann, D. (2005). Using Dublin Core, Dublin Core Metadata Initiative. http://dublincore.org/documents/usageguide/.

Hirschman, L., Colosimo, M., et al. (2005). Overview of BioCreAtIvE task 1B: normalized gene lists. *BMC Bioinformatics*, 6: S11. http://www.biomedcentral.com/1471-2105/6/S1/S11.

Hirschman, L., Yeh, A., et al. (2005). Overview of BioCreAtIvE: critical assessment of information extraction for biology. *BMC Bioinformatics*, 6: S1. http://www.biomedcentral.com/1471-2105/6/S1/S1.

Hiruki, T., Olson, D., (2001). An automated MeSH mapping tool to facilitate searching of the English-language web by Japanese users. *Technology and Health Care*, 9: 495–496.

Hochmuth, P. (2003). Speedy returns are Google's goal. *Network World*. 17–18. http://www.nwfusion.com/news/2003/0901google.html.

Hock, R. (2004). *The Extreme Searcher's Internet Handbook: A Guide for the Serious Searcher*. New York, NY. Information Today.

Hodge, J., Gostin, L., et al. (1999). Legal issues concerning electronic health information: privacy, quality, and liability. *Journal of the American Medical Association*, 282: 1466–1471.

Hoffmann, R., Krallinger, M., et al. (2005). Text mining for metabolic pathways, signaling cascades, and protein networks. *Science STKE*, 283: e21. http://stke.sciencemag.org/cgi/content/full/OC_sigtrans;stke.2832005pe21.

Hoffrage, U., Lindsey, S., et al. (2000). Communicating statistical information. *Science*, 290: 2261–2262.

Hole, W. and Srinivasan, S. (2000). Discovering missed synonymy in a large concept-oriented metathesaurus. *Proceedings of the AMIA 2000 Annual Symposium*, Los Angeles, CA. Hanley & Belfus. 354–358.

Hoover, J. (2007). The ultimate search engine. *Information Week*. Aug 4, 2007. http://www.informationweek.com/news/showArticle.jhtml?articleID=201202986.

Hopayian, K. (2001). The need for caution in interpreting high quality systematic reviews. *British Medical Journal*, 323: 681–684.

Hopewell, S., Clarke, M., et al. (2003). Handsearching versus Electronic Searching to Identify Reports of Randomized Trials. Update Software. http://www.cochrane.org/cochrane/mrabstr/mr000001.htm. Accessed.

Hopewell, S., McDonald, S., et al. (2003). Grey Literature in Meta-Analyses of Randomized Trials of Health Care Interventions. Update Software. http://www.cochrane.org/cochrane/mrabstr/mr000010.htm. Accessed.

Horowitz, G., Jackson, J., et al. (1983). PaperChase: self-service bibliographic retrieval. *Journal of the American Medical Association*, 328: 2495–2500.

Horsch, A., Prinz, M., et al. (2004). Establishing an international reference image database for research and development in medical image processing. *Methods of Information in Medicine*, 43: 409–412.

Horton, R. (2002). Postpublication criticism and the shaping of clinical knowledge. *Journal of the American Medical Association*, 287: 2843–2847.

Horton, R. (2003). 21st-century biomedical journals: failures and futures. *Lancet*, 362: 1510–1512.

Horton, R. (2004). A statement by the editors of The Lancet. *Lancet*, 363: 820–821.

Hotopf, M., Lewis, G., et al. (1997). Putting trials on trial: the costs and consequences of small trials in depression: a systematic review of methodology. *Journal of Epidemiology and Community Health*, 51: 354–358.

Hrachovec, J. and Mora, M. (2001). Reporting of 6-month vs 12-month data in a clinical trial of celecoxib. *Journal of the American Medical Association*, 286: 2398.

Hripcsak, G., Clayton, P., et al. (1996). Design of a clinical event monitor. *Computers and Biomedical Research*, 29: 194–221.

Hripcsak, G., Friedman, C., et al. (1995). Unlocking clinical data from narrative reports: a study of natural language processing. *Annals of Internal Medicine*, 122: 681–688.

Hripcsak, G. and Rothschild, A. (2005). Agreement, the F-measure, and reliability in information retrieval. *Journal of the American Medical Informatics Association*, 12: 296–298.

Hristovski, D., Peterlin, B., et al. (2005). Using literature-based discovery to identify disease candidate genes. *International Journal of Medical Informatics*, 74: 289–298.

Hsu, W., Long, L., et al. (2007). SPIRS: a framework for content-based image retrieval from large biomedical databases. *MEDINFO 2007 – Proceedings of the Twelfth World Congress on Health (Medical) Informatics*, Brisbane, Australia. IOS Press. 188–192.

Huang, X., Zhong, M., et al. (2005). York University at TREC 2005: Genomics track. *The Fourteenth Text REtrieval Conference Proceedings (TREC 2005)*, Gaithersburg, MD. National Institute for Standards and Technology. http://trec.nist.gov/pubs/trec14/papers/yorku-huang2.geo.pdf.

Hughes, C. (1998). Academic medical libraries' policies and procedures for notifying library users of retracted scientific publications. *Medical Reference Services Quarterly*, 17(2): 37–40.

Hull, D. (1994). Improving text retrieval for the routing problem using latent semantic indexing. *Proceedings of the 17th Annual International ACM SIGIR Conference on Research and Development in Information Retrieval*, Dublin, Ireland. Springer-Verlag. 282–291.

Hull, D. (1996). Stemming algorithms: a case study for detailed evaluation. *Journal of the American Society for Information Science*, 47: 70–84.

Hull, D. and Greffenstette, G. (1996). Querying across languages: a dictionary-based approach to multilingual information retrieval. *Proceedings of the 19th Annual International ACM SIGIR Conference on Research and Development in Information Retrieval*, Zurich, Switzerland. ACM Press. 49–57.

Humphrey, L., Chan, B., et al. (2002). Postmenopausal hormone replacement therapy and the primary prevention of cardiovascular disease. *Annals of Internal Medicine*, 137: 273–284.

Humphrey, S. (1988). Medindex system: medical indexing expert system. *Information Processing and Management*, 25: 73–88.

Humphrey, S. (1992). Indexing biomedical documents: from thesaural to knowledge-based systems. *Artificial Intelligence in Medicine*, 4: 343–371.

Humphreys, B. (2000). Electronic health record meets digital library: a new environment for achieving an old goal. *Journal of the American Medical Informatics Association*, 7: 444–452.

Humphreys, B., Lindberg, D., et al. (1998). The Unified Medical Language System: an informatics research collaboration. *Journal of the American Medical Informatics Association*, 5: 1–11.

Humphreys, B., McCray, A., et al. (1997). Evaluating the coverage of controlled health data terminologies: report on the results of the NLM/AHCPR large scale vocabulary test. *Journal of the American Medical Informatics Association*, 6: 484–500.

Hung, P., Johnson, S., et al. (2008). A multi-level model of information seeking in the clinical domain. *Journal of Biomedical Informatics*, 41(2): 357–370.

Hunter, L. and Cohen, K. (2006). Biomedical language processing: what's beyond PubMed? *Molecular Cell*, 21: 589–594.

Huth, E. (1989). The underused medical literature. *Annals of Internal Medicine*, 110: 99–100.

Huwiler-Muntener, K., Juni, P., et al. (2002). Quality of reporting of randomized trials as a measure of methodologic quality. *Journal of the American Medical Association*, 287: 2801–2804.

Hwang, W., Roh, S., et al. (2005). Patient-specific embryonic stem cells derived from human SCNT blastocysts. *Science*, 308: 1777–1783.

Hwang, W., Ryu, Y., et al. (2004). Evidence of a pluripotent human embryonic stem cell line derived from a cloned blastocyst. *Science*, 303: 1669–1674.

Ide, N., Loane, R., et al. (2007). Essie: a concept-based search engine for structured biomedical text. *Journal of the American Medical Informatics Association*, 14: 253–263.

Ingelfinger, F. (1969). Annual discourse: swinging copy and sober science. *New England Journal of Medicine*, 281: 526–532.

Ingelfinger, F. (1974). Peer review in biomedical publication. *American Journal of Medicine*, 56: 686–692.

Ingwersen, P. (1998). The calculation of web impact factors. *Journal of Documentation*, 54: 236–243.

Ingwersen, P. and Jarvelin, K. (2005). *The Turn – Integration of Information Seeking and Retrieval in Context*. Dordrecht, The Netherlands. Springer.

Insel, T., Volkow, N., (2003). Neuroscience networks: data-sharing in an information age. *PLoS Biology*, 1: E17.

Ioannidis, J. (1998). Effect of statistical significance of results on the time to completion and publication of randomized efficacy trials. *Journal of the American Medical Association*, 279: 281–286.

Ioannidis, J. (2005a). Contradicted and initially stronger effects in highly cited clinical research. *Journal of the American Medical Association*, 294: 218–228.

Ioannidis, J. (2005b). Why most published research findings are false. *PLoS Medicine*, 2(8): e124.

Ivanitskaya, L., O'Boyle, I., (2006). Health information literacy and competencies of information age students: results from the interactive online Research Readiness Self-Assessment (RRSA). *Journal of Medical Internet Research*, 8(2): e6. http://www.jmir.org/2006/2/e6/.

Ivics, Z., Hackett, P., et al. (1997). Molecular reconstruction of Sleeping Beauty, a Tc1-like transposon from fish, and its transposition in human cells. *Cell*, 91: 501–510.

Iyengar, S. and Greenhouse, J. (1988). Selection models and the file drawer problem. *Statistical Science*, 3: 109–135.

Jackson, P. and Moulinier, I. (2002). *Natural Language Processing for Online Applications: Text Retrieval, Extraction, and Categorization*. Amsterdam, Holland. Benjamin Johns Publishing.

Jacobs, A. (2004). New Entrez database: NLM Catalog. *NLM Technical Bulletin*. Sept–Oct, 2004. e2. http://www.nlm.nih.gov/pubs/techbull/so04/so04_entrez_cat.html.

Jadad, A., Cook, D., et al. (1998). Methodology and reports of systematic reviews and meta-analyses: a comparison of Cochrane reviews with articles published in paper-based journals. *Journal of the American Medical Association*, 280: 278–280.

Janes, J., Hill, C., et al. (2001). Ask-an-expert services analysis. *Journal of the American Society for Information Science and Technology*, 52: 1106–1121.

Jansen, B. (2005). Paid search as an information seeking paradigm. *Bulletin of the American Society for Information Science and Technology*, 32(2): 7–8. http://www.asis.org/Bulletin/Dec-05/jansen.html.

Jansen, B., Spink, A., et al. (1998). Real life information retrieval: a study of user queries on the web. *SIGIR Forum*, 32: 5–17.

Jansen, B., Zhang, M., et al. (2007). The effect of brand awareness on the evaluation of search engine results. *Conference on Human Factors in Computing Systems 2007*, San Jose, CA. ACM Press. http://ist.psu.edu/faculty_pages/jjansen/academic/pres/chi2007/jansen_branding_of_-search _engines.pdf.

Jarvelin, K. and Kekalainen, J. (2000). IR evaluation methods for retrieving highly relevant documents. *Proceedings of the 23rd Annual International ACM SIGIR Conference on Research and Development in Information Retrieval*, Athens, Greece. ACM Press. 41–48.

Jefferson, T., Wager, E., et al. (2002). Measuring the quality of editorial peer review. *Journal of the American Medical Association*, 287: 2786–2790.

Jensen, J. and Hersh, W. (2005). Manual query modification and data fusion for medical image retrieval. *Accessing Multilingual Information Repositories – 6th Workshop of the Cross-Language Evaluation Forum, CLEF 2005*, Vienna, Austria. Lecture Notes in Computer Science. Springer-Verlag 673–679. http://medir.ohsu.edu/~hersh/imageclef-OHSU-05.pdf.

Jensen, L., Saric, J., et al. (2006). Literature mining for the biologist: from information retrieval to biological discovery. *Nature Reviews – Genetics*, 7: 119–129.

Jerant, A. and Hill, D. (2000). Does the use of electronic medical records improve surrogate patient outcomes in outpatient settings? *Journal of Family Practice*, 49: 349–357.

Jiang, J. and Zhai, C. (2007). An empirical study of tokenization strategies for biomedical information retrieval. *Information Retrieval*, 10: 341–363.

Joachims, T. (2002a). Evaluating retrieval performance using clickthrough data. *Proceedings of the SIGIR Workshop on Mathematical/Formal Methods in Information Retrieval*, Tampere, Finland. ACM Press. http://www.cs.cornell.edu/People/tj/publications/joachims_02b.pdf.

Joachims, T. (2002b). Optimizing search engines using clickthrough data. *Proceedings of the ACM Conference on Knowledge Discovery and Data Mining*, Edmonton, Alberta, Canada. ACM Press. http://www.cs.cornell.edu/People/tj/publications/joachims_02c.pdf.

Joachims, T., Granka, L., et al. (2007). Evaluating the accuracy of implicit feedback from clicks and query reformulations in web search. *ACM Transactions on Information Systems*, 25: 7.

Joachims, T., Granka, L., et al. (2005). Accurately interpreting clickthrough data as implicit feedback. *Proceedings of the 28th International ACM SIGIR Conference on Research and Development in Information Retrieval*, Salvador, Brazil. ACM Press. 154–161.

Johnson, E., Sievert, M., et al. (1995). Retrieving research studies: a comparison of bibliographic and full-text versions of the New England Journal of Medicine. *Proceedings of the 19th Annual*

Symposium on Computer Applications in Medical Care, New Orleans, LA. Hanley & Belfus. 846–850.

Johnson, H., Wagner, M., et al. (2004). Analysis of web access logs for surveillance of influenza. *MEDINFO 2004 – Proceedings of the Eleventh World Congress on Medical Informatics*, San Francisco, CA. IOS Press. 1202–1206.

Johnson, S. (1996). Generic data modeling for clinical repositories. *Journal of the American Medical Informatics Association*, 3: 328–339.

Jollis, J., Ancukiewicz, M., et al. (1993). Discordance of databases designed for claims payment versus clinical information systems: implications for outcomes research. *Annals of Internal Medicine*, 119: 844–850.

Jones, M., Marsden, G., et al. (1999). Improving web interaction on small displays. *Proceedings of the 8th International World Wide Web Conference*, Toronto, Canada. http://www8.org/w8-papers/1b-multimedia/improving/improving.html.

Joyce, J., Rabe-Hesketh, S., et al. (1998). Reviewing the reviews: the example of Chronic Fatigue Syndrome. *Journal of the American Medical Association*, 280: 264–266.

Jüni, P., Rutjes, A., et al. (2002). Are selective COX 2 inhibitors superior to traditional non steroidal anti-inflammatory drugs? *British Medical Journal*, 324: 1287–1288.

Justice, A., Cho, M., et al. (1998). Does masking author identity improve peer review quality? A randomized controlled trial. *Journal of the American Medical Association*, 280: 240–242.

Kahle, B. (1997). Preserving the internet. *Scientific American*, 276(3): 82–83. http://www.archive.org/sciam_article.html.

Kahn, C. (2008). Effective metadata discovery for dynamic filtering of queries to a radiology image search engine. *Journal of Digital Imaging*: Epub ahead of print.

Kahn, C. and Thao, C. (2007). GoldMiner: a radiology image search engine. *American Journal of Roentgenology*, 188: 1475–1478.

Kaiser, J. (2008). Scientific publishing. Uncle Sam's biomedical archive wants your papers. *Science*, 319: 266.

Kalpathy-Cramer, J. and Hersh, W. (2007a). Automatic image modality based classification and annotation to improve medical image retrieval. *MEDINFO 2007 – Proceedings of the Twelfth World Congress on Health (Medical) Informatics*, Brisbane, Australia. IOS Press. 1334–1338.

Kalpathy-Cramer, J. and Hersh, W. (2007b). Medical image retrieval and automatic annotation: OHSU at ImageCLEF 2007. *Working Notes for the CLEF 2007 Workshop*, Budapest, Hungary. http://www.billhersh.info/imageclef-07-ohsu.pdf.

KamelBoulos, M., Maramba, I., et al. (2006). Wikis, blogs and podcasts: a new generation of web-based tools for virtual collaborative clinical practice and education. *BMC Medical Education*, 6: 41. http://www.biomedcentral.com/1472-6920/6/41.

Kan, M., McKeown, K., et al. (2001). Domain-specific informative and indicative summarization for information retrieval. *DUC 2001 – Workshop on Text Summarization*, New Orleans, LA. NIST. http://www-nlpir.nist.gov/projects/duc/pubs/2001papers/columbia_redo2.ps.

Kao, A. and Poteet, S. (2006). *Natural Language Processing and Text Mining*. New York, NY. Springer.

Kaplan, D. (2005). How to fix peer review. *The Scientist*, 19(11): 10. http://www.the-scientist.com/article/display/15501/.

Kassirer, J. (1992). Too many books, too few journals. *New England Journal of Medicine*, 326: 1427–1428.

Katcher, B. (2006). *Medline: A Guide to Effective Searching in PubMed and Other Interfaces*, Second Edition. San Francisco. Ashbury Press.

Kedar, I., Ternullo, J., et al. (2003). Internet based consultations to transfer knowledge for patients requiring specialised care: retrospective case review. *British Medical Journal*, 326: 696–699.

Keelan, J., Pavri-Garcia, V., et al. (2007). YouTube as a source of information on immunization: a content analysis. *Journal of the American Medical Association*, 298: 2482–2484.

Kempner, J., Perlis, C., et al. (2005). Forbidden knowledge. *Science*, 307: 854.

Kennedy, D. (2006). Editorial retraction. *Science*, 311: 335.

Kenney, A., Entlich, R., et al. (2006). E-Journal Archiving Metes and Bounds: A Survey of the Landscape. Washington, DC, Council on Library and Information Resources. http://www.clir.org/PUBS/reports/pub138/pub138.pdf.

Kenney, A., McGovern, N., et al. (2003). Google meets eBay – what academic librarians can learn from alternative information providers. *D-Lib Magazine*, 9(6). http://www.dlib.org/dlib/june03/kenney/06kenney.html.

Kent, A., Berry, M., et al. (1955). Machine literature searching VIII: Operational criteria for designing information retrieval systems. *American Documentation*, 6: 93–101.

Kessler, M. (1963). Bibliographic coupling between scientific papers. *American Documentation*, 14: 10–25.

Kim, J., Ohta, T., et al. (2003). GENIA corpus—semantically annotated corpus for bio-textmining. *Bioinformatics*, 19: i180–i182.

Kim, J., Ohta, T., et al. (2008). Corpus annotation for mining biomedical events from literature. *BMC Bioinformatics*, 9: 10. http://www.biomedcentral.com/1471–2105/9/10.

Kim, P., Eng, T., et al. (1999). Published criteria for evaluating health related web sites: review. *British Medical Journal*, 318: 647–649.

King, D. (1987). The contribution of hospital library information services to clinical care: a study of eight hospitals. *Bulletin of the Medical Library Association*, 75: 291–301.

Kingsland, L., Harbourt, A., et al. (1993). COACH: applying UMLS knowledge sources in an expert searcher environment. *Bulletin of the Medical Library Association*, 81: 178–183.

Kingsland, L., Syed, E., et al. (1992). COACH: an expert searcher program to assist Grateful Med users searching MEDLINE. *MEDINFO 92*, Geneva, Switzerland. North-Holland. 382–386.

Kishida, K. (2005). Technical issues of cross-language retrieval: a review. *Information Processing and Management*, 41: 433–456.

Kitts, B., LeBlanc, B., et al. (2005). Click fraud. *Bulletin of the American Society for Information Science and Technology*, 32(2): 20–23. http://www.asis.org/Bulletin/Dec-05/clickfraud.html.

Kjaergard, L., Villumsen, J., et al. (2001). Reported methodologic quality and discrepancies between large and small randomized trials in meta-analyses. *Annals of Internal Medicine*, 135: 982–989.

Klein, M., Ross, F., et al. (1994). Effect of online literature searching on length of stay and patient care costs. *Academic Medicine*, 69: 489–495.

Kleinberg, J. and Lawrence, S. (2001). The structure of the web. *Science*, 294: 1849–1850.

Knaus, D., Mittendorf, E., et al. (1994). Improving a basic retrieval method by links and passage level evidence. *Overview of the Third Text REtrieval Conference (TREC-3)*, Gaithersburg, MD. National Institute of Standards and Technology. 241–246.

Knight, E., Glynn, R., et al. (2000). Failure of evidence-based medicine in the treatment of hypertension in older patients. *Journal of General Internal Medicine*, 15: 702–709.

Kochen, C. and Budd, J. (1992). The persistence of fraud in the literature: The Darsee case. *Journal of the American Society for Information Science*, 43: 488–493.

Kock, N. (1999). A case of academic plagiarism. *Communications of the ACM*, 42(7): 96–104.

Koenemann, J., Quatrain, R., et al. (1994). New tools and old habits: the interactive searching behavior of expert online searchers using INQUERY. *Overview of the Third Text REtrieval Conference (TREC-3)*, Gaithersburg, MD. National Institute of Standards and Technology. 145–177.

Komatsoulis, G., Warzel, D., et al. (2007). caCORE version 3: implementation of a model driven, service-oriented architecture for semantic interoperability. *Journal of Biomedical Informatics*, 41(1): 106–123.

Koonce, T., Giuse, N., et al. (2004). Evidence-based databases versus primary medical literature: an in-house investigation on their optimal use. *Journal of the Medical Library Association*, 92: 407–411.

Koppel, M., Argamon, S., et al. (2002). Automatically categorizing written texts by author gender. *Literary and Linguistic Computing*, 17: 401–412.

Korn, D., Ehringhaus, S. (2006). Principles for strengthening the integrity of clinical research. *PLoS Clinical Trials*, 1: e1.

Korn, F. and Shneiderman, B. (1996). MeSHBROWSE: A Tool for Browsing Medical Terms. ftp://ftp.cs.umd.edu/pub/hcil/Reports-Abstracts-Bibliography/96–01html/96–01.html. Accessed: July 1, 2002.

Koster, M. (1996). A Method for Web Robots Control. San Francisco, America Online. http://www.robotstxt.org/norobots-rfc.txt.

Kotchen, T., Lindquist, T., et al. (2004). NIH peer review of grant applications for clinical research. *Journal of the American Medical Association*, 291: 836–843.

Kotchen, T., Lindquist, T., et al. (2006). Outcomes of National Institutes of Health peer review of clinical grant applications. *Journal of Investigative Medicine*, 54: 13–19.

Kousha, K. and Thelwall, M. (2007). Google scholar citations and Google Web/URL citations: a multi-discipline exploratory anlaysis. *Journal of the American Society for Information Science & Technology*, 58: 1055–1065.

Krallinger, M. and Valencia, A. (2005). Text-mining and information-retrieval services for molecular biology. *Genome Biology*, 6: 224. http://genomebiology.com/2005/6/7/224.

Kramer, M. and Feinstein, A. (1981). Clinical biostatistics: LIV. The biostatistics of concordance. *Clinical Pharmacology and Therapeutics*, 29: 111–123.

Krleza-Jeric, K., Chan, A., et al. (2005). Principles for international registration of protocol information and results from human trials of health related interventions: Ottawa statement (part 1). *British Medical Journal*, 330: 956–959.

Krovetz, R. and Croft, W. (1992). Lexical ambiguity and information retrieval. *ACM Transactions on Information Systems*, 10: 115–141.

Krupke, D., Naf, D., et al. (2005). The Mouse Tumor Biology Database: integrated access to mouse cancer biology data. *Experimental Lung Research*, 31: 259–270.

Kucera, H. and Francis, W. (1967). *Computational Analysis of Present-Day American English*. Providence, RI. Brown University Press.

Kuhn, T. (1962). *The Structure of Scientific Revolutions*. Chicago. University of Chicago Press.

Kunin, C., Tupasi, T., et al. (1973). Use of antibiotics – a brief exposition of the problem and some tentative solutions. *Annals of Internal Medicine*, 79: 555–560.

Kunst, H., Groot, D., et al. (2002). Accuracy of information on apparently credible websites: survey of five common health topics. *British Medical Journal*, 324: 581–582.

Kushniruk, A., Kan, M., et al. (2002). Usability evaluation of an experimental text summarization system and three search engines: implications for the reengineering of health care interfaces. *Proceedings of the AMIA 2002 Annual Symposium*, San Antonio, TX. Hanley & Belfus. 420–424.

Kwok, K., Grunfeld, L., et al. (1994). TREC-3 ad-hoc, routing retrieval, and thresholding experiments using PIRCS. *Overview of the Third Text REtrieval Conference (TREC-3)*, Gaithersburg, MD. National Institute of Standards and Technology. 247–255.

Lacoste, C., Lim, J., et al. (2007). Medical image retrieval based on knowledge-assisted text and image indexing. *IEEE Transactions on Circuits and Systems for Video Technology*, 17: 889–900.

Lafferty, J. and Zhai, C. (2001). Document language models, query models, and risk minimization for information retrieval. *Proceedings of the 24th Annual International ACM SIGIR Conference on Research and Development in Information Retrieval*, New Orleans, LA. ACM Press. 111–119.

Lagoze, C. and Van de Sompel, H. (2001). The open archives initiative: building a low-barrier interoperability framework. *Proceedings of the First ACM/IEEE-CS Joint Conference on Digital Libraries*, Roanoke, VA. ACM Press. 54–62.

Laine, C., Goldmann, D., et al. (2007). In the clinic. *Annals of Internal Medicine*, 146: 70.

Laine, C., Horton, R., et al. (2007). Clinical trial registration: looking back and moving ahead. *Journal of the American Medical Association*, 298: 93–94.

Laine, C., Proto, A., et al. (2001). A multi-journal authorship database: variation in author contributions by byline position. *Fourth International Congress on Peer Review in Biomedical Publication*, Barcelona, Spain. American Medical Association. http://www.ama-assn.org/public/peer/peerhome.htm.

Lalmas, M. and Tombros, A. (2007). Evaluating XML retrieval effectiveness at INEX. *SIGIR Forum*, 41(1): 40–57.

Lancaster, F. (1968). *Evaluation of the MEDLARS Demand Search Service*. Bethesda, MD. National Library of Medicine.

Lancaster, F. (1978). *Information Retrieval Systems: Characteristics, Testing, and Evaluation*. New York. Wiley.

Lancaster, F. and Warner, A. (1993). *Information Retrieval Today*. Arlington, VA. Information Resources Press.

Landauer, T. and Dumais, S. (1997). A solution to Plato's problem: the latent semantic analysis theory of the acquisition, induction, and representation of knowledge. *Psychological Review*, 104: 211–240.

Landauer, T. and Littman, M. (1990). Fully automatic cross-language document retrieval using latent semantic indexing. *Proceedings of the Sixth Annual Conference of the UW Centre for the New Oxford English Dictionary and Text Research*, Waterloo, Ontario. UW Centre for the New OED and Text Research. 31–38.

Langham, J., Thompson, E., et al. (1999). Identification of randomized controlled trials from the emergency medicine literature: comparison of hand searching versus MEDLINE searching. *Annals of Emergency Medicine*, 34: 25–34.

Langlotz, C. (2006). RadLex: a new method for indexing online educational materials. *Radiographics*, 26: 1595–1597.

Langville, A. and Meyer, C. (2006). *Google's PageRank and Beyond: The Science of Search Engine Rankings*. Princeton, NJ. Princeton University Press.

Lapinsky, S., Wax, R., et al. (2004). Prospective evaluation of an internet-linked handheld computer critical care knowledge access system. *Critical Care*, 8: R414–R421.

Larkey, L. and Croft, W. (1996). Combining classifiers in text categorization. *Proceedings of the 19th Annual International ACM SIGIR Conference on Research and Development in Information Retrieval*, Zurich, Switzerland. ACM Press. 289–297.

Law, D. (2006). Delivering open access: from promise to practice. *Ariadne*, 46. http://www.ariadne.ac.uk/issue46/law/.

Lawrence, S. (2001). Free online availability substantially increases a paper's impact. *Nature*, 411: 521.

Lawrence, S. and Giles, C. (1999). Accessibility and distribution of information on the web. *Nature*, 400: 107–109.

Lawrence, S., Giles, C., et al. (1999). Digital libraries and autonomous citation indexing. *Computer*, 32: 67–71.

Lebowitz, M. (1983). Memory based parsing. *Artificial Intelligence*, 21: 363–404.

Lee, K., Schotland, M., et al. (2002). Association of journal quality indicators with methodological quality of clinical research articles. *Journal of the American Medical Association*, 287: 2805–2808.

Lehmann, T., Güld, M., et al. (2004). Content-based image retrieval in medical applications. *Methods of Information in Medicine*, 43: 354–361.

Lei, J., Chen, E., et al. (2003). Development of infobuttons in a wireless environment. *Proceedings of the AMIA 2003 Annual Symposium*, Washington, DC. Hanley & Belfus. 906.

Leigh, T., Young, P., et al. (1993). Performances of family practice diplomates on successive mandatory recertification examinations. *Academic Medicine*, 68: 912–921.

Leonard, L. (1975). *Inter-indexer Consistency and Retrieval Effectiveness: Measurement of Relationships*. Ph.D. Thesis. University of Illinois.

Lesk, M. (2005). *Understanding Digital Libraries*, Second Edition. San Francisco, CA. Morgan Kaufmann.

Lesk, M. and Salton, G. (1968). Relevance assessments and retrieval system evaluation. *Information Storage and Retrieval*, 4: 343–359.

Levin, A. (2001). The Cochrane Collaboration. *Annals of Internal Medicine*, 135: 309–312.

Levy, S., Sutton, G., et al. (2007). The diploid genome sequence of an individual human. *PLoS Biology*, 5(10): e254.

Lewis, D. (1995). Evaluating and optimizing autonomous text classification systems. *Proceedings of the 18th Annual International ACM SIGIR Conference on Research and Development in Information Retrieval*, Seattle, WA. ACM Press. 246–254.

Lewis, D. (1996). The TREC-5 Filtering Track. *The Fifth Text REtrieval Conference (TREC-5)*, Gaithersburg, MD. National Institute of Standards and Technology. 75–96.

Lewis, D., Yang, Y., et al. (2004). RCV1: a new benchmark collection for text categorization research. *Journal of Machine Learning Research*, 5: 361–397.

Lexchin, J., Bero, L., et al. (2003). Pharamceutical industry sponsorship and research outcome and quality: systematic review. *British Medical Journal*, 326: 1167–1170.

Light, M., Qiu, X., et al. (2004). The language of bioscience: facts, speculations, and statements in between. *Proceedings of HLT-NAACL 2004 Workshop: BioLINK 2004, Linking Biological Literature, Ontologies and Databases*, Boston, MA. 17–24.

Lijmer, J., Mol, B., et al. (1999). Empirical evidence of design-related bias in studies of diagnostic tests. *Journal of the American Medical Association*, 282: 1061–1066.

Lilford, R., Braunholtz, D., et al. (2000). Trials and fast changing technologies: the case for tracker studies. *British Medical Journal*, 320: 43–46.

Lin, C. (2004). ROUGE: a package for automatic evaluation of summaries. *Proceedings of Text Summarization Branches Out Workshop*, Barcelona, Spain. Association for Computational Linguistics. http://www.isi.edu/~cyl/papers/WAS2004.pdf.

Lin, C. and Hovy, E. (2003). Automatic evaluation of summaries using n-gram co-occurrence statistics. *Proceedings of the 2003 Human Language Technology Conference (HLT-NAACL 2003)*, Edmonton, Alberta. North American Association for Computational Linguistics. http://www.isi.edu/~cyl/papers/NAACL2003.pdf.

Lin, J. and Wilbur, W. (2007). PubMed related articles: a probabilistic topic-based model for content similarity. *BMC Bioinformatics*, 8: 423. http://www.biomedcentral.com/1471–2105/8/423.

Lindberg, D. and Humphreys, B. (2005). 2015 – the future of medical libraries. *New England Journal of Medicine*, 352: 1067–1070.

Lindberg, D., Humphreys, B., et al. (1993). The Unified Medical Language System project. *Methods of Information in Medicine*, 32: 281–291.

Lindberg, D., Siegel, E., et al. (1993). Use of MEDLINE by physicians for clinical problem solving. *Journal of the American Medical Association*, 269: 3124–3129.

Ling, X., Jiang, J., et al. (2007). Generating gene summaries from biomedical literature: A study of semi-structured summarization. *Information Processing & Management*, 43: 1777–1791.

Link, A. (1998). US and non-US submissions: An analysis of reviewer bias. *Journal of the American Medical Association*, 280: 246–247.

Littenberg, B. (1992). Technology assessment in medicine. *Academic Medicine*, 67: 424–428.

Liu, H., Hu, Z., et al. (2006). BioThesaurus: a web-based thesaurus of protein and gene names. *Bioinformatics*, 22: 103–105.

Liu, K., Mitchell, K., et al. (2005). Automating tissue bank annotation from pathology reports – comparison to a gold standard expert annotation set. *Proceedings of the AMIA 2005 Annual Symposium*, Washington, DC. Hanley & Belfus. 460–464.

Los, R., vanGinneken, A., et al. (2005). OpenSDE: a strategy for expressive and flexible structured data entry. *International Journal of Medical Informatics*, 74: 481–490.

Loscalzo, J. (2006). The NIH budget and the future of biomedical research. *New England Journal of Medicine*, 354: 1665–1667.

Losee, R. (1990). *The Science of Information*. San Diego, CA. Academic Press.

Lovins, J. (1968). Development of a stemming algorithm. *Mechanical Translation and Computational Linguistics*, 11: 11–31.

Lovis, C., Chapko, M., et al. (2001). Evaluation of a command-line parser-based order entry pathway for the Department of Veterans Affairs electronic patient record. *Journal of the American Medical Informatics Association*, 8: 486–498.

Lu, Z., Cohen, K., et al. (2006). Finding GeneRIFs via gene ontology annotations. *Pacific Symposium on Biocomputing*, Maui, Hawaii. World Scientific. 52–63.

Luhn, H. (1957). A statistical approach to mechanized encoding and searching of literary information. *IBM Journal of Research and Development*, 1: 309–317.

Luhn, H. (1958). The automatic creation of literature abstracts. *IBM Journal of Research and Development*, 2: 159–165.

Lundeen, G., Tenopir, C., et al. (1994). Information needs of rural health care practitioners in Hawaii. *Bulletin of the Medical Library Association*, 82: 197–205.

Lussier, Y., Borlawsky, T., et al. (2006). Discovery of protein interaction networks shared by diseases. *Pacific Symposium on Biocomputing*, Maui, Hawaii. World Scientific. 76–87.

Lyman, P. and Varian, H. (2003). How Much Information. Berkeley, CA, University of California Berkeley. http://www.sims.berkeley.edu/research/projects/how-much-info-2003/.

Lyon, J., Giuse, N., et al. (2004). A model for training the new bioinformationist. *Journal of the Medical Library Association*, 92: 188–195.

MacCallum, C. (2007a). ONE for all: the next step for PLoS. *PLoS Biology*, 4: e401.

MacCallum, C. (2007b). When is open access not open access? *PLoS Biology*, 5: 2095–2097.

MacColl, J. (2006). Google challenges for academic libraries. *Ariadne*, 46. http://www.ariadne.ac.uk/issue46/maccoll/.

MacDonald, G. (2006). Congress's dilemma: When Yahoo in China's not Yahoo. *Christian Science Monitor*. Feb 14, 2006. http://www.csmonitor.com/2006/0214/p01s04-usfp.html.

Macleod, C., Chen, S., et al. (1987). Parsing unedited medical narrative, in Sager, N., Friedman, C. and Lyman, M., eds. *Medical Language Processing: Computer Management of Narrative Data*. Reading, MA. 163–173,Addison-Wesley.

MacMullen, W. and Denn, S. (2005). Information problems in molecular biology and bioinformatics. *Journal of the American Society for Information Science & Technology*, 56: 447–456.

Madden, M. and Fox, S. (2006). Finding Answers Online in Sickness and in Health. Washington, DC, Pew Internet & American Life Project. http://www.pewinternet.org/pdfs/PIP_Health_Decisions_2006.pdf.

Madlon-Kay, D. (1989). The weight of medical knowledge: still gaining. *New England Journal of Medicine*, 321: 908.

Maglott, D., Ostell, J., et al. (2007). Entrez Gene: gene-centered information at NCBI. *Nucleic Acids Research*, 35: D26–D31.

Magrabi, F., Coiera, E., et al. (2005). General practitioners' use of online evidence during consultations. *International Journal of Medical Informatics*, 74: 1–12.

Magrabi, F., Westbrook, J., et al. (2007). What factors are associated with the integration of evidence retrieval technology into routine general practice settings? *International Journal of Medical Informatics*, 76(10): 701–709.

Mailman, M., Feolo, M., et al. (2007). The NCBI dbGaP database of genotypes and phenotypes. *Nature Genetics*, 39: 1181–1186.

Mane, K. and Thakur, S. (2003). Oncosifter: A Customized Approach to Cancer Information. Bloomington, IN, Laboratory for Applied Informatics Research, Indiana University. http://vw.indiana.edu/ivira03/mane.pdf.

Mani, I. (2001). *Automatic Summarization*. Amsterdam. John Benjamins.

Mani, I. and Maybury, M. (1999). *Advances in Automatic Text Summarization*. Cambridge, MA. MIT Press.

Manola, F. and Miller, E. (2004). RDF Primer. Cambridge, MA, World Wide Web Consortium. http://www.w3.org/TR/rdf-primer/.

Mant, D. (1999). Can randomized trials inform clinical decisions about individual patients? *Lancet*, 353: 743–746.

Marcetich, J., Rappaport, M., et al. (2004). Indexing consistency in MEDLINE. *MLA 04 Abstracts*, Washington, DC. Medical Library Association. 10–11.

Marchionini, G. (1992). Interfaces for end-user information seeking. *Journal of the American Society for Information Science*, 43: 156–163.

Marchionini, G. (2006). Exploratory search: from finding to understanding. *Communications of the ACM*, 41(4): 41–46.

Marchionini, G., Wildemuth, B., et al. (2006). The Open Video Digital Library: a Mobius strip of research and practice. *Journal of the American Society for Information Science & Technology*, 57: 1629–1643.

Marcus, M., Santorini, B., et al. (1994). Building a large annotated corpus of English: the Penn Treebank. *Computational Linguistics*, 19: 313–330.

Marcus, R. (1983). An experimental comparison of the effectiveness of computer and humans as search intermediaries. *Journal of the American Society for Information Science*, 34: 381–404.

Markó, K., Schulz, S., et al. (2005). MorphoSaurus – design and evaluation of an interlingua-based, cross-language document retrieval engine for the medical domain. *Methods of Information in Medicine*, 44: 537–545.

Markoff, J. (2007). Searching for Michael Jordan? Microsoft Wants a Better Way. New York, NY. http://www.nytimes.com/2007/03/07/business/07soft.html. Accessed: March 7, 2007.

Marsh, E. and Sager, N. (1982). Analysis and processing of compact texts. *COLING 82: Proceedings of the Ninth International Conference on Computational Linguistics*. North-Holland. 201–206.

Marshall, J. (1992). The impact of the hospital library on decision making: the Rochester study. *Bulletin of the Medical Library Association*, 80: 169–178.

Martin, M., Kuhlman, D., et al. (2002). Federated digital rights management: a proposed DRM solution for research and education. *D-Lib Magazine*, 8: 7. http://www.dlib.org/dlib/july02/martin/07martin.html.

Masarie, F., Miller, R., et al. (1991). An interlingua for electronic exchange of medical information: using frames to map between clinical vocabularies. *Computers and Biomedical Research*, 24: 379–400.

Masys, D. (1992). An evaluation of the source selection elements of the prototype UMLS information sources map. *Proceedings of the 16th Annual Symposium on Computer Applications in Medical Care*, Baltimore, MD. McGraw-Hill. 295–298.

Masys, D., Welsh, J., et al. (2001). Use of keyword hierarchies to interpret gene expression patterns. *Bioinformatics*, 7: 319–326.

Matchar, D., Westermann-Clark, E., et al. (2005). Dissemination of Evidence-based Practice Center reports. *Annals of Internal Medicine*, 142: 1120–1125.

Mathis, Y., Huisman, L., et al. (1994). Mediated literature searches. *Bulletin of the Medical Library Association*, 69: 360.

Maviglia, S., Martin, M., et al. (2002). Usage of UpToDate at an academic medical center (abstract). *Journal of General Internal Medicine*, 17(Suppl): 204.

Maviglia, S., Yoon, C., et al. (2006). KnowledgeLink: impact of context-sensitive information retrieval on clinicians' information needs. *Journal of the American Medical Informatics Association*, 13: 67–73.

McAlister, F., Clark, H., et al. (1999). The medical review article revisited: has the science improved? *Annals of Internal Medicine*, 131: 947–951.

McAuley, L., Pham, B., et al. (2000). Does the inclusion of grey literature influence estimates of intervention effectiveness reported in meta-analyses? *Lancet*, 356: 1228–1231.

McCain, K., White, H., et al. (1987). Comparing retrieval performance in online databases. *Information Processing and Management*, 23: 539–553.

McCallum, A. (2005). Information extraction: distilling structured data from unstructured text. *ACM Queue*, 3(9). http://www.acmqueue.com/modules.php?name=Content&pa=showpage&-pid=350.

McCook, A. (2006). Is peer review broken? *The Scientist*, 20(2): 26–34. http://www.the-scientist.com/article/display/23061/.

McCray, A. (2005). Promoting health literacy. *Journal of the American Medical Informatics Association*, 12: 152–163.

McCray, A. and Aronson, A. (2002). Automated and Semi-Automated Indexing. *National Library of Medicine*. http://ii.nlm.nih.gov/resources/MTI_091102.pdf. Accessed: May 20, 2003.

McCray, A. and Gallagher, M. (2001). Principles for digital library development. *Communications of the ACM*, 44: 49–54.

McCray, A., Srinivasan, S., et al. (1994). Lexical methods for managing variation in biomedical terminologies. *Proceedings of the 18th Annual Symposium on Computer Applications in Medical Care*, Washington, DC. Hanley & Belfus. 235–239.

McCray, A. and Tse, T. (2003). Understanding search failures in consumer health information systems. *Proceedings of the AMIA 2003 Annual Symposium*, Washington, DC. Hanley & Belfus. 430–434.

McDonald, C. (1996). Medical heuristics: the silent adjudicators of clinical practice. *Annals of Internal Medicine*, 124: 56–62.

McEntyre, J. and Ostell, J., eds. (2005). *The NCBI Handbook*. Bethesda, MD. National Library of Medicine. http://www.ncbi.nlm.nih.gov/books/bv.fcgi?rid=handbook.TOC&depth=2.

McGhee, M. (2005). PubMed subject searching avoids conflicts with journal titles. *NLM Technical Bulletin*. Sept–Oct, 2005. e3. http://165.112.6.70/pubs/techbull/so05/so05_pm_exceptions.html.

McGregor, B. (2003). Medical indexing outside the National Library of Medicine. *Journal of the Medical Library Association*, 90: 339–341.

McHenry, R. (2004). The Faith-Based Encyclopedia. *Tech Central Station*. Nov 15, 2004. http://www.techcentralstation.com/111504A.html.

McIntosh, T. and Curran, J. (2007). Challenges for extracting biomedical knowledge from full text. *Proceedings of the Workshop on BioNLP 2007 (BioNLP)*, Prague, Czech Republic. Association for Computational Linguistics. http://www.aclweb.org/anthology-new/W/W07/W07–1023.pdf.

McKibbon, K. and Fridsma, D. (2006). Effectiveness of clinician-selected electronic information resources for answering primary care physicians' information needs. *Journal of the American Medical Informatics Association*, 13: 653–659.

McKibbon, K., Haynes, R., et al. (1990). How good are clinical MEDLINE searches? A comparative study of clinical end-user and librarian searches. *Computers and Biomedical Research*, 23 (6): 583–593.

McKibbon, K., Wilczynski, N., et al. (2004). What do evidence-based secondary journals tell us about the publication of clinically important articles in primary healthcare journals. *BMC Medicine*, 2: 33. http://www.biomedcentral.com/1741–7015/2/33.

McKibbon, K., Wilczynski, N., et al. (1995). The medical literature as a resource for health care practice. *Journal of the American Society for Information Science*, 46: 737–742.

McKiernan, G. (2003). New age navigation: innovative information interfaces for electronic journals. *The Serials Librarian*, 45: 87–123. http://www.public.iastate.edu/~gerrymck/New-Age.pdf.

McKinin, E., Sievert, M., et al. (1991). The MEDLINE/full-text research project. *Journal of the American Society for Information Science*, 42: 297–307.

McLellan, F. (2001). 1966 and all that – when is a literature search done? *Lancet*, 358: 646.

McNutt, R., Evans, A., et al. (1990). The effect of blinding on the quality of peer review. *Journal of the American Medical Association*, 263: 1371–1376.

Meadow, C. (1985). Relevance? *Journal of the American Society for Information Science*, 36: 354–355.

Meadow, C., Boyce, B., et al. (2007). *Text Information Retrieval Systems,* Third Edition. San Diego, CA. Academic Press.

Medlock, B. and Briscoe, T. (2007). Weakly supervised learning for hedge classification in scientific literature. *Proceedings of the 45th Annual Meeting of the Association of Computational Linguistics,* Prague, Czech Republic. Association for Computational Linguistics. 992–999. http://www.aclweb.org/anthology-new/P/P07/P07-1125.pdf.

Mendonça, E. and Cimino, J. (1999). Evaluation of the information sources map. *Proceedings of the AMIA 1999 Annual Symposium,* Washington, DC. Hanley & Belfus. 873–877.

Mendonça, E., Cimino, J., et al. (2001a). Using narrative reports to support a digital library. *Proceedings of the 2001 AMIA Annual Symposium,* Washington, DC. Hanley & Belfus. 458–462.

Mendonça, E., Cimino, J., et al. (2001b). Accessing heterogeneous sources of evidence to answer clinical questions. *Journal of Biomedical Informatics,* 34: 85–98.

Metaxas, P. and DeStefano, J. (2005). Web spam, propaganda and trust. *First International Workshop on Adversarial Information Retrieval on the Web,* Chiba, Japan. http://airweb.cse.lehigh.edu/2005/metaxas.pdf.

Meystre, S. and Haug, P. (2006). Natural language processing to extract medical problems from electronic clinical documents: performance evaluation. *Journal of Biomedical Informatics,* 39: 589–599.

Miles, A., Bentley, P., et al. (1997). Evidence-based medicine? Why all the fuss? This is why. *Journal of Evaluation in Clinical Practice,* 3: 83–86.

Miles, W. (1982). *A History of the National Library of Medicine: The Nation's Treasury of Medical Knowledge.* Bethesda, MD. U.S. Department of Health and Human Services.

Miller, M. (2007). *Googlepedia – The Ultimate Google Resource.* Indianapolis, IN. Que.

Miller, N., Kirby, M., (1988). MEDLINE on CD-ROM: end user searching in a medical school library. *Medical Reference Services Quarterly,* 7(3): 1–13.

Miller, N., Lacroix, E., et al. (2000). MEDLINEplus: building and maintaining the National Library of Medicine's consumer health web service. *Bulletin of the Medical Library Association,* 88: 11–17.

Miller, P. (1999). Z39.50 for all. *Ariadne,* 21. http://www.ariadne.ac.uk/issue21/z3950/.

Miller, P., Frawley, S., et al. (1995). Lessons learned from a pilot implementation of the UMLS information sources map. *Journal of the American Medical Informatics Association,* 2: 102–115.

Miller, R., Gieszczykiewicz, F., et al. (1992). CHARTLINE: providing bibliographic references relevant to patient charts using the UMLS Metathesaurus knowledge sources. *Proceedings of the 16th Annual Symposium on Computer Applications in Medical Care,* Baltimore, MD. McGraw-Hill. 86–90.

Mitchell, J., Aronson, A., et al. (2003). Gene indexing: characterization and analysis of NLM's GeneRIFs. *Proceedings of the AMIA 2003 Annual Symposium,* Washington, DC. Hanley & Belfus. 460–464.

Mitchell, J., Fun, J., et al. (2004). Design of genetics home reference: a new NLM consumer health resource. *Journal of the American Medical Informatics Association,* 11: 439–447.

Mitchell, J., Johnson, E., et al. (1992). Medical students using Grateful Med: analysis of failed searches and a six-month follow-up study. *Computers and Biomedical Research,* 25: 43–55.

Mitra, M., Singhal, A., et al. (1998). Improving automatic query expansion. *Proceedings of the 21st Annual International ACM SIGIR Conference on Research and Development in Information Retrieval,* Melbourne, Australia. ACM Press. 206–214.

Mobasheri, A., Airley, R., et al. (2004). Post-genomic applications of tissue microarrays: basic research, prognostic oncology, clinical genomics and drug discovery. *Histology and Histopathology,* 19: 325–335.

Moffat, A., Zobel, J., et al. (2005). Recommended reading for IR research students. *SIGIR Forum,* 39(2): 3–14. http://www.acm.org/sigir/forum/2005D/2005d_sigirforum_moffat.pdf.

Moher, D., Dulberg, C., et al. (1994). Statistical power, sample size, and their reporting in randomized controlled trials. *Journal of the American Medical Association,* 272: 122–124.

Moher, D., Jones, A., et al. (2001). Use of the CONSORT statement and quality of reports of randomized trials: a comparative before-and-after evaluation. *Journal of the American Medical Association*, 285: 2006–2007.

Moher, D., Pham, B., et al. (1998). Does quality of reports of randomised trials affect estimates of intervention efficacy reported in meta-analyses? *Lancet*, 352: 609–613.

Moher, D., Schulz, K., et al. (2001). The CONSORT statement: revised recommendations for improving the quality of reports of parallel-group randomized trials. *Annals of Internal Medicine*, 134: 657–662.

Moldovan, D., Pasca, M., et al. (2003). Performance issues and error analysis in an open-domain question answering system. *ACM Transactions on Information Systems*, 21(2): 133–154.

Molyneux, R. (1989). *ACRL University Library Statistics*. Chicago. Association of Research Libraries.

Montori, V., Devereaux, P., et al. (2005). Randomized trials stopped early for benefit: a systematic review. *Journal of the American Medical Association*, 294: 2203–2209.

Montori, V., Wilczynski, N., et al. (2004). Systematic reviews: a cross-sectional study of location and citation counts. *BMC Medicine*, 1: 2. http://www.biomedcentral.com/1741–7015/1/2.

Montori, V., Wilczynski, N., et al. (2005). Optimal search strategies for retrieving systematic reviews from Medline: analytical survey. *British Medical Journal*, 330: 68.

Mooers, C. (1951). Zatocoding applied to mechanical organisation of knowledge. *American Documentation*, 2: 20–32.

Moorman, P., Branger, P., et al. (2001). Electronic messaging between primary and secondary care: a four-year case report. *Journal of the American Medical Informatics Association*, 8: 372–378.

Morrison, P. (2007). Why are they tagging, and why do we want them to? *Bulletin of the American Society for Information Science and Technology*. Oct/Nov, 2007. http://www.asist.org/Bulletin/Oct-07/morrison.html.

Mothe, J. and Tanguy, L. (2005). Linguistic features to predict query difficulty. *Workshop on Predicting Query Difficulty – Methods and Applications*, Salvador, Brazil. http://www.haifa.il.ibm.com/sigir05-qp/papers/Mothe.pdf.

Mueller, P., Montori, V., et al. (2007). Ethical issues in stopping randomized trials early because of apparent benefit. *Annals of Internal Medicine*, 146: 878–881.

Mullen, T., Collier, N., et al. (2005). A baseline feature set for learning rhetorical zones using full articles in the biomedical domain. *ACM SIGKDD Explorations Newsletter*, 7(1): 52–58.

Müller, H., Deselaers, T., et al. (2007). Overview of the ImageCLEF 2007 medical retrieval and annotation tasks. *Working Notes for the CLEF 2007 Workshop*, Budapest, Hungary. http://www.billhersh.info/imageclefmed-07.pdf.

Müller, H., Deselaers, T., et al. (2006). Overview of the ImageCLEFmed 2006 medical retrieval and annotation tasks. *Evaluation of Multilingual and Multi-modal Information Retrieval – Seventh Workshop of the Cross-Language Evaluation Forum, CLEF 2006, Alicante, Spain*. Lecture Notes in Computer Science. Springer 595–608. http://www.clef-campaign.org/2006/working_notes/workingnotes2006/deselaersOCLEF2006.pdf.

Müller, H., Despont-Grosa, C., et al. (2006). Health care professionals' image use and search behaviour. *Proceedings of Medical Informatics Europe 2006*, Maastricht, Netherlands. 24–32. http://www.sim.hcuge.ch/medgift/publications/MIE2006_Mueller.pdf.

Müller, H., Geissbuhler, A., et al. (2004). Benchmarking image retrieval applications. *Proceedings of the Seventh International Conference on Visual Information Systems*, San Francisco, CA. http://www.sim.hcuge.ch/medgift/publications/visual2004.pdf.

Müller, H., Kenny, E., et al. (2004). Textpresso: an ontology-based information retrieval and extraction system for biological literature. *PLoS Biology*, 2: e309.

Müller, H., Michoux, N., et al. (2004). A review of content-based image retrieval systems in medical applications-clinical benefits and future directions. *International Journal of Medical Informatics*, 73: 1–23.

Mullner, M., Waechter, F., et al. (2005). How should abridged scientific articles be presented in journals? A survey of readers and authors. *Canadian Medical Association Journal*, 172: 203–205.

Mulrow, C. (1987). The medical review article: state of the science. *Annals of Internal Medicine*, 106: 485–488.

Mulrow, C., Cook, D., et al. (1997). Systematic reviews: critical links in the great chain of evidence. *Annals of Internal Medicine*, 126: 389–391.

Muramatsu, J. and Pratt, W. (2001). Transparent queries: investigating users' mental models of search engines. *Proceedings of the 24th Annual International ACM SIGIR Conference on Research and Development in Information Retrieval*, New Orleans, LA. ACM Press. 217–224.

Murphy, P. (1994). Reading ability of parents compared with reading level of pediatric patient education materials. *Pediatrics*, 93: 460–468.

Mynatt, B., Leventhal, L., et al. (1992). Hypertext or book: which is better for answering questions? *Proceedings of Computer-Human Interface*, 92: 19–25.

Nahin, A. (2003). Full author searching comes to PubMed. *NLM Technical Bulletin*. e4. http://165.112.6.70/pubs/techbull/mj05/mj05_full_author.html.

Nahin, A. (2005). My NCBI replaces the cubby: includes automatic e-mailing of search updates and filters. *NLM Technical Bulletin*. Jan–Feb, 2005. e3. http://www.nlm.nih.gov/pubs/techbull/jf05/jf05_myncbi.html.

Nakayama, T., Fukuhara, S., et al. (2003). Comparison between impact factors and citations in evidence-based practice guidelines. *Journal of the American Medical Association*, 290: 755–756.

Nakov, P., Schwartz, A., et al. (2004). BioText team experiments for the TREC 2004 genomics track. *The Thirteenth Text REtrieval Conference: TREC 2004*, Gaithersburg, MD. National Institute of Standards and Technology. http://trec.nist.gov/pubs/trec13/papers/ucal-berkeley.geo.pdf.

Namer, F. and Baud, R. (2007). Defining and relating biomedical terms: towards a cross-language morphosemantics-based system. *International Journal of Medical Informatics*, 76: 226–233.

Nankivell, C., Wallis, P., et al. (2001). Networked information and clinical decision making: the experience of Birmingham Heartlands and Solihull National Health Service Trust (Teaching). *Medical Education*, 35: 167–172.

Neal, D. (2007). Folksonomies and image tagging: seeing the future? *Bulletin of the American Society for Information Science and Technology*. Oct/Nov, 2007. http://www.asist.org/Bulletin/Oct-07/neal.html.

Nelson, S., Brown, S., et al. (2002). A semantic normal form for clinical drugs in the UMLS: early experiences with the VANDF. *Proceedings of the 2002 Annual AMIA Symposium*, San Antonio, TX. Hanley & Belfus. 557–561.

Nelson, S., Schopen, M., et al. (2000). An Interlingual Database of MeSH Translations. National Library of Medicine. http://www.nlm.nih.gov/mesh/intlmesh.html. Accessed: July 1, 2002.

Nelson, T. (1987). *Computer Lib,* Second Edition. Redmond, WA. Microsoft Press.

Nenkova, A. (2005). Automatic text summarization of newswire: lessons learned from the Document Understanding Conference. *Proceedings of the Twentieth National Conference on Artificial Intelligence and the Seventeenth Innovative Applications of Artificial Intelligence Conference*, Pittsburgh, PA. MIT Press. http://www1.cs.columbia.edu/nlp/papers/2005/nenkova_al_05.pdf.

Nenkova, A. and Passonneau, R. (2004). Evaluating content selection in summarization: the pyramid method. *Proceedings of the 2004 Human Language Technology Conference*, Boston, MA. North American Association for Computational Linguistics. 145–152. http://www.cs.columbia.edu/~ani/papers/pyramid.pdf.

Nicholson, D. (2006). An Evaluation of the Quality of Consumer Health Information on Wikipedia. Medical Informatics & Clinical Epidemiology. Capstone Thesis. Oregon Health & Science University. http://www.ohsu.edu/dmice/people/students/theses/2006/upload/Nicholson_CapstoneFinal06.pdf.

Nielsen, J. and Levy, J. (1994). Measuring usability: preference vs. performance. *Communications of the ACM*, 37: 66–75.

Nigg, H. and Radulsecu, G. (1994). Scientific misconduct in environmental science and toxicology. *Journal of the American Medical Association*, 272: 168–170.

Niu, Y. and Hirst, G. (2004). Analysis of semantic classes in medical text for question answering. *Workshop on Question Answering in Restricted Domains, 42nd Annual Meeting of the Association for Computational Linguistics*, Barcelona, Spain. Association for Computational Linguistics. http://ftp.cs.toronto.edu/pub/gh/Niu+Hirst-2004.pdf.

Niu, Y., Hirst, G., et al. (2003). Answering clinical questions with role identification. *Proceedings, Workshop on Natural Language Processing in Biomedicine, 41st annual meeting of the Association for Computational Linguistics*, Sapporo, Japan. Association for Computational Linguistics. http://ftp.cs.toronto.edu/pub/gh/Niu-etal-2003.pdf.

Niu, Y., Zhu, X., et al. (2006). Using outcome polarity in sentence extraction for medical question-answering. *Proceedings of the AMIA 2006 Annual Symposium*, Washington, DC. American Medical Informatics Association. 599–603. http://ftp.cs.toronto.edu/pub/gh/Niu-etal-2006.pdf.

Norman, G. (1999). Examining the assumptions of evidence-based medicine. *Journal of Evaluation in Clinical Practice*, 5: 139–147.

Norman, G. and Shannon, S. (1998). Effectiveness of instruction in critical appraisal (evidence-based medicine): a critical appraisal. *Canadian Medical Association Journal*, 158: 177–181.

Norris, S. and Atkins, D. (2005). Challenges in using nonrandomized studies in systematic reviews of treatment interventions. *Annals of Internal Medicine*, 142: 1112–1119.

Noruzi, A. (2006). Link spam and search engines. *Webology*, 3(1). http://www.webology.ir/2006/v3n1/editorial7.html.

Notess, G. (2006). *Teaching Web Search Skills: Techniques And Strategies Of Top Trainers*. Medford, NJ. Information Today.

Noy, N. and McGuinness, D. (2001). Ontology Development 101: A Guide to Creating Your First Ontology, Stanford University Knowledge Systems Laboratory. http://www.ksl.stanford.edu/people/dlm/papers/ontology101/ontology101-noy-mcguinness.html.

Nylenna, M., Riis, P., et al. (1994). Multiple blinded reviews of the same two manuscripts: effect of referee characteristics and publication language. *Journal of the American Medical Association*, 272: 149–151.

O'Mahony, B. (1999). Irish health care web sites: a review. *Irish Medical Journal*, 92: 334–337.

O'Neill, G. (2003). Gruber Winner Botstein Calls for Better Gene-naming System. Melbourne, Australia, XIX International Congress of Genetics. http://www.geneticsmedia.org/gruber_winner_botstein_calls_for_better_gene_name_system.htm.

O'Reilly, T. (2005). What Is Web 2.0? Sebastopol, CA, O'Reilly . http://www.oreillynet.com/pub/a/oreilly/tim/news/2005/09/30/what-is-web-20.html.

Oard, D. (1997). Alternative approaches for cross-language text retrieval. *AAAI Spring Symposium on Cross-Language Text and Speech Retrieval*, Palo Alto, CA. AAAI. http://www.ee.umd.edu/medlab/filter/sss/papers/oard/paper.html.

Ogbuji, U. (2003). Thinking XML: learning objects metadata. *IBM developerWorks*. Dec 2, 2003. http://www-128.ibm.com/developerworks/xml/library/x-think21.html.

Ogrinc, G., Headrick, L., et al. (2003). A framework for teaching medical students and residents about practice-based learning and improvement, synthesized from a literature review. *Academic Medicine*, 78: 1–9.

Olson, C., Rennie, D., et al. (2002). Publication bias in editorial decision making. *Journal of the American Medical Association*, 287: 2825–2828.

Olson, C., Rennie, D., et al. (2001). Association of industry funding with manuscript quality indicators. *Fourth International Congress on Peer Review in Biomedical Publication*, Barcelona, Spain. American Medical Association. http://www.ama-assn.org/public/peer/peerhome.htm.

Orio, N. (2006). Music retrieval: a tutorial and review. *Foundations and Trends in Information Retrieval*, 1: 1–90.

Osheroff, J. and Bankowitz, R. (1993). Physicians' use of computer software in answering clinical questions. *Bulletin of the Medical Library Association*, 81: 11–19.

Osheroff, J., Forsythe, D., et al. (1991). Physicians' information needs: analysis of questions posed during clinical teaching. *Annals of Internal Medicine*, 114: 576–581.

Overland, J., Hoskins, P., et al. (1993). Low literacy: a problem in diabetes education. *Diabetes Medicine*, 10: 847–850.

Pai, M., McCulloch, M., et al. (2004). Systematic reviews and meta-analyses: an illustrated, step-by-step guide. *National Medical Journal of India*, 17: 86–95.

Pakhomov, S., Hanson, P., et al. (2008). Automatic classification of foot examination findings using statistical natural language processing and machine learning. *Journal of the American Medical Informatics Association*, 15(2): 198–202.

Pakhomov, S., Weston, S., et al. (2007). Electronic medical records for clinical research: application to the identification of heart failure. *American Journal of Managed Care*, 13: 281–288.

Pandolfini, C., Impiccatore, P., et al. (2000). Parents on the web: risks for quality management of cough in children. *Pediatrics*, 105: 1–8.

Pao, M. (1986). An empirical examination of Lotka's law. *Journal of the American Society for Information Science*, 37: 26–33.

Pao, M. (1989). *Concepts of Information Retrieval*. Englewood, CO. Libraries Unlimited.

Pao, M. (1993). Perusing the literature via citation links. *Computers and Biomedical Research*, 26: 143–156.

Pao, M. and Worthen, D. (1989). Retrieval effectiveness by semantic and citation searching. *Journal of the American Society for Information Science*, 40: 226–235.

Paris, L. and Tibbo, H. (1998). Freestyle vs. Boolean: a comparison of partial and exact match retrieval systems. *Information Processing and Management*, 34: 175–190.

Park, J. and Hunting, S. (2003). *XML Topic Maps – Creating and Using Topic Maps for the Web*. Boston. Addison-Wesley.

Parker, L. and Johnson, R. (1990). Does order of presentation affect users' judgment of documents? *Journal of the American Society for Information Science*, 41: 493–494.

Paskin, N. (2006). *The DOI Handbook*. Oxford, England. International DOI Foundation. http://www.doi.org/handbook_2000/DOIHandbook-v4–4.pdf.

Patel, V., Evans, D., (1989). Biomedical knowledge and clinical reasoning, in Evans, D. and Patel, V., eds. *Cognitive Science in Medicine: Biomedical Modeling*. Cambridge, MA. MIT Press.53–112,

Patrick, T., Demiris, G., et al. (2004). Evidence-based retrieval in evidence-based medicine. *Journal of the Medical Library Association*, 92: 196–199.

Payne, P., Mendonça, E., et al. (2007). Conceptual knowledge acquisition in biomedicine: A methodological review. *Journal of Biomedical Informatics*, 40: 582–602.

Pennock, D., Flake, G., et al. (2002). Winners don't take all: characterizing the competition for links on the web. *Proceedings of the National Academy of Sciences*, 99: 5207–5211.

Perlis, R., Perlis, C., et al. (2005). Industry sponsorship and financial conflict of interest in the reporting of clinical trials in psychiatry. *American Journal of Psychiatry*, 162: 1957–1960.

Pestian, J. and Brew, C. (2007). The Computational Medicine Center's 2007 Medical Natural Language Processing Challenge. Cincinnati, OH, University of Cincinnati. http://www.computationalmedicine.org/challenge/cmcChallengeDetails.pdf.

Peters, D. and Ceci, S. (1982). Peer-review practices of psychological journals: the fate of published articles, submitted again. *Behavioral and Brain Sciences*, 5: 187–255.

Petticrew, M. (2001). Systematic reviews from astronomy to zoology: myths and misconceptions. *British Medical Journal*, 322: 98–101.

Pham, B., Platt, R., et al. (2001). Is there a "best" way to detect and minimize publication bias? An empirical evaluation. *Evaluation and the Health Professions*, 24: 109–125.

Pitkin, R., Branagan, M., et al. (1999). Accuracy of data in abstracts of published research articles. *Journal of the American Medical Association*, 281: 1110–1111.

Piwowar, H., Day, R., et al. (2007). Sharing detailed research data is associated with increased citation rate. *PLoS ONE*, 2(3). http://dx.doi.org/10.1371/journal.pone.0000308.

Plutchak, T. (2002). The informationist – two years later. *Journal of the Medical Library Association*, 90: 367–369.

Pluye, P. and Grad, R. (2004). How information retrieval technology may impact on physician practice: an organizational case study in family medicine. *Journal of Evaluation in Clinical Practice*, 10: 413–430.

Pluye, P., Grad, R., et al. (2005). Impact of clinical information-retrieval technology on physicians: a literature review of quantitative, qualitative and mixed methods studies. *International Journal of Medical Informatics*, 74: 745–768.

Politi, M., Han, P., et al. (2007). Communicating the uncertainty of harms and benefits of medical interventions. *Medical Decision Making*, 27: 681–695.

Pollitt, A. (1987). CANSEARCH: an expert systems approach to document retrieval. *Information Processing and Management*, 23: 119–136.

Ponte, J. and Croft, W. (1998). A language modeling approach to information retrieval. *Proceedings of the 21st Annual International ACM SIGIR Conference on Research and Development in Information Retrieval*, Melbourne, Australia. ACM Press. 275–281.

Poremsky, D. (2004). *Google and Other Search Engines*. Berkeley, CA. Peachpit Press.

Porter, M. (1980). An algorithm for suffix stripping. *Program*, 14: 130–137.

Powsner, S. and Miller, P. (1989). Linking bibliographic retrieval to clinical reports: Psychtopix. *Proceedings of the 13th Annual Symposium on Computer Applications in Medical Care*, Washington, DC. IEEE. 431–435.

Poynard, T., Munteanu, M., et al. (2002). Truth survival in clinical research: an evidence-based requiem? *Annals of Internal Medicine*, 136: 888–895.

Pratt, W. and Fagan, L. (2000). The usefulness of dynamically categorizing search results. *Journal of the American Medical Informatics Association*, 7: 605–617.

Pratt, W., Hearst, M., et al. (1999). A knowledge-based approach to organizing retrieved documents. *Proceedings of the 16th National Conference on Artificial Intelligence*, Orlando, FL. AAAI. 80–85.

Pratt, W. and Wasserman, H. (2001). QueryCat: automatic categorization of MEDLINE queries. *Proceedings of the 2001 AMIA Annual Symposium*, Washington, DC. Hanley & Belfus. 655–659.

Price, D. (1963). *Little Science, Big Science*. New York. Columbia University Press.

Price, D. (1965). Networks of scientific papers. *Science*, 149: 510–515.

Price, S. and Hersh, W. (1999). Filtering web pages for quality indicators: an empirical approach to finding high quality consumer health information on the World Wide Web. *Proceedings of the AMIA 1999 Annual Symposium*, Washington, DC. Hanley & Belfus. 911–915.

Price, S., Hersh, W., et al. (2002). SmartQuery: context-sensitive links to medical knowledge sources from the electronic patient record. *Proceedings of the 2002 Annual AMIA Symposium*, San Antonio, TX. Hanley & Belfus. 627–631.

Purcell, G., Donovan, S., et al. (1998). Changes to manuscripts during the editorial process: characterizing the evolution of a clinical paper. *Journal of the American Medical Association*, 280: 227–228.

Pyysalo, S., Ginter, F., et al. (2007a). BioInfer: a corpus for information extraction in the biomedical domain. *BMC Bioinformatics*, 8: 50. http://www.biomedcentral.com/1471–2105/8/50.

Pyysalo, S., Ginter, F., et al. (2007b). On the unification of syntactic annotations under the Stanford dependency scheme: a case study on BioInfer and GENIA. *Proceedings of the ACL BioNLP'07 Workshop*, Prague, Czech Republic. Association for Computational Linguistics. http://www.it.utu.fi/BioInfer/files/pyysalo_et_al_on_the_unification.pdf.

Quint, B. (1992). The last librarians: end of a millennium. *Canadian Journal of Information Science*, 17: 33–40.

Rabenback, L., Viscoli, C., et al. (1992). Problems in the conduct and analysis of randomized controlled trials. *Archives of Internal Medicine*, 152: 507–512.

Rada, R. (2007). Retractions, press releases and newspaper coverage. *Health Information and Libraries Journal*, 24: 210–215.

Radev, D., Jing, H., et al. (2000). Centroid-based summarization of multiple documents: sentence extraction, utility-based evaluation, and user studies. *NAACL-ANLP 2000 Workshop on Automatic Summarization*, Seattle, WA. http://tangra.si.umich.edu/~radev/papers/cacm05.pdf.

Radev, D., Otterbacher, J., et al. (2005). NewsInEssence: summarizing online news topics. *Communications of the ACM*, 48(10): 95–98.

Radev, D., Teufel, S., et al. (2003). Evaluation challenges in large-scale document summarization. *Proceedings of the 41st Annual Meeting of the Association for Computational Linguistics*, Sapporo, Japan. Association for Computational Linguistics. 375–382.

Rafkind, B., Lee, M., et al. (2006). Exploring text and image features to classify images in bioscience literature. *HLT-NAACL 2006 Workshop: Linking Natural Language Processing and Biology: Towards Deeper Biological Literature Analysis (BioNLP'06)*, New York, NY. http://www.dbmi.columbia.edu/homepages/yuh9001/BioNLP-image.pdf.

Rainie, L. and Shermak, J. (2005). Search Engine Use November 2005. Washington, DC, Pew Internet & American Life Project. http://www.pewinternet.org/pdfs/PIP_SearchData_1105.pdf.

Raja, A. and Singer, P. (2004). Transatlantic divide in publication of content relevant to developing countries. *British Medical Journal*, 329: 1429–1430.

Ramsey, P., Carline, J., et al. (1991). Changes over time in the knowledge base of practicing internists. *Journal of the American Medical Association*, 266: 1103–1108.

Raychaudhuri, S., Chang, J., et al. (2002). Associating genes with gene ontology codes using a maximum entropy analysis of biomedical literature. *Genome Research*, 12: 203–214.

Readings, B. (1994). Caught in the net: notes from the electronic underground. *Surfaces*, 4: 9–10.

Rebholz-Schuhmann, D., Arregui, M., et al. (2008). Text processing through web services: calling Whatizit. *Bioinformatics*, 24: 296–298.

Redman, P., Kelly, J., et al. (1997). Common ground: the HealthWeb project as a model for internet collaboration. *Bulletin of the Medical Library Association*, 85: 325–330.

Rees, A. (1966). The relevance of relevance to the testing and evaluation of document retrieval systems. *Aslib Proceedings*, 18: 316–324.

Rees, A. and Schultz, D. (1967). *A Field Experimental Approach to the Study of Relevance Assessments in Relation to Document Searching*. Cleveland, OH, Center for Documentation and Communication Research, Case Western Reserve University.

Refinetti, R. (1991). In defense of the least publishable unit. *The FASEB Journal*, 4: 128–129.

Reid, M., Lachs, M., et al. (1995). Use of methodologic standards in diagnostic test research: getting better but still not good. *Journal of the American Medical Association*, 274: 645–651.

Rekapalli, H., Cohen, A., et al. (2007). A comparative analysis of retrieval features used in the TREC 2006 Genomics Track passage retrieval task. *Proceedings of the AMIA 2007 Annual Symposium*, Chicago, IL. American Medical Informatics Association.

Rennie, D. (1997). Thyroid storm. *Journal of the American Medical Association*, 277: 1238–1243.

Resiel, J. and Shneiderman, B. (1987). Is bigger better? The effects of display size on program reading, 113–122, in Salvendy, G., ed. *Social, Ergonomic and Stress Aspects of Work with Computers*. Amsterdam. Elsevier Sciencex.

Resnick, M. and Vaughan, M. (2006). Best practices and future visions for search user interfaces. *Journal of the American Society for Information Science & Technology*, 57: 781–787.

Richardson, C., Resnick, P., et al. (2002). Does pornography-blocking software block access to health information on the internet? *Journal of the American Medical Association*, 288: 2887–2894.

Richardson, R. and Smeaton, A. (1995). Automatic word sense disambiguation in a KBIR application. *New Review of Document and Text Management*, 1: 299–319.

Richardson, S. and Powell, A. (2004). Exposing information resources for e-learning – Harvesting and searching IMS metadata using the OAI protocol for metadata harvesting and Z39.50. *Ariadne*, 34. http://www.ariadne.ac.uk/issue34/powell/.

Richardson, W. and Wilson, M. (2002). Textbook desciprtions of disease – where's the beef? *ACP Journal Club*, 137: A11–A12.

Riesenberg, L. and Dontineni, S. (2001). Review of reference inaccuracies. *Fourth International Congress on Peer Review in Biomedical Publication*, Barcelona, Spain. American Medical Association. http://www.ama-assn.org/public/peer/peerhome.htm.

Rinaldi, F., Dowdall, J., et al. (2004). Answering questions in the genomics domain. *ACL 2004 Workshop on Question Answering in Restricted Domains*, Barcelona, Spain. Association for Computational Linguistics. http://www.ifi.unizh.ch/cl/rinaldi/OntoGene-RAW/papers/bionlp. pdf.

Roberts, P. (1999). Scholarly publishing, peer review, and the internet. *First Monday*, 4. http:// firstmonday.org/issues/issue4_4/proberts/.

Roberts, P. (2006). Mining literature for systems biology. *Briefings in Bioinformatics*, 7: 399–406. http://bib.oxfordjournals.org/cgi/rapidpdf/bbl037v1.

Roberts, P. and Hayes, W. (2008). Information needs and the role of text mining in drug development. *Pacific Symposium on Biocomputing*, Big Island, Hawaii. World Scientific. 592–603.

Robertson, S. and Hull, D. (2000). The TREC-9 Filtering Track final report. *The Ninth Text REtrieval Conference (TREC-9)*, Gaithersburg, MD. National Institute of Standards and Technology. 25–40.

Robertson, S. and Soboroff, I. (2001). The TREC 2001 Filtering Track report. *The Tenth Text REtrieval Conference (TREC 2001)*, Gaithersburg, MD. National Institute of Standards and Technology. 26–37. http://trec.nist.gov/pubs/trec10/papers/filtering2_track.pdf.

Robertson, S. and Thompson, C. (1990). Weighted searching: the CIRT experiment. *Informatics 10: Prospects for Intelligent Retrieval*, York. ASLIB. 153–166.

Robertson, S. and Walker, S. (1994). Some simple effective approximations to the 2-Poisson model for probabilistic weighted retrieval. *Proceedings of the 17th Annual International ACM SIGIR Conference on Research and Development in Information Retrieval*, Dublin, Ireland. Springer-Verlag. 232–241.

Robertson, S., Walker, S., et al. (1998). Okapi at TREC-7: automatic ad hoc, filtering, VLC, and interactive track. *The Seventh Text REtrieval Conference (TREC-7)*, Gaithersburg, MD. National Institute of Standards and Technology. 253–264.

Robertson, S., Walker, S., et al. (1994). Okapi at TREC-3. *Overview of the Third Text REtrieval Conference (TREC-3)*, Gaithersburg, MD. National Institute of Standards and Technology. 109–126.

Robertson, W., Leadem, E., et al. (2001). Design and implementation of the National Institute of Environmental Health Sciences Dublin Core Metadata schema. *Proceedings of the International Conference on Dublin Core and Metadata Applications 2001*, Tokyo, Japan. National Institute of Informatics (NII). http://www.nii.ac.jp/dc2001/proceedings/product/paper-29.pdf.

Rochon, P., Bero, L., et al. (2002). Comparison of review articles published in peer-reviewed and throwaway journals. *Journal of the American Medical Association*, 287: 2853–2856.

Röhle, T. (2007). Desperately seeking the consumer: personalized search engines and the commercial exploitation of user data. *First Monday*, 12(9). http://www.firstmonday.org/issues/ issue12_9/rohle/.

Rose, L. (1998). Factors Influencing Successful Use of Information Retrieval Systems by Nurse Practitioner Students. School of Nursing. M.S. Thesis. Oregon Health Sciences University.

Rose, L., Crabtree, K., et al. (1998). Factors influencing successful use of information retrieval systems by nurse practitioner students. *Proceedings of the AMIA 1998 Annual Symposium*, Orlando, FL. Hanley & Belfus. 1067.

Rosenblatt, B., Trippe, B., et al. (2002). *Digital Rights Management - Business and Technology*. New York. M&T Books.

Rosenbloom, S., Geissbuhler, A., et al. (2005). Effect of CPOE user interface design on user-initiated access to educational and patient information during clinical care. *Journal of the American Medical Informatics Association*, 12: 458–473.

Rosenbloom, S., Giuse, N., et al. (2005). Providing evidence-based answers to complex clinical questions: evaluating the consistency of article selection. *Academic Medicine*, 80: 109–114.

Rosenbloom, S., Miller, R., et al. (2006). Interface terminologies: facilitating direct entry of clinical data into electronic health record systems. *Journal of the American Medical Informatics Association*, 13: 277–288.

Rosenbloom, S., Miller, R., et al. (2008). A model for evaluating interface terminologies. *Journal of the American Medical Informatics Association*, 15: 65–76.

Rosenthal, D., Robertson, T., et al. (2005). Requirements for digital preservation systems: a bottom-up approach. *D-Lib Magazine*, 11(1). http://www.dlib.org/dlib/january05/rosenthal/01rosenthal.html.

Rosenthal, R. (1979). The "file drawer problem" and tolerance for null results. *Psychological Bulletin*, 86: 638–641.

Ross, J., Gross, C., et al. (2006). Effect of blinded peer review on abstract acceptance. *Journal of the American Medical Association*, 295: 1675–1680.

Rothenberg, J. (1999). Ensuring the Longevity of Digital Information. RAND Corporation. http://www.clir.org/pubs/archives/ensuring.pdf. Accessed: July 1, 2002.

Rothschild, J., Lee, T., (2002). Clinician use of a palmtop drug reference guide. *Journal of the American Medical Informatics Association*, 9: 223–229.

Roto, V. (2006). Search on mobile phones. *Journal of the American Society for Information Science & Technology*, 57: 834–837.

Roush, W. (2005). The infinite library. *Technology Review*. May, 2005. http://www.technologyreview.com/articles/05/05/issue/feature_library.asp.

Rowlands, I. and Nicholas, D. (2005). New Journal Publishing Models: An International Survey of Senior Researchers. London, England. Centre for Information Behaviour and the Evaluation of Research. http://www.ucl.ac.uk/ciber/ciber_2005_survey_final.pdf.

Royle, J., Blythe, J., et al. (1995). Literature search and retrieval in the workplace. *Computers in Nursing*, 13: 25–31.

Rubin, D., Lewis, S., et al. (2006). National Center for Biomedical Ontology: advancing biomedicine through structured organization of scientific knowledge. *OMICS*, 10: 185–198.

Rubin, J. (1994). *Handbook of Usability Testing: How to Plan, Design, and Conduct Effective Tests*. New York. Wiley.

Rubin, R. (2004). *Foundations of Library and Information Science*, Second Edition. New York, NY. Neal-Schuman.

Ruch, P. (2006). Automatic assignment of biomedical categories: toward a generic approach. *Bioinformatics*, 22: 658–664.

Rui, Y., Huang, T., et al. (1999). Image retrieval: past, present and future. *Journal of Visual Communication and Image Representation*, 10: 1–23.

Ruiz, M. and Aronson, A. (2007). User-centered Evaluation of the Medical Text Indexing (MTI) System. Bethesda, MD, National Library of Medicine. http://0-ii.nlm.nih.gov.catalog.llu.edu/resources/MTIEvaluation-Final.pdf.

Rusbridge, C. (2006). Excuse me… some digital preservation fallacies? *Ariadne*, 46. http://www.ariadne.ac.uk/issue46/rusbridge/.

Sackett, D., Richardson, W., et al. (2000). *Evidence-Based Medicine: How to Practice and Teach EBM*. New York, NY. Churchill Livingstone.

Sadowski, Z., Alexander, J., et al. (1999). Multicenter randomized trial and a systematic overview of lidocaine in acute myocardial infarction. *American Heart Journal*, 137: 792–798.

Safran, C., Bloomrosen, M., et al. (2007). Toward a national framework for the secondary use of health data: an American Medical Informatics Association white paper. *Journal of the American Medical Informatics Association*, 14: 1–9.

Sager, N., Friedman, C., et al. (1987). *Medical Language Processing: Computer Management of Narrative Data*. Reading, MA. Addison-Wesley.

Sager, N., Lyman, M., et al. (1994). Natural language processing and the representation of clinical data. *Journal of the American Medical Informatics Association*, 1: 142–160.

Saha, S., Saint, S., et al. (2003). Impact factor: a valid measure of journal quality? *Journal of the Medical Library Association*, 91: 42–46.

Salamone, S. (2004). LSID: an informatics lifesaver. *BIO-IT World*. Jan, 2004. 38–42. http://www.bio-itworld.com/archive/011204/lsid.html.

Salton, G. (1970). Automatic processing of foreign language documents. *Journal of the American Society for Information Science*, 21: 187–194.

Salton, G. (1972). A new comparison between conventional indexing (MEDLARS) and automatic text processing (SMART). *Journal of the American Society for Information Science*, 23(2): 75–84.

Salton, G. (1991). Developments in automatic text retrieval. *Science*, 253: 974–980.

Salton, G. and Buckley, C. (1988). Term-weighting approaches in automatic text retrieval. *Information Processing and Management*, 24: 513–523.

Salton, G. and Buckley, C. (1990). Improving retrieval performance by relevance feedback. *Journal of the American Society for Information Science*, 41: 288–297.

Salton, G. and Buckley, C. (1991). Global text matching for information retrieval. *Science*, 253: 1012–1015.

Salton, G., Buckley, C., et al. (1990). On the application of syntactic methodologies in automatic text analysis. *Information Processing and Management*, 26: 73–92.

Salton, G., Fox, E., et al. (1983). Extended Boolean information retrieval. *Communications of the ACM*, 26: 1022–1036.

Salton, G. and Lesk, M. (1965). The SMART automatic document retrieval system: an illustration. *Communications of the ACM*, 8: 391–398.

Salton, G. and McGill, M. (1983). *Introduction to Modern Information Retrieval*. New York. McGraw-Hill.

Sanderson, M. (1994). Word sense disambiguation and information retrieval. *Proceedings of the 17th Annual International ACM SIGIR Conference on Research and Development in Information Retrieval*, Dublin, Ireland. Springer-Verlag. 142–151.

Sanderson, R., Young, J., et al. (2005). SRW/U with OAI. *D-Lib Magazine*, 11(2). http://www.dlib.org/dlib/february05/sanderson/02sanderson.html.

Santaguida, P., Helfand, M., (2005). Challenges in systematic reviews that evaluate drug efficacy or effectiveness. *Annals of Internal Medicine*, 142: 1066–1072.

Saracevic, T. (1975). Relevance: a review of and a framework for the thinking on the notion in information science. *Journal of the American Society for Information Science*, 26: 321–343.

Saracevic, T. and Kantor, P. (1988a). A study in information seeking and retrieving. II. Users, questions, and effectiveness. *Journal of the American Society for Information Science*, 39: 177–196.

Saracevic, T. and Kantor, P. (1988b). A study of information seeking and retrieving. III. Searchers, searches, and overlap. *Journal of the American Society for Information Science*, 39: 197–216.

Saracevic, T., Kantor, P., et al. (1988). A study of information seeking and retrieving. I. Background and methodology. *Journal of the American Society for Information Science*, 39: 161–176.

Sawaya, G., Guirguis-Blake, J., et al. (2007). Update on the methods of the U.S. Preventive Services Task Force: estimating certainty and magnitude of net benefit. *Annals of Internal Medicine*, 147: 871–875.

Sayers, E. (2005). PubChem: an entrez database of small molecules. *NLM Technical Bulletin*. e2. http://165.112.6.70/pubs/techbull/jf05/jf05_pubchem.html.

Sayers, E. and Wheeler, D. (2007). Building customized data pipelines using the entrez programming utilities (eUtils), in Airozo, D., Al-Ubaydli, M., Sayers, E. and Wheeler, D., eds. *NCBI Short Courses*. Bethesda, MD. National Library of Medicine. http://www.ncbi.nlm.nih.gov/books/bookres.fcgi/coursework/chapter_eutils.pdf.

Scargle, J. (2000). Publication bias: the "file-drawer" problem in scientific inference. *Journal of Scientific Exploration*, 14: 91–106.

Scarpa, T. (2006). Research funding: peer review at NIH. *Science*, 311: 41.

Schacher, L. (2001). Clinical librarianship: its value in medical care. *Annals of Internal Medicine*, 134: 717–720.

Schamber, L., Eisenberg, M., et al. (1990). A re-examination of relevance: toward a dynamic, situational definition. *Information Processing and Management*, 26: 755–776.

Scherer, R. and Langenberg, P. (2001). Full publication of results initially presented in abstracts: revisited. *Fourth International Congress on Peer Review in Biomedical Publication*, Barcelona, Spain. American Medical Association. http://www.ama-assn.org/public/peer/peerhome.htm.

Schleimer, S., Wilkerson, D., et al. (2003). Winnowing: local algorithms for document fingerprinting. *Proceedings of the 2003 ACM SIGMOD International Conference on Management of Data*, San Diego, CA. ACM Press. 76–85.

Schlein, A. (2004). Find it online, Fourth Edition: *The Complete Guide to Online Research*. Tempe, AZ. Facts on Demand Press.

Schmidt, H., Norman, G., et al. (1990). A cognitive perspective on medical expertise: theory and implications. *Academic Medicine*, 65: 611–621.

Scholer, F., Williams, H., et al. (2004). Query association surrogates for web search. *Journal of the American Society for Information Science*, 55: 637–650.

Schroter, S. (2006). Importance of free access to research articles on decision to submit to the BMJ: survey of authors. *British Medical Journal*, 332: 394–396.

Schroter, S. and Tite, L. (2006). Open access publishing and author-pays business models: a survey of authors' knowledge and perceptions. *Journal of the Royal Society of Medicine*, 99: 141–148.

Schroter, S., Tite, L., et al. (2006). Differences in review quality and recommendations for publication between peer reviewers suggested by authors or by editors. *Journal of the American Medical Association*, 295: 314–317.

Schroter, S., Tite, L., et al. (2005). Perceptions of open access publishing: interviews with journal authors. *British Medical Journal*, 330: 756.

Schuemie, M., Weeber, M., et al. (2004). Distribution of information in biomedical abstracts and full-text publications. *Bioinformatics*, 20: 2597–2604.

Schulz, K., Chalmers, I., et al. (1994). Assessing the quality of randomization from reports of controlled trials published in obstetrics and gynecology journals. *Journal of the American Medical Association*, 272: 125–128.

Schulz, K., Chalmers, I., et al. (1995). Empirical evidence of bias: dimensions of methodological quality associated with estimates of treatment effects in controlled trials. *Journal of the American Medical Association*, 273: 408–412.

Schulz, S. and Hahn, U. (2000). Morpheme-based, cross-lingual indexing for medical document retrieval. *International Journal of Medical Informatics*, 58: 87–99.

Schutze, H. and Pedersen, J. (1995). Information retrieval based on word senses. *Proceedings of the 4th Annual Symposium on Document Analysis and Information Retrieval*, Las Vegas, NV. University of Nevada, Las Vegas. 161–175.

Schuyler, P., McCray, A., et al. (1989). A test collection for experimentation in bibliographic retrieval. *MEDINFO 89 – Proceedings of the Sixth Congress on Medical Informatics*, Singapore. North-Holland. 910–912.

Schwartz, K., Northrup, J., et al. (2003). Use of on-line evidence-based resources at the point of care. *Family Medicine*, 35: 251–256.

Schwartz, L. and Woloshin, S. (2004). The media matter: a call for straightforward medical reporting. *Annals of Internal Medicine*, 140: 226–228.

Schwartz, L., Woloshin, S., et al. (2002). Media coverage of scientific meetings: too much, too soon? *Journal of the American Medical Association*, 287: 2859–2863.

Sebastiani, F. (2005). Text categorization, 109–129, in Zanasi, A., ed. *Text Mining and its Applications*. Southampton, UK. WIT Press. http://nmis.isti.cnr.it/sebastiani/Publications/TM05.pdf.

Sedrakyan, A. and Shih, C. (2007). Improving depiction of benefits and harms: analyses of studies of well-known therapeutics and review of high-impact medical journals. *Medical Care*, 45: S23–S28.

Seki, K., Costello, J., et al. (2004). TREC 2004 Genomics Track experiments at IUB. *The Thirteenth Text Retrieval Conference: TREC 2004*, Gaithersburg, MD. National Institute of Standards and Technology. http://trec.nist.gov/pubs/trec13/papers/indianau-seki.geo.pdf.

Seki, K. and Mostafa, J. (2007). Discovering implicit associations between genes and hereditary diseases. *Pacific Symposium on Biocomputing*, Maui, Hawaii. World Scientific. 316–327.

Self, P., Filardo, T., et al. (1989). Acquired immunodeficiency syndrome (AIDS) and the epidemic growth of its literature. *Scientometrics*, 17: 49–60.

Séror, A. (2006). A case analysis of INFOMED: The Cuban National Health Care Telecommunications Network and Portal. *Journal of Medical Internet Research*, 8(1): e1. http://www.jmir.org/2006/1/e1/.

Service, R. (2006a). Columbia lab retracts key catalysis papers. *Science*, 311: 1533.

Service, R. (2006b). Researchers raise new doubts about 'bubble fusion' reports. *Science*, 311: 1532–1533.

Sewell, W. and Teitelbaum, S. (1986). Observations of end-user online searching behavior over eleven years. *Journal of the American Society for Information Science*, 37(4): 234–245.

Shannon, C. and Weaver, W. (1949). *The Mathematical Theory of Communication*. Urbana, IL. University of Illinois Press.

Shatkay, H., Chen, N., et al. (2006). Integrating image data into biomedical text categorization. *Bioinformatics*, 22: e446–e453.

Shaughnessy, A., Slawson, D., et al. (1994). Becoming an information master: a guidebook to the medical information jungle. *Journal of Family Practice*, 39: 489–499.

Shearer, B., Seymour, A., (2001). Bringing the best of medical librarianship to the patient team. *Journal of the Medical Library Association*, 90: 22–31.

Sheffield, C. (2006). e-Learning Object Portals: a new resource that offers new opportunities for librarians. *Medical Reference Services Quarterly*, 25(4): 65–74.

Shekelle, P., Ortiz, E., et al. (2001). Validity of the Agency for Healthcare Research and Quality clinical practice guidelines: how quickly do guidelines become outdated? *Journal of the American Medical Association*, 286: 1461–1467.

Shelstad, K. and Clevenger, F. (1996). Information retrieval patterns and needs among practicing general surgeons: a statewide experience. *Bulletin of the Medical Library Association*, 84: 490–497.

Sheridan, S., Pignone, M., et al. (2003). A randomized comparison of patients' understanding of number needed to treat and other common risk reduction formats. *Journal of General Internal Medicine*, 18: 884–892.

Sherman, C. and Price, G. (2001). *The Invisible Web: Uncovering Information Sources Search Engines Can't See*. Chicago. Independent Publishers Group.

Shiffman, R., Brandt, C., et al. (1999). A design model for computer-based guideline implementation based on information management services. *Journal of the American Medical Informatics Association*, 6: 99–103.

Shipman, J., Cunningham, D., et al. (2002). The informationist conference: report. *Journal of the Medical Library Association*, 90: 458–464.

Shneiderman, B. (1987). User interface design and evaluation for an electronic encyclopedia, 207–223, in Slavendy, G., ed. *Cognitive Engineering in the Design of Human-Computer Interaction and Expert Systems*. Amsterdam. Elsevier Science.

Shneiderman, B. and Plaisant, C. (2005). *Designing the User Interface: Strategies for Effective Human-Computer Interaction*, Fourth Edition. Reading, MA. Addison-Wesley.

Shojania, K. and Bero, L. (2001). Taking advantage of the explosion of systematic reviews: an efficient MEDLINE search strategy. *Effective Clinical Practice*, 4: 157–162.

Shojania, K., Sampson, M., et al. (2007). How quickly do systematic reviews go out of date? A survival analysis. *Annals of Internal Medicine*, 147: 224–233.

Shon, J. and Musen, M. (1999). The low availability of metadata elements for evaluating the quality of medical information on the World Wide Web. *Proceedings of the AMIA 1999 Annual Symposium*, Washington, DC. Hanley & Belfus. 945–949.

Shuchman, M. and Wilkes, M. (1997). Medical scientists and health news reporting: a case of miscommunication. *Annals of Internal Medicine*, 126: 976–982.

Sievert, M., Patrick, T., et al. (2001). Need a bloody nose be a nosebleed? or, lexical variants causing surprising results. *Bulletin of the Medical Library Association*, 89: 68–71. http://pubmedcentral.gov/articlerender.fcgi?artid=31706.

Silberg, W., Lundberg, G., et al. (1997). Assessing, controlling, and assuring the quality of medical information on the internet: caveat lector et viewor – let the reader and viewer beware. *Journal of the American Medical Association*, 277: 1244–1245.

Silverstein, F., Faich, G., et al. (2000). Gastrointestinal toxicity with celecoxib vs nonsteroidal anti-inflammatory drugs for osteoarthritis and rheumatoid arthritis: the CLASS study: a randomized controlled trial. *Journal of the American Medical Association*, 284: 1247–1255.

Silverstein, F., Simon, L., et al. (2001). Reporting of 6-month vs 12-month data in a clinical trial of celecoxib – In reply. *Journal of the American Medical Association*, 286: 2399–2400.

Sim, I. and Detmer, D. (2005). Beyond trial registration: a global trial bank for clinical trial reporting. *PLoS Medicine*, 2(11): e65.

Singhal, A. (2004). Challenges in Running a Commercial Web Search Engine. Mountain View, CA, Google. http://www.research.ibm.com/haifa/Workshops/searchandcollaboration2004/papers/haifa.pdf.

Singhal, A., Buckley, C., et al. (1996). Pivoted document length normalization. *Proceedings of the 19th Annual International ACM SIGIR Conference on Research and Development in Information Retrieval*, Zurich, Switzerland. ACM Press. 21–29.

Sintchenko, V., Coiera, E., et al. (2004). Comparative impact of guidelines, clinical data, and decision support on prescribing decisions: an interactive web experiment with simulated cases. *Journal of the American Medical Informatics Association*, 11: 71–77.

Sioutos, N., deCoronado, S., et al. (2007). NCI Thesaurus: a semantic model integrating cancer-related clinical and molecular information. *Journal of Biomedical Informatics*, 40: 30–43.

Slack, W., Lewis, D., et al. eds. (2005). *Consumer Health Informatics: Informing Consumers and Improving Health Care*. New York, NY. Springer.

Slawson, D., Shaughnessy, A. et al. (2005). Teaching evidence-based medicine: should we be teaching information management instead? *Academic Medicine*, 80: 685–689.

Smalheiser, N. and Swanson, D. (1998). Using ARROWSMITH: a computer-assisted approach to formulating and assessing scientific hypotheses. *Computer Methods and Programs in Biomedicine*, 57: 149–153.

Smeaton, A. (2005). Large scale evaluations of multimedia information retrieval: the TRECVid experience. *The 4th International Conference on Image and Video Retrieval (CIVR 2005)*, Singapore. Lecture Notes in Computer Science. Springer-Verlag 11–17.

Smeaton, A., Over, P., et al. (2006). Evaluation campaigns and TRECVid. *Proceedings of the 8th ACM SIGMM International workshop on Multimedia Information Retrieval*, Santa Barbara, California. ACM Press. http://twentyone.tpd.tno.nl/mmts/papers/mir710-Smeaton.pdf.

Smeulders, A., Worring, M., (2000). Content-based image retrieval at the end of the early years. *IEEE Transactions on Pattern Analysis and Machine Intelligence*, 22: 1349–1380.

Smith, A. (1999). A tale of two web spaces: comparing sites using web impact factors. *Journal of Documentation*, 55: 577–592.

Smith, C., Ganschow, P., et al. (2000). Teaching residents evidence-based medicine skills: a controlled trial of effectiveness and assessment of durability. *Journal of General Internal Medicine*, 15: 710–715.

Smith, L., Rindflesch, T., et al. (2004). MedPost: a part-of-speech tagger for biomedical text. *Bioinformatics*, 14: 2320–2321.

Smith, R. (2003). Medical journals and pharmaceutical companies: uneasy bedfellows. *British Medical Journal*, 326: 1202–1205.

Smith, R. (2005). Medical journals are an extension of the marketing arm of pharmaceutical companies. *PLoS Medicine*, 2(5): e138.

Smith, R. and Roberts, I. (1997). An amnesty for unpublished trials. *British Medical Journal*, 315: 622.

Smith, S. (1994). *The Jordan Rules*. New York, NY. Pocket Books.

Sneiderman, C., Demner-Fushman, D., et al. (2007). Knowledge-based methods to help clinicians find answers in MEDLINE. *Journal of the American Medical Informatics Association*, 14: 772–780.

Soboroff, I. (2002). Do TREC web collections look like the web? *SIGIR Forum*, 36(2): 23–31. http://www.sigir.org/forum/F2002/soboroff.pdf.

Soboroff, I., Nicholas, C., et al. (2001). Ranking retrieval systems without relevance judgments. *Proceedings of the 24th Annual International ACM SIGIR Conference on Research and Development in Information Retrieval*, New Orleans, LA. ACM Press. 66–73.

Soergel, D. (1997). Multilingual thesauri in cross-language text and speech retrieval. *AAAI Spring Symposium on Cross-Language Text and Speech Retrieval*, Palo Alto, CA. AAAI. http://www.ee.umd.edu/medlab/filter/sss/papers/soergel.ps.

Sollins, K. and Masinter, L. (1994). Functional Requirements for Uniform Resource Names. *Internet Engineering Task Force*. http://www.w3.org/Addressing/rfc1737.txt. Accessed: July 1, 2002.

Soualmia, L. and Darmoni, S. (2005). Combining different standards and different approaches for health information retrieval in a quality-controlled gateway. *International Journal of Medical Informatics*, 74: 141–150.

Sox, H., Blatt, M., et al. (1988). *Medical Decision Making*. Boston, MA. Butterworths.

Sox, H. and Rennie, D. (2006). Research misconduct, retraction, and cleansing the medical literature: lessons from the Poehlman case. *Annals of Internal Medicine*, 144: 609–613.

Sparck-Jones, K. (2006). What's the value of TREC – is there a gap to jump or a chasm to bridge? *SIGIR Forum*, 40(1): 10–20. http://www.acm.org/sigir/forum/2006J/2006j_sigirforum_sparck_jones.pdf.

Sparck-Jones, K. and Sakai, T. (2001). Generic summaries for indexing in IR. *Proceedings of the 24th Annual International ACM SIGIR Conference on Research and Development in Information Retrieval*, New Orleans, LA. ACM Press. 190–198.

Spath, M. and Buttlar, L. (1996). Information and research needs of acute-care clinical nurses. *Bulletin of the Medical Library Association*, 84: 112–116.

Spink, A., Jansen, B., et al. (2002). From e-sex to e-commerce: web search changes. *Computer*, 35: 107–109.

Spitzer, V., Ackerman, M., et al. (1996). The visible human male: a technical report. *Journal of the American Medical Informatics Association*, 3: 118–130.

Srinivasan, P. (1996a). Optimal document-indexing vocabulary for MEDLINE. *Information Processing and Management*, 32: 503–514.

Srinivasan, P. (1996b). Query expansion and MEDLINE. *Information Processing and Management*, 32: 431–444.

Srinivasan, P. (1996c). Retrieval feedback in MEDLINE. *Journal of the American Medical Informatics Association*, 3: 157–168.

Srinivasan, P. (2004). Text mining: generating hypotheses from MEDLINE. *Journal of the American Society for Information Science & Technology*, 55: 396–413.

Srinivasan, P. and Libbus, B. (2004). Mining MEDLINE for implicit links between dietary substances and diseases. *Bioinformatics*, 20: i290–i296.

Stafford, R., Furberg, C., et al. (2004). Impact of clinical trial results on national trends in alpha-blocker prescribing, 1996–2002. *Journal of the American Medical Association*, 291: 54–62.

Staggers, N. and Mills, M. (1994). Nurse-computer interaction: staff performance outcomes. *Nursing Research*, 43: 144–150.

Stein, H., Nadkarni, P., et al. (2000). Exploring the degree of concordance of coded and textual data in answering clinical queries from a clinical data repository. *Journal of the American Medical Informatics Association*, 7: 42–54.

Stein, L., Mungall, C., et al. (2002). The generic genome browser: a building block for a model organism system database. *Genome Research*, 12: 1599–1610.

Steinberger, R., Pouliquen, B., et al. (2006). The JRC-Acquis: a multilingual aligned parallel corpus with 20+ languages. *Proceedings of the 5th International Conference on Language*

Resources and Evaluation (LREC'2006), Genoa, Italy. 2142–2147. http://langtech.jrc.it/Documents/0605_LREC_JRC-Acquis_Steinberger-et-al.pdf.

Steinbrook, R. (2005). Gag clauses in clinical-trial agreements. *New England Journal of Medicine*, 352: 2160–2162.

Steinbrook, R. (2006). Searching for the right search – reaching the medical literature. *New England Journal of Medicine*, 354: 4–7.

Sterling, T. (1959). Publication decisions and their possible effects on inferences drawn from tests of significance – or vice versa. *Journal of the American Statistical Association*, 54: 30–34.

Stern, J. and Simes, R. (1997). Publication bias: evidence of delayed publication in a cohort study of clinical research projects. *British Medical Journal*, 315: 640–645.

Stevens, R., Goble, C., et al. (2001). A classification of tasks in bioinformatics. *Bioinformatics*, 17: 180–188.

Stossel, T. (1985). Reviewer status and review quality: experience of the Journal of Clinical Investigation. *New England Journal of Medicine*, 312: 658–659.

Straus, S., Richardson, W., et al. (2005). *Evidence Based Medicine: How to Practice and Teach EBM*, Third Edition. New York, NY. Churchill Livingstone.

Strivens, M. and Eppig, J. (2004). Visualizing the laboratory mouse: capturing phenotype information. *Genetica*, 122: 89–97.

Stross, J. and Harlan, W. (1979). The dissemination of new medical information. *Journal of the American Medical Association*, 241: 2622–2624.

Stross, J. and Harlan, W. (1981). Dissemination of relevant information on hypertension. *Journal of the American Medical Association*, 246: 360–362.

Stroup, D., Berlin, J., et al. (2000). Meta-analysis of observational studies in epidemiology: a proposal for reporting. *Journal of the American Medical Association*, 283: 2008–2012.

Strouse, R. (2004). Content User Profile: Update On Scientists. Burlingame, CA, Outsell http://content.outsellinc.com/coms2/summary_0245–888_ITM.

Strzalkowski, T., Lin, F., et al. (1999). Evaluating natural language processing techniques in information retrieval, 113–146, in Strzalkowski, T., ed. *Natural Language Information Retrieval*. Dordrecht, The Netherlands. Kluwer.

Stumpf, W. (1980). "Peer" review. *Science*, 207: 822–823.

Suarez-Almazor, M., Belseck, E., et al. (2000). Identifying clinical trials in the medical literature with electronic databases: MEDLINE alone is not enough. *Controlled Clinical Trials*, 21: 476–487.

Sun, Y., Zhuang, Z., et al. (2007). Determining bias to search engines from robots.txt. *2007 IEEE/WIC/ACM International Conference on Web Intelligence*, Fremont, CA. http://clgiles.ist.psu.edu/papers/WI2007-robots.txt.pdf.

Swan, R. and Allan, J. (1998). Aspect windows, 3-D visualization, and indirect comparisons of information retrieval systems. *Proceedings of the 21st Annual International ACM SIGIR Conference on Research and Development in Information Retrieval*, Melbourne, Australia. ACM Press. 173–181.

Swanson, D. (1977). Information retrieval as a trial-and-error process. *Library Quarterly*, 47: 128–148.

Swanson, D. (1986). Two medical literatures that are logically but not bibliographically connected. *Perspectives in Biology and Medicine*, 30: 7–18.

Swanson, D. (1988a). Historical note: information retrieval and the future of an illusion. *Journal of the American Society for Information Science*, 39: 92–98.

Swanson, D. (1988b). Migraine and magnesium: eleven neglected connections. *Perspectives in Biology and Medicine*, 31: 526–557.

Swanson, D. and Smalheiser, N. (1997). An interactive system for finding complementary literatures: a stimulus to scientific discovery. *Artificial Intelligence*, 91: 183–203.

Tait, J., ed. (2005). *Charting a New Course: Natural Language Processing and Information Retrieval*. Dordrecht, The Netherlands. Springer.

Tanabe, L., Scherf, U., et al. (1999). MedMiner: an Internet text-mining tool for biomedical information, with application to gene expression profiling. *Biotechniques*, 27: 1210–1214, 1216–1217.

Tanabe, L. and Wilbur, W. (2002). Tagging gene and protein names in biomedical text. *Bioinformatics*, 18: 1124–1132.

Tanenbaum, S. (1994). Knowing and acting in medical practice: the epistemological politics of outcomes research. *Journal of Health Politics, Policy and Law*, 19: 27–44.

Tang, H. and Ng, J. (2006). Googling for a diagnosis—use of Google as a diagnostic aid: internet based study. *British Medical Journal*, 333: 1143–1145.

Tang, P., Newcomb, C., et al. (1997). Meeting the information needs of patients: results from a patient focus group. *Proceedings of the 1997 AMIA Annual Fall Symposium*, Nashville, TN. Hanley & Belfus. 672–676.

Tapscott, D. and Williams, A. (2006). *Wikinomics – How Mass Collaboration Changes Everything*. New York, NY. Portfolio.

Tatsioni, A., Bonitsis, N., et al. (2007). Persistence of contradicted claims in the literature. *Journal of the American Medical Association*, 298: 2517–2526.

Taylor, H. and Leitman, R. (2001). The Increasing Impact of eHealth on Physician Behavior. http://www.harrisinteractive.com/news/newsletters/healthnews/HI_HealthCareNews2001Vol1_iss31.pdf. Accessed: November 13, 2001.

Taylor, R. and Giles, J. (2005). Cash interests taint drug advice. *Nature*, 437: 1070–1071.

Tenopir, C. (1985). Full text database retrieval performance. *Online Review*, 9(2): 149–164.

Teufel, S. and Moens, M. (2002). Summarizing scientific articles: experiments with relevance and rhetorical status. *Computational Linguistics*, 28: 409–445.

Thelwall, M. (2000). Extracting macroscopic information from web links. *Journal of the American Society for Information Science*, 52: 1157–1168.

Thelwall, M. (2003). What is this link doing here? Beginning a fine-grained process of identifying reasons for academic hyperlink creation. *Information Research*, 8: 3. http://informationr.net/ir/8–3/paper151.html.

Thelwall, M. and Harries, G. (2004). Do the web sites of higher rated scholars have significantly more online impact? *Journal of the American Society for Information Science & Technology*, 55: 149–159.

Theodosiou, T., Angelis, L., et al. (2007). Gene functional annotation by statistical analysis of biomedical articles. *International Journal of Medical Informatics*, 76: 601–613.

Thomas, D., Rosenbloom, K., et al. (2007). The ENCODE project at UC Santa Cruz. *Nucleic Acids Research*, 35: D663–D667.

Thomas, O. and Willett, P. (2000). Webometric analysis of departments of librarianship and information science. *Journal of Information Science*, 26: 421–428.

Thurow, S. (2007). *Search Engine Visibility*, Second Edition. Berkeley, CA. Peachpit Press.

Tibbo, H. (2001). Archival perspectives on the emerging digital library. *Communications of the ACM*, 44(5): 69–70.

Tierney, W., Miller, M., et al. (1993). Physician inpatient order writing on microcomputer workstations: effects on resource utilization. *Journal of the American Medical Association*, 269: 379–383.

Timpka, T. and Arborelius, E. (1990). The GP's dilemmas: a study of knowledge need and use during health care consultations. *Methods of Information in Medicine*, 29: 23–29.

Tooker, J. (2004). ACP Comments on Proposed NIH Public Access Policy. Philadelphia, PA, American College of Physicians. http://www.acponline.org/hpp/nih_open.htm.

Torvik, V. and Smalheiser, N. (2007). A quantitative model for linking two disparate sets of articles in MEDLINE. *Bioinformatics*, 23: 1658–1665.

Torvik, V., Weeber, M., et al. (2005). A probabilistic similarity metric for Medline records: a model for author name disambiguation. *Journal of the American Society for Information Science & Technology*, 56: 140–158.

Tramer, M., Reynolds, D., et al. (1997). Impact of covert duplicate publication on meta-analysis: a case study. *British Medical Journal*, 315: 635–640.

Tran, D., Dubay, C., et al. (2004). Applying task analysis to describe and facilitate bioinformatics tasks. *MEDINFO 2004 – Proceedings of the Eleventh World Congress on Medical Informatics*, San Francisco, CA. IOS Press. 818–822.

Troyanskaya, O. (2005). Putting microarrays in a context: integrated analysis of diverse biological data. *Briefings in Bioinformatics*, 6: 34–43.

Trueswell, R. (1969). Some behavioral patterns of library users: the 80/20 rule. *Wilson Library Bulletin*, 43: 458–461.

Trumble, J., Anderson, M., et al. (2007). A Systematic Evaluation of Evidence Based Medicine Tools for Point-of-Care Houston, TX, Texas Health Science Libraries Consortium. http://ils. mdacc.tmc.edu/THSLC_SCC2006_EBM.zip.

Tuason, O., Chen, L., et al. (2004). Biological nomenclatures: a source of lexical knowledge and ambiguity. *Pacific Symposium on Biocomputing*, Kona, Hawaii. World Scientific. 238–249.

Tunis, S., Stryer, D., et al. (2003). Practical clinical trials – increasing the value of clinical research for decision making in clinical and health policy. *Journal of the American Medical Association*, 290: 1624–1632.

Turner, E. (2004). A taxpayer-funded clinical trials registry and results database. *PLoS Medicine*, 1: 180–182.

Turner, E., Matthews, A., et al. (2008). Selective publication of antidepressant trials and its influence on apparent efficacy. *New England Journal of Medicine*, 358: 252–260.

Turpin, A. and Hersh, W. (2001). Why batch and user evaluations do not give the same results. *Proceedings of the 24th Annual International ACM SIGIR Conference on Research and Development in Information Retrieval*, New Orleans, LA. ACM Press. 225–231.

Turpin, A. and Hersh, W. (2004). Do clarity scores for queries correlate with user performance? *Proceedings of the Fifteenth Australasian Database Conference (ADC2004)*, Dunedin, New Zealand. Australian Computer Society. 85–91. http://crpit.com/confpapers/CRPITV27Turpin. pdf.

Turpin, A. and Scholer, F. (2006). User performance versus precision measures for simple search tasks. *Proceedings of the 29th Annual International ACM SIGIR Conference on Research and Development in Information Retrieval*, Seattle, WA. ACM Press. 11–18.

Turtle, H. (1994). Natural language vs. Boolean query evaluation: a comparison of retrieval performance. *Proceedings of the 17th Annual International ACM SIGIR Conference on Research and Development in Information Retrieval*, Dublin, Ireland. Springer-Verlag. 212–220.

Turtle, H. and Croft, W. (1991). Evaluation of an inference network-based retrieval model. *ACM Transactions on Information Systems*, 9: 187–222.

Tybaert, S. and Rosov, J. (2004). MEDLINE data changes – 2004. *NLM Technical Bulletin*. Nov–Dec, 2003. e6. http://www.nlm.nih.gov/pubs/techbull/nd03/nd03_med_data_changes. html.

Tyrväinen, P. (2005). Concepts and a design for fair use and privacy in DRM. *D-Lib Magazine*, 11 (2). http://www.dlib.org/dlib/february05/tyrvainen/02tyrvainen.html.

Udvarhelyi, I., Colditz, G., et al. (1992). Cost-effectiveness and cost-benefit analyses in medical literature. *Annals of Internal Medicine*, 116: 238–244.

Umefjord, G., Sandström, H., et al. (2008). Medical text-based consultations on the internet: a 4-year study. *International Journal of Medical Informatics*, 77: 114–121.

Unger, K. and Couzin, J. (2006). Scientific misconduct – even retracted papers endure. *Science*, 312: 40–41.

Urquhart, J. and Bunn, R. (1959). A national loan policy for science serials. *Journal of Documentation*, 15: 21–25.

Uruqhart, C. and Crane, S. (1994). Nurses' information-seeking skills and preceptions of information sources: assessment using vignettes. *Journal of Information Science*, 20: 237–246.

Uzuner, O., Goldstein, I., et al. (2008). Identifying patient smoking status from medical discharge records. *Journal of the American Medical Informatics Association*, 15: 14–24.

Uzuner, O., Luo, Y., et al. (2007). Evaluating the state-of-the-art in automatic de-identification. *Journal of the American Medical Informatics Association*, 14: 550–563.

Vandenbroucke, J. (2001). In defense of case reports and case series. *Annals of Internal Medicine*, 134: 330–334.

Van de Sompel, H. and Lagoze, C. (1999). The Santa Fe Convention of the Open Archives Initiative. *D-Lib Magazine*, 5. http://www.dlib.org/dlib/february00/vandesompel-oai/02vande-sompel-oai.html.

Van de Sompel, H., Nelson, M., et al. (2004). Resource harvesting within the OAI-PMH framework. *D-Lib Magazine*, 10(12). http://www.dlib.org/dlib/december04/vandesompel/12vande-sompel.html.

vanNieuwenhoven, C., Buskens, E., et al. (2001). Relationship between methodological trial quality and the effects of selective digestive decontamination on pneumonia and mortality in critically ill patients. *Journal of the American Medical Association*, 286: 335–340.

vanRijsbergen, C. (1979). *Information Retrieval*. London, England. Butterworth.

vanRooyen, S., Godlee, F., et al. (1998). Effect of blinding and unmasking on the quality of peer review: a randomized trial. *Journal of the American Medical Association*, 280: 234–237.

vanRooyen, S., Goldbeck-Wood, S., et al. (2001). What makes an author? A comparison between what authors say they did and what editorial guidelines require. *Fourth International Congress on Peer Review in Biomedical Publication*, Barcelona, Spain. American Medical Association. http://www.ama-assn.org/public/peer/peerhome.htm.

Veenstra, R. (1992). Clinical medical librarian impact on patient care: a one-year analysis. *Bulletin of the Medical Library Association*, 80: 19–22.

Venema, A., vanGinneken, A., et al. (2007). Is OpenSDE an alternative for dedicated medical research databases? An example in coronary surgery. *BMC Medical Informatics & Decision Making*, 7: 31. http://www.biomedcentral.com/1472-6947/7/31.

Venter, J., Adams, M., (2001). The sequence of the human genome. *Science*, 291: 1304–1351.

Villanueva, P., Piero, S., et al. (2003). Accuracy of pharmaceutical advertisements in medical journals. *Lancet*, 361: 27–32.

Vinayagam, A., König, R., et al. (2004). Applying support vector machines for gene ontology based gene function prediction. *BMC Bioinformatics*, 5: 116. http://www.biomedcentral.com/1471-2105/5/116.

Vise, D. and Malseed, M. (2005). *The Google Story*. New York, NY. Delacorte Press.

Vizenor, L., Bodenreider, O., et al. (2006). Enhancing biomedical ontologies through alignment of semantic relationships: exploratory approaches. *Proceedings of the AMIA 2006 Annual Symposium*, Washington, DC. American Medical Informatics Association. 804–808.

Vogelstein, F. (2005). Search and destroy. *Fortune*. May 2, 2005. http://money.cnn.com/magazines/fortune/fortune_archive/2005/05/02/8258478/.

Volmink, J., Siegfried, N., et al. (2004). Research synthesis and dissemination as a bridge to knowledge management: the Cochrane Collaboration. *Bulletin of the World Health Organization*, 82: 778–783.

vonElm, E., Altman, D., et al. (2007). The Strengthening the Reporting of Observational Studies in Epidemiology (STROBE) statement: guidelines for reporting observational studies. *Annals of Internal Medicine*, 147: 573–577.

vonElm, E., Costanza, M., et al. (2003). More insight into the fate of biomedical meeting abstracts: a systematic review. *BMC Medical Research Methodology*, 3: 12. http://www.biomedcentral.com/1471-2288/3/12.

vonElm, E., Poglia, G., et al. (2004). Different patterns of duplciate publication: an analysis of articles used in systematic reviews. *Journal of the American Medical Association*, 291: 974–980.

Voorhees, E. (1993). Using WordNet to disambiguate word senses for text retrieval. *Proceedings of the 16th Annual International ACM SIGIR Conference on Research and Development in Information Retrieval*, Pittsburgh, PA. ACM Press. 171–180.

Voorhees, E. (1994). Query expansion using lexical-semantic relations. *Proceedings of the 17th Annual International ACM SIGIR Conference on Research and Development in Information Retrieval*, Dublin, Ireland. Springer-Verlag. 61–69.

Voorhees, E. (1998). Variations in relevance judgments and the measurement of retrieval effectiveness. *Proceedings of the 21st Annual International ACM SIGIR Conference on Research and Development in Information Retrieval*, Melbourne, Australia. ACM Press. 315–323.

Voorhees, E. (2005). Question answering in TREC, 233–257, in Voorhees, E. and Harman, D., eds. *TREC – Experiment and Evaluation in Information Retrieval*. Cambridge, MA. MIT Press.

Voorhees, E. (2006). The TREC 2005 robust track. *SIGIR Forum*, 40(1): 41–48. http://www.acm.org/sigir/forum/2006J/2006j_sigirforum_voorhees.pdf.

Voorhees, E. and Harman, D., eds. (2005). *TREC: Experiment and Evaluation in Information Retrieval*. Cambridge, MA. MIT Press.

Wager, E. and Middleton, P. (2001). Reference accuracy in peer-reviewed journals: a systematic review. *Fourth International Congress on Peer Review in Biomedical Publication*, Barcelona, Spain. American Medical Association. http://www.ama-assn.org/public/peer/peerhome.htm.

Wager, E., Parkin, E., et al. (2006). Are reviewers suggested by authors as good as those chosen by editors? Results of a rater-blinded, retrospective study. *BMC Medicine*, 4: 13. http://www.biomedcentral.com/1741–7015/4/13.

Walczuch, N., Fuhr, N., et al. (1994). Routing and ad-hoc retrieval with the TREC-3 collection in a distributed loosely federated environment. *Overview of the Third Text REtrieval Conference (TREC-3)*, Gaithersburg, MD. National Institute of Standards and Technology. 135–144.

Walji, M., Sagaram, S., et al. (2004). Efficacy of quality criteria to identify potentially harmful information: a cross-sectional survey of complementary and alternative web sites. *Journal of Medical Internet Research*, 6(2): e21. http://www.jmir.org/2004/2/e21/.

Walker, C., McKibbon, K., et al. (1991). Problems encountered by clinical end users of MEDLINE and Grateful Med. *Bulletin of the Medical Library Association*, 79: 67–69.

Wallingford, K., Humphreys, B., et al. (1990). Bibliographic retrieval: a survey of individual users of MEDLINE. *M.D. Computing*, 7: 166–171.

Wang, P. (1994). A Cognitive Model of Document Selection of Real Users of Information Retrieval Systems. College of Library and Information Services. Ph.D. Thesis. University of Maryland.

Wang, Y., Addess, K., et al. (2007). MMDB: annotating protein sequences with Entrez's 3D-structure database. *Nucleic Acids Research*, 35: D298–D300.

Wang, Y. and Liu, Z. (2007). Automatic detecting indicators for quality of health information on the web. *International Journal of Medical Informatics*, 76: 575–582.

Ward, J. (2005). Gene indexing and entrez gene. *NLM Technical Bulletin*. e6. http://165.112.6.70/pubs/techbull/ma05/ma05_gene.html.

Wartik, S., Fox, E., et al. (1992). Hashing algorithms, 293–362, in Frakes, W. and Baeza-Yates, R., eds. *Information Retrieval: Data Structures and Algorithms*. Englewood Cliffs, NJ. Prentice-Hall.

Wasserman, H. and Wang, J. (2003). An applied evaluation of SNOMED CT as a clinical vocabulary for the computerized diagnosis and problem list. *Proceedings of the AMIA 2003 Annual Symposium*, Washington, DC. Hanley & Belfus. 699–703.

Watson, R. and Richardson, P. (1999). Identifying randomized controlled trials of cognitive therapy for depression: comparing the efficiency of Embase, Medline, and PsycINFO bibliographic databases. *British Journal of Medical Psychology*, 72: 535–542.

Waxman, H. (2005). The lessons of Vioxx – drug safety and sales. *New England Journal of Medicine*, 352: 2576–2578.

Weeber, M., Kors, J., et al. (2005). Online tools to support literature-based discovery in the life sciences. *Briefings in Bioinformatics*, 6: 277–286.

Weeber, M., Vos, R., et al. (2003). Generating hypotheses by discovering implicit associations in the literature: a case report of a search for new potential therapeutic uses for thalidomide. *Journal of the American Medical Informatics Association*, 10: 252–259.

Weiner, J., Parente, S., et al. (1995). Variation in office-based quality – a claims-based profile of care provided to Medicare patients with diabetes. *Journal of the American Medical Association*, 273: 1503–1508.

Weise, F. (2004). Being there: library as place. *Journal of the Medical Library Association*, 92: 6–13.

Weiss, S., Indurkhya, N., et al. (2005). *Text Mining: Predictive Methods for Analyzing Unstructured Information.* New York, NY. Springer.

West, R. (1996). Impact factors need to be improved. *British Medical Journal*, 313: 1400.

Westbrook, J. (1960). Identifying significant research. *Science*, 132: 1229–1234.

Westbrook, J., Coiera, E., et al. (2005). Measuring the impact of online evidence retrieval systems using critical incidents and journey mapping. *Studies in Health Technology and Informatics*, 116: 533–538.

Westbrook, J., Gosling, A., et al. (2004). Do clinicians use online evidence to support patient care? A study of 55,000 clinicians. *Journal of the American Medical Informatics Association*, 11: 113–120.

Westbrook, J., Gosling, A., et al. (2005). The impact of an online evidence system on confidence in decision making in a controlled setting. *Medical Decision Making*, 25: 178–185.

Wheeler, D., Barrett, T., et al. (2007). Database resources of the National Center for Biotechnology Information. *Nucleic Acids Research*, 35: D5–D12.

Whitely, W., Rennie, D., et al. (1994). The scientific community's response to evidence of fraudulent publication: the Robert Slutsky case. *Journal of the American Medical Association*, 272: 170–173.

Wiesman, F., vandenHerik, H., et al. (2004). Information retrieval by metabrowsing. *Journal of the American Society for Information Science and Technology*, 55: 565–578.

Wilbur, W., Kim, W., et al. (2006). Spelling correction in the PubMed search engine. *Information Retrieval*, 9: 543–564.

Wilbur, W., Rzhetsky, A., et al. (2006). New directions in biomedical text annotation: definitions, guidelines and corpus construction. *BMC Bioinformatics*, 7: 356. http://www.biomedcentral.com/1471–2105/7/356.

Wilbur, W. and Yang, Y. (1996). An analysis of statistical term strength and its use in the indexing and retrieval of molecular biology texts. *Computers in Biology and Medicine*, 26: 209–222.

Wilczynski, N., Garg, A., et al. (2007). A method for defining a journal subset for a clinical discipline using the bibliographies of systematic reviews. *MEDINFO 2007 – Proceedings of the Twelfth World Congress on Health (Medical) Informatics*, Brisbane, Australia. IOS Press. 721–724.

Wilczynski, N., Morgan, D., et al. (2005). An overview of the design and methods for retrieving high-quality studies for clinical care. *BMC Medical Informatics and Decision Making*, 5: 20. http://www.biomedcentral.com/1472–6947/5/20.

Wilczynski, N., Walker, C., et al. (1995). Reasons for the loss of sensitivity and specificity of methodologic MeSH terms and text words in MEDLINE. *Proceedings of the 19th Annual Symposium on Computer Applications in Medical Care*, New Orleans, LA. Hanley & Belfus. 436–440.

Wildemuth, B., de Bliek, R., et al. (1995). Medical students' personal knowledge, searching proficiency, and database use in problem solving. *Journal of the American Society for Information Science*, 46: 590–607.

Wildemuth, B. and Moore, M. (1995). End-user search behaviors and their relationship to search effectiveness. *Bulletin of the Medical Library Association*, 83: 294–304.

Wilkes, M., Doblin, B., et al. (1992). Pharmaceutical advertisements in leading medical journals: experts' assessments. *Annals of Internal Medicine*, 116: 912–919.

Wilkinson, R. and Fuller, M. (1996). Integration of information retrieval and hypertext via structure, 257–271, in Agosti, M. and Smeaton, A., eds. *Information Retrieval and Hypertext.* Norwell, MA. Kluwer.

Williams, D., Counselman, F., et al. (1996). Emergency department discharge instructions and patient literacy: a problem of disparity. *American Journal of Emergency Medicine*, 14: 19–22.

Williamson, J. (1990). Information Needs of Qualified Nurses in Bloomsbury Health Authority. M.Phil. Thesis. University of London.

Williamson, J., German, P., (1989). Health science information management and continuing education of physicians. *Annals of Internal Medicine*, 110: 151–160.

Willinsky, J. (2005). The unacknowledged convergence of open source, open access, and open science. *First Monday*, 10: 8. http://www.firstmonday.org/issues/issue10_8/willinsky/.

Winker, M., Flanagin, A., et al. (2000). Guidelines for medical and health information sites on the internet: principles governing AMA web sites. *Journal of the American Medical Association*, 283: 1600–1606.

Wishart, D., Knox, C., et al. (2006). DrugBank: a comprehensive resource for in silico drug discovery and exploration. *Nucleic Acids Research*, 34: D668–672.

Wishart, D., Tzur, D., et al. (2007). HMDB: the Human Metabolome Database. *Nucleic Acids Research*, 35: D521–D526.

Witten, I. and Bainbridge, D. (2003). *How to Build a Digital Library*. San Francisco. Morgan Kaufmann.

Wood, F., Wallingford, K., et al. (1997). Transitioning to the internet: results of a National Library of Medicine user survey. *Bulletin of the Medical Library Association*, 85: 331–340.

Woods, W. (1970). Transition network grammars for natural language analysis. *Communications of the ACM*, 13: 591–602.

Wright, J., Perry, T., et al. (2001). Reporting of 6-month vs 12-month data in a clinical trial of celecoxib. *Journal of the American Medical Association*, 286: 2398–2399.

Wu, M., Fuller, M., et al. (2000). Using clustering and classification approaches in interactive retrieval. *Information Processing and Management*, 37: 459–484.

Wu, M., Fuller, M., et al. (2001). Searcher performance in question answering. *Proceedings of the 24th Annual International ACM SIGIR Conference on Research and Development in Information Retrieval*, New Orleans, LA. ACM Press. 375–381.

Xie, H., Wasserman, A., et al. (2002). Large-scale protein annotation through gene ontology. *Genome Research*, 12: 785–794.

Xu, H., Fan, J., et al. (2007). Gene symbol disambiguation using knowledge-based profiles. *Bioinformatics*, 23: 1015–1022.

Yang, J., Cohen, A., et al. (2007). Automatic summarization of mouse gene information by clustering and sentence extraction from MEDLINE abstracts. *Proceedings of the AMIA 2007 Annual Symposium*, Chicago, IL. American Medical Informatics Association.

Yang, J., Cohen, A., et al. (2008). GICSS: gene information clustering and summarization by sen-tence extraction from MEDLINE abstracts. *Bioinformatics*: in press.

Yang, K., Maglaughlin, K., et al. (2000). Passage feedback with IRIS. *Information Processing and Management*, 37: 521–541.

Yang, Y. (1999). An evaluation of statistical approaches to text categorization. *Information Retrieval*, 1: 67–88.

Yang, Y. and Chute, C. (1994). An example-based mapping method for text categorization and retrieval. *ACM Transactions on Information Systems*, 12: 252–277.

Yeh, A., Hirschman, L., et al. (2003). Evaluation of text data mining for database curation: lessons learned from the KDD Challenge Cup. *Bioinformatics*, 19: i331–i339.

Yeh, A., Morgan, A., et al. (2005). BioCreAtIvE Task 1A: gene mention finding evaluation. *BMC Bioinformatics*, 6: S2. http://www.biomedcentral.com/1471-2105/6/S1/S2.

Yu, H. and Agichtein, E. (2003). Extracting synonymous gene and protein terms from biological literature. *Bioinformatics*, 19: i340–i349.

Yu, H., Kim, W., et al. (2007). Using MEDLINE as a knowledge source for disambiguating abbreviations and acronyms in full-text biomedical journal articles. *Journal of Biomedical Informatics*, 40: 150–159.

Yu, H. and Lee, M. (2006). Accessing bioscience images from abstract sentences. *Bioinformatics*, 22: e547–e556.

Yu, H., Lee, M., et al. (2007). Development, implementation, and a cognitive evaluation of a definitional question answering system for physicians. *Journal of Biomedical Informatics*, 40: 236–251.

Yu, L. (2007). *Introduction to the Semantic Web and Semantic Web Services*. Boca Raton, FL/ West Palm Beach, FL. Chapman & Hall/CRC.

Zarin, D., Ide, N., et al. (2007). Issues in the registration of clinical trials. *Journal of the American Medical Association*, 297: 2112–2120.

Zarin, D., Tse, T., et al. (2005). Trial Registration at ClinicalTrials.gov between May and October 2005. *New England Journal of Medicine*, 353: 2779–2787.

Zeng, Q. and Cimino, J. (1997). Linking a clinical system to heterogenous information resources. *Proceedings of the 1997 AMIA Annual Fall Symposium*, Nashville, TN. Hanley & Belfus. 553–557.

Zerhouni, E. (2003). The NIH Roadmap. *Science*, 302: 63–64, 72. http://www.sciencemag.org/ feature/plus/nihroadmap.pdf.

Zerhouni, E. (2004). Access to Biomedical Research Information. Bethesda, MD, National Institutes of Health.http://library.cpmc.columbia.edu/hsl/pdfs/NIH_access_report.pdf.

Zerhouni, E. (2007). Translational research: moving discovery to practice. *Clinical Pharmacology and Therapeutics*, 81: 126–128.

Zhai, C. and Lafferty, J. (2004). A study of smoothing methods for language models applied to information retrieval. *ACM Transactions on Information Systems*, 22: 179–214.

Zhao, J. and Resh, V. (2001). Internet publishing and transformation of knowledge processes. *Communications of the ACM*, 44(12): 103–110.

Zheng, Z., Brady, S., et al. (2005). Applying probabilistic thematic clustering for classification in the TREC 2005 Genomics Track. *The Fourteenth Text REtrieval Conference Proceedings (TREC 2005)*, Gaithersburg, MD. National Institute for Standards and Technology. http://trec. nist.gov/pubs/trec14/papers/queensu.geo.pdf.

Zhou, L. and Hripcsak, G. (2007). Temporal reasoning with medical data—a review with emphasis on medical natural language processing. *Journal of Biomedical Informatics*, 40: 183–202.

Zhou, L., Parsons, S., et al. (2008). The evaluation of a temporal reasoning system in processing clinical discharge summaries. *Journal of the American Medical Informatics Association*, 15: 99–106.

Zhou, X., Hu, X., et al. (2007). Topic signature language models for ad hoc retrieval. *IEEE Transactions on Knowledge and Data Engineering*, 19: 1276–1287.

Ziman, J. (1969). Information, communication, knowledge. *Nature*, 224: 318–324.

Zins, C. (2007a). Classification schemes of information science: 28 scholars map the field. *Journal of the American Society for Information Science & Technology*, 58: 645–672.

Zins, C. (2007b). Conceptions of information science. *Journal of the American Society for Information Science & Technology*, 58: 335–350.

Zins, C. (2007c). Conceptual approaches for defining "data", "information", and "knowledge". *Journal of the American Society for Information Science & Technology*, 58: 479–493.

Zins, C. (2007d). Knowledge map of information science. *Journal of the American Society for Information Science & Technology*, 58: 526–535.

Zobel, J. (1998). How reliable are the results of large-scale information retrieval experiments? *Proceedings of the 21st Annual International ACM SIGIR Conference on Research and Development in Information Retrieval*, Melbourne, Australia. ACM Press. 307–314.

Zobel, J. and Moffat, A. (1998). Exploring the similarity space. *SIGIR Forum*, 32: 18–34.

Zweigenbaum, P. (2003). Question answering in biomedicine. *European Chapter of the Association for Computational Linguistics Workshop on Natural Language Processing for Question Answering*, Budapest, Hungary. Association for Computational Linguistics. http://staff.science. uva.nl/~mdr/NLP4QA/05zweigenbaum.pdf.

Index

Printed in the United States of America